Brunnstrom's
Clinical
Kinesiology

Brunnstrom's Clinical Kinesiology

Fifth Edition

Revised by

Laura K. Smith, PhD, PT
Professor (Retired), Department of Physical Therapy
School of Allied Health Sciences
The University of Texas Medical Branch
Galveston, Texas

Elizabeth Lawrence Weiss, PhD, PT
Professor, Director—New Orleans Campus
Department of Physical Therapy
LSU Medical Center
New Orleans, Louisiana

L. Don Lehmkuhl, PhD, PT
Associate Professor of Physical Medicine and Rehabilitation
Baylor College of Medicine
Houston, Texas

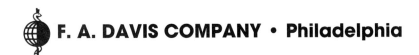 **F. A. DAVIS COMPANY • Philadelphia**

F. A. Davis Company
1915 Arch Street
Philadelphia, PA 19103

Printed in the United States of America

Last digit indicates print number: 10 9 8 7 6 5

Publisher: Jean-François Vilain
Developmental Editor: Crystal S. McNichol
Production Editor: Jessica Howie Martin
Cover Designer: Steven R. Morrone

As new scientific information becomes available through basic and clinical research, recommended treatments and drug therapies undergo changes. The authors and publisher have done everything possible to make this book accurate, up to date, and in accord with accepted standards at the time of publication. The authors, editors, and publisher are not responsible for errors or omissions or for consequences from application of the book, and make no warranty, expressed or implied, in regard to the contents of the book. Any practice described in this book should be applied by the reader in accordance with professional standards of care used in regard to the unique circumstances that may apply in each situation. The reader is advised always to check product information (package inserts) for changes and new information regarding dose and contraindications before administering any drug. Caution is especially urged when using new or infrequently ordered drugs.

Library of Congress Cataloging-in-Publication Data
Smith, Laura K., 1923–
  Brunnstrom's clinical kinesiology. — 5th ed. / revised by Laura
K. Smith, Elizabeth Weiss, L. Don Lehmkuhl.
      p.   cm.
  Rev. ed. of: Brunnstrom's clinical kinesiology. 4th ed. / revised
by L. Don Lehmkuhl and Laura K. Smith.
    ISBN 0-8036-7916-5 (hardcover : alk. paper)
    1. Kinesiology. 2. Applied kinesiology. I. Weiss, Elizabeth.
II. Lehmkuhl, L. Don, 1930–. Brunnstrom's clinical kinesiology.
III. Title.
    [DNLM: 1. Muscles—physiology. 2. Muscle Contraction.
3. Movement. 4. Joints—physiology.   WE 500 S654b 1996]
QP303. B78   1996
612.7′4—dc20
DNLM/DLC
for Library of Congress   95-4491
                                                        CIP

Preface to the Fifth Edition

Signe Brunnstrom's astute analysis of muscle activity and her emphasis on palpation of living anatomy and clinical observations are continued in the fifth edition of *Brunnstrom's Clinical Kinesiology*. Revisions in Chapters 1 to 3, which cover kinematics, kinetics, and muscle physiology and neurophysiology, have been made to clarify concepts. Figures have been added, and material has been reorganized for reader convenience. New material is presented on end-feels of normal passive joint motion and the effects of pressure on tissues. The title of Chapter 4 has been changed to "Muscle Activity and Strength" to better reflect the content. Additional information is presented on isometric, concentric, eccentric, and elastic forces of muscles. Theories on the different myofilament mechanisms for these contractions are discussed. A section on quantitative muscle force testing, reproducibility, and neural adaptation has been added to assist in evaluation of measurements of muscle strength.

Major revisions and additions have been made in the chapters on joint areas (Chaps. 5 to 11). The sections on joints and their soft tissue structures have been expanded, and new figures have been added to improve visualization. Functional characteristics of joints, such as end-feels of passive motion, accessory motion, and joint forces, are included. The sections on muscles have been combined to reduce redundancies and expanded to include all of the muscles of the area. Attachments for the muscles of the neck and back, the temporomandibular joint, the muscles of the hand, and the intrinsic muscles of the foot are presented to remind students that all muscles are important, even though the functions may not be well understood. Analysis of muscles in functional activities has been expanded and is emphasized in three chapters—Chapter 7 ("Shoulder Complex") for the upper extremity, Chapter 10 ("Ankle and Foot") for the lower extremity, and Chapter 11 ("Head, Neck, and Trunk") for the trunk and extremities. Each of the chapters on joint areas (Chaps. 5 to 11) now contains a biomechanical problem with a diagram to illustrate forces in a functional activity. Chapter 12, "Standing and Walking," has been updated and expanded. Figures on photographic techniques for studying gait have been moved to Chapter 12 from Chapter 1. Figures have been added to help the reader visualize the normal displacements occurring in walking. The section on muscle activity in the gait cycle has been expanded to include information on kinesiologic electromyography and activity of all of the muscles in the gait cycle.

Clinical applications are described throughout the text to illustrate the use of kinesiologic principles in the evaluation and understanding of abnormal movement.

Material in the appendices of the fourth edition has been deleted or transferred to appropriate areas in the text. The appendix "Summary Ranges of Joint Motion" has been expanded into a table and moved to Chapter 1. Laboratory activities have been revised, expanded, and placed at the end of each chapter.

A sketch of Signe Brunnstrom's life and her great legacy to physical and occupational therapists follows the Preface to the First Edition. It was written by her biographer, Jay Schleichkorn.

Laura K. Smith
Elizabeth Lawrence Weiss
L. Don Lehmkuhl

Preface
to the
First Edition

Kinesiology—broadly defined as the science of human motion—has ramifications reaching into many fields of study, such as anatomy, physiology, mechanics, physics, mathematics, orthopedics, neurology, pathology and psychology. To be of practical value, a textbook dealing with such a vast subject must be geared to the specific needs of the groups for which it is intended, in the present case the members of medical, paramedical and physical education professions. Because the background requirements and the curricula for students who prepare to enter these professions include subjects closely related to kinesiology, the task at hand was to supplement, not duplicate, the contents of other courses. A certain amount of overlap between courses in anatomy and kinesiology was inevitable. However, throughout the preparation of this book an effort was made to present a minimum of anatomical details while emphasizing the function of skeletal and neuromuscular structures. Both the text and the illustrations aim at developing the student's skill in palpating anatomical structures in the living, a skill which is invaluable in dealing with patients.

Much of the contents of this book has been used over the years by the author in teaching kinesiology to students of physical therapy and occupational therapy. The writing of the book originated with a teaching grant from the Office of Vocational Rehabilitation which enabled the author to prepare a mimeographed laboratory manual to serve as a study aid for students of physical therapy and occupational therapy at College of Physicians and Surgeons, Columbia University. The original manual was then revised and enlarged to include material on certain aspects of pathological motor behavior. The clinical aspects of kinesiology were given emphasis to meet the needs of workers in the field of rehabilitation of the physically handicapped.

Although basic kinesiology is concerned with normal motion of individuals with intact neuromuscular systems, the inclusion of selected pathological cases seemed justifiable and desirable. The effect of loss of specific muscles or muscle groups on movement is particularly well demonstrated in individuals having certain types of peripheral nerve injuries; since the paralysis in this group is specific, illustrations have been drawn mainly from these patients. The motor behavior of patients with upper motoneuron lesions was not included because, to be of value, such a discussion would have to be too lengthy to fit into the framework of this publication.

The section on erect posture, although brief, is intended to present the most important mechanical principles governing the balance of body segments in the upright position. These principles may also serve as a rationale for evaluating the difficulties arising from disorders of the lower extremities, as in persons with paraplegia, lower extremity amputations, poliomyelitis, and the like. By implication, some understanding of the basic principles of bracing and of lower extremity prosthetics should also be derived, although the latter subjects have not been dealt with specifically.

Originally, the author did not intend to discuss human locomotion, but did so at the request of professional personnel who felt that, without a chapter on locomotion, a textbook of kinesiology would be incomplete. Justice cannot be done to this subject in one short chapter, hence the locomotion chapter must be looked upon as an introduction only. For the benefit of those who wish to go deeper into the study of locomotion, references to scientific material are given.

In preparing this book, the author was many times tempted to discuss the application of kinesiology to various therapeutic training procedures employed by physical therapists and occupational therapists. Such follow up of the basic material, however, does not belong in this publication—special courses are offered to deal with therapeutic applications.

The book has fulfilled its purpose if the reader gains a basic knowledge and appreciation of human motion and if, to some extent, it opens scientific vistas which call for further exploration and investigation.

ACKNOWLEDGEMENTS FOR THE FIRST EDITION

The author is happy to acknowledge the valuable assistance she has received from colleagues and professional friends in the preparation of this book, and to extend to them her sincere thanks for their efforts and interest:

To Dr. Herbert O. Elftman, Associate Professor of Anatomy, College of Physicians and Surgeons, Columbia University, for reading the manuscript and for giving so generously of his time and effort. Thanks to his constructive criticism, errors have been corrected, questionable statements clarified, and much irrelevant material eliminated. It has been a privilege, indeed, to have Dr. Elftman take an active interest in this publication.

To Dr. Robert E. Darling, Professor of Physical Medicine and Rehabilitation, for his support and encouragement.

To Professor Mary E. Callahan, Director, Courses for Physical Therapy, and to Professor Marie Louise Franciscus, Director, Courses for Occupational Therapy, for their interest and assistance. To Professors Ruth Dickinson, R.P.T., and Martha E. Schnebly, O.T.R., co-instructors in Kinesiology, who have tested and evaluated the material under actual teaching conditions, and who have assisted in numerous ways.

To Dr. T. Campbell Thompson, for the permission to use photographs taken at Hospital for Special Surgery.

The author also wishes to extend her thanks to the young man who patiently served as a model for a great many photographs in this book and to Mr. Crew, of the Crew Photo Studio, Carmel, New York, for his splendid cooperation.

Signe Brunnstrom

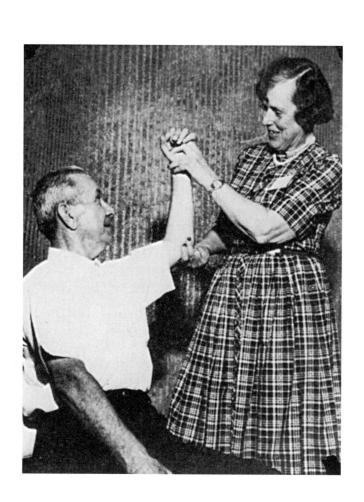

Biographical Sketch of Signe Brunnstrom, 1898-1988

Anna Signe Sofia Brunnstrom was born at Karlberg Castle (the Swedish Military Academy) in Stockholm, Sweden, on January 1, 1898. She was the second daughter of Captain Edvin Brunnstrom and his wife Hedwig. She died in Darien Convalescent Center, Darien, Connecticut, on February 21, 1988. During the 90 years of her life, she served in many capacities. She was a master clinician, scholar, translator, researcher, educator, author, lecturer, mentor, traveler, and humanitarian. Her reputation as a physical therapist was known worldwide.

At age 16, she entered Uppsala College, where she studied sciences, history, geography, and gymnastics. In 1917, she passed the required examination to enter the Royal Institute for Gymnastics in Stockholm. The Institute was founded by fencing master Per Henrik Ling in 1813. Ling developed a system of medical gymnastics, called "Swedish exercises" as they spread across Europe and later into the United States. His exercises were unusual at the time because hands-on resistance or assistance was applied by the therapist. Ling's techniques became the foundation for many of the treatment approaches that Miss Brunnstrom would use in her future work. At the Institute, she excelled in calisthenics and graduated on May 30, 1919, with the title of "Gymnastikdirektor."

In 1920, Miss Brunnstrom went to Berne, Switzerland, to work with a physical therapist. A year later, she established her own "Sjugymnastik Institute" in Lucerne. There she gained a reputation as a therapist treating disabled children with scoliosis and poliomyelitis. She also established an evening program for working women in need of remedial exercise.

She left Switzerland in 1927 and traveled to New York City, where she accepted a position in exercise therapy at the Hospital for the Ruptured and Crippled (later to be renamed the Hospital for Special Surgery). Fourteen Scandinavians worked in the physiotherapy department, and Miss Brunnstrom became the person to whom they all looked for advice as a generous and patient friend. To make ends meet during the depression years, Miss Brunnstrom became a physical training instructress in the gymnasium of the Metropolitan Life Insurance Company. There she applied her ideas about physical education for working women and started special remedial exercise classes. She worked for Metropolitan on and off for 20 years and also offered "Swedish massage" to private patients, received referrals from physicians, and taught exercise classes at New York University.

In 1931, Miss Brunnstrom was admitted to Barnard College, where she took nine credits in chemistry and three credits in English. Recognizing that she could successfully handle American university work, she then enrolled at New York University, where as a part-time student she earned a master's degree in physical education and a master of arts degree in education.

On November 26, 1934, at age 36, Anna Signe Sofia Brunnstrom became a citizen of the United States of America and officially had her name changed to Signe Brunnstrom.

Only 6 years after she came to New York, her first article in English, "Faulty Weight Bearing with Special Reference to Position of the Thigh and Foot" (Physiother. Rev. 15 (3), 1935), was published. This article was the forerunner of 22 clinical articles; several book chapters; three voluminous research reports; numerous abstracts and book reviews (including many translations of classic European work); several films; and three major textbooks on prosthetic training, kinesiology, and hemiplegia movement therapy. She also read and translated the works of major European and American scientists and brought them to the kinesiology literature. These scientists included Blix, Borelli, Bethe and Franke, Braune and Fisher, Elfman, Duchenne, Fick, Inman, Marey, Magus, and the Weber brothers.

Signe Brunnstrom remains one of the most productive contributors to the body of physical therapy knowledge. Through her students and writings, she has left a great legacy to practicing physical and occupational therapists.

In 1938, Miss Brunnstrom was appointed an instructor of therapeutic exercise at New York University. She taught there until 1942 and later in 1948, when she joined the faculty of the Institute for Rehabilitation Medicine as a research associate working on a suction socket study sponsored by the Veterans Administration and NYU.

In the spring of 1941, with the United States still not drawn into World War II, Miss Brunnstrom applied through the American Red Cross to serve as a civilian physical therapist in a military hospital. She was assigned to the physical therapy department at Sheppard Field, Texas, with the Army Air Corps. She left Texas 2 years later, hoping to enlist in the US Army Medical Specialist Corps, but was refused because of her age (she was 45). She then enlisted in the US Navy, and in 1943 reported to the Navy Hospital at Mare Island, California, as the officer in charge of physical therapy. It was there, while working with a young naval medical officer, Dr. Henry Kessler, that she made major contributions to the rehabilitation of amputees. After the war, Dr. Kessler founded the well-known Kessler Institute of Rehabilitation in West Orange, New Jersey. Miss Brunnstrom was discharged from the Navy in 1946 with the rank of lieutenant.

After the war, Miss Brunnstrom participated in prosthetic research at the University of California and New York University. In addition, she was Director of Professional Education at the Kessler Institute. She was also a clinical consultant at the Burke Foundation, White Plains, New York, the New York State Rehabilitation Hospital at West Haverstraw, and the Veterans Administration; and a visiting instructor at Stanford University in California. In 1951, she was awarded a Fullbright Lectureship to Greece, where she worked on developing a school of physical therapy and trained aides to carry out amputee exercise programs. Throughout this time, Miss Brunnstrom was in great demand to conduct continuing education courses, seminars, and workshops.

From 1955 through 1971, one of Miss Brunnstrom's many professional activities was teaching kinesiology to physical and occupational therapy students at the College of Physicians and Surgeons, Columbia University, New York. A teaching grant from the US Office of Vocational Rehabilitation enabled her to prepare a laboratory manual for the students. The manual was developed into the textbook *Clinical Kinesiology*, which was published in 1962. This was the first American kinesiology text to be written for physical and occupational therapy students. Before this time, most kinesiology textbooks were oriented to physical education and athletic activities.

Signe Brunnstrom received numerous honors and awards, including the U. S. Navy Medal of Merit in 1945, the Marian Williams Research Award presented by the American Physical Therapy Association (APTA) in 1965, the University Citation of the State University of New York at Buffalo (equivalent to an honorary doctorate) in 1973, and an appointment to honorary membership in the Union of Swedish Physical Therapists in 1974. In 1987, the Board of Directors of APTA renamed the Award for Excellence in Clinical Teaching in her honor. The award is now known as the Signe Brunnstrom Award for Excellence in Clinical Teaching.

Jay Schleichkorn, PhD, PT

CONTENTS

Chapter 3   **Aspects of Muscle Physiology and Neurophysiology**   **69**

CHAPTER 1

Mechanical Principles: Kinematics

Kinesiology, the study of motion, developed from the fascination of human beings with animal motion: How does a person walk? How do fish swim? How do birds fly? What are the limits of muscular strength? From the quest for answers to these questions, the science of motion evolved, combining theories and principles from anatomy, physiology, psychology, anthropology, and mechanics. The application of mechanics to the living human body is called **biomechanics**. Mechanics may be further subdivided into **statics,** which is concerned with bodies at rest or in uniform motion, and **dynamics,** which treats bodies that are accelerating or decelerating. Because most of the motion with which physical and occupational therapists deal therapeutically is slow and lacks rapid accelerations, the concepts from mechanics applicable to clinical practice can be gained using principles from statics.

The purpose of studying clinical kinesiology is to understand the forces acting on the human body and to manipulate these forces in treatment procedures so that human performance may be improved and further injury may be prevented. Although humans have always been able to see and feel their postures and mo-

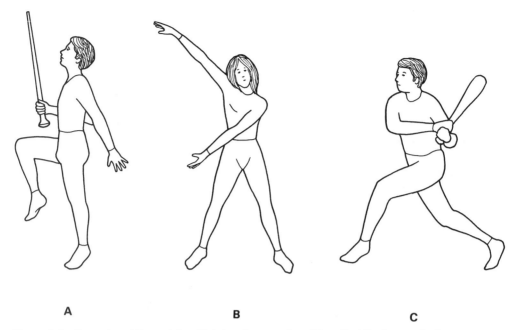

Figure 1–1   Examples of the variety of joint and segment positions that the human body can assume: (*A*) demonstrates flexion and extension positions of joints, (*B*) emphasizes lateral motions of abduction and adduction, and (*C*) illustrates rotation. A view of these positions in three dimensions is even more complex.

tions, the forces affecting motion (gravity, muscle tension, external resistance, and friction) are never seen and seldom felt. Where these forces act in relation to positions and movements of the body in space is fundamental to the ability to produce human motion and to modify it.

The human body can assume many diverse positions that appear difficult to describe or classify (Fig. 1–1). **Kinematics** is the science of the motion of bodies in space. This may include the movement of a single point on the body (such as the center of gravity), position of several segments (such as the upper extremity), or position of a single joint or motions that occur between adjacent joint surfaces. Kinematics applies the rectangular coordinate system to describe the body in space. This subject is further subdivided into **osteokinematics**, which is concerned with the movements of the bones, and **arthrokinematics**, which addresses the movements occurring between joint surfaces.

PLANAR CLASSIFICATION OF POSITION AND MOTION (OSTEOKINEMATICS)

To define joint and segment motions and to record the location in space of specific points on the body, a reference point is required. In kinesiology, the three-dimensional rectangular coordinate system is used to describe anatomic relationships of the body. The standard **anatomic body position** is defined as standing erect with the head, toes, and palms of the hands facing forward and with the fingers extended. Three imaginary planes are arranged perpendicular to each other through the body, with their axes intersecting at the center of gravity of the body

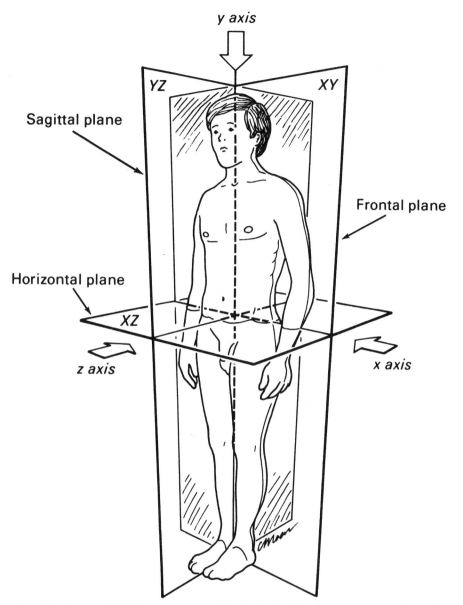

Figure 1–2 The three cardinal planes and axes of the body standing at ease. (A person is considered to be in the standard anatomic position when standing with the palms facing forward.)

(a point slightly anterior to the second sacral vertebra). These planes are called the **cardinal planes** of the body (Fig. 1–2).

Frontal Plane

The frontal plane (coronal, or XY plane) is parallel to the frontal bone and divides the body into front and back parts. Motions that occur in this plane are defined as **abduction** and **adduction**. Abduction is a position or motion of the segment away from the midline, regardless of which segment moves. Abduction of the hip (Fig. 1–3) occurs when either the thigh segment moves away from the midline or

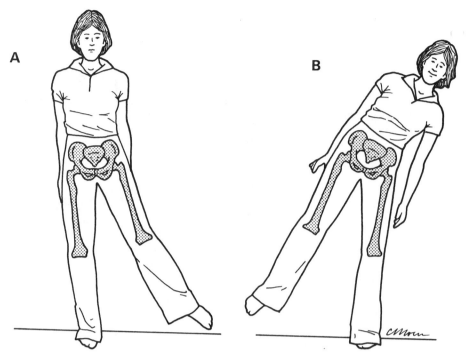

Figure 1–3   Abduction of the left hip. (*A*) Femur abducted on the pelvis. (*B*) Pelvis abducted on the femur.

the pelvic segment approaches the thigh, as in tilting to the side while standing on one leg. Adduction is a position or motion toward the midline. Motions of abduction and adduction occur around the z axis.

Sagittal Plane

The sagittal plane (midsagittal, or YZ plane) is vertical and divides the body into right and left sides. Photographically, this is a side view. Joint motions occurring in the sagittal plane are defined as **flexion** and **extension.** Flexion indicates that two segments approach each other; for example, flexion of the elbow may be accomplished by flexion of the forearm on the arm or by flexion of the arm on the forearm, as in a pull-up. Extension occurs when two segments move away from each other. If extension goes beyond the anatomic reference position, it is called **hyperextension.** Motions of flexion and extension pivot around the x axis.

Horizontal Plane

The horizontal plane (transverse, or XZ plane) divides the body into upper and lower parts and is like a view from above. Rotations occur in this plane around the vertical y axis. **Internal rotation** (inward or medial rotation) is a transverse rotation oriented to the anterior surface of the body. Internal rotation of the hip brings points marked on the anterior surface of the pelvis and femur closer together regardless of which of the segments moves. **Pronation** is the term used for internal rotation of the forearm. **External rotation** (outward or lateral rotation) is in the opposite direction and is oriented to the posterior surface of the body. **Supination** is the term used at the forearm and is the reference point for the anatomic position.

Special Cases

Sagittal, frontal, and horizontal planes may be laid through points other than the center of gravity of the body, but these are **secondary planes.** For example, it may be convenient to lay three planes through the center of a joint, such as the hip joint, for determination of body points in relation to such a joint.

Definitions for motions of the digits require placing the coordinate system on the extremity. In the hand, the sagittal plane is centered through the third segment; in the foot, the sagittal plane is centered through the second segment. Motion or position away from the reference segment is called abduction, and motion toward the segment is called adduction. At the wrist, the motion of abduction is frequently referred to as **radial deviation** (toward the radius), and adduction is called **ulnar deviation.** In the anatomic position, the foot is at a right angle to the leg in the sagittal plane. By convention (general acceptance), movement of the dorsum of the foot toward the tibia is called **dorsiflexion**, and movement of the sole of the foot away from the tibia is called **plantar flexion.**

The thumb is also a special case because it is normally rotated 90 degrees from the plane of the hand. Thus, motions of flexion and extension occur in the frontal plane, and abduction and adduction occur in the sagittal plane (see Fig. 6–21).

Goniometry

Goniometry (Gr. *gonia,* angle, and *metron,* measure) is an application of the coordinate system to a joint to measure the degrees of motion present in each plane of a joint. The goniometer, which is a protractor with two arms hinged at the origin, represents the plane. It is placed parallel to the two body segments to be measured and with the axis of the joint and the axis of the goniometer superimposed (Fig. 1–4). Thus, the position of the segments in the plane can be recorded. When joints have motions in several planes, as in the shoulder (flexion, abduction, and rotation), the goniometer is moved to each plane and axis for measurement. For details on the techniques of goniometry, the reader is referred to the comprehensive text by Norkin and White (1995).

Even though degrees of joint motion may be measured, communicating the result of the measurement is a problem because two systems of recording exist. The system presented in this book uses 0 degrees as the reference point for the standard anatomic position (extension, adduction, and neutral rotation). Motions or positions of flexion, abduction, and internal and external rotation are recorded as they move toward 180 degrees. The second system uses 180 degrees as the reference point for the standard anatomic position and records flexion, abduction, and the rotations as they approach 0 degrees. Thus, the same position of the elbow is reported in the first system as 120 degrees and in the second as 60 degrees. This is very confusing. Failure to identify the system being used can have serious consequences in interpretation of patient records.

Although many textbooks provide values for normal range of motion, standardized normal tables according to age, sex, body build, and type of motion (active or passive) have not been established. Thus, the most accurate measurement of normal motion is the patient's opposite extremity if it is present and unim-

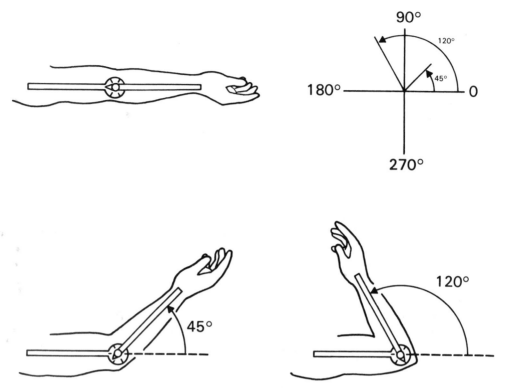

Figure 1–4 Application of a goniometer to measure the position of the elbow in the sagittal plane. The stationary arm of the goniometer is aligned parallel to the long axis of the subject's arm. The moving arm of the goniometer is aligned parallel to the long axis of the forearm, and the axis of the goniometer is placed over the axis of the elbow joint.

paired. The following goniometric values may be used as guidelines to the approximate normal joint range of motion in the adult (Table 1–1). **The values in bold type are round numbers that are convenient to remember in estimating the amount of normal motion present.** The values in parentheses are the range of *average* normal motion reported in several sources (American Academy of Orthopaedic Surgeons, 1965; Departments of the Army and Air Force, 1968; Kendall, Kendall, and Wadsworth, 1971; Daniels and Worthingham, 1972; Gerhardt and Russe, 1975; Kapandji, 1982, 1987). For details of positioning and landmarks for the measurements, the original references should be consulted.

Normal individual ranges of motion vary with bony structure, muscular development, body fat, ligamentous integrity, gender, and age. Thin persons and those with loose ligaments may have more range of motion than those who have greater muscular development or who are obese. Dubs and Gschwend (1988) measured index finger hyperextension in over 2000 people and found wide variability, from 100 degrees to 10 degrees. Joint laxity was greater in females than in males and decreased with age. Males showed a more rapid decrease in adolescence and a greater overall decrease. The range of motion in some joints of infants and children may differ markedly from the average adult values. These differences are marked in the hips. Details of joint motion variability and ranges of motion for body parts are described in Chapters 5 through 11.

Table 1-1 Summary Ranges of Joint Motion

SHOULDER	flexion **0°** to **180°** (150° to 180°) extension **0°** hyperextension **0°** to **45°** (40° to 60°) abduction **0°** to **180°** (150° to 180°) internal rotation **0°** to **90°** (70° to 90°) external rotation **0°** to **90°** (80° to 90°)
ELBOW	flexion **0°** to **145°** (120° to 160°) extension **0°**
FOREARM	supination from midposition **0°** to **90°** (80° to 90°) pronation from midposition **0°** to **80°** (70° to 80°)
WRIST	neutral when the midline between flexion and extension is 0° and when forearm and third metacarpal are in line flexion **0°** to **90°** (75° to 90°) extension **0°** to **70°** (65° to 70°) radial abduction **0°** to **20°** (15° to 25°) ulnar abduction **0°** to **30°** (25° to 40°)
FINGERS	MCP flexion **0°** to **90°** (85° to 100°) MCP hyperextension **0°** to **20°** (0° to 45°) MCP abduction **0°** to **20°** MCP adduction **0°** PIP flexion **0°** to **120°** (90° to 120°) DIP flexion **0°** to **90°** (80° to 90°) IP extension **0°**
THUMB	MCP flexion **0°** to **45°** (40° to 90°) MCP abduction and adduction (NEGLIGIBLE) IP flexion **0°** to **90°** (80° to 90°)
HIP	flexion **0°** to **120°** (110° to 125°) hyperextension **0°** to **10°** (0° to 30°) abduction **0°** to **45°** (40° to 55°) adduction **0°** (30° to 40° across midline) external rotation **0°** to **45°** (40° to 50°) internal rotation **0°** to **35°** (30° to 45°)
KNEE	flexion **0°** to **120°** (120° to 160°) extension **0°**
ANKLE	neutral with foot at a right angle to the leg and knee flexed plantar flexion **0°** to **45°** (40° to 50°) dorsiflexion **0°** to **15°** (10° to 20°) inversion and eversion (see Chapter 10).
TOES	MTP flexion **0°** to **40°** (30° to 45°) MTP hyperextension **0°** to **80°** (50° to 90°) MTP abduction (present) IP flexion **0°** to **60°** (50° to 80°) IP extension **0°**

The values in bold type are round numbers that are convenient to remember in estimating the amount of normal
  motion present. The values in parentheses are the ranges of *average* normal motion reported in several sources.
KEY:
  DIP = distal interphalangeal joint
   IP = interphalangeal joint
 MCP = metacarpophalangeal joint
 MTP = metatarsophalangeal joint
  PIP = proximal interphalangeal joint
SOURCES: American Academy of Orthopaedic Surgeons, 1965; Departments of the Army and Air Force, 1968;
  Kendall, Kendall, and Wadsworth, 1971; Daniels and Worthingham, 1972; Gerhardt and Russe, 1975; and
  Kapandji, 1982 and 1987.

Normal End-Feel

When a normal joint is moved passively to the end of its range of motion, resistance to further motion is felt by the examiner. This resistance is called the **end-feel** or the **physiologic end-feel**. The resistance is described as hard, firm, or soft. A hard or bony end-feel is felt when the motion is stopped by contact of bone on bone, as in elbow extension. A firm or springy end-feel is one in which the limitation is from ligamentous, capsular, or muscle structures. Wrist flexion is an example. A soft end-feel occurs with contact of adjacent soft tissues such as the arm and forearm when the elbow is flexed fully.

Pathologic end-feels occur at a different place in the range of motion or have an end-feel that is not characteristic of the joint. An empty end-feel is a pathologic type denoting pain on motion but absence of resistance.

ROTARY AND TRANSLATORY MOTION

The shape and congruency of articulating joint surfaces determine the movements permitted at various joints. Movements are described as occurring around an axis or a pivot point, identified in mechanical terms as **rotary motion, angular motion,** or **rotation.** Rotary motions take place about a fixed or relatively fixed axis. These motions are called rotary because every point on a segment adjacent to the joint follows the arc of a circle, the center of which is the joint axis. Thus, in flexion and extension of the elbow, the bones of the forearm (or the bone of the upper arm or both) rotate about the axis of the elbow joint. Individual points on the segment move at different velocities, the velocity of each point being related to its distance from the axis of motion. Thus, if the arm swings forward and backward at the shoulder, the velocity (in centimeters per second) of the hand is greater than that of the elbow and far greater than that of a point on the upper portion of the arm that lies close to the center of rotation. (Note, however, that the angular velocity, that is, degrees per second, is the same for all points on the rotating segment.)

In mechanics, the term **translatory motion** is used to describe movement of a body in which **all of its parts** move in the same direction with equal velocity. Thus, any point on the body can be used to describe the path of the total body. Translatory motion may either be in a straight line (linear) or follow a curve (curvilinear). There are few examples of true translatory motions in the human body; these usually involve passive transport of the body in a vehicle such as a wheelchair, stretcher, or car. In walking, the trunk and the body as a whole move in a forward direction, but this is not a true translatory motion because the body segments move with different velocities. Nevertheless, it is an example of how multiple rotary motions of limb segments can produce a "relative" translatory movement of the body as a whole. In the upper extremity, combinations of rotary motions at the shoulder, elbow, radioulnar, and wrist joints permit the hand to move freely in space, taking a translatory path.

Degrees of Freedom

The ability of the body to transform stereotyped angular motions of joints into more efficient curvilinear motion of parts can be appreciated by using the concept of **degrees of freedom** of motion. (Reuleaux, 1875; Fisher, 1907). This term is commonly used in bioengineering literature and should be differentiated from the meaning of the same term when it is used in discussions of statistics.

Joints have been classified according to the number of planes in which their segments move or the number of primary axes they possess. Joints that move in one plane possess one axis and have one degree of freedom. Examples are the interphalangeal and elbow joints, which possess motion of flexion and extension around a transverse (x) axis, and the radioulnar joints, which permit supination and pronation around a longitudinal (y) axis. Any one point on the moving segment is restricted to a predetermined arc of motion in a single plane.

If a joint has two axes, the segments can move in two planes, and the joint is said to possess **two degrees of freedom of motion.** Examples are the metacarpophalangeal joints of the hand and the radiocarpal joint of the wrist, which permit flexion-extension around a transverse axis and abduction-adduction around a sagittal axis.

Ball-and-socket joints such as the hip joint, which permit flexion-extension, abduction-adduction, and transverse rotation, are said to possess **three degrees of freedom.** Movements take place about three main axes, all of which pass through the joint's center of rotation (in the case of the hip joint, the axes pass through the center of the head of the femur). At the hip, the axis for flexion-extension has a transverse direction, the axis for abduction-adduction has a sagittal direction, and the axis for transverse rotation courses longitudinally from the center of the hip joint to the center of the knee joint. The glenohumeral joint of the shoulder is another example of a joint with three degrees of freedom.

By well-coordinated, successive combinations of the movement components, a **circumduction** motion is performed during which the moving segment follows the surface of a cone and the tip of the segment traces a circular path. Circumduction is characteristic of joints with two and three degrees of freedom but cannot take place in joints with one degree of freedom.

Three degrees of freedom of motion are the maximum number that a single joint can possess in planar motion. It is through the summation of the degrees of freedom of two or more joints that parts of the body may gain sufficient degrees of freedom to produce smooth translations of the body and curvilinear motions. In actuality there are six degrees of freedom, with the additional three coming from the small but important motions of distraction and translatory glides, which are discussed later in this chapter under Accessory Motions.

Kinematic Chains

A combination of several joints uniting successive segments constitutes a **kinematic chain.** Successively, the more **distal segments can have higher degrees of freedom than do proximal ones.** For example, from the thoracic wall to the finger, at least 19 degrees of freedom in planar motions can be identified (Steindler, 1955). Such freedom of motion constitutes the mechanical basis for performance of skilled manual activities and the versatility of the upper extremity. In the lower extremity and trunk, the 25 or more degrees of freedom between the pelvis and the toe not only permit the foot to adjust to an irregular or slanting surface but also allow the body's center of gravity to be maintained within the small base of support of the planted foot.

Debating the **exact** number of degrees of freedom in a kinematic chain is an exercise in futility. For example, identifying each motion of the intercarpal joints of the wrist and the intertarsal joints of the foot is extremely complex and sometimes variable.

Open and Closed Kinematic Chains

In an open kinematic chain, the distal segment of the chain moves in space, whereas in a closed kinematic chain, the distal segment is fixed, and proximal parts move (Steindler, 1955). In the upper extremity, open-chain motion occurs when reaching or bringing the hand to the mouth, and closed-chain motion occurs when performing a chin-up. Movement of one segment in closed-chain motion requires all the segments to move. In open-chain motions segments can move independently or not at all.

Planar classifications of motion imply that the proximal segment is fixed and the distal segment moves. Although this open-chain type of motion is important in human motion, it is only **one** type. Equally important are closed-chain motions that occur when the distal segment is fixed and the proximal segment moves, and when both segments move. An example is sitting down in a chair (Fig. 1–5). Here the leg moves forward on the fixed foot (dorsiflexion), the thigh approaches the leg (knee flexion), and the thigh approaches the pelvis (hip flexion). Walking and stairclimbing are examples of alternation of closed-chain motion during the support phase of the extremity and open-chain motion during the swing phase. When a person uses the armrest of a chair to assist in coming to the standing position (or performs a push-up in a wheelchair), the hand is fixed and the forearm moves in relation to the hand, the arm moves away from the forearm (elbow extension), and the arm moves toward the trunk (shoulder adduction). Other clinical examples of closed-chain motion in the upper extremity include crutch-walking and elevating the body using an overbed trapeze. Both open and closed kinematic chain motions can be seen to occur in different segments during body motion as in Figures 1–1 and 1–3.

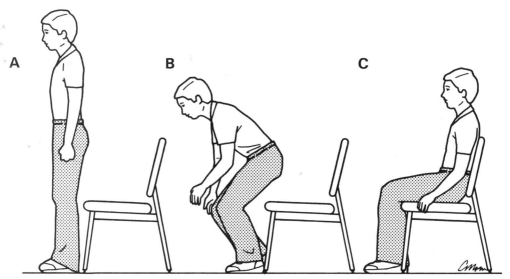

A   B   C

Figure 1–5 Closed kinematic chain motion of the ankle, knee, and hip joints as the subject moves from the standing to the sitting position.

Clinical Applications

The rectangular coordinate system is a method of communication used to define, describe, and document complex body positions and motions. Normal motions and postures are not so stereotyped but rather combine planes and axes. The multiple degrees of freedom of body segments permit a wide selection of movement patterns. Thus there are many ways to perform a given task such as writing, eating, throwing a ball, or getting into and out of an automobile. In the simple movement of rising from a supine to a standing position, 21 different combinations of the arm, leg, and head-trunk components have been documented in healthy young adults (Van Sant, 1988).

Goniometry is a valuable clinical measurement to describe the positions of joints in movement and to record the available range of motion in joints. Pathologic limitations of motion in a joint, such as edema, pain, or soft tissue shortening, can restrict normal function. The large number of degrees of freedom in a kinematic chain is an advantage used to maintain function. The person who cannot fully pronate the forearm can accomplish hand function by compensatory increases in wrist, elbow, shoulder, and even trunk motions. A person with a stiff knee can walk using compensatory motions of the ankle, hip, back, or the opposite lower extremity. Such compensation, however, is always at a price of increased energy expenditure for the activity at the same speed. Years of compensatory use may result in repetitive microtrauma and dysfunction in the compensating joint structures.

Limitation of additional degrees of freedom in a kinematic chain further increases impairment and decreases the options for function. Sometimes even loss of one degree of freedom can be severely disabling as would occur in a finger joint of a professional typist, violinist, or baseball pitcher.

ARTHROKINEMATICS

Arthrokinematics is concerned with the movement of the articular surfaces in relation to the direction of movement of the distal extremity of the bone (osteokinematics). Although human joints have been compared with geometric shapes and mechanical joints such as the hinge, pivot, plane, sphere, and cone, the exquisite motions and capabilities of human joints exceed any joint that humans have made. Normally, human joints retain their functional capacities beyond the organic life span of the human being (70 to 100 years). The phenomenal superiority of human joints as compared with man-made joints is due not only to the physiologic capacities of biologic joints, such as low coefficient of friction, presence of sensation and proprioceptive feedback, and dynamic growth responses to wear and use, but also to the mechanical complexities of human joints.

Ovoid and Sellar Joint Surfaces

The surfaces of movable joints are not flat, cylindric, conic, or spheric; they are ovoid (egg-shaped), a shape in which the radius of curvature varies from point to point (MacConaill and Basmajian, 1969). The ovoid articular surfaces of two bones form a convex-concave paired relationship (Fig. 1–6). The concave-convex

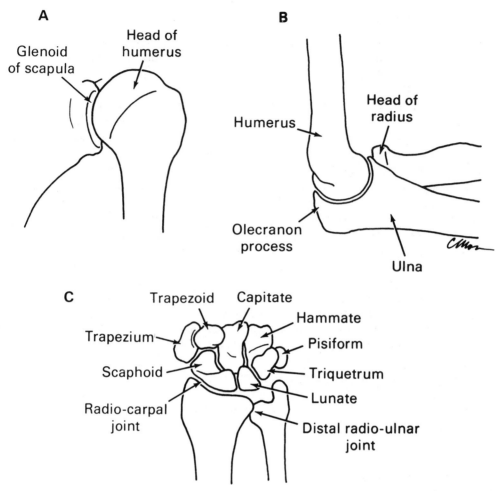

Figure 1–6   Examples of concave-convex relationships of joint surfaces redrawn from radiographs. (*A*) Glenohumeral joint of the shoulder (anterior-posterior view). (*B*) Ulnohumeral joint of the elbow (lateral view). (*C*) Radiocarpal and intercarpal joints of the wrist (anterior-posterior view).

joint relationship may range from "nearly planar," as in the carpal and tarsal joints, to "nearly spheroid," as in the glenohumeral and hip joints. In engineering, the convex curvature is called the male component, and the concave curvature is called the female component. The center of rotation is in the convex component at some distance from the joint surface.

Some joints have both convex and concave surfaces on each articulating bone (Fig. 1–7). These are called **sellar** (L., saddle) joints because they resemble the matching of a rider in a saddle (reciprocal reception). Examples of sellar joints include the carpometacarpal joint of the thumb, the elbow, the sternoclavicular joint, and the ankle (talocrural joint).

In most cases, the ovoid surface of one bone in a pair is larger than its companion, as seen in the glenohumeral joint (see Fig. 1–6), the knee (Fig. 1–8), and the interphalangeal joint (Fig. 1–9). This phenomenon of the biologic joint permits a large range of motion with an economy of articular surface and reduction in the size of the joint.

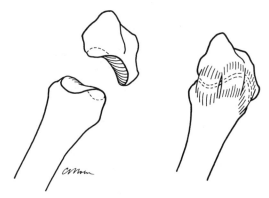

Figure 1–7 Sellar joint with concave and convex surfaces of each bone (carpometacarpal joint of the thumb).

Movements of Joint Surfaces

Arthrokinematically, when a joint moves, three types of motion can occur between the two surfaces: (1) rolling or rocking, (2) sliding or gliding, and (3) spinning (MacConaill and Basmajian, 1969). In a pure rolling motion such as a ball rolling on a table, each subsequent point on one surface contacts a new point on the other surface (see Fig. 1–8). In sliding and spinning, the same point on one surface contacts new points on the mating surface. Most normal joint movement has some combination of rolling, sliding, and spinning. The knee joint shows this most clearly. If there were only a rolling of the condyles of the femur on the tibial plateau, the femur would roll off the tibia and the

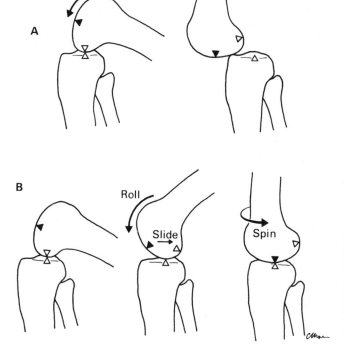

Figure 1–8 Movements of joint surfaces. (*A*) Pure rolling or hinge motion of the femur or the tibia would cause joint dislocation. (*B*) Normal motion of the knee demonstrates a combination of rolling, sliding, and spinning in the last 20 degrees of extension (terminal rotation of the knee).

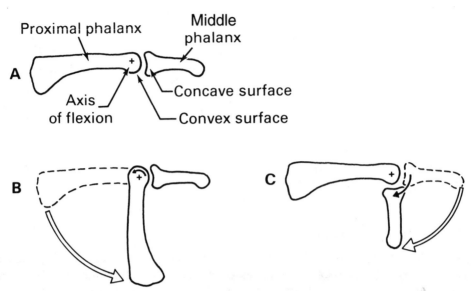

Figure 1–9   Lateral view of the proximal interphalangeal joint of the index finger (A) in extension and (B,C) in flexion. When the bone with the convex joint surface moves into flexion (B), the joint surface moves in an opposite direction to the motion of the shaft of the bone. When the bone with the concave joint surface moves into flexion (C), the joint surface moves in the same direction as the shaft of the bone.

knee would dislocate (see Fig. 1–8A). Instead, when the femur is extended on the fixed tibia, as in rising from a seated to a standing position, the femoral condyles roll and slide so that they are always in contact with the tibial condyles (see Fig. 1–8B). In the last part of knee extension, the femur spins (internally rotates on the tibia).

The combination of roll, slide, and spin thus permits a large range of motion while using a small articular surface. If joints possessed only one of these motions, the range of motion would be limited or joint surfaces would need to be larger to accomplish the same range of motion.

Joint Axes

Because of the incongruity of joint surfaces and the motions of roll, slide, and spin, animal joint axes are complex. The axis does not remain stationary, as in a mechanical hinge joint, but moves as the joint position changes, usually following a curved path (see Fig. 9–3). The largest movement of the axes occurs in the knee, elbow, and wrist. In addition, the joint axes are seldom exactly perpendicular to the long axes of the bones but are frequently oblique. This is particularly noticeable when the little finger is flexed into the palm. The tip of the finger points to the base of the thumb rather than to the base of the fifth metacarpal. When the elbow is extended from full flexion with the forearm in supination, the forearm laterally deviates 0 to 20 degrees. This is called the **carrying angle** and is usually larger in women than in men (see Fig. 5–1).

These oblique axes and changing positions of the joint centers create problems and necessitate compromise when mechanical appliances and joints are applied to the body, as in goniometry, orthotics, and exercise equipment. Mechanical appliances usually have a fixed axis of motion that is perpendicular to the moving part. When the mechanical and anatomic parts are coupled, perfect alignment can occur at only one point in the range of motion. At other points in the range of motion, the mechanical appliance may bind and cause pressure on the body part, or it may force the human joint in abnormal directions. Thus, the placement of mechanical joints is critical where large ranges of motion are desired. The search continues for mechanical joints that more nearly approximate the complexity of human joints.

Convex-Concave Relationships

The arthrokinematic movement of joint surfaces relative to the movement of the shaft of the bones (osteokinematics) follows convex-concave principles. If the bone with the convex joint surface moves on the bone with the concavity, the convex joint surfaces move in the **opposite** direction to the bone segment (see Fig. 1–9). If the bone with the concavity moves on the convex surface, the concave articular surfaces moves in the **same** direction as the bone segment. The proximal interphalangeal joint of the index finger is used as an example in Figure 1–9. Flexion can occur with movement of either the proximal or middle phalanx. When flexion occurs by movement of the proximal phalanx, points on this convex surface move in an opposite direction to the shaft of the moving bone (see Fig. 1–9B). On the other hand, if the concave surface of the middle phalanx moves on the fixed proximal phalanx, the joint surface moves in the **same** direction as the moving bone. The articular cartilages experience flexion as **either** a dorsal motion of the convex proximal phalanx **or** a volar motion of the concave middle phalanx. Thus, arthrokinematically, the planar motion of shoulder abduction is either a downward motion of the humeral head on the glenoid fossa when the humerus is moving upward, or an upward movement of the glenoid on the humeral head when the scapula is moving as in a handstand (closed kinematic chain). Knee extension is an anterior movement of the concave tibial plateau on the femur or a posterior movement of the femoral condyles on the tibia.

Close-Packed and Open-Packed Positions

The ovoid surfaces of joint pairs match each other perfectly in only one position of the joint. This point of congruency (coinciding exactly) is called the **close-packed position** (MacConaill and Basmajian, 1969). In this position, (1) the maximum area of surface contact occurs, (2) the attachments of the ligaments are farthest apart and under tension, (3) capsular structures are taut, and (4) the joint is mechanically compressed and difficult to distract (separate). In all other positions, the ovoid joint surfaces do not fit perfectly but are incongruent and called **open-packed,** or **loose-packed.** The ligamentous and capsular structures are slack, and the joint surfaces may be distracted several millimeters (Fig. 1–10B). Loose-packed positions allow the necessary motions of spin, roll, and slide and may decrease joint friction.

The close-packed position usually occurs at one extreme in the range of motion. This is in full extension at the elbow, wrist, hip, and knee; dorsiflexion at the ankle; and flexion at the metacarpophalangeal joints. In these positions, the joint

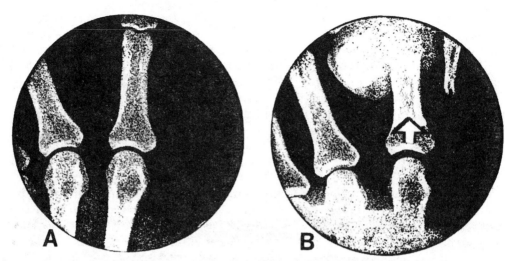

Figure 1–10   Radiograph of the metacarpophalangeal joint of the index finger (*A*) at rest and (*B*) at the limit of long-axis distraction. The relationship of the articulating surfaces of the bones in (*B*) should be compared with their relationship with the joint at rest. *Arrow* indicates the direction of pull by the examiner. (From Mennell, JM: *Joint Pain: Diagnosis and Treatment Using Manipulative Techniques*. Little, Brown & Co, Boston, 1964, p 33, with permission.)

has great mechanical stability with reduction in need for muscle forces to maintain the position. When the metacarpophalangeal joints are in 90 degrees of flexion, lateral motion (abduction) cannot occur. This is an advantage in gripping where muscle forces can be channeled to finger flexion rather than needing some of the force to keep the fingers from spreading. During standing, the hips and knees are in their close-packed positions of extension. In humans, this permits erect standing with little or no contraction of the muscles of the hips or knees and results in an economy of energy expenditure.

Accessory Motions

In addition to angular motions such as flexion or abduction, joint surfaces can be moved passively a few millimeters in translatory motion. These small motions are called **accessory movements** (Maitland, 1970) or joint play (Mennell, 1964). An example is distraction or separation of joint surfaces at the metacarpophalangeal joint (see Fig. 1–10). In addition to distraction, the surfaces of freely movable joints may undergo lateral glide, anterior-posterior glide, and rotation. Accessory motions cannot be performed voluntarily by the subject but rather require relaxation of muscles and the application of passive movement by an examiner. These small motions are essential for normal pain-free joint function and are performed by therapists in both the evaluation and treatment of joint motion problems. The importance of the presence of accessory motions can be appreciated in the arthrokinematic example of glenohumeral joint abduction. If the necessary distal movement of the head of the humerus on the glenoid fossa were not present, elevation of the hand would be severely restricted ("frozen shoulder"). The greater tuberosity may strike the acromion process instead of sliding beneath it. Striking the acromion process (and adjacent soft tissues) would produce additional injury and pain.

Mennell (1964) defines the condition of loss of normal joint play (movement) that is accompanied by pain as joint dysfunction. He describes a vicious cycle that occurs: "1) When a joint is not free to move, the muscles that move it cannot be free to move it, 2) muscles cannot be restored to normal if the joints which they move are not free to move, 3) normal muscle function is dependent on normal joint movement, and 4) impaired muscle function perpetuates and may cause deterioration in abnormal joints."

Clinical Applications

Application of arthrokinematic principles is basic to the assessment of the integrity of joint structures and use of joint mobilization techniques in the treatment of hypomobile or painful soft tissues. Normally, ligaments and capsular structures limit passive accessory motions in open-packed positions. If a ligament has been severed or stretched out, the accessory motion that the ligament controls will be excessive or hypermobile. If the structures are in an acute inflammatory stage, the accessory motion will be painful and hypomobile.

Many angular joint motions, such as flexion and extension, occur by an exquisite coordination of several joints. The wrist, for example, has 12 or more articulations in the intercarpal and radiocarpal joints (see Fig. 1–6C). In a person with pain and limitation of wrist flexion, localization of the lesion may be made by evaluation of the accessory movements at each of these articulations.

Joint surface relationships are of extreme importance when motion of the joint is limited and exercise is being used to increase motion. If, for example, interphalangeal joint flexion is limited (as may occur with scar tissue formation of the skin, capsule, tendon, or ligaments), the normal downward movement of the phalanx into a position of flexion cannot occur (see Fig. 1–9C). When the concave base of the phalanx cannot move down, a force applied distally on the phalanx may pry the joint so that some structures are overstretched and others are compressed (Fig. 1–11C). This could result in further injury to joint structures. Attention should be paid to gaining downward movement of the phalanx by applying the force close to the joint and in line with normal joint surface movements (Fig. 1–11B).

Figure 1–11 A normal interphalangeal joint (*A*) in extension and (*B*) in flexion, showing the base of the middle phalanx moving down on the head of the proximal phalanx and eventually under the head. (*C*) Application of a distal stretching force to a joint with limited motion. The base of the middle phalanx is pried away from, and compressed against, the proximal joint surface in an abnormal manner.

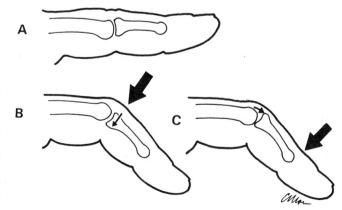

Laboratory Activities

Following all of the chapters are suggested laboratory activities that are presented as a guide to further study of material using visual, tactile, and kinesthetic practice. The activities are designed to aid in learning principles and internalizing anatomic details. Many of the activities are basic to needed clinical skills and knowledge. With supervised practice the student should be able to:

1. Describe and demonstrate normal range of motion of joints and their normal end-feels.
2. Describe the location and magnitude of the forces of gravity, external resistance, friction, muscles, and joints on human postures and motions.
3. Identify by palpation normal anatomic structures of the human body such as bony prominences, joint spaces, ligaments, tendons, and muscles.
4. Demonstrate joint stability in close-packed positions and joint mobility in open-packed positions.
5. Elicit isolated contractions of muscles by applying anatomic knowledge and principles of positioning, stabilization, palpation, and resistance.
6. Perform open- and closed-chain motions. Describe joint motions, muscles activated, and types of muscle contractions.
7. Analyze functional activities such as grip, pinch, pushing, pulling, lifting, lowering, push-ups, pull-ups, sitting down and standing up, ascending and descending stairs, propelling a manual wheelchair, and crutch-walking. Describe joint motions, muscles activated, and type of muscle contraction for each.
8. Describe the oscillations, motions, and major muscle activity in normal walking.

MATERIALS AND EQUIPMENT

For laboratory study you will need the following:
1. A disarticulated bone set and access to a skeleton
2. A comprehensive anatomy textbook
3. A partner
4. Suitable laboratory attire to permit exposure to body segments
5. Some additional simple equipment will be identified within the units of study
6. Availability of electronic equipment such as electromyographs, dynamometers, balance meters, video taping, or a gait laboratory permit excellent laboratory illustration of muscle activities in exercise and function, muscle forces, joint motions, and movements of the center of gravity in function and gait analysis

MECHANICAL PRINCIPLES: KINEMATICS

1. With a partner, perform and observe motions in all the planes. Observe from the front while your partner performs frontal plane motions at the neck, trunk,

shoulder, elbow, wrist, fingers, hip, knee, ankle, and toes. Identify the direction of the axis of motion. Repeat for motions in the sagittal plane, viewing from the side, and in the horizontal plane, viewing from above.

2. With a partner or a group, lead an active range of motion dance. Call out the motion and the approximate degrees of motion as they are listed in Table 1–1.

3. With a partner or a small group, figure out and demonstrate closed-chain functional activities or potential exercises for the shoulder, elbow, wrist, hip, knee, and ankle.

4. Perform normal joint motions using a disarticulated bone set to observe the convex-concave principles. Note the directions of the articular surface and the shaft when the bone with the convex surface is moved and when the bone with the concave surface is moved. (If disarticulated bones are not available, an articulated skeleton can be used.)

5. Have your partner sit at a table or desk so that the forearm and palm are supported and the fingers are hanging over the edge. The examiner should sit in front or to the side of the subject and should hold the second metacarpal (index finger) between the thumb and fingers of one hand and the first phalange of the index finger with the other hand. The subject **must** relax the forearm and hand throughout the following exercises:

   a. **Convex-concave principles**—Hold the metacarpal still and passively move the phalange from flexion to extension several times. Visualize the directions of motion of the articular surface and the shaft. Then hold the phalange still and move the metacarpal into flexion and extension to visualize movements (see Fig. 1–9).

   b. **Close-packed and open-packed position**—Hold the metacarpal still and move the phalange. Notice that in extension of the joint, abduction and adduction are present, but in 90 degrees of flexion, the joint is stable (close-packed position).

   c. **Accessory motions**—Keep the metacarpal stabilized so that it cannot move, keep the joint in an open-packed position, and keep the subject relaxed while gently performing the following passive motions.
   Distraction: Gently pull the phalange distally 1 to 2 mm. Subject can palpate the joint space with the other forefinger (see Fig. 1–10).
   Rotation: Gently twist the phalange in each direction.
   Anterior and posterior glides: The examiner's thumb must be on the dorsal surface of the base of the phalange and forefinger on the palmar surface. The phalange is moved passively up and down without any angular motion (ie, flexion or extension). Note that these motions cannot be performed actively by the subject and that they cannot be performed passively in the close-packed position or if the subject is not relaxed.

CHAPTER 2

Mechanical Principles: Kinetics

Kinetics, a branch of dynamics, deals with **forces that produce, arrest, or modify motion of bodies** as a whole or of individual segments. In applying principles of kinetics, the clinician is particularly concerned with the forces exerted by gravity, muscles, friction, and external resistances. These primary forces lead in turn to joint compression, joint distraction, and pressures on the surfaces of the body.

THEORIES OF MOTION

For more than 1500 years, the theories of Aristotle (384–322 BC) were used to explain how objects moved. The natural state was considered to be rest. Motion required a mover such as a horse pulling a wagon. When the mover stopped, the motion also stopped. Aristotelian theorists, however, had to give special properties to air and water to explain the movement of the arrow after it left the bowstring and the movement of the boat when the oars were out of the water. The missing element of this theory was the effect of the force of friction on motion. Even now, it is difficult to create a friction-free environment or to envision what motion would be like in the absence of friction. By experimentation and deduction, Galileo (1564–1642) concluded that an external force was required to change the velocity of motion but that no force was needed to maintain motion. A very smooth block set in motion on a very smooth surface would continue in motion indefinitely if it did not meet resistance. Galileo's discoveries and those of others contributed to Newton's (1642–1727) development of the three laws of motion that form the current basis for mechanics and biomechanics.

The formulas used in mechanics to describe Newton's Laws are simple, such as force equals mass times acceleration ($F = ma$), and the definitions can be memorized easily. However, understanding and applying the laws in the study of human motion are difficult because the forces are never seen, seldom felt, and difficult to define.

FORCES

A simple way to conceptualize force is to think of a **push (compression) or a pull (tension)**. Such pushing and pulling can be visualized in the tug of war (Fig. 2–1). If both teams pull on the rope with the same force, no movement of the rope occurs. The system is balanced, or in a state of **equilibrium.** Movement occurs if the forces are unbalanced as one team pulls harder or one team slips. Both teams also are exerting pushing forces with their legs on the ground and the ground is pushing back on their feet—**action and reaction.** To produce these forces, each boy is exerting his maximal pulling or pushing forces at every joint between his hands and feet. In addition, the boys are leaning backward to add the effects of the pull of gravity on their body mass to the rope. The importance of frictional forces at the hands and feet can be seen as well, for if a hand or foot slips, the force produced on the rope by that boy is lost to the team.

Therapeutically, four primary sources of force are of major concern:

- **Gravity** or weight of body parts and attachments such as splints, casts, eating utensils, books, or weights
- **Muscles,** which can produce forces on the bone segments by active contraction or by being passively stretched
- **Externally applied resistances** such as exercise pulleys, manual resistance, doors, or windows
- **Friction,** which can provide stability if optimum, retard motion if excessive, and lead to instability if inadequate

Application of these primary forces may, in turn, lead to three secondary consequences of considerable clinical importance:

- Joint compression
- Joint distraction
- Pressure (force per unit area) on body tissues

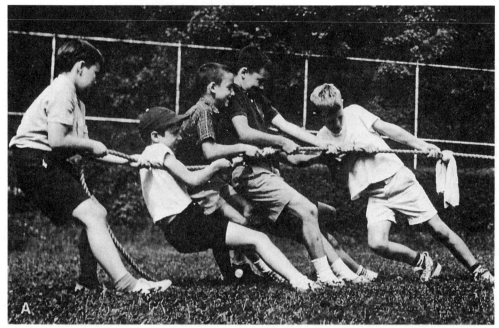

Figure 2–1 Forces at equilibrium in a tug-of-war. (From Strong, A, and Ubell, E: *The World of Push and Pull*. Atheneum, New York, 1964, pp 2–3, with permission).

Force Conventions

Forces are vector quantities, which have both magnitude and direction, as opposed to scalar quantities, which have magnitude only (6 books or 12 vertebrae). Vector forces can be expressed both graphically and mathematically (Fig. 2–2). Graphically, force vectors are represented by an arrow. The tail of the arrow represents the point of attachment of the force on another body. The arrowhead indicates the direction of the force. The shaft is the line of action of the force, and its length is drawn to a scale representing the magnitude of the force. The force system is located in space by placement on the rectangular coordinate system, with forces directed up or to the right given a positive (+) sign, and forces directed to the left or down given a negative (−) sign. The magnitudes of the forces are expressed in pounds, newtons (N), or dynes (Table 2–1).

The graphic and mathematic representations provide visualization and simplification of the abstract and complex forces occurring in postures and motions. An understanding of where and how forces act provides a basis for therapeutically modifying or altering forces to reduce pain, restore motion, and increase function.

Newton's Laws of Motion

The three fundamental laws governing motion are I, equilibrium; II, mass and acceleration; and III, action and reaction. The third law will be discussed first because it is helpful to understand the behavior of a single force before considering multiple forces.

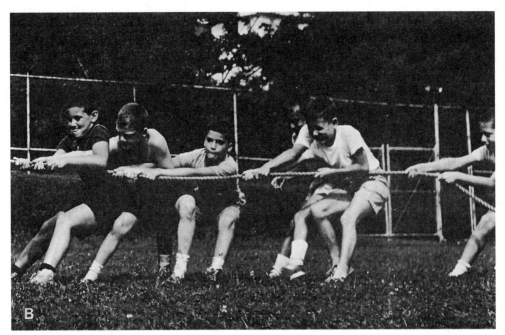

Figure 2–1 (*Continued*)

Action and Reaction (Newton's Third Law)

Each of the forces acting on a body or part arises from another body. Thus, forces do not act in isolation but rather as an interactive pair where the two bodies come in contact. In the tug of war, at equilibrium the boys push on the ground and the ground pushes back with an equal and opposite force (see Fig. 2–1). A weight held in the hand creates a 10-lb (44 N) force on the hand, and the hand resists the weight with a 10-lb force. A muscle pulls on a bone, and the bone reacts with an equal and opposite force as seen in Figure 2–3. Newton's third law of motion states that **for every action force there is an equal and opposite reaction force.** Thus, whenever two bodies are in contact, they exert equal and opposite forces on

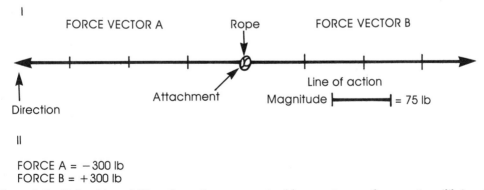

Figure 2–2 (*I*) Graphic and (*II*) mathematic components of force vectors on the rope at equilibrium in the tug-of-war (see Fig. 2–1).

Table 2-1   Systems Commonly Used to Express Weights and Measures

System	Mass	Force	Distance	Torque	Time
B.E.	slug	pound	foot	lb-ft	sec
MKS	kg	Newton	meter	N-m	sec
cgs	gram	dyne	cm	dyne-cm	sec

B.E. = British Engineering (foot, pound, sec); MKS = meter, kilogram, second; cgs = centimeter, gram, second

each other. The state of motion of a body depends on the forces acting on that body rather than on the forces it may exert on other bodies. This concept can be seen and felt in a situation of decreased friction, such as on ice skates. If the skater pushes against a fixed object, the skater is pushed in the opposite direction.

Equilibrium (Newton's First Law)

Fundamental in Newtonian mechanics is that Aristotle's natural state is equilibrium (L. *aequilibrare,* to balance). In a state of equilibrium, the sum of the forces acting on the body is zero or balanced. In the tug of war (see Fig. 2–1), many large forces exist, but the system is at rest or in static equilibrium because all the forces on the right side equal those on the left side. A hockey puck resting on an ice rink is in equilibrium because the weight or force of the puck upon the ice is balanced by an equal force of the ice upon the puck. After the puck has been struck (accelerated), it is again in equilibrium and moves in a particular direction and at a particular velocity until other forces are impressed upon it. Friction between the ice–puck interface decelerates the velocity of the puck, and collision with a stick or wall changes the direction and velocity.

Newton's first law, the law of inertia, states, "Every body persists in its state of rest or of uniform motion in a straight line unless it is compelled to change that state by forces impressed on it" (Resnick and Halliday, 1960). In simpler terms, it can be said that a force is required to start a motion, to change direction or speed of a motion, and to stop a motion.

Translatory applications of this law can be disastrous when a person is being transported in a wheelchair, on a stretcher, or in an automobile and the vehicle is

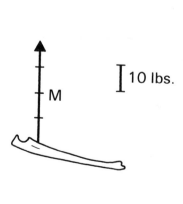

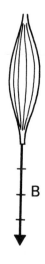

Figure 2–3 Vector representation of the force of the brachialis muscle (M) contraction on the bone and of the force of the bone (B) on the muscle. M could be considered the action force and B the reaction force or vice versa, depending on the circumstances.

stopped suddenly. If the person is not attached to the vehicle (eg, by a seat belt), the body continues forward until stopped by another force. Fractured femurs are common injuries to patients who are thrown out of wheelchairs in this manner. Seat belts or restraining straps are recommended, and frequently required, to prevent injuries caused by abrupt stops of wheelchairs and stretchers, as well as of automobiles. Whiplash injuries to the neck from rear-end collisions of automobiles occur because the automobile seat and the person's body are impelled forward as a unit, while the unsupported head remains at rest. The violent stretching of the neck structures then produces a force to rapidly "whip" the head and neck into flexion, with resulting injury to both posterior and anterior structures of the head and neck.

Clinical applications of the law of equilibrium affecting angular motion at a joint are found in the lower extremity during the swing phase of walking. Not only is a force required to start the thigh moving (hip flexors) but also to stop the leg (hamstring muscles). The terminal velocity of the foot in normal walking is approximately 15 miles per hour. The magnitude of this stopping force can be appreciated when walking barefooted in the dark and striking the toes against a rock, chair leg, or bedpost. Persons with above-knee amputations, on the other hand, do not have muscles to stop the swing of the prosthetic leg. The problem of permitting the leg to swing without overswinging requires careful adjustment of the frictional forces in the joint of the artificial knee.

Mass and Acceleration (Newton's Second Law)

The same force or forces acting on different bodies cause the bodies to move differently. The property of a body that resists change in motion or equilibrium is defined as **inertia.** Newton's second law of motion states: **The acceleration (a) of a body is proportionate to the magnitude of the resultant forces (F) on it and inversely proportionate to the mass (m) of the body.** As an equation, this is written:

$$a \propto \frac{F}{m}$$

More simply stated, a greater force is required to move (or stop the motion of) a large mass than a small one. In the tug of war (see Fig. 2–1) the boy at the left end is using this law advantageously to his team.

Application of this law is demonstrated in the movement of body segments in response to muscle contraction. When a muscle contracts, it shortens and produces the same amount of force at its proximal and distal attachments (origin and insertion). Thus, **either one or both** segments may move. This can be seen in a subject performing a sit-up. The hip flexor muscles (iliopsoas) attach to the trunk and to the femur; thus the part with the least mass moves when the muscles contract forcefully. Individuals with relatively light mass in their lower extremities have difficulty performing a sit-up because the lower extremities elevate. Stabilization of the lower extremities is needed to perform the desired motion. Other clinical applications of the law of inertia are seen with changes in the mass of segments. When the mass is increased, as in walking with heavy boots or a cast on the leg, greater muscle force is needed to start and stop the leg swing. In patients with muscle weakness (inability to develop adequate muscle force), one of the important considerations is to keep the mass of appliances (such as splints and adapted equipment) as light as possible to reduce the muscle force requirements.

WEIGHT The basic equation describing the relationship among acceleration, force, and mass can also be written as F = ma. With this equation, the concept of weight can be differentiated from mass. Weight (W) is the effect of the acceleration of gravity (g) on a mass. Thus, the equation for weight is W = mg. Weight, then, is a force and is expressed in pounds, newtons, or dynes. Mass is expressed in slugs, kilograms, or grams (see Tables 2–1 and 2–2). The weight of a body varies with its location from the center of the earth, whereas the mass (inertia) always remains the same. This difference is of importance in therapeutic exercise and space kinesiology for the understanding of a human's ability to move and perform work in a gravity-reduced environment. When an astronaut in space reaches forward or attempts to push a lever or door, the body moves in the opposite direction from the work because there is insufficient weight to stabilize the body. To stabilize the body, toeholds and clamps are needed.

Clinically, several methods are used to reduce the effect of weight on body segments. Body parts may be positioned and supported to move in a plane parallel to the earth to decrease the effect of gravity and thus permit motion by weak muscles. Movement in this plane is frequently called "gravity-free," "gravity-eliminated," or "gravity-minimized" motion. The weight of the body or segments may be suspended from above by slings and springs or supported from below, thereby permitting weak muscles to exercise or painful joints to be unloaded (Kelsey and Tyson, 1994). Another weightless environment is the therapeutic pool, where Archimedes' principle of buoyancy is used—**a body submerged in a liquid is buoyed up by a force equal to the weight of the liquid displaced.** Weak muscles that cannot overcome the effects of gravity can perform graded underwater exercises, and painful joints can be unloaded of weight to permit pain-free exercise and walking.

FORCE VECTOR DIAGRAMS Newton's third law of action and reaction provides a method to visualize all the forces acting on a body or a segment. The paired action and reaction forces act on different bodies. Thus, the state of motion of a particular body depends on the forces acting on it rather than on the forces it may exert on another body. If one wishes to estimate the forces acting on the forearm when

Table 2-2 Conversion Factors

Mass

1 slug (sg)	= 14.59 kilograms (kg)
1 gram (gm)	= 0.001 kilogram (kg)

Force

1 pound (lb)	= 4.448 newtons (N)
1 newton (N)	= 0.225 pound (lb)
1 dyne	= 0.00001 newton (N)
1 pound (lb)	= 0.45 kilogram (kg)*
1 kilogram (kg)*	= 2.2 pound (lb)

Distance

1 foot (ft)	= 0.3048 meter (m)
1 inch (in)	= 2.54 centimeters (cm)
1 centimeter (cm)	= 0.01 meter (m)

Torque (bending moment)

1 foot-pound (ft-lb)	= 1.356 newton-meters (N-m)
1 dyne-centimeter (dyne-cm)	= 0.0000001 newton-meter (N-m)

*The kilogram is a unit of mass, but it is commonly used as a unit of force instead of the correct unit, newton.

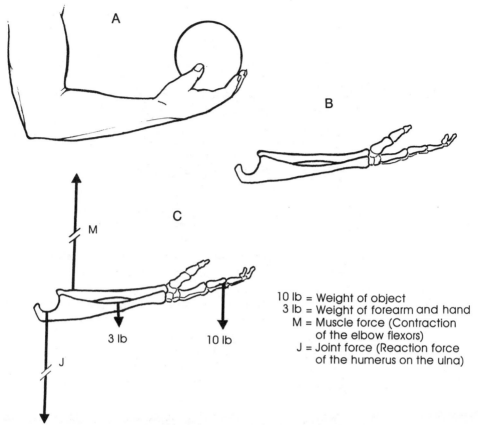

10 lb = Weight of object
3 lb = Weight of forearm and hand
M = Muscle force (Contraction
of the elbow flexors)
J = Joint force (Reaction force
of the humerus on the ulna)

Figure 2-4 Forces on the forearm when holding a 10-lb weight in the hand. (*A*) Anatomic representation, (*B*) line drawing of the isolated forearm, and (*C*) vector representation of the forces exerted by the removed structures and gravity.

holding a weight in the hand (Fig. 2–4A) the forearm is represented in isolation with a simple line drawing (see Fig. 2–4B). All the structures touching it are omitted and replaced by their force vectors (see Fig. 2–4C). The vectors are labeled with force units if known or with symbols if their magnitude is unknown. Later measurement of anatomic distances permits calculation of the magnitude of the unknown forces (see Levers later in this chapter).

In engineering, these diagrams are called space diagrams, or free body diagrams.

Composition of Forces

Frequently, several forces act simultaneously on a body (Fig. 2–5). To simplify and better visualize the magnitude and direction of such multiple forces, the process of composition of forces is used. By adding or subtracting two or more forces, their combined effect can be shown by a single resultant force. This resultant force is the simplest force (or force system) that can produce the same effect as all the forces acting together. If two or more forces act along a line or parallel lines, the forces can be added to find the single resultant force. In Figure 2–6, the weights of the leg and the exercise apparatus form a linear force system that causes distraction of the knee joint. The magnitude of the distracting force can be found by

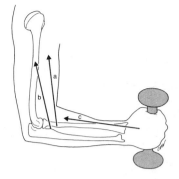

Figure 2–5   Vector representation of forces developed by (*A*) the biceps brachialis, (*B*) the brachialis, and (*C*) a combination of the brachioradialis, extensor carpi radialis longus, and extensor carpi radialis brevis muscles when the subject lifts an exercise weight with the hand and forearm.

graphic composition of forces (drawing the force vectors to scale) or by algebraic composition of forces (see Fig. 2–6D) using the formula that the resultant force (R) is equal to the sum of the individual forces (R = ΣF). In both methods, the resultant force is the same and has the same effect on the femur as the three original forces do together. In this problem, the resultant is equal and opposite to the forces of the joint ligaments, fascia, and capsule.

Similar procedures can be used to find the resultant force in a linear force system when the forces act in opposite directions, as occurs when applying a 25-lb (111 N) traction force to the cervical structures with the subject sitting upright (Fig. 2–7). In this case, the upward force on the cervical spine is only 15 lb (67 N).

Force Acting at Angles

The resultant force of vector forces in the same plane acting at angles to each other cannot be found by simple addition or subtraction but must be found graphically or trigonometrically. If two forces are pulling from the same point, the resultant force can be found graphically by constructing a parallelogram (Fig. 2–8).

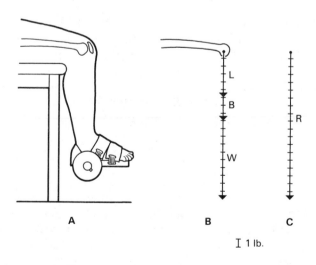

A

B   **C**

Ⅰ 1 lb.

D

Figure 2–6   Forces acting at the knee joint when the subject is sitting with an exercise boot and weight on the foot. (*A*) Anatomic diagram. (*B*) Free body diagram of the forces on the femur. (*C*) Graphic composition of the resultant force. (*D*) Algebraic composition of the resultant force (negative sign indicates that the direction of the force is down).

R = ΣF
R = –L – B –W
R = –6 lbs. –3 lbs. –10 lbs.
R = –19 lbs.

L = weight of leg and foot = 6 lbs.
B = weight of boot = 3 lbs.
W = weights = 10 lbs.
R = resultant force = 19 lbs.

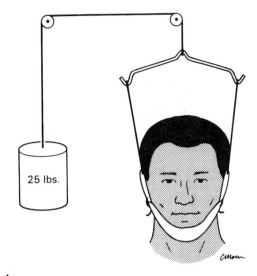

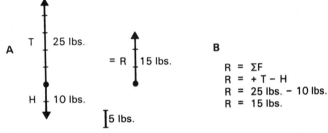

Figure 2–7 (*A*) Graphic and (*B*) algebraic solutions for the force applied to the head and neck structures when an upward force of 25 lb is applied to the head, which weighs 10 lb.

T = traction force (25 lbs.)
H = weight of head (10 lbs.)

R = ΣF
R = + T – H
R = 25 lbs. – 10 lbs.
R = 15 lbs.

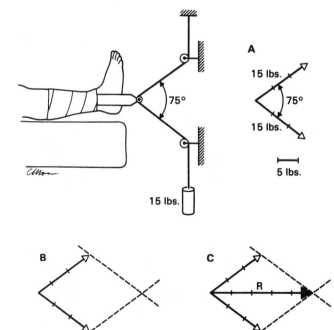

Figure 2–8 Parallelogram method of finding the resultant traction force on the leg. (*A*) The force vectors acting on the leg are drawn to scale. (*B*) Lines are drawn parallel to each force vector from the arrowhead of the other vector to form a parallelogram. (*C*) The resultant force is the diagonal from the origin of the forces. The magnitude can be found by measuring the length of the action line.

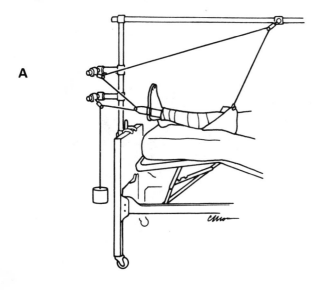

A

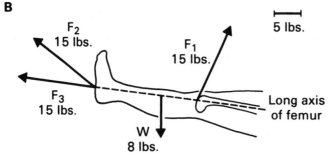

B

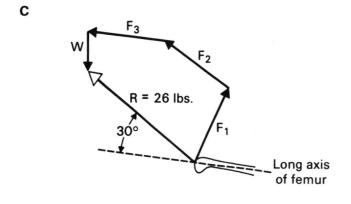

C

Figure 2–9 (A) Polygon method for composition of forces using Russell traction, which applies a distraction force on the femur. (A) Fifteen pounds of weight are suspended on the weight carrier. The leg, foot, and footpiece weigh 8 lb. (B) Scale diagram of the forces acting on the femur. (C) The force vectors are connected serially, according to their angle and direction. The open side of the polygon is the single resultant force. In this case, the traction force on the femur is 26 lb and is acting at a 30-degree angle from the long axis of the femur. Realignment of the pulleys is needed to bring the resultant force in line with the long axis of the femur.

The resultant force is the diagonal of the parallelogram, not the sum of the two forces. Note that, as the angle between the two forces increases, the resultant force decreases, reaching a minimum when the forces are on the same line and acting in opposite directions, when the angle becomes 180 degrees. Conversely, as the angle between the forces becomes smaller, the resultant force increases. When the angle becomes zero, the forces are on the same line, and the resultant force is the sum of the two forces. Thus, in the leg traction example, if the patient moves toward the head of the bed, the angle between the ropes becomes smaller, and the traction force increases. If the patient moves toward the foot of the bed, the angle between the ropes becomes larger, and the traction force decreases. The same effects occur if someone moves the fixed pulleys on the bedpost farther apart or closer together.

Other examples of forces acting at angles to each other occur in muscles where parts may have different lines of pull. Examples include contraction of the upper and lower trapezius to result in adduction of the scapula, and contraction of the two heads of the gastrocnemius with a resultant force on the tendon of Achilles.

When more than two forces are acting, the resultant force can be obtained graphically by forming a polygon. One force vector is drawn to scale and placed in its proper direction. Subsequent vectors are drawn in the same manner, and the tail of each vector is placed at the tip of the previous vector (Fig. 2–9). This process forms a polygon that is open on one side. The resultant force closes the polygon. Measurement of the magnitude and the angle of the resultant force shows the single effect of the diverse forces.

In actuality, the parallelogram method for two forces is a special case of the polygon method. Instead of drawing a parallelogram, one could draw the second force tail from the tip of the first. Closing the triangle forms the resultant force. Algebraic solutions of the resultant force for the triangle and polygon can be found using the cosine law of trigonometry (LeVeau, 1977).

LEVERS

A machine that operates on the principle of a rigid bar being acted on by forces that tend to rotate the bar about its pivot point is called a **lever**. In biomechanics, the principles of the lever are used to visualize the more complex system of forces that produce rotary motion in the body. By reducing these forces to their simplest form of three resultant forces, approximate magnitudes of forces and displacement of segments can be found, and the basis for therapeutic manipulation of forces can be better understood.

The three forces of the mechanical lever are the axis A (or pivot), the weight W (or resistance R), and the moving (or holding) force F (Fig. 2–10). The perpendicular distance from the pivot point (or center of rotation) to the line of action of the weight is called the weight arm. The perpendicular distance from the holding force to the axis is called the force arm.

Mechanical advantage (MA) of the lever refers to the ratio between the length of the force arm and the length of the weight arm. The equation is:

$$MA = \frac{\text{Force Arm Length}}{\text{Weight Arm Length}}$$

The ratios for the lever systems shown in Figure 2–10 would be: I = 1, II = 2, and III = 0.5. The higher the number, the greater the mechanical advantage. An increase in the length of the force arm or a decrease in the length of the weight arm (or resistance arm) results in greater mechanical advantage, thus facilitating the task to be performed.

In angular motions or postures of the body, the bone or segment is the lever,

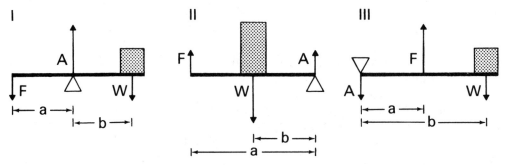

Figure 2–10 Vector diagrams of the first-class, second-class, and third-class levers. Classification is according to the positions of the weight and force in relation to the axis. A = axis or fulcrum; W = weight or resistance; F = moving or holding force; a = force arm distance; b = weight or resistance arm distance.

and the axis is usually at the joint. Muscle contraction is the holding or moving force, and the resistance is the weight of the part, body segments, or applied resistances (Fig. 2–11). Different positions of these forces on the lever arm give different advantages for motion and work. The operation of levers provides either force or excursion advantages.

First-Class Lever

First-class levers, such as the seesaw or balance scale, may be used to gain either force or distance, depending on the relative lengths of the force arm and the weight arm. This principle is used in the forearm trough of the ball-bearing feeder

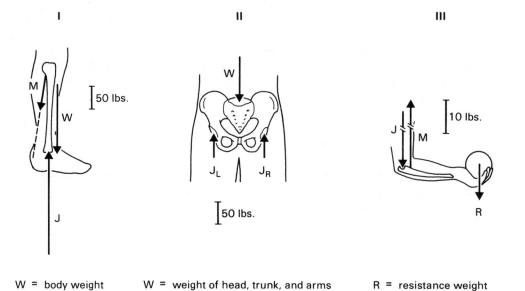

W = body weight	W = weight of head, trunk, and arms	R = resistance weight
M = soleus muscle	J_L = joint force (left)	M = elbow flexor muscles
J = joint force	J_R = joint force (right)	J = joint force

Figure 2–11 Anatomic examples of the three lever systems. (*I*) Forces at the ankle when standing on one foot. (*II*) Forces on the pelvis when standing on both feet. (*III*) Forces on the forearm when holding a weight in the hand (weight of forearm is neglected). The break in vectors (J and M in [*III*]) indicates that their magnitude is not drawn to scale.

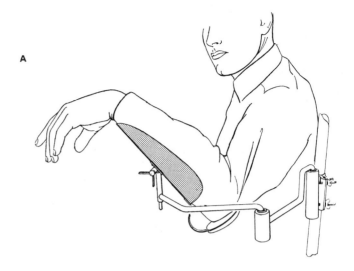

A

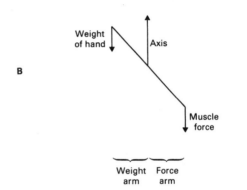

B

Figure 2–12 (*A*) Ball-bearing forearm orthosis (feeder) used by patients who have severe muscle weakness of the elbow and shoulder. (*B*) The trough is an example of a first-class lever system. With careful placement of the axis to gain the proper weight arm and force arm distances, patients with very little muscle strength can feed and groom themselves. (Adapted from Licht, S, and Kamenetz, H: *Orthotics Etcetera.* Elizabeth Licht, Pub, 1966, p 219).

(Fig. 2–12) by moving the axis proximally or distally. In the body, the first-class lever system is frequently used for maintaining postures or balance (see Fig. 2–11 I). An example is found at the atlanto-occipital joint (axis), where the head (weight) is balanced by neck extensor muscle force. The same principle occurs at the intervertebral joints in sitting or standing, where the weight of the trunk is balanced by the erector spinae muscle forces acting on the vertebral axis. This type of lever arrangement is commonly used in orthotics to apply a support or correctional force to body parts (Fig. 2–13) and is frequently called the three-point system for applying a force.

Second-Class Lever

Second-class levers provide a force advantage such that large weights can be supported or moved by a smaller force. The wheelbarrow and the use of a crowbar for prying are mechanical examples of this type of leverage. In the body, there are limited examples of the second-class lever. The forces on the floor when a person is standing on both feet are an example, as are the forces at the pelvis in bilateral stance (see Fig. 2–11II). The only muscle example is the pull of the brachioradialis and the wrist extensors to maintain the position of elbow flexion. Normally, however, these muscles do not act in this isolated manner. Some patients with muscu-

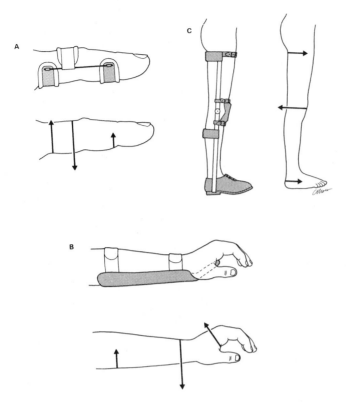

Figure 2–13 Examples of static positioning orthoses and the forces they exert on the body part. (*A*) Interphalangeal extension splint. (*B*) Cock-up splint to maintain wrist extension. (*C*) Knee-ankle-foot orthosis (KAFO) to prevent knee flexion.

lar dystrophy who have paralysis of the biceps brachii and brachialis muscles can use the brachioradialis and wrist extensors to hold the elbow in a position of flexion. If anything heavy is held in the hand, however, the system changes to a third-class lever, and the brachioradialis and wrist extensor muscle forces cannot maintain the position.

Third-Class Lever

The third-class lever is most common in the human body. In this type of leverage, the weight arm is always longer than the force arm, and the mechanical advantage may be 0.1 or even lower. This arrangement is designed for producing speed of the distal segment and for moving a small weight a long distance. Thus, in the human body, a small amount of shortening of a muscle such as the brachialis causes a large arc of motion of the hand. This type of leverage is found in most open-chain motions of the extremities: the deltoid acting on the glenohumeral joint, the flexor digitorum superficialis at the interphalangeal joints, the extensor carpi radialis at the wrist, the anterior tibialis at the ankle joint, and the biceps-brachialis at the elbow (see Fig. 2–11III).

All three types of levers demonstrate that what is gained in excursion is lost in force and, conversely, **what is gained** in force is lost in distance.

The classification of levers as first, second, or third class solely depends on the relationships among the axis, weight, and force. If the axis is central, the class is I; if the weight is central, the class is II; and if the force is central, the class is III. Frequently, such categories do not exist. The orthotic applications in Figure 2–13 are three-point force systems. It would be a useless exercise to try to classify these lever systems. More important than memorization of the lever systems is recognition of the commonalities of the placement, directions, and magnitude of the three forces. Review of the force vector diagrams in Figures 2–10 through 2–13 shows that all have a large central force in one direction flanked by two smaller forces in the opposite direction.

Static Equilibrium

In the fundamental Newtonian equation $F = ma$, F represents the sum or resultant of **all the forces** acting on the body of interest. When that body is not moving, it is in the state of static equilibrium and acceleration is zero ($\Sigma F = 0$). Static equilibrium equations for the forces on the three-lever systems in Figure 2–10 can be written in the following manner (using positive and negative signs for direction):

$$\Sigma F = 0$$

$$
\begin{array}{llll}
\text{I} & A - F - W = 0 & \text{or} & A = F + W \\
\text{II} & A + F - W = 0 & & A = -F + W \\
\text{III} & -A + F - W = 0 & & A = F - W \\
\end{array}
$$

Thus if two of the forces are known, the unknown third force can be calculated.

Statics is a special case of dynamics where acceleration is zero. In this text, the simpler equations of static equilibrium are used to illustrate the magnitude of the forces occurring clinically. In the majority of therapeutic activities, movement is very slow and does not have rapid accelerations as in activities such as throwing, running, or diving. Clinical concepts can be gained by examining these slow movements and postures at selected points in the range of motion (see Fig. 2–14).

For example, it can be shown that, in standing, the force between the joint surfaces at the ankle (eg, the force on the tibia from the talus when standing on one leg) is greater than the superincumbent body weight (weight of segments above the joint). Referring to Figure 2–11I, we see that the center-of-gravity line (W) of the body falls not through the ankle joint, but slightly anterior to the lateral malleolus. The axis of motion (or potential motion) is the ankle joint (J). The person is prevented from falling forward at the ankle (dorsiflexion) by contraction of the soleus muscle (M), whose proximal attachment is on the tibia and distal attachment is on the calcaneus. Using a body weight of 150 lb (667 N) and positive signs for upward forces and negative signs for downward forces, the equation would be:

$$\Sigma F = 0$$
$$-M + J - W = 0$$
$$-M + J - 150 \text{ lb} = 0$$
$$J = 150 \text{ lb} + M$$

The compression force on the ankle is 150 lb plus the force the muscle must exert to maintain the position. Calculation of the magnitude of the muscle and joint forces, however, requires the use of lever arm distances and torques.

While this text is limited to statics, students of kinesiology are encouraged to pursue the study of dynamics (LeVeau, 1977). Dynamics addresses kinematic characteristics of motion such as displacement, velocity, and acceleration and the kinetic effects of acceleration, momentum, work, and energy.

TORQUE

Torque (τ), or moment of a force, is the product of a force times the perpendicular distance (d) from its line of action to the axis of motion (or potential motion). The equation is $\tau = F \perp d$. Torque is the expression of the effectiveness of a force in turning a lever system. A common example is represented by attempts to open a door that is stuck. One may push or pull at the center of the door with all the force that can be mustered and not open the door. If, however, this same force is applied as far as possible from the door hinges (axis), the force is more effective in opening the door (increased length of the force arm). Using a simple mechanical lever, such as the seesaw, a 50-lb (222 N) child can balance a 100-lb (445 N) child if the lever arm distance for the 50-lb child is twice the length of the lever arm distance for the 100-lb child. Extending this principle further, the resistance of the 100-lb child could be balanced by fingertip pressure if the force lever arm were very long. It is told that Archimedes (287–212 BC), in reference to this principle stated, "Give me a place to stand and I will move the earth."

Torque principles are used by therapists in testing the strength of muscles (manual muscle testing) and in applying manual resistive exercise. For example, in testing the strength of the elbow flexors, the therapist prefers to apply resistance at the wrist rather than in the middle of the forearm. In each case, the torque produced by the patient's elbow flexors is the same. The force that the therapist applies, however, is approximately one-half less at the wrist than at the mid-forearm because of the longer resistance arm. This lower force provides the therapist with better control and discrimination of the torque produced by the patient.

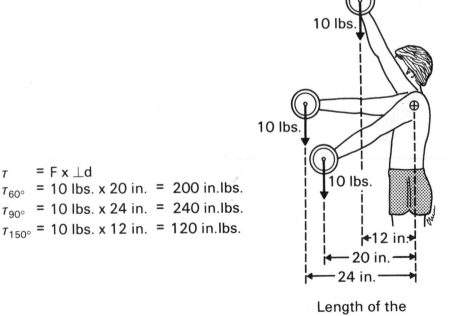

$$\tau = F \times \perp d$$
$$\tau_{60°} = 10 \text{ lbs.} \times 20 \text{ in.} = 200 \text{ in.lbs.}$$
$$\tau_{90°} = 10 \text{ lbs.} \times 24 \text{ in.} = 240 \text{ in.lbs.}$$
$$\tau_{150°} = 10 \text{ lbs.} \times 12 \text{ in.} = 120 \text{ in.lbs.}$$

Length of the resistance arms

Figure 2–14 Variation of the resistance torque at the shoulder when a 10-lb weight is held in the hand and the shoulder is flexed to 60, 90, and 150 degrees.

In Figure 2–14, the subject is shown holding an exercise weight in the hand with the shoulder in three positions of flexion. At the shoulder, the torque produced by the weight varies with the perpendicular distance from the line of action of the force (weight) to the joint center. The perpendicular distance is then the resistance arm. Thus, the torque produced by the weight increases as the hand is brought away from the body, and reaches the maximum at 90 degrees of shoulder flexion. The torque then decreases again as shoulder flexion continues. Only when the line of action of a force is perpendicular to the lever arm is the distance the same as the actual lever arm, as it is at 90° in Figure 2–14. (Later, procedures for resolution of forces provide for use of a perpendicular component of the force whereby the actual lever arm length can be used.)

Clinically, torque reduction is emphasized in lifting and carrying to prevent strain or injury to the person lifting. For example, in the two- or three-person lift and transfer of a patient from bed to stretcher or wheelchair, instructions include sliding the patient close to the edge of the bed (and to the bodies of the lifters) before attempting to lift the patient. The next instruction is to lift and quickly roll the patient toward the lifters' chests. The moves of first sliding and then rolling the patient bring the patient's center of gravity closer to the center of gravity of the lifters, thus reducing the torque and likelihood of injury from excessive strain.

At equilibrium when no motion or acceleration of the body is occurring, the torque of the resistance force equals the torque of the holding force: force times the force arm equals resistance times the resistance arm. In the lever examples in Figure 2–10, the equation is $F \times a = W \times b$ for each type of lever. The general formula is derived from Newton's first law. If a body is in equilibrium, the sum of the resultant forces equals zero and therefore the sum of the torques must also be balanced and equal to zero. The formula for torque at equilibrium is $\Sigma\tau = 0$. This formula permits understanding and calculation of the magnitude of muscle and joint compression forces, which cannot be measured directly.

Parallel Force Systems

A parallel force system occurs when all of the forces acting on the segment are applied at a 90-degree angle as in the levers (see Fig. 2–10), the forearm (see Fig. 2–4), and the orthotic applications (see Fig. 2–13A and C). The static equilibrium formulas for torque ($\Sigma\tau = 0$) and force ($\Sigma F = 0$) permit development of algebraic equations to find the unknown forces. As an example, the forces on the forearm in the free body diagram (see Fig. 2–4) are placed on the coordinate system (Fig. 2–15) with the joint force (J) at the origin of the system. Measured lever arm distances are added. The torque produced by each force ($\tau = F \times \perp d$) is substituted into the equilibrium formula ($\Sigma\tau = 0$). Then positive and negative signs are assigned. **In the torque equation, these signs show the turning effect of the force on the coordinate system and not the direction of the force.** If a torque produces or tends to produce a clockwise motion of the coordinate system, the sign is positive. If a torque tends to produce a counterclockwise motion, a negative sign is assigned. The equation is then solved for the magnitude of the muscle force (69 lb). Once we know the value of M, the joint compression force of 56 lb is calculated using the formula for forces ($\Sigma F = 0$). The placement of one of the unknown forces on the origin of the coordinate system (eg, J) reduces the lever arm distance to zero. The force then has no turning effect on the system, exerts

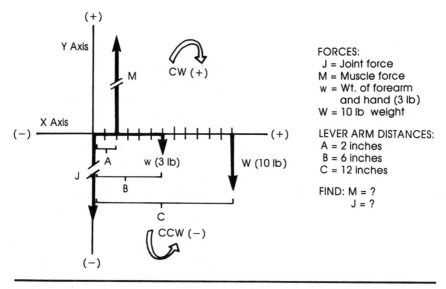

FORCES:
J = Joint force
M = Muscle force
w = Wt. of forearm
      and hand (3 lb)
W = 10 lb weight

LEVER ARM DISTANCES:
A = 2 inches
B = 6 inches
C = 12 inches

FIND: M = ?
          J = ?

I. FORMULAS NEEDED TO FIND M:

$$\tau = F \times \perp d$$
$$\Sigma\tau = 0$$

CALCULATIONS:
$$\tau J + [-\tau M] + \tau w + \tau W = 0$$
$$[J \times 0] - [M \times 2 \text{ in}] + [3 \text{ lb} \times 6 \text{ in}] + [10 \text{ lb} \times 12 \text{ in}] = 0$$
$$-[M \times 2 \text{ in}] + [18 \text{ in-lb}] + [120 \text{ in-lb}] = 0$$
$$-M \times 2 \text{ in} = -138 \text{ in-lb}$$
$$M = \frac{138 \text{ in-lb}}{2 \text{ in}}$$

$$\boxed{M = 69 \text{ lb}}$$

II. FORMULA NEEDED TO FIND J:

$$\Sigma F = 0$$

CALCULATIONS:
$$-J + M - w - W = 0$$
$$-J + 69 \text{ lb} - 3 \text{ lb} - 10 \text{ lb} = 0$$
$$-J = -56 \text{ lb}$$

$$\boxed{J = 56 \text{ lb}}$$

Figure 2–15 Coordinate system with vector diagram for calculating the forces on the forearm when holding a 10-lb weight in the hand (see Fig. 2–4 for the free body diagram). The force J has been placed at the origin of the coordinate system. Lever arm distances have been measured and stated in the nearest whole number. Formulas and calculations for solving the problem are provided. Note that the positive and negative signs for the direction of a force are negative to the left and down and positive to the right and up, while the directions of a torque are positive for clockwise motion and negative for counterclockwise motion (or potential motion).

no torque, and is conveniently eliminated from the equation leaving only one unknown value (M).

This problem can be solved as well by placing the muscle force at the origin of the coordinate system using appropriate distances and new signs. This problem could not be solved, however, if the weight were placed at the origin because the equation would contain two unknown values.

Biologically, there probably are no strictly parallel force systems. Nevertheless, the model provides estimates and concepts of the magnitudes of the forces occurring in motions and postures. The forces calculated for the forearm in Figure 2–15 illustrate the use of a third-class lever system in the body where very large forces must be generated by muscles and joints to hold or move a small distally placed resistance. In the shoulder flexion diagram (see Fig. 2–14), the torque of the resistance varies with the weight arm distance and is at a maximum of 20 ft-lb when the extremity is horizontal. At equilibrium, the shoulder flexor muscles also must produce an equal torque at each position ($\Sigma\tau = 0$). The force arm of the muscles is, however, only a few inches long. Thus the muscles must exert great forces (more than 10 times that of the weight) to hold the weight at the 2-ft distance.

On the other hand, the use of the first-class lever system illustrates energy efficiency with smaller muscle forces used to support larger resistances. An example is standing on one foot (Fig. 2–16). Calculations show that a body weight of 150 lb

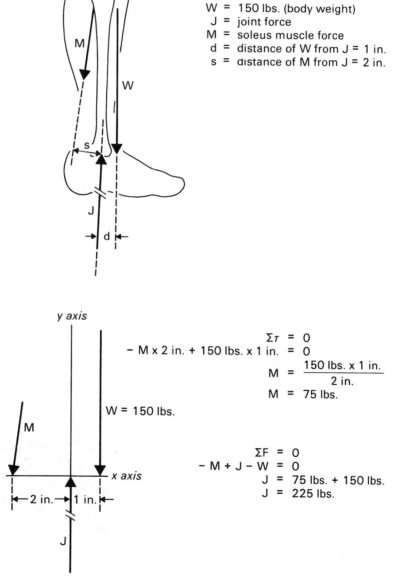

W = 150 lbs. (body weight)
J = joint force
M = soleus muscle force
d = distance of W from J = 1 in.
s = distance of M from J = 2 in.

$$\Sigma\tau = 0$$
$$- M \times 2 \text{ in.} + 150 \text{ lbs.} \times 1 \text{ in.} = 0$$
$$M = \frac{150 \text{ lbs.} \times 1 \text{ in.}}{2 \text{ in.}}$$
$$M = 75 \text{ lbs.}$$

W = 150 lbs.

$$\Sigma F = 0$$
$$- M + J - W = 0$$
$$J = 75 \text{ lbs.} + 150 \text{ lbs.}$$
$$J = 225 \text{ lbs.}$$

Figure 2–16 Diagram and equations for the forces on the tibia during unilateral stance with approximate calculations of the magnitudes of the muscle (M) and joint compression (J) forces. This is not a true parallel force system because M is at a slight angle to J and W.

can be prevented from turning the system by a counterforce of 75 lb. Only one half the force is needed because of the long (2-inch) lever arm of the calcaneus. The joint compression force of the tibia on the talus is 225 lb, which exceeds the superincumbent weight of the body. If the person sways forward slightly so that the line of the center of gravity falls 2 inches in front of the ankle center, the muscle force increases to 200 lb and the joint compression force increases to 300 lb.

The ankle problem illustrates the principle that lengthening or shortening the lever arm distance of one force in a system causes changes in the magnitude of other forces. Shortening of a lever arm can increase the forces applied to the body and thereby increase pressure. Figure 2–17 illustrates the forces applied by a forearm splint designed to provide dynamic assistance to finger extension (by a rubber band). Shortening the forearm lever arm in C increases all three forces and the resulting pressures. Another clinical example is that of the three orthotic forces needed to keep the knee extended (see Fig. 2–13C). Examination of Figure 2–18A shows that the posterior thigh band lever arm has been shortened and that the anterior knee force is divided between the anterior cuffs above and below the knee. This configuration does not provide sufficient forces to maintain knee extension in the person with muscle paralysis in the lower extremities. This lady is "sitting" on the posterior thigh band, the anterior knee forces are not sufficient to prevent knee flexion, and she cannot achieve standing balance without holding on with her hands. In Figure 2–18B, she is shown with a lengthened lever arm for the thigh band and an additional anterior cuff close to the knee to help maintain knee

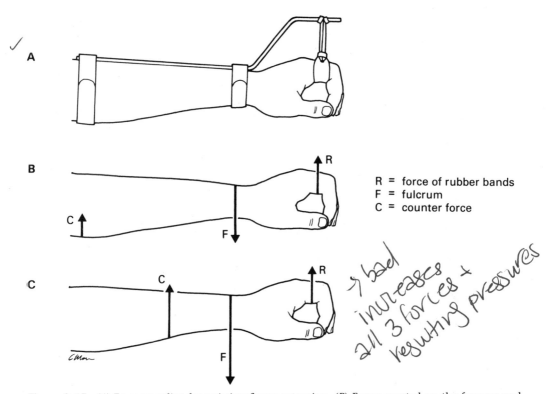

R = force of rubber bands
F = fulcrum
C = counter force

Figure 2–17 (A) Forearm splint for assisting finger extension. (B) Forces exerted on the forearm and hand. (C) Increase in counterforce C (and consequently in F) when the forearm lever arm is reduced in length.

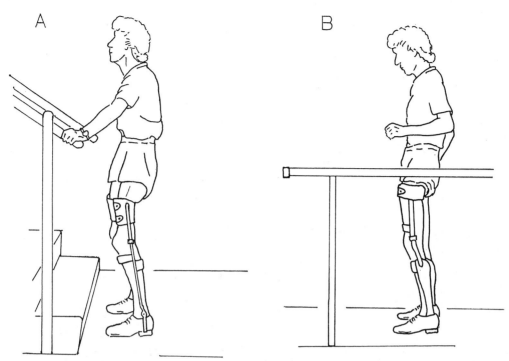

Figure 2–18 Subject with lower extremity muscle paralysis standing in long leg braces (knee-ankle-foot orthoses) to keep the knees extended. (*A*) The posterior thigh band is too low, causing the subject to "sit" in the braces with resulting increased forces (and tissue pressure) at the thigh and knee. The knee is flexed and the subject lacks standing balance. (*B*) Decreased forces and pressures result from correct position of the thigh band. The knee is extended and balance is achieved.

extension. She is able to achieve standing balance without use of the hands, and tissue pressures, especially on the posterior thigh, have been reduced.

Resolution of Forces

Many of the forces that occur in or on the body are applied at angles to the segment rather than in a linear or parallel system, as in previous examples. Figure 2–19 shows an example in which the forces (W, M, and J) are neither parallel to each other nor perpendicular to the lever arm. **Resolution of a force** into two component forces is used (1) to visualize the effect of such angular forces on the body, (2) to determine the torque produced by the forces, and (3) to calculate the magnitude of unknown muscle and joint forces. The process is based on the principle that any number can be represented by two or more different numbers (eg, 7 can be represented by 6 + 1 or 5 + 2). Thus, any vector can be represented by two or more vectors. Resolution of a force vector is the division of the vector into two or more **component vectors** whose combined magnitudes and directions produce the same effect as the original force (Fig. 2–20). In biomechanics, two rectangular components are drawn from the point of the original force so that two right triangles are formed, with the original force as the common hypotenuse. The rectangular (right angle) components are formed, first, by drawing a line of action perpendicular to the x (or y) axis of the coordinate system and, second, by drawing a line of action parallel to the x (or y) axis. The magnitudes of the two component forces

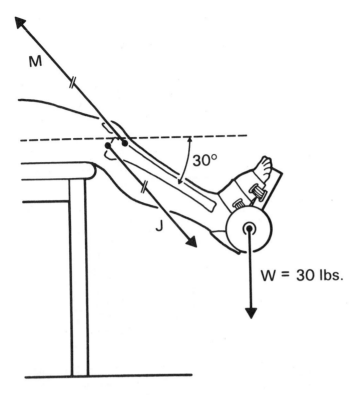

Figure 2–19   Forces acting on the leg (tibia) when the seated subject has an exercise weight on the foot and the knee is in 30 degrees of flexion. (The weight of the leg and foot has been omitted in this example.)

are found by drawing lines parallel to the component forces that intersect at the arrowhead of the original **force.**

In Figure 2–21, the coordinate system has been placed on the leg so that the x axis coincides with the long axis of the tibia. The quadriceps muscle force (M) and the resistance force (W) have been resolved into their rectangular components. The **perpendicular component** (M or W) is called the **rotary component** or the **rotary force.** It is that part of the original force (M or W) that is effective in causing rotary motion of the segment around the axis (or maintaining a posture or resisting a motion). In the example, the quadriceps muscle (M), with a line of pull at an acute angle

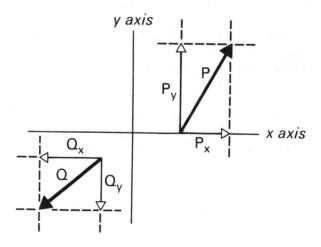

Figure 2–20   Resolution of force vectors P and Q into two components (P_y and P_x, Q_y and Q_x), the combined magnitude and direction of which produce the same effect as the original force.

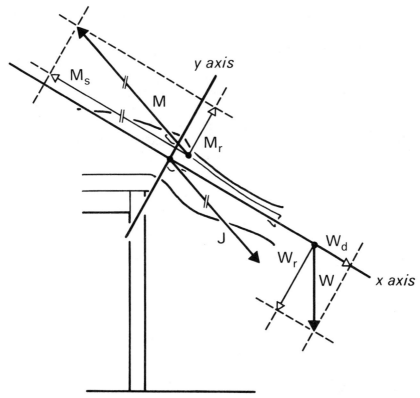

Figure 2–21 Resolution of the resistance (W) and muscle (M) forces from Figure 2–19 into rectangular components. The rotary components (W_r and M_r) are perpendicular to the long axis of the segment. The stabilizing component of the muscle force (M_s) and the distracting component of the weight (W_d) are parallel to the long axis of the segment. (The weight of the leg and foot has been omitted from this diagram.)

to the tibia, must produce a relatively large force in order to create a sufficient rotary component (M_r) to maintain the knee in extension. Conversely, the weight (W) acting at an acute angle to the long axis of the segment resists extension of the knee— not with the full force of 30 lb, but with the smaller rotary component W_r. **Only when** the weight acts at a 90-degree angle (perpendicular) to the segment is the rotary force the same magnitude as the weight. Since the rotary component is perpendicular to the long axis, the measurement of distances to calculate torque ($\tau = F{\perp}d$) is simplified. In this case, torque of the weight (or muscle force) can be found by multiplying the rotary component (W_r) by the actual weight arm distance of the lever.

The parallel component of the original force causes either compression or distraction of the joint surfaces, depending on the direction of the component. In the example shown in Figure 2–21, a large part of the tension produced by the quadriceps muscle (M) is directed toward the femur and is causing the tibia to be compressed against the femur. This component (M_s) is called the stabilizing or joint compression component of the muscle force (M). On the other hand, the parallel component of the weight (W_d) causes separation of the joint surfaces and is called the distracting component. The magnitudes of both the distracting and stabilizing components of the force can vary from 0 to 100 percent of the total force, depending on joint position, but the magnitudes are inversely related, with one approaching 0 percent as the other approaches 100 percent.

Examples of the effect of different angles of application of a force are illustrated in Figure 2–22 with the rubber band finger extension sling. If the band is attached proximally (to an outrigger), the force applied to gaining extension is not the full force of the band (A) but rather only the perpendicular rotary component. The parallel component (F_s) is causing joint compression. If the point of attachment is moved forward, the rotary component increases (B). Only when the sling is attached at a right angle (C) is the total force of the rubber band applied to gain extension. If the patient later develops the ability to increase the range of extension (D), but the outrigger has not been adjusted, the rotary component of the force again decreases, and the parallel component causes a distraction at the joint.

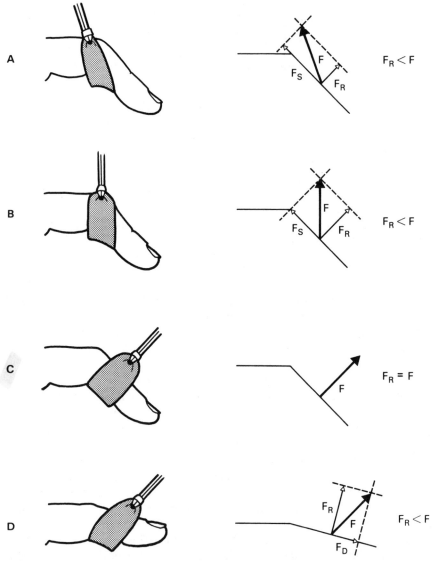

Figure 2–22 Resolution of the force (F) of a sling (attached to an outrigger hand splint) for gaining interphalangeal joint extension. In (A) and (B), the line of pull is incorrect; in (C), the outrigger is adjusted to gain the correct perpendicular line of pull; in (D), the range of motion has increased and the line of pull is again incorrect.

Laws of the Right Triangle

The rectangular components of the force are used to take advantage of the laws of the right triangle so that the magnitudes of the torques and unknown muscle and joint forces can be calculated. The rectangular components (with their parallel sides) form two right triangles, with the original force as the hypotenuse (Fig. 2–23). The ratios of the sides and hypotenuse of the right triangle are always the same for the same angle. The relationship is expressed by the Pythagorean theorem: the square of the hypotenuse of a right triangle is equal to the sum of the squares of the two sides. The ratio of the sides to the angle is expressed by the trigonometric functions sine (sin), cosine (cos), and tangent (tan). Table 2–3 lists the values of common trigonometric functions. For example, the value of 0.500 for the sine of a 30-degree angle means that the opposite side is one-half the length (magnitude) of the hypotenuse. Thus, if the values of one side and one angle are known (or two sides), the remaining sides and angles can be found.

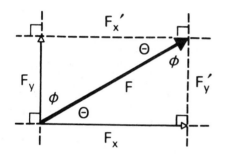

F = original force

F_x F_y = rectangular components of F

F_x' F_y' = parallels to F_x F_y

θ ϕ = acute angles formed by F with F_x and F_y

□ = 90°

Relationships

Pythagorean theorum

$$F^2 = F_x{}^2 + F_y{}^2$$

$$F = \sqrt{F_x{}^2 + F_y{}^2}$$

Angles

$$90° + \theta + \phi = 180°$$
$$\theta + \phi = 90°$$
$$90° - \theta = \phi$$

Sides

$$F_x = F_x'$$

$$F_y = F_y'$$

Trigonometric Functions

$$\sin\theta = \frac{F_y}{F} \qquad F_y = F\sin\theta$$

$$\cos\theta = \frac{F_x}{F} \qquad F_x = F\cos\theta$$

$$\tan\theta = \frac{F_y}{F_x}$$

Figure 2–23 Resolution of a force into rectangular components with the geometric relationships of the sides and angles of the resulting right triangles.

Table 2–3 Useful Trigonometric Functions and Ratios of Common Angles (for Other Angles, the Reader Should Refer to Tables of Natural Trigonometric Functions)

Angle	sin	cos	tan
0°	0.000	1.000	0.000
10°	0.174	0.985	0.176
20°	0.342	0.940	0.364
30°	0.500	0.866	0.577
45°	0.707	0.707	1.000
60°	0.866	0.500	1.732
70°	0.940	0.342	2.747
80°	0.985	0.174	5.671
90°	1.000	0.000	∞

Calculation of Muscle and Joint Forces

The forces that occur in muscles and between joint surfaces usually cannot be measured directly in the living human subject. This information can be gained indirectly by use of the equilibrium formulas ($\Sigma F = 0$ and $\Sigma\tau = 0$), composition and resolution of forces, and the trigonometric ratios of the right triangle. An example of this process is illustrated in Figure 2–24, which demonstrates how to find the magnitude of the unknown quadriceps muscle and knee joint compression forces when the subject is sitting and extending the knee with a 30-lb weight on the foot (see Fig. 2–19). In Figure 2–21, this example has been placed on the coordinate system with the origin coinciding with the unknown joint force, and in Figure 2–24, each of the three forces (W, M, and J) has been resolved into perpendicular components. The diagram has been labeled and the measured weight, angles, and distances recorded. The approximate magnitudes of the muscle force (M = 380 lb) and joint force (J = 350 lb), as well as the direction of the joint force ($\alpha = 17$ degrees), are found using the equilibrium formulas and trigonometric ratios. The following equations are arranged to show a step-by-step solution to the same problem. They illustrate the details of the relationships and provide solutions or explanations to parts of the problem, such as the rotary force of the weight, the torque of the resistance, or the muscle force.

The rotary component (W_r) of the 30-lb weight must first be found; use the formula for resolution of forces:

$$W_r = W \cos 30$$
$$W_r = 30 \text{ lb} \times 0.866$$
$$W_r = 26 \text{ lb}$$

To find the torque produced by the weight (τ_w), use the formula for torque:

$$\tau_w = W_r \times d$$
$$\tau_w = 26 \text{ lb} \times 20 \text{ in}$$
$$\tau_w = 520 \text{ in-lb}$$

To find the torque that the muscle must produce (τ_m), use the equilibrium formula:

$$\Sigma\tau = 0$$
$$\tau_w - \tau_m = 0$$
$$\tau_m = \tau_w$$
$$\tau_m = 520 \text{ in-lb}$$

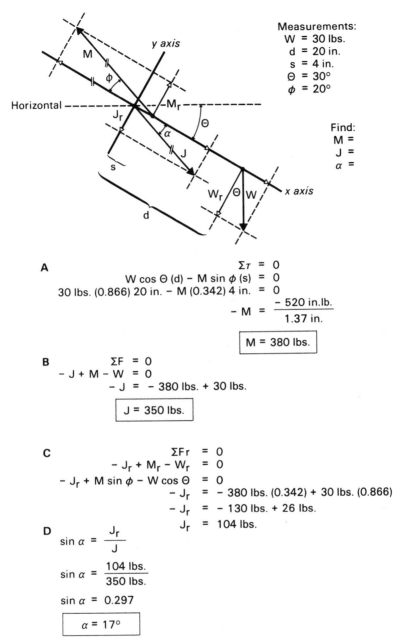

Measurements:
W = 30 lbs.
d = 20 in.
s = 4 in.
Θ = 30°
φ = 20°

Find:
M =
J =
α =

A

$$\Sigma_T = 0$$
$$W \cos \Theta (d) - M \sin \phi (s) = 0$$
$$30 \text{ lbs. } (0.866) \ 20 \text{ in. } - M (0.342) \ 4 \text{ in. } = 0$$
$$-M = \frac{-520 \text{ in.lb.}}{1.37 \text{ in.}}$$

$$\boxed{M = 380 \text{ lbs.}}$$

B

$$\Sigma F = 0$$
$$-J + M - W = 0$$
$$-J = -380 \text{ lbs. } + 30 \text{ lbs.}$$

$$\boxed{J = 350 \text{ lbs.}}$$

C

$$\Sigma Fr = 0$$
$$-J_r + M_r - W_r = 0$$
$$-J_r + M \sin \phi - W \cos \Theta = 0$$
$$-J_r = -380 \text{ lbs. } (0.342) + 30 \text{ lbs. } (0.866)$$
$$-J_r = -130 \text{ lbs. } + 26 \text{ lbs.}$$
$$J_r = 104 \text{ lbs.}$$

D

$$\sin \alpha = \frac{J_r}{J}$$

$$\sin \alpha = \frac{104 \text{ lbs.}}{350 \text{ lbs.}}$$

$$\sin \alpha = 0.297$$

$$\boxed{\alpha = 17°}$$

Figure 2–24 Trigonometric solution for the magnitude of the muscle and joint forces as well as the angle of the joint force when the seated subject is holding a 30-lb weight on the foot and the knee is at 30 degrees of flexion (see Fig. 2–19). Force vectors are placed on the coordinate system and resolved into components, as in Figure 2–21. Angles and distances are determined and labeled. The problem is solved by using the two equilibrium formulas and trigonometric ratio. The angle and the distance of the patellar tendon attachment were measured from radiographs. The angle of knee flexion and the distance of the weight from the joint center were measured on the subject. (This simplified equation introduces a 7-lb error in the value of J. A more accurate equation requires finding J_x as well as J_r and then using the Pythagorean theorem to find $J = \sqrt{J_r{}^2 + J_x{}^2}$.

To find the force in the muscle (M), the rotary component M_r must first be found. To find the magnitude of the rotary component of the muscle (M_r), use the formula for torque:

$$\tau_m = M_r \times s$$
$$M_r = \tau_m \div s$$
$$M_r = 520 \text{ in-lb} \div 4 \text{ in}$$
$$M_r = 130 \text{ lb}$$

To find the muscle force (M), use trigonometric functions of the right triangle:

$$\sin 20° = M_r \div M$$
$$M = M_r \div \sin 20°$$
$$M = 130 \text{ lb} \div 0.342$$
$$M = 380 \text{ lb}$$

To find the approximate magnitude of the joint force (J), use the equilibrium formula:

$$\Sigma F = 0$$
$$-J + M - W = 0$$
$$-J = -380 \text{ lb} + 30 \text{ lb}$$
$$J = 350 \text{ lb}$$

To find the angle of application for J, one of the components of J must be found. If, at equilibrium, the sum of the forces is zero, then the sum of the rectangular components must also be zero. To find the magnitude of J component, use the equilibrium formula $\Sigma F_x = 0$ or $\Sigma F_y = 0$.

$$\Sigma F_y = 0$$
$$-J_r + M_r - W_r = 0$$
$$-J_r = -M_r + W_r$$
$$-J_r = -130 \text{ lb} + 26 \text{ lb}$$
$$J_r = 104 \text{ lb}$$

To find the angle of the joint force, use trigonometric functions and find the degree of the angle in a table of sines and cosines.

$$\sin \alpha = J_r \div J$$
$$\sin \alpha = 104 \text{ lb} \div 350 \text{ lb}$$
$$\sin \alpha = 0.297$$
$$\alpha = 17°$$

If this problem were repeated with the knee in full extension, the rotary component of the weight (W_r) would be larger, thus increasing the torque of the weight (τ_w) as well as the torque of the muscle (τ_m), the muscle force (M), and the joint force (J). Conversely, if the angle between the horizontal and the tibia were increased to 60 degrees, the values of W_r, τ_w, τ_m, M and J would all be less.

Note that the weight of the leg and foot was omitted in this problem (see Fig. 2–23). The weight of the leg and foot (w) is approximately 9 lb acting at its center of gravity 8 inches from the origin of the coordinate system in a vertical direction. When this force is added, the corrected equilibrium equations are:

A.
$$\Sigma \tau = 0$$
$$30 \text{ lb } (0.866) \, 20 \text{ in} + 9 \text{ lb } (0.866) \, 8 \text{ in} - M \, (0.342) \, 4 \text{ in} = 0$$
$$M = 425 \text{ lb}$$

B.
$$\Sigma F = 0$$
$$-J + 425 \text{ lb} - 30 \text{ lb} - 9 \text{ lb} = 0$$
$$J = 386 \text{ lb}$$

The vector equation $\Sigma F = 0$ has been used to simplify equations for finding the joint forces (J) and introduces a 2 percent error into this problem. The correct equation requires finding both of the components of J and then using the Pythagorean theorem: $J = \sqrt{Jx^2 + Jy^2}$. When this is done, J is found to be 357 lb when the weight of the leg is neglected and 396 lb when the weight of the leg is included.

For examples of calculations in other activities, positions, and joint areas and for calculation of forces in dynamics, the reader is referred to LeVeau (1992), Frankel and Nordin (1989), and Soderberg (1986).

CLINICAL APPLICATIONS OF STATICS

Weight and the Center of Gravity

The action line of the force vector of the weight of a body is always vertical and is located at the center of gravity of the body. The center of gravity is defined as the single point of a body about which every particle of its mass is equally distributed ($\Sigma\tau = 0$). If the body were suspended (or supported) at this point, the body would be perfectly balanced. Each body behaves as if its entire mass were acting or being acted upon at its center of gravity.

Stable, Unstable, and Neutral Equilibrium

If the center of gravity of a body is disturbed slightly and the body tends to return the center of gravity to its former position, the body is said to be in **stable equilibrium.** Examples include attempting to turn a brick over or pushing on a person who is sitting in a rocking chair. If the center of gravity does not tend to return but seeks a new position, the body falls. The body is then in a state of **unstable equilibrium,** such as may occur if a person sitting on a narrow-based stool leans forward. **Neutral equilibrium** is demonstrated by a rolling ball or a person being propelled in a wheelchair. When the center of gravity is displaced it remains at the same level; that is, it neither falls nor returns to its former position.

The degree of stability (resistance to being overthrown) of a body depends on four factors: (1) **the height of the center of gravity above the base of support,** (2) **the size of the base of support,** (3) **the location of the gravity line within the base of support,** and (4) **the weight of the body.** Stability is enhanced by a low center of gravity, a wide base of support, the gravity line at the center of the support, and heavy weight. The size of, and the positions taken by, a football lineman promote stability and resistance to being overthrown. Instability, on the other hand, is enhanced by a high center of gravity, narrow base of support, and light weight as exemplified by the positions and moves of football running backs.

Calculation of the Center of Gravity of the Body

The concept of center of gravity of a solid object, such as a brick or a ball, is not difficult to visualize. The human body, however, has many irregularly shaped segments. As the positions of the segments change, so does the center of gravity of the body as a whole. A patient with muscle weakness can collapse in a fraction of a second if the gravity line is allowed to move outside the base of support. Knowledge of where and how the force of gravity acts on the body (and its segments) is important clinically to facilitate motion, alter exercise loads, balance parts, and prevent falls.

The **center of gravity of the adult human in the anatomic position has been found to be slightly anterior to the second sacral vertebra** (Braune and

Fischer, 1984), or approximately 55 percent of a person's height (Hellebrandt et al, 1938). The horizontal plane through this point can be found experimentally using a long board supported at one end by a bathroom scale and supported at the other end by blocks (Fig. 2–25). Triangular strips of wood are placed between the plank and the supports to act as "knife edges." The distance between the edges is measured. Then the subject, who has been previously weighed, lies down on the board with all of the body positioned between the knife edges to form a second-class lever system. The values for (1) the scale reading, (2) the subject's weight, and (3) the distance between the knife edges can be entered into the equilibrium formula $\Sigma\tau = 0$ to find **the distance from the axis (A)** that the weight is centered. The distance is the center of gravity in the horizontal plane and can be marked on the subject with chalk before the subject moves from the board.

The center-of-gravity mark usually falls near the level of the anterior-superior spines of the ilium. Variations in body proportions and weight distribution cause

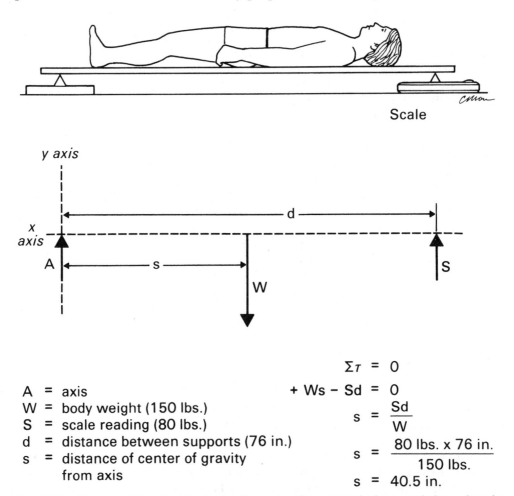

$$\Sigma\tau = 0$$

A = axis $+ Ws - Sd = 0$

W = body weight (150 lbs.)

S = scale reading (80 lbs.) $s = \dfrac{Sd}{W}$

d = distance between supports (76 in.)

s = distance of center of gravity $s = \dfrac{80 \text{ lbs.} \times 76 \text{ in.}}{150 \text{ lbs.}}$

     from axis $s = 40.5 \text{ in.}$

Figure 2–25 Experimental method for finding the center of gravity in the horizontal plane when the subject is in the anatomic position. The vector diagram is placed on the coordinate system with the axis (A) at the origin and the board on the x axis. The weight of the board is eliminated from the equation by placing the scale on zero before the subject lies down.

alterations in the location of this point. It is usually found to be slightly higher in men than in women, because men tend to have broader shoulders, while women tend to have broader hips. Patients with above-knee amputations will have a high center of gravity and may be in unstable equilibrium in a conventional wheelchair unless compensatory weights are placed on the footrests.

Any change from the anatomic position causes the center of gravity to move. If the arms are folded on the chest or raised overhead, the center of gravity rises. If the subject flexes the head, trunk and hips, the center of gravity moves toward the feet. The relatively high center of gravity in humans places the erect person in a position of unstable equilibrium. Only a small force is needed to cause displacement of the body and to initiate walking. Falling of the body is prevented by an intact and automatic neuromuscular system, which places a base of support (the extended leg) under the center of gravity. Thus, walking can be described as a sequence of disturbing and catching the center of gravity. Uncertainty in the person's ability to control and balance the body may cause the subject to protectively lower the center of gravity, even though this may require greater energy or promote further loss of balance. For example, the novice snow skier sits back rather than leans forward. People who attempt to walk in a dark and unfamiliar place usually tend to flex at the hips and knees, as do patients who are unsure or frightened. The therapist is responsible for providing both the physical and psychological support to help patients learn to take advantage of their center of gravity in performing motor tasks safely and effectively.

Base of Support

For static stability, the center of gravity of a body must project within the base of support. The frontal and sagittal plane projections of the center of gravity to the base of support in an upright subject also can be found by using the board-and-scale method. A piece of paper is lightly taped to the board. The subject, who has been previously weighed, stands on the paper facing the axis, and the feet are outlined on the paper with a pen. The calculations are made using the formula in Figure 2–25, and the **distance from the axis** is marked on the paper to locate the frontal plane projection. To locate the sagittal plane projection, the paper with the outlined feet is turned 90 degrees on the board. The subject places the feet into the outline and stands in the same posture as before, and the calculations are repeated. Intersection of the two lines indicates the projection of the center of gravity to the base of support. The projection is found near the center of the outlined base of support, if the subject has been standing erect with weight evenly distributed on both feet. When the subject is facing the axis and leans forward (or rises up on the toes), the center of gravity moves forward, but it always remains within the base of support (Fig. 2–26). When the subject is facing at a right angle to the axis (sagittal plane) and bears more weight on one leg, the center of gravity shifts toward that foot. If the subject stands on one leg, the center of gravity projects within the weight-bearing foot. Balance on this smaller base of support increases the demand on the neuromuscular system, as can be seen by the increased muscle contractions about the ankle and knee. Lateral balance on one leg becomes a major task because the safety zone for stability of side-to-side sway is limited.

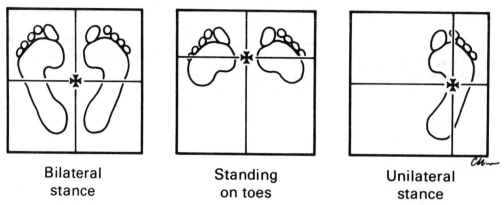

Bilateral stance   **Standing on toes**   **Unilateral stance**

Figure 2–26   Sagittal and frontal plane projections of the center of gravity to the base of support in the erect subject.

CLINICAL APPLICATIONS   A common problem of patients with hemiplegia* is the inability to move the body's center of gravity over the foot of the involved lower extremity. These patients state that they "can move the bad leg forward but cannot move the good leg!" When they are supporting their weight on the "good" (unaffected) extremity, it is, of course, impossible to pick it up and move it forward. Only after patients learn to bear the body weight on the affected extremity can they move the unaffected extremity forward. Another problem of patients with hemiplegia in moving their center of gravity over the base of support is that of coming to the standing position from a chair. As illustrated in Figure 2–27, the center of gravity of the seated subject falls beneath the chair. To

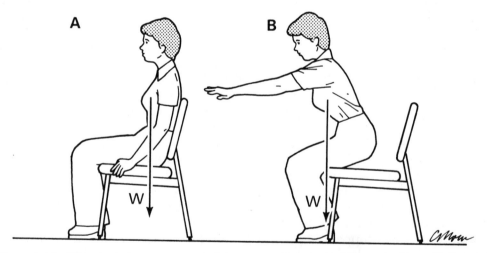

Figure 2–27   (A) Sagittal plane projections of the center of gravity in the seated subject. (B) To stand up, the subject must move the center of gravity of the body forward over the base of support formed by the feet.

*Hemiplegia (Gr. *hemi-*, half; plus *plege*, a stroke). Paralysis or paresis of one side of the body, usually caused by interruption of blood flow to a region of the brain containing nerve cells that control movement of muscles.

stand up, the center of gravity of the body must first be moved forward so that it projects beneath the feet. Patients with hemiplegia, however, frequently push the body backward and upward when trying to stand up. Instead, they should be taught to move forward over the feet to bring the center of gravity over the new base of support. When this occurs, the patient is in a position to stand up.

Increased stability is gained by broadening the base of support. In the presence of diminished muscle strength or poor coordination, crutches, canes, and walkers may provide stability for the patient. The patient must learn, however, to shift the body's center of gravity so that the assistive device or a lower extremity can be lifted and moved forward.

A wide base of support is also advantageous in lifting and carrying. This principle is exemplified by weight lifters as well as by therapists transferring the patient with paralysis from bed to wheelchair. In preparation for the lift and transfer, therapists will place their feet in a wide anterior-posterior stance so that the weight can be placed primarily on one foot at the initiation of the lift and shifted to the other foot at the end of the lift. Although the patient's weight may be moved the distance of a meter, the therapist provides stability to the system by containing the weight between both feet. If the therapist kept the feet together and "walked" the patient to the wheelchair, the patient and the therapist would be in a condition of unstable equilibrium, leading to a likely fall by the patient or therapist as well as a potential injury to both.

Centers of Gravity and Weights of Segments

The center of gravity of the body as a whole is the sum of the centers of gravity of individual segments ($\Sigma\tau = 0$). Knowledge of the location of the segmental centers of gravity and the approximate weight of the segments is clinically useful in adjusting exercise loads, applying traction, and balancing parts of the body.

Approximate locations of the individual centers of mass and weight of body segments are given in Figure 2–28 and Table 2–4. Body segment parameters have been determined on cadavers by Dempster and Clauser (1955), McConville and Young (1969), and Braune and Fischer (1984). For specific details, the reader is referred to the original studies or to the reviews by LeVeau (1977) and Drillis and associates (1958).

The center of gravity of the extended upper extremity is just above the elbow joint, and that of the extended lower extremity is just above the knee joint. The arm, forearm, thigh, and leg are larger proximally, and thus their individual centers of gravity lie closer to the proximal end. This point is approximately $^4/_9$ (45 percent) of the length of the segment, measured from the proximal end.

A change in the position of individual segments causes a change in the position of the center of gravity of the extremity and the body as a whole. When the extremity is flexed, the center of gravity moves proximally and to a point on a line between individual segment centers (Fig. 2–29). Deliberate movement of the center of gravity of segments is frequently used in therapeutic exercise to alter the resistive torque (weight times its perpendicular distance to the axis of motion) of an extremity. Shoulder flexion against gravity is easier to perform when the elbow is flexed than when the elbow is extended. The sit-up is easiest to perform when the arms are at the sides, and it becomes progressively more difficult as the arms are folded on the chest or the hands placed behind the head. Changing the torque of

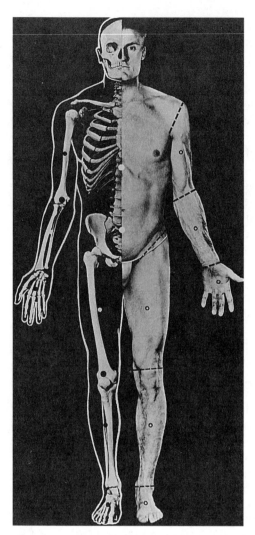

Figure 2–28 Location of center of gravity in major body segments of a man weighing 150 lb (see also Table 2–4). (From Williams, M, and Lissner, HR: *Biomechanics of Human Motion*. WB Saunders, Philadelphia, 1962, p 14, with permission.)

the lower extremities provides a method for altering the difficulty of abdominal muscle exercises. In the supine position, these muscles contract to stabilize the pelvis when the legs are raised. The resistance that the abdominal muscles must meet is reduced by flexing the lower extremities before lifting the legs, and the resistance is further reduced by raising only one leg. The magnitude of the decrease in torque is illustrated in Figure 2–29. Although the weight of the single extremity is the same in both positions, the center of gravity has moved from 15 inches (37 cm) from the hip joint axis to 8 inches (20 cm); therefore, the torque has been reduced from 360 in-lb (40.6 N) to 192 in-lb (21.7 N). This decrease in torque not only reduces the stabilization force required on the abdominal muscles but also reduces the force that the hip flexor muscles must produce to raise the leg.

The center of gravity of the head, arms, and trunk (HAT as described by Elftman, 1955) is located anterior to the border of the 11th thoracic vertebra and just below the xiphoid process of the sternum. The weight of HAT is approximately equal to 60 percent of the body weight. In Figure 2–30, note the increased distance from the hip joint to the line of the center of gravity of HAT as forward inclina-

Table 2-4 Average Weight of Body Segments and Anatomic Location of Center of Gravity of Individual Body Segments of a Man Weighing 150 lb

Segment Weights and Percentage of Total Body Weight	Approximate Anatomic Location of Centers of Gravity
Head: 10.3 lb (6.9%)	*Head.* In sphenoid sinus, 4 mm beyond anterior inferior margin of sella. (On lateral surface, over temporal fossa on or near nasion-inion line.)
Head and neck: 11.8 lb (7.9%)	*Head and neck.* On inferior surface of basioccipital bone or within bone 23 ± 5 mm from crest of dorsum sellae. (On lateral surface, 10 mm anterior to supratragal notch above head of mandible.)
Head, neck, and trunk: 88.5 lb (59.0%)	*Head, neck, and trunk.* Anterior to 11th thoracic vertebra.
UPPER LIMB. JUST ABOVE ELBOW JOINT.	
Arm: 4.1 lb (2.7%)	*Arm.* In medial head of triceps, adjacent to radial groove; 5 mm proximal to distal end of deltoid insertion.
Forearm: 2.4 lb (1.6%)	*Forearm.* 11 mm proximal to most distal part of pronator teres insertion; 9 mm anterior to interosseus membrane.
Hand: 0.9 lb (0.6%) *Upper limb:* 7.3 lb (4.9%) *Forearm and hand:* 3.3 lb (2.2%)	*Hand* (in rest position). On axis of metacarpal III, usually 2 mm deep to volar skin surface. 2 mm proximal to proximal transverse palmar skin crease, in angle between proximal transverse and radial longitudinal crease.
LOWER LIMB. JUST ABOVE KNEE JOINT.	
Thigh: 14.5 lb (9.7%)	*Thigh.* In adductor brevis muscle (or magnus or vastus medialis), 13 mm medial to linea aspera, deep to adductor canal, 29 mm below apex of femoral triangle, and 18 mm proximal to most distal fibers of adductor brevis.
Leg: 6.8 lb (4.5%)	*Leg.* 35 mm below popliteus, at posterior part of posterior tibialis; 16 mm above proximal end of Achilles tendon; 8 mm posterior to interosseus membrane.
Foot: 2.1 lb (1.4%) *Lower limb:* 23.4 lb. (15.6%) *Leg and foot:* 9.0 lb. (6.0%)	*Foot.* In plantar ligaments, or just superficial in adjacent deep foot muscles; below proximal halves of second and third cuneiform bones. On a line between ankle joint center and ball of foot in plane of metatarsal II.
ENTIRE BODY. ANTERIOR TO SECOND SACRAL VERTEBRA.	

SOURCE: Williams, M and Lissner, HR: *Biomechanics of Human Motion.* WB Saunders, Philadelphia, 1962, p 15, with permission.

tion is increased. This position requires increasingly more force in the back and hip extensor muscles to support the weight of the trunk. In patients with paralysis of the hip musculature (paraplegia and quadriplegia), control of the center of gravity of HAT is essential for stability in sitting. Although momentary sitting balance may be achieved, the patient is in a position of unstable equilibrium. Stability of HAT for functional use of the hands then requires an additional external force. In a wheelchair, this may be gained by leaning against the backrest or holding onto parts of the chair (Fig. 2–31). Wheelchair fitting requires consideration not only of stability of the trunk in the sitting position but also of control and stability in other positions of function. As illustrated in Figure 2–31, a high-back chair can provide greater stability when sitting, but the high back may prohibit hooking the elbow or wrist around the handles to control the trunk when reaching forward.

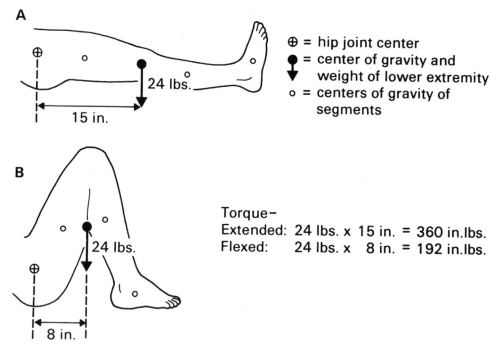

⊕ = hip joint center
● = center of gravity and
   weight of lower extremity
o = centers of gravity of
   segments

Torque–
Extended: 24 lbs. x 15 in. = 360 in.lbs.
Flexed: 24 lbs. x 8 in. = 192 in.lbs.

Figure 2–29   Alteration of the torque of the lower extremity by changing the position of individual segments.

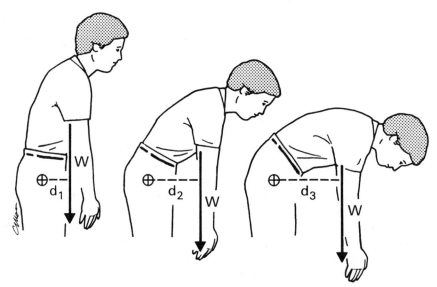

Figure 2–30   Distance (d_1, d_2, d_3) from the center of the hip joint to the center-of-gravity line of the head, arms, and trunk (HAT) increases as forward inclination increases.

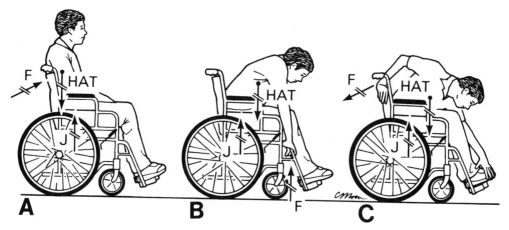

Figure 2–31 Methods of stability and control of the center of gravity of the head, arms, and trunk (HAT) in a person with a cervical spinal cord transection, in which J = the force supporting the body at the center of the base of support and F = the counterforce needed to maintain equilibrium. (*A*) Sitting with the support of the backrest. (*B*) Leaning forward on passively "locked" elbows and using the scapular muscles. (*C*) Hooking the wrist around the handlebar and using the elbow flexors to lower and raise the trunk.

Applied Weights and Resistances

Clinically, the external resistances encountered by the body include the forces produced by casts, braces (orthoses), books, plates of food, pulleys, dumbbells, crutches, doors, exercise equipment, or manual resistance by a therapist. Although these forces may be small, they are usually applied distally on the extremity and, therefore, exert relatively large torques that the muscles must match. Knowledge of the behavior of these forces and their rectangular components permits their manipulation and adaptation for therapeutic purposes. For example, if the objective is to give resistive exercise to a particular muscle, a resistive torque should be selected that most nearly matches the torque that the muscle is capable of developing. If, however, the objective is to assist functional use of a weak muscle, the resistance torque should be made as small as possible.

Applied weights such as dumbbells or books behave in the same manner as weights of body segments because gravity always pulls downward in a vertical direction. The maximum resistance torque of the weight occurs when the extremity or segment is horizontal. In this position, the perpendicular distance from the action line of the force to the axis of motion is the longest (see Fig. 2–14); or alternatively, the rotary component of the weight is equal to the weight vector. At all other points in the range of motion, the resistance torque is less. The two alternative methods for calculating torque are shown in Figure 2–32. The first method uses the magnitude of the force (weight or muscle contraction) times the measured perpendicular distance from the line of action of the force to the axis of motion (see Fig. 2–14). The second method uses the resolution of forces to find the rotary component of the force times the measured distance from the point of attachment of the force to the axis of motion. In each method, the distance is perpendicular to the force or the rotary component, and the resulting torque is the same. The method selected is the one for which distances and angles are most readily obtained.

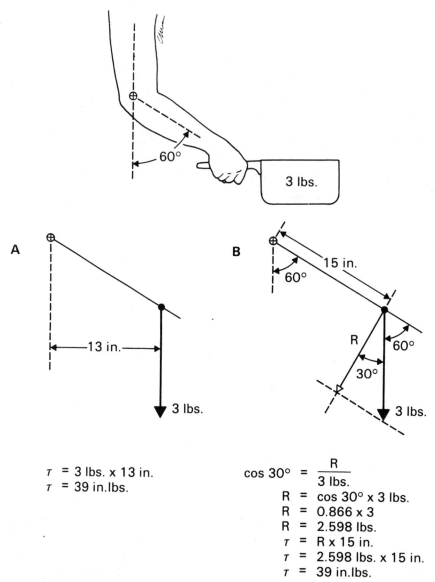

$$\tau = 3 \text{ lbs.} \times 13 \text{ in.}$$
$$\tau = 39 \text{ in.lbs.}$$

$$\cos 30° = \frac{R}{3 \text{ lbs.}}$$
$$R = \cos 30° \times 3 \text{ lbs.}$$
$$R = 0.866 \times 3$$
$$R = 2.598 \text{ lbs.}$$
$$\tau = R \times 15 \text{ in.}$$
$$\tau = 2.598 \text{ lbs.} \times 15 \text{ in.}$$
$$\tau = 39 \text{ in.lbs.}$$

Figure 2–32   Alternative methods for calculating torque, using, as an example, the effect on the elbow of a 3-lb weight held in the hand. (*A*) The force times the perpendicular distance from its action line to the axis of elbow motion. (*B*) The rotary component of the force times the distance from its attachment to the axis of motion. The same methods may be used for other forces, such as muscle contraction and applied resistances. In this example, if it were desired to find the torque in several positions of the elbow, (*B*) would be more convenient.

Distractive Component of Weights

Weights applied to the extremities frequently exert traction on joint structures, which may or may not be therapeutically desirable. The magnitude of the traction force is the distractive component of the resistive force and is found by resolution of forces. Thus, if the elbow in Figure 2–32 were in extension, the weight would be acting entirely as a distracting force and would not have a rotary component. Codman's pendulum exercises for reducing limitation of shoulder motion are based on this effect (Zohn and Mennell, 1976). The subject holds a weight in the hand, bends over, and flexes at the hips, thus placing the shoulder in a position of flexion. The extremity is swung as a pendulum so that the hand describes larger and larger circles within the pain-free range. The distracting component of the weight promotes the downward movement of the head of the humerus on the glenoid fossa so that shoulder flexion and abduction may occur.

In some pathologic conditions, the effect of the distracting component of a weight is unwanted because it may cause pain and further damage to joint structures. For example, in ligamentous injuries to the knee, weights attached to the foot for the purpose of applying strengthening exercises to the knee extensor muscles may be contraindicated (see Figs. 2–6 and 2–19). In such cases, a resistance method is used that has only a rotary component. This is accomplished by applying the resistance force perpendicular to the long axis of the segment, as can be done manually by the therapist or by using equipment designed to eliminate the distractive component of the resistive force such as isokinetic dynamometers (see Fig. 4–2).

Externally applied forces, which may occur with manual resistance, exercise pulleys, crutch-walking, propelling a wheelchair, or opening a door, do not act in a vertical direction as do weights attached to the body. Instead, the forces exert effects that vary according to their particular angle of application and have either distracting or stabilizing components. In pulley systems, the angle of application changes in different parts of the range of motion (Fig. 2–33). Each change in the angle (or direction) of the force causes a change in the magnitude of the rotary component of the force. Consequently, the resistance torque will vary at different points of the range of motion.

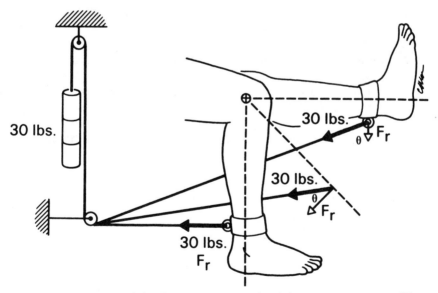

Figure 2–33 Vector diagram of the decreasing magnitude of the rotary component (F_r) or resistive force to knee extension in a pulley system when the knee is at (1) 0 degrees, (2) 45 degrees, and (3) 90 degrees of flexion. The rotary component (F_r) of the 30-lb force in the pulley system is found using the formula $\cos \theta = F_r/30$ lb, or $F_r = \cos \theta \times 30$ lb:

	Knee angle	θ	$\cos \theta \times 30$ lb	=	F_r
(1)	0°	60°	0.5 × 30 lb		15 lb
(2)	45°	30°	0.86 × 30 lb		24 lb
(3)	90°	0°	1.0 × 30 lb		30 lb

Pulleys

Pulleys are frequently used in exercise and traction equipment to change the direction of a force or to increase or decrease the magnitude of a force (see Figs. 2–8, 2–9, and 2–33).

SINGLE FIXED PULLEY   The line of action of a force may be changed by means of a pulley (Fig. 2–34). A force (F), acting in a downward direction, is used to move a weight in an upward direction. Such a single fixed pulley does not provide any mechanical advantage to the force but only changes its direction. This principle is illustrated by the cervical traction example (see Fig. 2–7).

MOVABLE PULLEY   If a weight is attached to a movable pulley (Fig. 2–35), half of the weight is supported by the rope attached to the stationary hook, and half by the rope on the other side of the pulley. Therefore, the mechanical advantage of the force (F) is 2. The rope, however, must be moved twice the distance that the weight is raised, and what is gained in force is lost in distance. The fixed pulley in the illustration serves only to change the direction of the force but gives no mechanical advantage. The movable pulley is not represented in the body but may be convenient to use for exercise equipment. The leg traction systems in Figures 2–8 and 2–9 are examples. The pulley at the foot can be considered "movable," and the pulleys on the bedpost fixed. Since the pulley at the foot receives the force from two parts of the rope, this pulley in turn exerts greater than 15 lb of traction on the leg. In the exercise system in Figure 2–33, the two fixed pulleys change only the direction of the force. Some systems, however, have a movable pulley on the weight pan, as in Figure 2–35, which reduces the exercise force to one-half of the weight.

ANATOMIC PULLEYS   In the body, several structures are called pulleys because they have properties of the single pulley. Tendons may be deflected from their straight course by bony prominences or soft tissues. This occurs in the leg, where the peroneal and long toe flexor tendons descend distally on the posterior aspect of the leg to go behind and around the malleoli to form attachments in the foot and toes. A pulley also may provide a mechanical advantage to the muscle by lifting the tendon away from the joint axis (increased force arm distance). An example is in the quadriceps and patellar tendons, which not only change the direction of pull as the knee flexes but also improve the force arm distance because of the interposed patella.

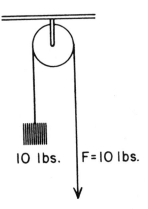

10 lbs.   F = 10 lbs.

Figure 2–34 Fixed pulley. Change of direction of force, but no mechanical advantage.

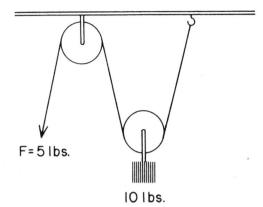

Figure 2–35 Movable pulley. Mechanical advantage for force.

Another pulley system involving the tendons of the long finger flexors is found on the palmar side of the phalanges. When the flexor digitorum profundus and superficialis contract, their tendons rise from the joint axes. The tendons are held down by seven pulley-like loops that also cause deflection of the tendons with movement. These structures can be seen in Figure 6–20 covering the flexor digitorum profundus tendon on the palmar surface. In the lateral view in Figure 6–12, the pulleys have been removed, showing slack in the tendons, requiring considerably more tendon excursion to provide movement.

Muscle Forces and Leverage

Anatomically, muscles may be diverted by a pulley mechanism around a condyle; in biomechanics, however, the muscle force vector is straight. The line of action is usually from the immediate point of attachment of the muscle to the bone and extends into space according to the magnitude of the force (see Figs. 2–16 and 2–19). The vector may, however, be placed at some point along the line of pull of the muscle. In either case, the vector is straight and does not follow the anatomic directions of the entire muscle.

Mechanically, the greater the perpendicular distance between the action line of the muscle and the joint center (force arm distance), the greater the torque produced by the muscle at that joint. This principle is sometimes called the **leverage factor** of muscles. Bony processes thus play an important role in providing force arm distances for the muscles and in increasing the angle of attachment of tendon to bone.

The calcaneus provides a 2-inch lever arm distance for the gastrocnemius-soleus muscles (see Fig. 2–16). The neck of the femur places the hip abductor muscles several inches away from the hip joint. The condyles of the phalanges increase the force arm distances of the finger flexors. The patella raises the line of pull of the quadriceps muscle from the knee joint axis. Small changes in these processes, as may occur with disease, injury, or surgery, can cause marked changes in the torque that a muscle can produce.

The first step in analyzing leverage factors of muscles is to identify at any single joint all the axes about which rotary movements occur. Following this, the relationship (distance) of each muscle action line to each axis can be visualized and the movement capabilities of those muscles clarified. If a muscle crosses one joint that permits one degree of freedom of movement, and if this muscle runs directly

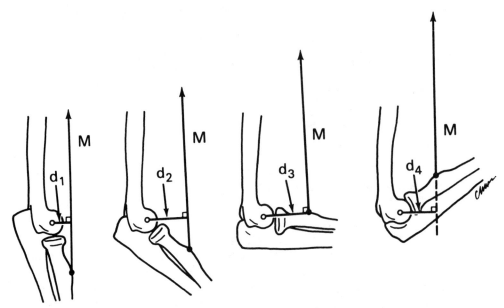

Figure 2–36 Changes in the force arm distance (d) for the biceps brachii muscle in four positions of elbow flexion. The maximum muscle torque occurs at the greatest lever arm distance (d_3, when attachment of the muscle to the bone is perpendicular; see Fig. 4-14).

between its attachments (i.e., its direction is not changed by bony processes or other means), its line of action is comparatively simple to define. Complexity of analysis of the line of action increases in instances where muscles possess widespread attachments and where joints permit increased degrees of freedom of movement.

The leverage principle is an important consideration in a muscle whose force arm distance changes as movement occurs, for its torque output also varies at different points in the range of motion. A prime example of changing leverage in a muscle is the biceps brachii acting as an elbow flexor (Fig. 2–36). When the elbow is in extension, the action line of the muscle is closest to the joint center. As the elbow is flexed toward 90 degrees, the action line moves away from the joint center and then begins to return as the elbow reaches 120 degrees of flexion. Thus, **for the same force of muscle contraction, the biceps muscle produces the most torque at 90 degrees of elbow flexion.** The muscle is least effective as an elbow flexor when the elbow is in extension. Although the leverage factor affects the torque output of all muscles, the effect varies with the muscle, joint, and motion. The biceps brachii, brachioradialis, and hamstring muscles show this effect more than muscles such as the triceps brachii, deltoid, or gastrocnemius-soleus, where the perpendicular distance to the joint axis shows minimal changes throughout the range of motion.

Inverse Actions of Muscles

In joints with a large range of motion, however, muscles can produce inverse actions. That is, a muscle may be able to produce opposite actions from different positions in the range of motion depending on where the line of action falls in relation to the axes of motion. Inverse actions occur with the adductor muscles at the hip joint. When the hip is flexed, the adductor muscles can act as hip extensors (as in climbing a ladder). Conversely, when the hip is in extension, the adductor muscles may act as hip flexors. In the upper extremity, the wrist extensors cross the elbow joint and are attached on the lateral epicondyle of the humerus. When the elbow is in extension, the wrist extensors pass posteriorly to the elbow joint axis, and the muscles act as elbow extensors. When the elbow is flexed, however, the line of action of the wrist extensors is considerably anterior to the elbow axis, and these muscles become elbow flexors.

Mechanical Disadvantage of Muscles

Muscle attachments and action lines lie close to joint axes, and most muscle tendons attach to bones at an acute angle. Consequently, muscles have short force arm distances and a mechanical disadvantage relative to the more distally placed resistances. Muscles must generate large forces to match or overcome the resistance torques. As an example, the subject illustrated in Figure 2–37 is shown pressing down with the hand on a scale that registers 20 lb (89 N). To maintain this position and to keep the elbow from flexing, the triceps brachii muscle must exert a force of 222 lb (987 N)! Although presented as a problem of statics, the forces at the elbow are similar to those that are found in dynamic activities such as sanding wood, cutting a tough steak, or pushing up from an armchair.

If, in Figure 2–37, the olecranon process of the ulna were reduced in length by only ¼ inch (0.6 cm) and if the muscle could still generate 222 lb of force, the force recorded by the scale would be reduced from 20 to 15 lb. In the hand, changes in force arm distances of even a few millimeters can affect function markedly. This occurs frequently in rheumatoid arthritis, where the extensor digitorum tendons may move down between the metacarpal heads.

Joint Forces

Forces occur in joints secondary to the primary forces of muscle contraction, gravity, external resistance, and friction. Understanding the causes and the results of these joint forces forms a major basis for the rationale of therapeutic exercise and physical rehabilitation. The primary forces may produce joint distraction, as when holding a suitcase in the hand, applying traction (see Fig. 2–7), or placing exercise weights on a dependent extremity (see Fig. 2–6). In these cases, tension is placed on the ligaments and joint capsules. Most activities, however, produce compression of joint surfaces. Compression is readily appreciated in weight-bearing joints in sitting, standing, or walking. What is not always appreciated by able-bodied persons is the magnitude of joint compression forces that occur with these activities, as well as those forces that occur with active muscle contraction and functional activities. In rotary motions or postures of the body, one end of the bone (near its joint surface) serves as the fulcrum or axis of the lever system (see Figs. 2–10 and 2–11). The joint force (J) is the reaction force of the mating joint surface. In the elbow extension problem (see Fig. 2–37), J represents the force on the distal end of the humerus. The calculations show this joint force to be 239 lb (1063 N)! In joint pathologies such as arthritis, function is lost because such large compressive forces cause excruciating pain. To illustrate this effect, the elbow problem in Figure 2–37 can be calculated, assuming that the subject can tolerate only a 20-lb force at the joint. Placement of the origin of the coordinate system at the muscle

A

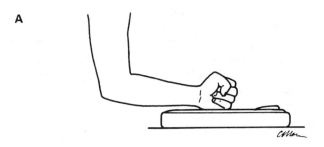

B

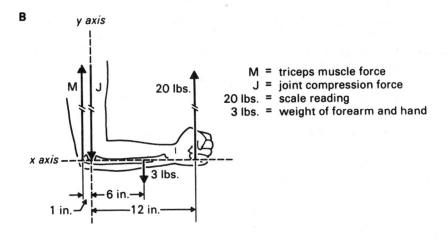

M = triceps muscle force
J = joint compression force
20 lbs. = scale reading
3 lbs. = weight of forearm and hand

C Calculation of triceps muscle force:

$$\Sigma_T = 0$$
$$+ (M \times 1 \text{ in.}) + (3 \text{ lbs.} \times 6 \text{ in.}) - (20 \text{ lbs.} \times 12 \text{ in.}) = 0$$
$$+ M = \frac{+ 240 \text{ in.lb.} - 18 \text{ in.lb.}}{1 \text{ in.}}$$
$$M = 222 \text{ lbs.}$$

D Calculation of joint compression force:

$$\Sigma F = 0$$
$$+ 222 \text{ lbs.} - J - 3 \text{ lbs.} + 20 \text{ lbs.} = 0$$
$$- J = - 239 \text{ lbs.}$$
$$J = 239 \text{ lbs.}$$

Figure 2–37 Example of the magnitudes of muscle and joint forces that occur with a moderate distal resistance. (*A*) Subject sitting and pressing down on a scale that records a force of 20 lb. (*B*) Diagram of the forces on the forearm and the lever arm distances placed on the coordinate system with the joint force (J) at the origin. (*C*) Equilibrium formula and calculations of the force of the triceps brachii muscle (M). (*D*) Equilibrium formula and calculations to find the joint compression force (J).

force (M) permits calculation of the small amount of force (F) the subject could exert on the scale:

$$\Sigma\tau = 0$$
$$(20 \text{ lb} \times 1 \text{ in}) + (3 \text{ lb} \times 7 \text{ in}) - (F \times 13 \text{ in}) = 0$$
$$F = \frac{20 \text{ in-lb} + 21 \text{ in-lb}}{13 \text{ in}}$$
$$F = 3.2 \text{ lb}$$

Although the amount of joint compression force developed in this parallel force system is large, it is frequently even greater because most muscles attach at an acute angle to the bone rather than at a right angle (see Fig. 2–21). To produce an effective rotary component, the muscle must generate a relatively large force, which in turn creates a large stabilization component. The quadriceps muscle tendon attaches at a 20-degree angle to the tibia, and a large part of the muscle force generated compresses the tibial plateau against the femoral condyles. In Figure 2–24, a quadriceps muscle force of 380 lb is required to produce the rotary component of 130 lb needed to hold the distal 30 lb weight. The stabilizing component of the muscle force, however, is 357 lb!

CLINICAL APPLICATIONS

Stretching Versus Joint Mobilization

Passive stretching in an attempt to increase joint motion after fractures, surgery, or joint pathologies has long been considered contraindicated by many therapists and orthopedists. Biomechanically, there are sound reasons for this caution. When force is placed on the distal end of a bone, that force is exerted on a long lever arm and has a high mechanical advantage over the limiting or injured joint structures. This force can be amplified 10 to 20 times in the joint area. If, for example, in passive stretching of a knee or an elbow, the therapist pulls with a force of only 10 lb (4.5 kg) applied 10 inches (25 cm) from the joint center, this is the same as applying a force of 50 lb 2 inches from the joint center or 100 lb 1 inch away. Forces of these magnitudes readily cause additional trauma to healing tissues. In addition, such distally placed forces do not reproduce normal joint motions; instead, they may cause levering of joints and abnormal motions (see Fig. 1–11).

On the other hand, mobilizations or passive movements of joint surfaces following normal accessory motions and arthrokinematic principles are frequently indicated in pathologic conditions to relieve pain and restore normal joint motions. Some biomechanical commonalities of the basic mobilization techniques are that:

- The direction of the applied force follows the normal arthrokinematics of that joint.
- The magnitude of the force is carefully controlled to be gentle and compatible with the underlying pathology. "No forceful movement must ever be used and no abnormal movement must ever be used" (Mennell, 1964).
- Motions of the joint surfaces are small, ranging from barely perceptible to a few millimeters in distance.

Achievements of such precision and control are gained by using very short force arms. In most instances, the force is applied at the head (or base) of the bone that forms the joint.

Pressure

To simplify biomechanical problems, forces are depicted as acting at their mid-point on a body. The tissues of the body, however, could not tolerate the pressures created by these point forces. In most cases the application of forces on the skin, muscles, joint surfaces, and bones is over a larger area to reduce pressure.

Pressure is a function of the applied force per unit area ($P = F/A$) and is reported in pounds per square inch (PSI) or kilograms per square centimeter. Thus, if a 10-lb force is applied to a body over an area of 1 square inch, the pressure is 10 PSI, but if the same force is applied over an area of 2 square inches, the pressure is reduced to 5 PSI. Pressure in liquids, such as blood in the arteries and veins, is recorded in millimeters of mercury (Hg). One PSI is approximately equal to 50 mm Hg and is about the magnitude of the pressure it takes to cause occlusion of arterioles (60 to 30 mm Hg) and capillaries (30 to 10 mm Hg) at the level of the heart. When segments are dependent, as are the feet in standing, these pressures are increased by hydrostatic pressure. This pressure can be felt and the effects seen when one presses down on the fingernail and blanches (occludes) the capillary beds.

Skin, muscles, fasciae, ligaments, cartilage, and bone respond to optimal applications of pressure with normal growth and functional hypertrophy. For example, the skin on the soles of the feet becomes thicker and tougher with weight bearing and walking. If, however, the person is subjected to bedrest for several months, the thick skin on the sole of the foot sluffs off and the skin becomes thin and soft like a baby's foot. On the other hand, excessive pressure causes tissue injury, including inflammation, pain, blisters, corns, calluses, "stone bruises," ulcers, wounds, and fractures. The length of time that a pressure is applied to the tissue is also a determining factor in injury. A low pressure such as 1 PSI applied over many hours can lead to necrosis of tissue. This can occur from something as innocuous as a wrinkle in the sock or a tight shoe in people who have conditions that include loss of sensation (spinal cord severance, spina bifida, peripheral nerve injuries, diabetes, and Hansen's disease).

Principles of decreasing pressure therapeutically are to **decrease the magnitude of the force, increase the area of application, and decrease the time of application.** Usually only one or possibly two of these factors can be changed and still maintain functionality. Examples of decreasing the magnitude of a force can be done with orthotics by increasing the force arm length (see Figs. 2–17 and 2–18). Avoiding point pressures by distributing the force over larger areas can be done using convoluted foam mattress covers and waterbeds for sleeping, or air-cell cushions for sitting and closed-cell foam shoe inserts for walking. Decreasing the time that the force is applied requires such things as a wearing schedule for a prosthesis or frequent body weight shifts to relieve seating pressures.

Laboratory Activities

MECHANICAL PRINCIPLES: KINETICS

1. Determine the center of gravity in the horizontal plane for one or two female subjects and one or two male subjects. The method is described under Calculation of the Center of Gravity of the Body and illustrated in Figure 2–25. You

will need a **strong** board that is wide enough to support the supine subject and is one foot longer than the tallest subject, a bathroom scale and an equivalent height board for the axis, two pieces of triangular wood (about 18 inches long) for the points of the axis and scale forces, and a tape measure to measure the distance between the axis and the scale forces and the distances from the axis to a point on the subject's body that can be marked by chalk. Two scales may be used but only one is necessary. Why is this?

2. Determine the projection of the center of gravity within the base of support. The method is described under Base of Support and illustrated in Figure 2–26. The same equipment can be used as in exercise number 1 with the addition of some large sheets of wrapping paper and some cellophane tape, or the measurements may be done on a smaller board (about 18 by 36 inches). Bizarre results, such as finding the center of gravity outside the base of support, are usually due to errors in measuring d (the distance between supports) and measuring s (the support) from the scale instead of from the axis. As you become familiar with the method, just observe the scale and the movement of the center of gravity while the subject carefully shifts weight to one side, rises on toes, moves arms forward, and so on.

3. Levers and forces: Make a 3-point lever system using a board about 40 inches long and 6 inches wide. Mark the center of the board and 6-inch intervals on either side. Support the board on either end 18 inches from the center by triangular pieces of wood on bathroom scales (as in exercise number 1) and zero the scales.

   Place a 10-lb round or square weight on the center of the board. Call the force on the left A, the one in the center B, and the one in the right C. Draw a free body diagram of the lever (remove the scales and weight and replace with force vectors), and label the force vectors with their letters and with the known forces (round numbers).

   Add 10 more pounds at the center of the lever. What is the relationship of the forces between A, B, and C? Write this as an equation using positive and negative signs, and then substitute the pound values of the forces to check it. Move the weight B to the right 6 inches. Does this relationship still hold? Move the weight back to the center and move the scale C in 6 inches. Same relationship? Notice that change in the magnitude of one force or change in the length of a force arm produces changes in the magnitude of the other two forces but the sum of the forces remains (equilibrium equation: $\Sigma F = 0$).

4. Torques and unknown forces: Use the same lever system as in number 3. Consider scale A as the fulcrum (or joint force) at the origin of the coordinate system. Cover the meter on scale A. Place a 10-lb weight on the center of the lever. Calculate the torque exerted by weight B and calculate the torque exerted by scale C. Repeat for a 20-lb weight. What is the relationship between the two torques? Write the equilibrium equation for this relationship.

5. Press down on a scale with your fist as hard as you can as illustrated in Figure 2–37A. To record elbow extension muscle force only and to keep the problem in a parallel force system, the subject needs to keep the elbow flexed at a right angle. Make a free body diagram of the forces, and label the unknown forces with letters and the known forces with pounds. Measure the distance from the joint center to the center of force on the hand, and use 1 inch for the muscle force arm. Write the equilibrium equation for torque and solve for the mus-

cle force. Then write the equilibrium equation for force and solve for the joint force. Why are the muscle and joint forces so large compared to the force of the hand on the scale? (If you wish to add the force of the hand and forearm, it is 2.2 percent of body weight. You will find that with maximum forces such as these, addition of the forearm weight has little effect.)

6. Why is it impossible to do the following party tricks without cheating:
   A. Stand with back and heels touching a wall and bend forward from the hips to touch the floor. Return to the upright position without falling or moving the feet.
   B. Stand facing the edge of an open door with nose and abdomen touching the edge, the feet straddling the door, and the hands to the sides. Attempt to rise up on the toes.
   Observe what body motions occur to keep the center of gravity within the base of support when these activities are performed without the impediments.

7. Describe the movements of the body's center of gravity from sitting to standing.

CHAPTER 3

Aspects of Muscle Physiology and Neurophysiology

Purposeful movement is a fundamental characteristic of human behavior. Movement is achieved biomechanically by contraction of skeletal muscles acting within a system of levers and pulleys formed by bones, tendons, and ligaments. A person's individuality is expressed by the pattern of muscular contractions that produces facial expressions, body postures, performance of fine motor skills such as typing or playing a musical instrument, and accomplishment of gross motor activities (eg, walking and running). The individual with an intact neuromusculoskeletal system has a remarkable ability to develop just the right amount of muscle contraction needed to perform an endless variety of motor tasks—from placing a contact lens in one's eye to carrying a heavy load of textbooks to class.

Each skeletal muscle (or group of muscles) exhibits properties that permit the muscle to achieve, within wide limits, the requirements placed on it. Skeletal muscles demonstrate great variability in properties. For example, **speed** of movement may be a desirable quality in activities such as running or playing a piano, but so is **economy of energy** in maintaining posture. Muscles must shorten sufficiently to provide a full **range of movement** at the joints over which the muscles cross, yet the muscles must generate sufficient **power** to move a load at each end of the range. Muscles must sometimes function for **long periods** without fatiguing and at other times must provide **maximal efforts** of **great force** for only a few seconds.

An elaborate nervous system provides fine control of muscle contractions over a wide range of lengths, tensions, speeds, and loads. The nervous system is very complex and has numerous functions, including memory, thought processes, emotion, and behavior, as well as various sensory and motor functions. One part of the nervous system, the **central nervous system (CNS)**, is composed of the brain and spinal cord. A second portion of the nervous system, the **peripheral nervous system**, is composed of receptors and effectors of the body, peripheral ganglia, and neuronal processes that connect the peripheral nervous system to the CNS.

Sensory portions of the nervous system are designed to provide accurate and timely information (in the form of sensory nerve impulses) about the status of each part of the body and the state of the environmental surroundings. Incoming sensory information, along with information previously stored in the brain, is used by other parts of the nervous system, including the motor system. The motor portion of the nervous system sends instructions (in the form of motor nerve impulses) to selected muscles or groups of muscles to produce desired movements. Thus, the end product—desired movement—is achieved through the collaborative interaction and coordination of the motor and sensory systems. The interaction involves numerous anatomic, physiologic, biochemical, and biomechanical factors. These factors include the ability of muscles to develop **graded** amounts of active **tension;** the ability of the cardiovascular, respiratory, and digestive systems to provide the ingredients that "fuel" the contractile process, and the ability of the nervous system to **perceive** what is happening and to **regulate** the rate and amount of contraction needed to accurately **move** certain body parts while **stabilizing** other parts.

Owing to the "micro" and "macro" complexities of human movement, a multidisciplinary approach is necessary to understand movement. Anatomists and physiologists study motor function to determine which structures are responsible for producing movements at particular joints as well as the neural circuits used to control specific muscles. Anthropologists study motor function among different species and cultures as an indicator of evolutionary development. Physical educators teach persons how to perform relatively complex motor skills that serve as the foundation for various sports and recreational activities, and members of health professions study motor function as a basis for detecting deviations in human movement and to assist in finding solutions to restore functional abilities as much as possible. The more one understands about the characteristics and basic principles of operation of the systems that support and sustain motor behavior, the more effective one can be in assessing impairments of motor function and in suggesting possible solutions to clinical problems.

The material in this chapter may serve as a review for those who have previously studied the anatomy and physiology of the neuromuscular system. For those who have not had the benefit of such courses, sufficient detail is included to emphasize the most important concepts. Additionally, vocabulary is defined to provide a basis for understanding the subject matter that follows. Textbooks on human physiology and neuroscience may be consulted for a more complete explanation of the functions of the neuromuscular system.

STRUCTURE OF SKELETAL MUSCLE

Organization of Muscles

Skeletal muscles (Fig. 3–1A) are composed of muscle fibers that are organized into bundles. Each bundle of muscle fibers is termed a **fasciculus** (see Fig. 3–1B). **Myofilaments** comprise **myofibrils,** which in turn are grouped together to form **muscle fibers.** The length of a muscle fiber varies from a few millimeters (mm) to 60 or 70 centimeters (cm), and the diameter of an individual muscle fiber is 50 to 100 micrometers (μm).* Each fiber has a covering or membrane, the **sarcolemma,** and is composed of a gelatin-like substance, **sarcoplasm** (see Fig. 3–1C). Hundreds of contractile myofibrils and other important structures, such as mitochondria and the sarcoplasmic reticulum, are imbedded in the sarcoplasm (Fig. 3–2). Mitochondria serve as "tiny factories" where metabolic processes occur. The **contractile myofibril** (see Fig. 3–1D) is composed of units, and each unit is referred to as a **sarcomere,** the portion between two **Z lines.** An interesting feature of skeletal muscle fibers is the appearance of striations (for this reason, skeletal muscle is often referred to as "striated" muscle). The striations are alternate bands of light and dark light-refractive materials that, when viewed under a microscope, are seen to be al-

---

*1 micrometer $= 10^{-6}$ meter, or one-millionth of a meter.

SKELETAL MUSCLE

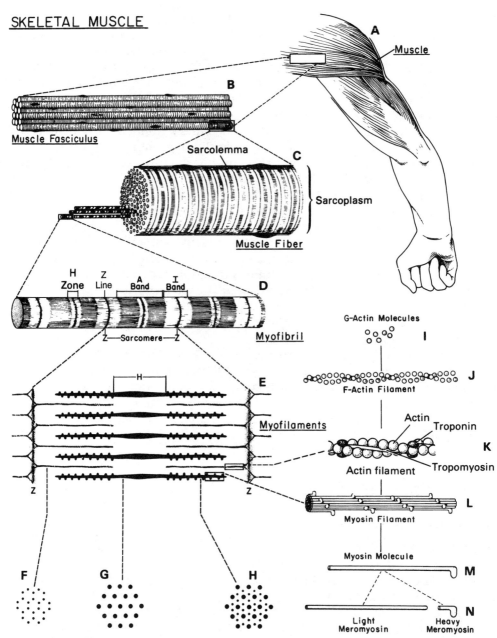

Figure 3–1 Diagram of the organization of skeletal muscle at rest, from (*A*) the gross to (*E*) the molecular levels. (*F*), (*G*), and (*H*) are cross sections of the myofibrils at the levels indicated. (*I–N*) are diagrams of the composition of the myofilaments. (Adapted from Bloom, W, and Fawcett, DW: *A Textbook of Histology*, ed 10. WB Saunders, Philadelphia, 1975, p 306.)

ternately **lighter** and **darker** bands (see Figs. 3–1D and 3–2). Each myofibril, in turn, contains many **myofilaments**. The myofilaments are fine threads of two protein molecules, **actin** (thin filaments) and **myosin** (thick filaments; see Fig. 3–1E).

The darker band in skeletal muscles, referred to as the anisotropic or **A band**, contains both **actin** and **myosin** filaments (see Fig. 3–1D,H). **A bands** have a relatively isotropic middle zone, the **H zone**, that contains only **myosin** filaments (see Fig. 3–1D,G). The lighter band in skeletal muscles, designated as the isotropic

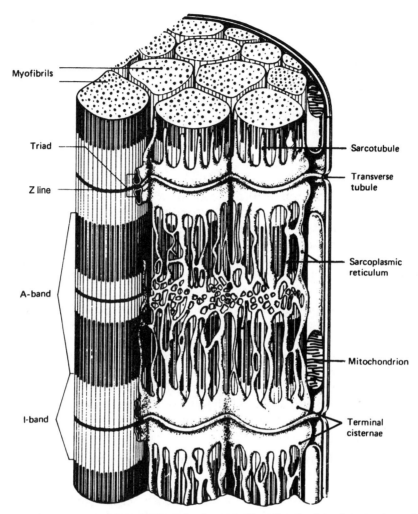

Figure 3–2 Endoplasmic reticulum of the skeletal muscle fiber. Sketch of the fine structure of part of a muscle fiber based on an electron micrograph. The cell membrane *(right)* invaginates at the level of each Z line, sending transverse tubules across the interior of the fiber. Between the Z lines and parallel to the myofibrils runs the sarcoplasmic reticulum, of which saclike enlargements (the terminal cisternae) adjoin the transverse tubules. A cross section through a transverse tubule and an adjacent terminal cisterna reveals a configuration known as a triad *(upper left)*. (From Bloom, W, and Fawcett, DW: *A Textbook of Histology,* ed. 10. WB Saunders, Philadelphia, 1975, with permission.)

or **I band**, contains only **actin** filaments and is bisected transversely by a **Z line** (see Figs. 3–1D,F and 3–2). One end of each actin myofilament within the I band is attached to the Z line. As will be described in more detail in subsequent sections, muscles develop tension and shorten through electrochemical reactions between actin and myosin filaments.

The thin **actin** filaments of the I bands are comprised of actin, tropomyosin, and troponin (see Fig. 3–1K). The basic building block of actin is a globular molecule, designated as **G-actin**, which is about 5.5 nanometers (nm)* in diameter (see Fig. 3–1I). In muscle, G-actin molecules are polymerized (linked together) to form a long fibrous strand, referred to as **F-actin.** Two strands of F-actin are twisted

---

*1 nanometer = 10^{-9} meter, or one-billionth of a meter.

about each other (see Fig. 3–1J) to form part of the actin filament. Another filamentous protein, **tropomyosin**, is about 40 nm long. Two strands of tropomyosin are twisted around the double coil of F-actin in such a way as to lie in the hollows of the twisted actin (see Fig. 3–1K). **Troponin**, another globular protein, binds to a specific region of the tropomyosin filament, to give one troponin globule per 40 nm of tropomyosin filament (see Fig. 3–1K). An important function of troponin is believed to be based on its enormous avidity for calcium ions (Ca^{++}), a property that is considered when discussing the activation of the contractile process. This complex array of G-actin, F-actin, tropomyosin, and troponin comprises the actin filaments in the sarcomere.

Myosin filaments (see Fig. 3–1L) are thicker than actin filaments and are composed of myosin molecules that form a rod about 150 nm long and 1.5 to 2.0 nm in diameter (see Fig. 3–1M). Under certain conditions, the myosin molecule can be split into two fragments, one about twice the weight of the other. The lighter-weight fragment (light meromyosin) is a straight rod that is responsible for the self-aggregation properties of myosin (see Fig. 3–1N). The heavier fragment (heavy meromyosin) is shaped like the lower one-fourth of a hockey stick (see Fig. 3–1N). The heavy meromyosin fragment exhibits enzyme-like qualities capable of splitting adenosine triphosphate (ATP) into adenosine diphosphate (ADP) and phosphate (PO_4) plus energy. The significance of this reaction is discussed in the section dealing with the energetics of muscle contraction.

Within the sarcomere unit, the thick filaments have small projections of heavy meromyosin extending transversely from the long axis of the filament in a helical pattern (see Fig. 3–1L). Transverse processes of the myosin filaments are repeated approximately every 43 nm and are believed to interact with specific sites on the actin filament to produce relative motion between the two types of filament.

Structural Basis for Muscle Contraction and Relaxation

Investigators using light and electron microscopy have observed relaxed and contracted states of muscle tissue. The length of each serially repeating **sarcomere unit** is approximately 2.5 μm when the muscle is **relaxed** (Fig. 3–3A). The length of each sarcomere **decreases** to about 1.5 μm when the muscle is **fully contracted** (see Fig. 3–3B,C). In contrast, the sarcomere unit may be **increased** to about 3.0 μm when the muscle is **stretched** (see Fig. 3–3D).

The sarcomere is bounded on each end by a Z line (see Figs. 3–1D and 3–2). Widths of individual A bands do not change during contraction. The I band, however, does become more narrow, and the H zone within the A band is obliterated. These findings suggest that muscles contract by the free ends of the actin filaments sliding toward each other into the central H zone of the A bands. As the actin filaments move toward each other, the **Z lines** are pulled **closer** together so that the I bands shorten (Fig. 3–3A–C). Although the amount of shortening of each sarcomere unit is small, for example, 0.5 to 1.0 μm, the shortening of several thousands of sarcomere units linked in series can produce a reduction of several centimeters in the overall length of the muscle. For example, a muscle fiber 10 cm in length (such as many fibers in the biceps brachii muscle of adults) would have approximately 40,000 sarcomere units lined up end to end.* If **each** of the 40,000

---

*1 cm = 10^4 μm = 10,000 μm; thus, the 10 cm muscle fiber = 100,000 μm in length. 100,000 μm divided by 2.5 μm per sarcomere = 40,000 sarcomere units.

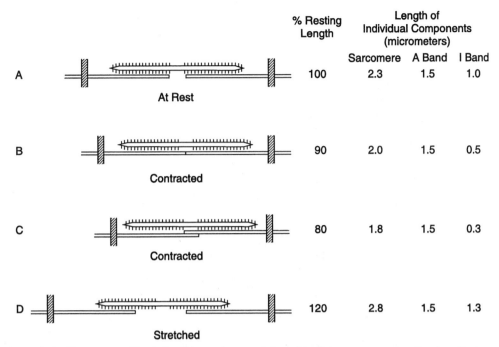

	% Resting Length	Length of Individual Components (micrometers)		
		Sarcomere	A Band	I Band
A	100	2.3	1.5	1.0
At Rest				
B	90	2.0	1.5	0.5
Contracted				
C	80	1.8	1.5	0.3
Contracted				
D	120	2.8	1.5	1.3
Stretched				

Figure 3–3 The structural basis for changes in muscle length: (*A*) A sarcomere at resting length showing changes (*B, C*) in arrangement of filaments under various degrees of contraction and (*D*) when stretched. Relative changes in length of the sarcomere are indicated on the *left*, and the approximate lengths (in micrometers) of the sarcomere, the A band, and the I band are listed on the *right*. Note the constancy of the A band length. (Adapted from Schottelius, BA, and Schottelius, DD: *Textbook of Physiology*, ed 17. CV Mosby, St. Louis, 1973, p 87.)

sarcomere units were **shortened** by 1 μm, the ends of the entire muscle fiber would be brought 40,000 μm (or 4 cm) closer together. Thus, an overall shortening of 40 percent of the length of the muscle would occur.

The concept that actin and myosin filaments slide past each other during muscle contraction is termed the **sliding filament** theory of muscle contraction (Hanson and Huxley, 1953; Huxley, 1969). The specific way in which actin filaments are drawn past myosin filaments to develop muscle tension and muscular shortening is uncertain. Investigators using electron microscopy suggest that a regular array of transverse processes extend from each myosin filament (see Fig. 3–1E,L) to link up with six actin filaments surrounding each myosin filament (see Fig. 3–1H). When chemical energy is available following stimulation of the muscle fiber, an interaction occurs between the myosin transverse processes (cross-bridges) and active sites on the actin filaments. Interaction of the cross-bridges on myosin processes with the actin filament results in movement of the actin filaments into the H zone. However, the active sites on the actin filament are partially shielded by troponin. Two major events, therefore, are required for the mechanical linkages between actin and myosin filaments to produce shortening of the sarcomeres and, thus, contraction of the muscle:

- A specific stimulus triggers the uncovering of an active site on the actin filament to allow coupling of the two filaments.
- Chemical reactions provide energy for the development of active tension.

A. Descending (motor) pathway

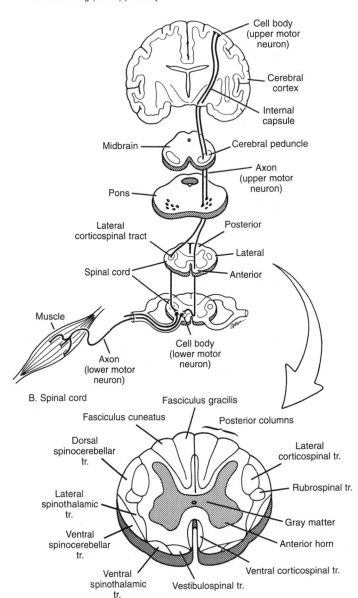

Cell body
(upper motor
neuron)

Cerebral
cortex

Internal
capsule

Midbrain

Cerebral peduncle

Axon
(upper motor
neuron)

Pons

Lateral
corticospinal tract

Posterior

Lateral

Spinal cord

Anterior

Muscle

Cell body
(lower motor
neuron)

Axon
(lower motor
neuron)

B. Spinal cord

Fasciculus gracilis

Fasciculus cuneatus

Posterior columns

Dorsal
spinocerebellar
tr.

Lateral
corticospinal tr.

Lateral
spinothalamic
tr.

Rubrospinal tr.

Gray matter

Ventral
spinocerebellar
tr.

Anterior horn

Ventral
spinothalamic
tr.

Vestibulospinal tr.

Ventral corticospinal tr.

Figure 3–4 Major structures involved in the transmission of impulses to activate skeletal muscle fibers. (*A*) Central and peripheral components of the descending (motor) pathways from the cerebral cortex to the spinal cord and to muscles. (*B*) Cross section of the spinal cord at the thoracic level, illustrating the central gray matter and the peripheral white matter with ascending and descending tracts. Note that structures and tracts exist on both the left and right sides; for simplicity, however, only one side is illustrated. tr. = tract.

EXCITATION OF NERVE AND SKELETAL MUSCLE FIBERS

All living cells are surrounded by membranes formed by a continuous phospholipid bilayer. Embedded throughout the membrane are proteins with various characteristics. Both nervous and muscular tissue are excitable; that is, their membranes can be depolarized. Furthermore, the depolarization can be propagated along the membrane of the nerve or muscle. A neuron (nerve cell) that innervates skeletal muscle and the skeletal muscle itself are not only excitable but also possess membrane characteristics that ensure that the excitation that occurs generates

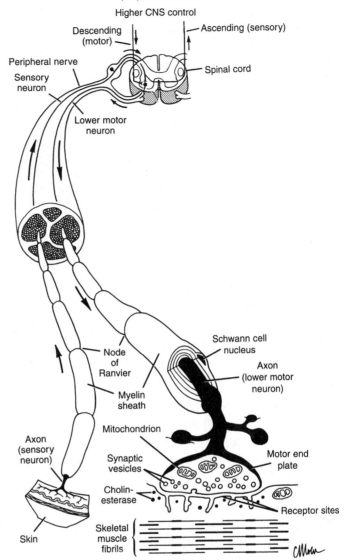

C. Some connections of peripheral nerve fibers

Figure 3–4 (*Continued*) (*C*) Peripheral nerve fibers are enlarged to illustrate sensory and motor components.

an **action potential.** Action potentials are propagated with no changes in **amplitude (intensity),** regardless of how great the distance over which the action potential must travel to reach its target. Further discussion of membrane and action potentials and depolarization are presented in subsequent sections of the present chapter.

The stimulus that produces muscle contraction may be electrical, mechanical, chemical, or thermal. The stimulus usually is chemical in origin, arises in the nervous system, and is conducted to each muscle fiber by a nerve fiber. The stimulus for excitation is a wave of electrochemical activity that moves rapidly along nerve and muscle fibers and is associated with local changes in the electrical potential of each of the fibers. General anatomic features of the neural pathways for conducting nerve impulses from the brain to individual muscle fibers are illustrated schematically in Figure 3–4. Axons of upper motor neurons located in the cerebral cortex of the brain descend to the spinal cord and form axonal bundles referred to as the corticospinal pathways or tracts (the term "tract" is used to describe a group of axons with common origin, function, and termination). Corticospinal tracts are located in either the lateral or the ventral (anterior) portions of the spinal cord (see Fig. 3–4A) and are referred to as the lateral or ventral corticospinal tract, respectively. The axons of the corticospinal tracts make synaptic contact (usually via interneurons) with lower motor neurons situated in gray matter in the ventral horn of the spinal cord. Each lower motor neuron innervates and controls the activity of a set of muscle fibers within a muscle.

A cross-section of a thoracic segment of the spinal cord and the locations of major motor and sensory tracts are illustrated in Figure 3–4B. The name of a tract often indicates the general origin and destination of the axons within the tract. For example, axons in the corticospinal tract descend from the cerebral cortex and terminate within the spinal cord. Likewise, the spinocerebellar tracts convey sensory impulses from their point of entry into the spinal cord to the cerebellum. General features of the connections between a nerve and a muscle are illustrated in Figure 3–4C. An enlarged sketch of the major links in the nerve-to-muscle pathway is included to show more anatomic detail. The function of each of the links is considered in more detail in subsequent portions of the present chapter.

Membrane Potential

Differences in electrical potential exist across the membranes of living cells. Fluids bathing the inside and outside of each cell contain charged particles (ions) dissolved in solution. Metabolic processes occur in every cell to produce a net difference in the concentration of positive and negative ions between the inside and outside of each cell (Fig. 3–5A). Two factors are responsible for the ability of a cell to maintain a potential difference across its membrane:

- The cell membrane is relatively impermeable to certain ions (however, permeability of the membrane to an ion can be increased transiently by certain chemical substances released by nerve endings, as is discussed later).
- The cell can actively move ions across the membrane to maintain a required resting potential.

The potential inside a cell membrane is measured relative to the fluid just outside the membrane (see Fig. 3–5). Under resting conditions, the membrane potential (**resting potential**) is **negative** and becomes **positive** during an **action potential**. Nerve cells, muscle cells, and sensory receptors maintain a more negative **resting potential** (-60 to -80 mV) between the inside and outside of the membrane than do other types of cells. Nerve cells and muscle cells also are excitable and are capable of transmitting electrochemical impulses along their membranes.

Action Potential

A stimulus (electrical, mechanical, chemical, or thermal) of sufficient strength applied to an excitable cell can cause the cell membrane to become more permeable to certain ions in the region where the stimulus is applied. The increase in permeability results in a rapid exchange of positive and negative ions across the membrane that were previously separated by the membrane. The rapid exchange of positive and negative ions is referred to as **depolarization**. An **action potential** depolarizes the membrane and establishes a difference in electrical potential be-

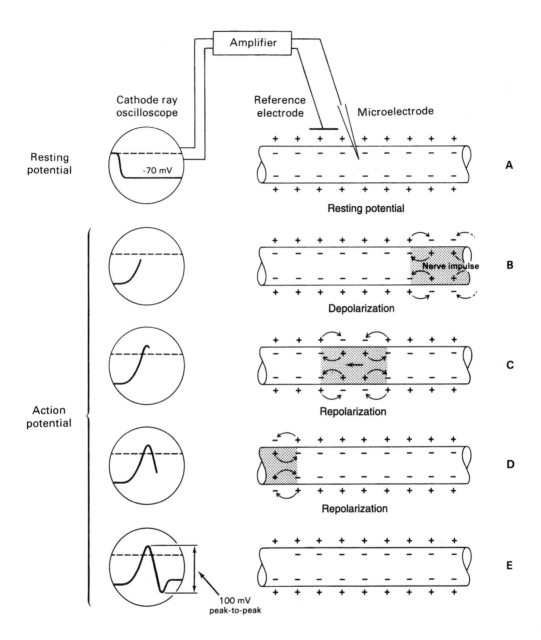

Figure 3–5 Generation of an action potential. A microelectrode can be introduced into an excitable cell to record (*A*) the resting potential (−70 mV) as well as (*B–E*) changes in transmembrane potential associated with the spread of an action potential along the cell membrane. The difference in electric potential "seen" by the two electrodes (one outside and one inside the cell) (*A*) is amplified electronically and displayed on the cathode ray oscilloscope on the *left* (*A–E*). Once a small region of membrane is depolarized, local electric currents flow, depolarizing adjacent regions of the membrane. Very soon after being depolarized, the membrane again becomes impermeable to most ions, and the resting potential is re-established (repolarization [*C, D*]). The dynamics of the passive and active migration of ions across the membrane actually result in some overshoot of the action potential above the zero line and below the average resting potential of −70 mV. Thus, the peak-to-peak amplitude (*E*) of the action potential is of the order of 100 mV.

tween active and inactive regions of the membrane, resulting in current flow between the two regions (see Fig. 3–5). The flow of current between adjacent regions serves to excite the polarized region ahead of the current, with the result that this region now contributes a greatly amplified electric signal, capable of spreading to the next region and exciting it also. Thus, the action potential is propagated. An action potential transmitted over a nerve fiber is referred to as a nerve impulse, whereas an action potential conducted over a muscle fiber is designated as a muscle impulse.

Immediately after depolarization, an active process, termed **repolarization**, begins in the cell membrane to re-establish the resting membrane potential. The advancing wave of depolarization coupled with repolarization is referred to as an action potential. Amplitudes and shapes of action potentials vary from one type of cell to another (Fig. 3–6A–D). Note in Figure 3–6 that the nerve impulse (A) is very

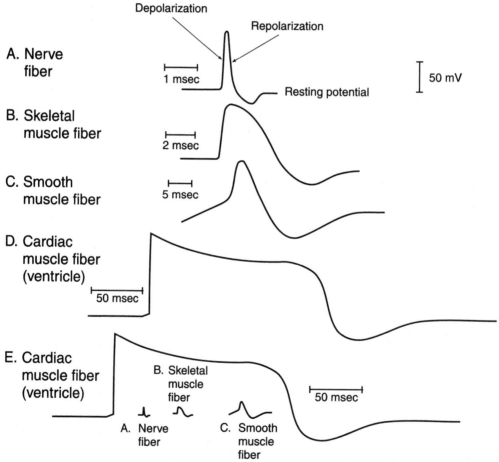

Figure 3–6   Examples of action potentials in different types of excitable cells. (*A*) Nerve impulse. (*B*) Skeletal muscle fiber impulse. (*C*) Smooth muscle fiber impulse. (*D*) Cardiac muscle fiber impulse. Note that amplitudes and shapes of action potentials vary from one type of cell to the next. The nerve impulse (*A*) is a very rapid event, lasting about 1 msec. The skeletal muscle impulse (*B*) lasts about 5 to 10 times as long as the nerve impulse, and the cardiac muscle impulse (*D*) lasts as long as 200 to 300 msec. Note the different time calibrations in (*A–D*). In (*E*), the action potentials of each type of excitable cell illustrated in (*A–C*) are superimposed on the largest action potential, the cardiac muscle fiber, to demonstrate the approximate size of each impulse to compare the action potentials as if they were recorded using a similar time calibration.

rapid and lasts approximately 1 msec, whereas the skeletal muscle (B) and smooth muscle (C) impulses last about 5 to 10 times as long as the nerve impulse. The cardiac muscle fiber impulse (C) lasts even longer, about 200 to 300 msec. To illustrate variations in amplitudes, shapes, and velocities of impulses of different fiber types, the impulses are superimposed schematically on the cardiac muscle fiber impulse (see Fig. 3–6E). Along one cell, however, action potentials are propagated with no change in amplitude.

Neurotransmission

Neurons send "control signals" to other neurons (or to muscles) by releasing small amounts of chemicals termed **neurotransmitters.** Each time a nerve impulse arrives at the synapse (Gr. *synapsis,* a connection), that is, at the junction between nerves or at the junction between a motor neuron and a muscle fiber, neurotransmitters are released at the synapse. Physiologically, the chemical synapse between two neurons may be either excitatory or inhibitory. **Excitatory** synapses cause **depolarization** of the postsynaptic membrane, thus tending to make a neuron upon which it synapses fire one or more nerve impulses. In contrast, **inhibitory** synapses result in a **hyperpolarization** (more negative potential) of the postsynaptic membrane that tends to keep the postsynaptic neuron inactive. Action potentials of inhibitory impulses are the same as those of facilitatory impulses except that the chemical transmitter released at the presynaptic ending of an inhibitory neuron produces hyperpolarization of the postsynaptic membrane rather than depolarization (Burt, 1993). Further discussion of neurotransmitters is found in the section on neural modification of excitability.

Transmission of Impulses From Nerves to Skeletal Muscle Fibers: Myoneural Junction

The nervous system regulates the activity of muscle fibers by sending control signals in the form of action potentials. Conversion of a nerve impulse to a muscle impulse, however, occurs through a complicated process. The nerve fiber branches at its end to form a motor end-plate, which adheres tightly to the muscle fiber but which does not lie within the muscle fiber membrane (see Fig. 3–4C). The junction formed is a type of synapse referred to as the **myoneural** (Gr. *mye,* muscle) **junction.** The end-plate of the motor neuron contains mitochondria that synthesize (manufacture) a neurotransmitter, **acetylcholine.** Molecules of acetylcholine are stored in small vesicles located in the presynaptic ending of motor neurons. The arrival of a nerve impulse at the myoneural junction causes release of acetylcholine from some of the vesicles. When freed from storage in the vesicles, acetylcholine diffuses rapidly across the short distance between the motor end-plate and muscle fiber membrane. Acetylcholine then interacts with receptor sites on the muscle fiber membrane. The interaction **increases** the **permeability** of the muscle cell membrane to ions in the fluid bathing the junction. Movement of the ions into the muscle cell **depolarizes** the muscle fiber (postjunctional) membrane and triggers a muscle action potential that is propagated along the muscle fiber by an electrochemical mechanism similar to that responsible for the propagation of a nerve impulse.

After causing an increase in permeability of the postjunctional membrane to ions, acetylcholine is rapidly **inactivated** by an enzyme, cholinesterase (see Fig. 3–4C). Ordinarily, cholinesterase is present in the fluid bathing the synaptic space and begins immediately to split acetylcholine. The very short time that acetylcholine remains in contact with the muscle fiber membrane, about 2 msec, is usually sufficient to excite the muscle fiber, and yet the rapid inactivation of acetylcholine by cholinesterase prevents re-excitation after the muscle fiber has repolarized from the first action potential.

Conduction of Muscle Impulses to the Interior of the Muscle Fiber: Endoplasmic Reticulum

Change in electrical potential in the immediate vicinity of actin and myosin filaments triggers a process that leads to shortening of each sarcomere. Thus, a muscle action potential must be conveyed throughout the entire muscle fiber as effectively as possible. The interior of a muscle fiber contains two interlaced systems of tubes that play an important role in excitation of muscle fibers and in the coupling of excitation to contraction (see Fig. 3–2). One system, the **transverse tubular system (T system)**, speeds the transmission of a muscle action potential to all portions of the muscle fiber. The other system, the **sarcoplasmic reticulum (SR)**, has been implicated in the storage and release of calcium ions during the contractile process. The two systems, the transverse tubular system and the sarcoplasmic reticulum, together are referred to as the **endoplasmic reticulum** (see Fig. 3–2).

Excitation-Contraction Coupling

Energy must be supplied to myofilaments to cause movement of the actin filaments toward the center of the A bands. Energy for this purpose is available from molecules of adenosine triphosphate (ATP), which are coupled to myosin crossbridges. The energy is actually provided by the action of myosin when molecules of ATP are split into adenosine diphospate (ADP) and a phosphate group (PO_4). The enzymatic ATP-splitting property of myosin, termed myosin ATPase activity, is stimulated by calcium. The essentials of the splitting of ATP for energy may be expressed by an equation.*

Sliding Filament Theory of Muscle Contraction

A sequential series of events is hypothesized to explain how sliding filaments develop tension and shorten (Fig. 3–7). Projections of heavy meromyosin, termed **cross-bridges**, are located on the myosin myofilaments. At rest, the cross-bridges are not coupled with actin myofilaments (see Fig. 3–7A). Also at rest, calcium is stored in the SR, and the ATP molecules are coupled near the end of each crossbridge (see Fig. 3–7A). Potential reactive sites on actin myofilaments are covered by troponin and, therefore, are not available to the myosin cross-bridges.

As a pulse of depolarization descends the T tubules, quantities of calcium are released from storage sites in the SR. Some of the calcium ions interact with troponin, causing a deformation in the shape of the troponin molecule (see Fig. 3–7B). The changes in shape caused by the interaction of calcium with troponin

---

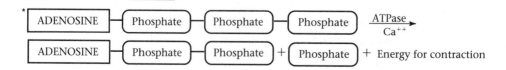

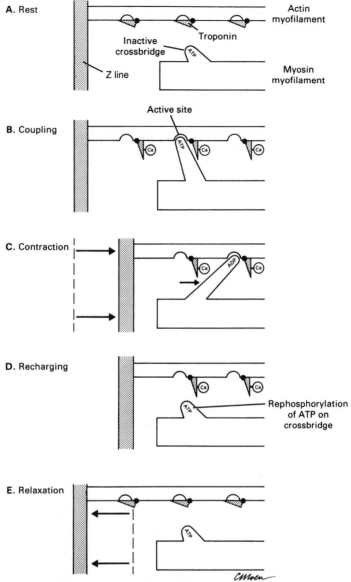

Figure 3–7 The hypothesized sequential series of reactions between active sites on actin and myosin filaments that pull the actin filament (and attached Z line) past the myosin filament to produce shortening of the sarcomere. The recovery process is also illustrated. Many repetitions of the cycle at a large percentage of the active sites are needed to produce a strong contraction. (*A*) Rest. Cross-bridges project from a myosin myofilament but are not coupled with an actin myofilament. Adenosine triphosphate (ATP) is attached near the head of the cross-bridge; troponin covers the active sites on the actin myofilament; calcium ions are stored in the sarcoplasmic reticulum. (*B*) Coupling. Arrival of the muscle action potential depolarizes the sarcolemma and T tubules; calcium ions are released and react with troponin; change in the shape of the troponin-calcium complex uncovers active sites on actin; a cross-bridge couples with an adjacent active site, thereby linking myosin and actin myofilaments. (*C*) Contraction. Linkage of a cross-bridge and an active site triggers adenosine triphosphatase (ATPase) activity of myosin; ATP splits to adenosine disphosphate (ADP) + PO_4 + energy; the reaction produces a transient flexion of the cross-bridge; the actin myofilament is pulled a short distance past the myosin myofilament; Z lines are moved closer together. (*D*) Recharging. The cross-bridge uncouples from the active site and retracts; ATP is replaced on the cross-bridge. The recoupling, flexion, uncoupling, retraction, and recharging processes are repeated hundreds of times per second. (*E*) Relaxation. Cessation of excitation occurs; calcium ions are removed from the vicinity of the actin myofilament and are returned to storage sites in the sarcoplasmic reticulum; troponin returns to its original shape, covering active sites on the actin myofilament; actin and myosin myofilaments return to rest state.

appear to uncover an active site on the thin actin filament that electrostatically attracts the myosin cross-bridge. Linkage between the myosin cross-bridge and an active site on the actin filament forms an actin-myosin cross-bridge. The actin-myosin crossbridge, in turn, triggers the ATPase activity of myosin and results in splitting ATP into ADP plus phosphate and energy. The splitting of ATP produces transient "flexion" of the cross-bridge (see Fig. 3–7C), which pulls the actin filament a short distance before the linkage is broken and another molecule of ATP is coupled to the end of the cross-bridge (see Fig. 3–7D). Once recharged with ATP, the cross-bridge can react with another active site to pull the actin filament a little farther past the myosin filament. The recoupling, flexion, uncoupling, retraction, and recharging processes are repeated hundreds of times each second.

The strength of contraction (active tension) of individual myofibrils appears to depend on the average number of links between actin and myosin at any given instant. Likewise, release of calcium from the SR depends on the presence of an action potential in the sarcolemma. As soon as the sarcolemma repolarizes, calcium begins to re-enter the SR. Thus, if the muscle cell is depolarized at a frequency exceeding the time course of calcium reuptake, the concentration of calcium in the sarcoplasm will increase. Increases in the concentration of calcium in turn lead to the formation of greater numbers of cross-bridges (until troponin is saturated with calcium) and contributes to greater tension developed during some contractions.

Energy must be spent to maintain active tension in the muscle. Energy is required even in the absence of overall shortening of the muscle, such as occurs when the muscle is attempting, unsuccessfully, to lift an excessively heavy load. In the latter case, an absence of external work, as defined by physics, is being accomplished.

Muscle Relaxation

Once depolarization of the muscle fiber has ended (5 to 10 msec), the intracellular concentration of calcium drops very quickly, and relaxation occurs (see Fig. 3–7E). The rapid drop in intracellular calcium appears to be the result of an active "pumping" of calcium ions from the region of the myofilaments back into storage sites in the SR. The exact nature of the pumps is unknown, but metabolic energy is required to transport calcium across the membrane into the SR. Active transport of calcium against a concentration gradient continues until the concentration of calcium remaining in the intracellular fluid bathing the myofilaments reaches a very low level under resting conditions. Removal of calcium ions from the vicinity of the actin myofilaments results in the troponin returning to its original shape, thus covering the active sites on the actin myofilament. The actin and myosin myofilaments are returned to their "resting," relaxed state. Thus, interaction between actin and myosin myofilaments ceases because of an insufficient concentration of intracellular calcium.

ENERGY SOURCES FOR MUSCLE CONTRACTION

Muscle cells, like other living cells in the body, expend energy (even when at rest) to support the metabolic processes required for maintenance of life. When a muscle contracts, chemical energy (derived from the breakdown of ATP) is converted to mechanical energy, thereby increasing the need for more chemical energy. The ultimate source of energy for metabolic processes is ATP. Energy becomes available for metabolic work through chemical reactions in the mitochondria that oxidize food materials. Because the body cannot store as large a supply of oxygen as it can food materials, metabolically active cells depend upon a constant supply of oxygen from the respiratory and cardiovascular systems. However, muscle cells are unique with respect to the use of oxygen. In muscle, oxygen serves as an indirect source of energy. The direct source of energy for muscle contraction is ATP. A series of chemical reactions involving stored materials serves to replenish the supply of ATP as it is used for contraction. Oxygen, however, is the key molecule in the production of ATP.

Anaerobic Metabolism

Enough ATP is stored in each skeletal muscle to provide the chemical energy for performing only two or three strong contractions of the muscle. Because the reactions do not require expenditure of oxygen, the processes are referred to as **anaerobic** (Gr. *a*, without, and *aero*, air) **metabolism.** The chemical equation for the reaction is:

$$ATP \xrightarrow{\text{ATPase}} ADP + PO_4 + Energy$$

With addition of energy from the breakdown of another high-energy compound, phosphocreatine ($CrPO_4$) to creatine (Cr) and phosphate (PO_4), the by-products of the original reaction can be used to regenerate the supply of ATP, that is,

$$CrPO_4 \longrightarrow Cr + PO_4 + Energy$$
$$ADP + PO_4 + Energy \longrightarrow ATP$$

A relatively large reservoir of phosphocreatine can provide energy for muscle contractions over a period of 20 to 30 seconds. Regeneration of phosphocreatine is accomplished partly through the breakdown of glucose to lactic acid. Supplies of glucose are replenished quickly by the breakdown of glycogen from storage depots in muscles and in the liver—a process termed **glycolysis.** Energy derived from the chain of reactions is capable of regenerating sufficient ATP to support vigorous muscle contractions for approximately 30 seconds.

Aerobic Metabolism

Ultimately, chemical energy reserves for muscle contraction are restored by oxidative metabolism of fats, carbohydrates, and proteins in the mitochondria of muscle fibers. Carbohydrate, fat, and protein molecules are mobilized from storage sites in the body; enzymes split the large molecules into smaller units that can be oxidized in a series of chemical reactions termed the **tricarboxylic acid cycle** (Krebs cycle). Oxygen is used at the terminal point of the electron transport chain that is driven by the products of the Krebs cycle. Specifically, oxygen serves as the final electron acceptor where the reaction end products are carbon dioxide, water, and ATP. The end products are used for restoration and maintenance of energy stores **or** are released in respiration.

Use of energy from anaerobic chemical reactions to power the contractile process for the first few minutes of strenuous physical exertion produces an oxygen debt that is repaid by continuing oxidative (aerobic) metabolism at a relatively high rate for several minutes after cessation of the exercise. The size of the oxygen debt constitutes a limiting factor for the continuation of exercise. The rate of buildup of the debt depends on the severity of the exercise. Once the maximum oxygen debt has been attained, the rate of energy expenditure cannot exceed the rate of energy production through oxidative metabolism. In addition to the rate at which chemical reactions proceed through the tricarboxylic acid cycle, other factors limit the steady-state performance of a person, such as the adequacy of operation of the respiratory and cardiovascular systems in supplying oxygen to the active cells **and** in removing the end products of metabolism.

Efficiency of Muscular Work

The relative efficiency of the muscular system in performing mechanical work (output per unit of energy put into the muscular system) has been calculated to be approximately 20 to 25 percent. This means that lifting a particular load a certain distance requires four to five times as much chemical energy as might be expected if **all** of the energy were directed at moving the load. The additional energy shows up as heat. When muscles are exercised vigorously, considerable heat is produced, and special physiologic mechanisms are set into motion to regulate the body temperature.

The rate at which energy is being expended in the body to sustain life (resting level) or to support physical activity can be measured either by monitoring the rate of heat production or by monitoring the uptake of oxygen from the air being breathed. Expressed in terms of heat production, a typical resting level of energy expenditure is approximately 1 Calorie per minute for a young adult weighing 70 kg (154 lb).* Total energy expenditure for 24 hours is approximately 1500 Calories to maintain the cellular processes of the body at rest (resting metabolic rate). Walking at 5 km per hour (3.1 miles per hour) increases the energy expenditure to about 5 Calories per minute, and climbing a flight of stairs rapidly increases the energy expenditure to about 8 Calories per minute.

Expressed in terms of oxygen consumption, the same person described above would use about 0.2 liter of oxygen per minute at rest, 1 liter per minute walking at 5 km per hour, and 1.6 liters of oxygen per minute climbing stairs. Measurements in trained athletes have yielded a maximum rate of oxygen consumption of approximately 6 liters per minute.

Metabolic equivalent (MET) is another term used to describe energy requirements for various activities. MET is an approximate multiple of the resting metabolic rate. One MET is arbitrarily defined as the resting oxygen consumption of an individual. The average value at rest is 3.5 mL of oxygen per kilogram of body weight per minute. The energy cost of any additional activity is then expressed as some multiple of the resting metabolic rate. For example, the energy cost of walking 5 km per hour would be expressed as 5 METs. The relative energy costs of various activities are listed in Table 3–1. The energy cost of any particular activity can vary considerably, depending on the intensity with which the activity is pursued (see also Passmore and Durnin, 1955).

---

*One Calorie, or large calorie (Cal), is the amount of heat required to raise the temperature of 1 kg (2.2 lb) of water 1°C. Calorie is the unit commonly used to express the energy content of food that is eaten. One small calorie (cal) is the amount of heat required to raise the temperature of 1 gm of water 1°C (1 Calorie = 1000 calories). Many people writing in newspapers and popular magazines erroneously use the lower-case spelling of the unit, but they usually mean the Calorie (word beginning with an upper-case letter). The Calorie is sometimes referred to as a kilocalorie.

Table 3–1 Approximate Energy Cost in METs*
During Various Activities

Activities	METs
Self-Care Activities	
Supine rest	1.0
Sitting relaxed	1.0
Standing relaxed	1.5
Eating	1.5
Dressing, undressing	2.0
Washing hands, face	2.0
Wheelchair propulsion	2.0
Showering	3.5
Using bedpan	4.0
Locomotion Activities	
Walk 2.0 mph	2.0
Walk 2.5 mph	3.5
Walk 3.0 mph	3.0
Walk 3.5 mph	4.0
Walk downstairs	4.5
Walk with crutches/braces	6.5
Walk upstairs (eight 9-inch steps)	
11 steps/min	3.3
22 steps/min	5.4
33 steps/min	8.0
Recreational and Work Activities	
Back packing	5–11
Bed exercise (arm movement, supine or sitting)	1–2
Bicycling (pleasure or to work)	3–8
Bowling	2–4
Cleaning windows	2–4
Conditioning exercises (calisthenics)	3–8
Crutch-walking†	2–8
Dancing (social and square)	3–7
Football, touch	6–10
Golf	
Using power cart	2–3
Walking (carrying a bag or pulling a cart)	4–7
Handball	8–12
Hiking, cross-country	3–7
Jogging, 5 mph	7–8
Making beds	2–4
Paddleball (or racquetball)	8–12
Pushing a power mower	3–5
Propelling a wheelchair	2–5
Stair climbing	4–8
Swimming	4–8
Table tennis	3–5
Tennis	4–9
Volleyball	3–6

*METs represent metabolic equivalents. One MET is an approximate
multiple of the resting metabolic rate and is arbitrarily defined as the
resting oxygen consumption of the individual. The average value at rest
is 3.5 mL of oxygen per kg of body weight per minute. Energy cost of
any additional activity is then expressed as some multiple of the resting
metabolic rate.
†An important consideration for crutch-walking is the energy cost per
meter walked.

MUSCLE FIBER TYPES

To most efficiently perform various functions, three different types of skeletal
muscle fiber exist: type I, type IIA, and type IIB. Some investigators have described
more than three types of muscle fibers (Burke, 1981) but, for the purpose of this

text, only the three main types of muscle fibers are discussed. Each type of fiber has different properties, and the majority of skeletal muscles contain a **mixture** of all three types, with the proportion of one type greater than the others.

The first type of fiber (**type I**) is dark (like the dark meat of a chicken*) because it contains large numbers of mitochondria and a high concentration of myoglobin (muscle hemoglobin that stores oxygen). Type I also is referred to as **slow-twitch**, or **slow oxidative (SO)**. The second type of fiber (**type IIB**) is pale (like the white meat of a chicken*) because it contains fewer mitochondria and only small amounts of myoglobin. Type IIB muscle fibers, also termed **fast-twitch** or **fast glycolytic (FG)**, are larger in diameter than type I muscle fibers. Type IIB fibers also develop greater **force** of contraction and complete a single twitch in a significantly **shorter** time than type I muscle fibers. Type IIB fibers, however, **fatigue** more quickly than type I.

When samples of muscle are sectioned and stained with appropriate chemicals to reveal the presence of specific classes of enzymes, the mitochondria of **type I** muscle fibers are found to have an abundance of **oxidative** enzymes (associated with **aerobic** metabolism). In contrast, **type IIB** muscle fibers are found to have a preponderance of **glycolytic** enzymes (associated with **anaerobic** metabolism) in their mitochondria. Thus, muscle fibers may be classified on the basis of appearance (anatomic and histologic) and functional (physiologic) characteristics. Slow-twitch muscle fibers, **type I**, are **fatigue-resistant** and fast-twitch muscle fibers, **type IIB**, have a tendency to **fatigue rather quickly.** For most purposes, the terms slow-twitch (SO) type I and fast-twitch (FG) type IIB muscle fibers are used to describe the two **extremes.**

The third type of fiber, **type IIA**, is referred to as **fast oxidative-glycolytic (FOG)** and is **intermediate** in characteristics such as color, numbers of mitochondria, size, speed of contraction, and rate of fatigue. Table 3–2 summarizes the characteristics of each fiber type.

Table 3–2   Characteristics of Skeletal Muscle Fibers Based on Physical and Metabolic Properties

Property	Muscle Fiber Type		
	Type I Slow-Twitch SO	Type IIA Intermediate FOG	Type IIB Fast-Twitch FG
Muscle fiber diameter	Small	Intermediate	Large
Color	Red (dark)	Red	White (pale)
Myoglobin content	High	High	Low
Mitochondria	Numerous	Numerous	Few
Oxidative enzymes	High	Intermediate	Low
Glycolytic enzymes	Low	Intermediate	High
Glycogen content	Low	Intermediate	High
Myosin ATPase activity	Low	High	High
Major source of ATP	Oxidative phosphorylation	Oxidative phosphorylation	Glycolysis
Speed of contraction	Slow	Intermediate	Fast
Rate of fatigue	Slow	Intermediate	Fast

SO = slow oxidative; FG = fast glycolytic; FOG = fast oxidative-glycolytic.
SOURCE: Burke, RE and Edgerton, VR: Motor unit properties and selective involvement in movement. Exer Sport Sci Rev 3:31, 1975, adapted with permission.

---

*A different situation exists in birds in flight.

Human trunk and limb muscles contain various proportions of the three types of muscle fibers. In addition, some investigators suggest that the proportions of fast-twitch and slow-twitch muscle fibers in a particular muscle vary from subject to subject (Gollnick et al., 1972; Johnson et al., 1973; Edgerton et al., 1975; Thorstensson, 1976). However, despite subject-to-subject variation, the proportion of slow-twitch (type I) fibers is high in the human soleus muscle in the leg (as great as 85 percent of the fibers) and low in the orbicularis oculi of the eyeball (10 percent). The proportion of slow-twitch fibers in representative muscle groups ranked in descending order is as follows: soleus, adductor pollicis, tibialis anterior, biceps femoris, peroneus longus, deltoid, gastrocnemius, biceps brachii, quadriceps, sternocleidomastoid, triceps brachii, and orbicularis oculi (Johnson et al, 1973). The degree to which a particular muscle exhibits physiologic characteristics of contracting slowly and tonically (sustained contraction) and of resisting fatigue can be expected to follow the same distribution. In reverse order, beginning with the orbicularis oculi muscle, the muscles listed above exhibit physiologic characteristics of contracting briskly and phasically (brief contraction) and yet of fatiguing quickly.

THE MOTOR UNIT

Large motor neurons that constitute the link to the pathway of motor response are located either in the brainstem (for the muscles of the face and head) or in the spinal cord (for the muscles of the neck, trunk, and extremities). Specifically, the motor neurons in the spinal cord are located in the gray matter of the ventral (anterior) horns (see Fig. 3–4A–C). An individual motor neuron, together with its axon and all of the muscle fibers that are innervated by the motor neuron, comprise the **motor unit.** Various types of motor neurons exist. The majority, if not all, of the neurons that innervate **skeletal muscles** are the A, **alpha** (α), classification. The term α **motor neuron,** therefore, often is used. Motor commands are carried from the neuronal cell bodies over peripheral nerve fibers and then are transmitted across the neuromuscular junction (the synapse between the nerve and the muscle). The number of muscle fibers innervated by a single motor nerve fiber varies from as few as 5 (in some eye muscles, which have fine control) to as many as 1000 or more (in large muscles such as the gastrocnemius of the leg, which does not require as fine an amount of control). The term **innervation ratio** is used to describe the average number of muscle fibers per motor unit in a given muscle. The innervation ratio is determined by dividing the number of muscle fibers by the number of large motor axons innervating that particular muscle. The number of motor units and the average number of muscle fibers per motor unit are summarized in Table 3–3.

As the term "motor unit" implies, all muscle fibers within a given motor unit contract or relax almost simultaneously; that is, it is impossible for some muscle fibers of a motor unit to contract while other fibers in the same motor unit are relaxed. Also, if the nerve activates the muscle fibers of a motor unit sufficiently that the muscle fibers contract, those fibers will contract maximally. The principle described is known as the **all-or-none law.** The law, however, applies only to individual motor units. Physiologic mechanisms do exist for fine gradation of the force of contraction of the muscle as a whole.

Table 3–3 Number of Motor Units, Motor Fibers, and Muscle Spindles
Per Motor Unit in Human Muscle

Muscle	Number of α Motor Axons	Number of Muscle Fibers		Number of Muscle Spindles	
		Per Muscle × 10³	Average Per Motor Unit	Per Muscle	Per Motor Unit
Biceps brachii	774	580	750	320	0.4
Brachioradialis	330	130	390	65	0.2
First dorsal interosseus	119	41	340	34	0.3
First lumbrical	98	10	110	53	0.6
Opponens pollicis	133	79	595	44	0.3
Masseter	1020	1000	980	160	0.2
Temporalis	1150	1500	1300	217	0.2
Gastrocnemius medius	580	1000	1720	80	0.1
Tibialis anterior	445	270	610	284	0.6

SOURCE: Adapted from Buchthal, F, and Schmalbruch, H: Motor unit of mammalian muscle. *Physiol Rev* 60:95, 1980.

Gradation of Strength of Muscle Contraction

Increased strength of contraction of a muscle, as a whole, occurs in three ways:

- By **initially** activating motor neurons with the smallest innervation ratio, thereby activating few muscle fibers
- By **increasing** the **number** of motor units activated simultaneously (recruitment)
- By **increasing** the **frequency** of stimulation of individual motor units, thereby increasing the percentage of time that each active muscle fiber is developing maximum tension

The **size principle of recruitment** describes the fact that the **smallest** motor neurons are the **first** to be recruited and the **largest** motor neurons are recruited **last** (Henneman, 1981). Small motor neurons participate in most functional activities because small motor neurons tend to innervate slow-twitch, type I muscle fibers that fatigue slowly. Only when contractions requiring greater strength are attempted do the largest fast-twitch motor units become active.

NERVE FIBERS

Peripheral Neurons

Neurons have many different shapes and sizes depending on their location in the nervous system and the functions for which the neurons are responsible. Characteristics of a sensory and a motor neuron are depicted in Figure 3–8. A typical neuron consists of a cell body (containing the nucleus), several short radiating processes (dendrites), and one long process (the axon) that terminates in twig-like branches and may have branches (collaterals) projecting along its course. The axon, together with its covering (sheath), forms the nerve fiber. Large motor and sensory nerves are wrapped with a covering containing a white lipid substance, myelin (an insulating material). The myelin sheath forms regular indentations

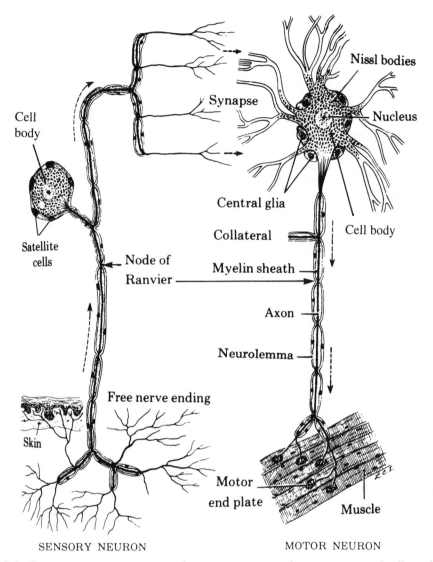

SENSORY NEURON   MOTOR NEURON

Figure 3–8 Diagrammatic representation of a sensory neuron and a motor neuron. Satellite cells and central glia cells are supporting cells that surround the nerve cell body. Synaptic connections between the terminal processes of the sensory neuron and the dendrites of the motor neuron are not shown. (From King, BG, and Showers, MJ: *Human Anatomy and Physiology*, ed 6. WB Saunders, Philadelphia, 1969, p 59, with permission.)

along its length, known as nodes of Ranvier (named after a French histologist, Louis Ranvier, 1835–1922).

A peripheral nerve trunk is composed of many nerve fibers that are bound together by supporting connective tissue (see Fig. 3–4C). Functionally, peripheral nerves contain one or more of the following classes of fibers:

1. **Motor fibers** conduct nerve impulses **from the spinal cord to skeletal muscle fibers** for the control of voluntary muscular activity. Their cell bod-

ies are located in the gray matter of the spinal cord and brain stem. Motor fibers often are referred to as **efferent** (L. *ex*, out, plus *ferre*, to carry) nerve fibers.

2. **Sensory fibers** carry impulses arising **from** various receptors in the skin, muscles, and special sense organs **to the CNS**, where the impulses are interpreted. Sensory nerves often are referred to as **afferent** (L. *ad*, to, plus *ferre*, to carry) nerve fibers, and their cell bodies lie in special ganglia.

3. **Autonomic fibers** are concerned with the involuntary control of glandular activities and smooth muscles, including smooth muscles surrounding arterioles and venules within muscles. Comprehensive explanations of the autonomic nervous system may be found in physiology and neuroscience textbooks.

Classification of Motor and Sensory Nerve Fibers on the Basis of Axonal Diameter

When histologists and anatomists began studying the characteristics of the nervous system, neurons supplying various motor and sensory structures in the body were classified on the basis of the **diameter** of their axons. The **largest** axons were labeled **type A** and the **smallest** fibers were referred to as **type C;** those of **intermediate** diameter thus were referred to as **type B.** A and B fibers are myelinated, whereas C fibers are unmyelinated. Subdivision of the type A category is convenient and also is based on fiber diameter. Type A subdivisions include **type A alpha (α), type A beta (β), type A gamma (γ), and type A delta (δ).**

The **speed** at which a nerve impulse travels along the length of an axon is related to the diameter of the axon. **Larger** axons conduct impulses at a **faster velocity.** Adding a myelin sheath causes the axon to conduct an impulse even faster. The largest myelinated axons (type A α with a diameter of 20 μm) conduct an impulse at a maximum velocity of approximately 120 M per second. The longest motor axons are those extending from the lumbar segments of the spinal cord to muscles in the foot—a distance of approximately 1 M in an adult of average height. A minimum of 8 msec (0.008 second), therefore, is needed for a nerve impulse to travel the length of the largest motor axon. The largest sensory axons are also of the A α type. Consequently, a similar amount of time is needed for a sensory impulse to travel from a receptor in the foot to the spinal cord. The **average** conduction velocity of large motor and sensory fibers in a peripheral nerve ranges from 50 to 70 M per second. Thus, at least 28 msec are necessary for a nerve impulse to travel the 2-M reflex arc from a sensory receptor in the foot to a motor cell in the spinal cord and back to a muscle in the foot. To this must be added:

- The time needed to generate the action potential in the sensory receptor (1 to 5 msec)
- The time required to transmit the signal across the synapse between the sensory ending and the motor cell (0.5 msec)
- The amount of time to transmit the signal throughout the sarcotubular system of the muscle (1 to 5 msec)
- The time to activate the contractile apparatus (1 to 2 msec)
- The amount of time required to produce shortening of the muscle (10 to 300 msec)

The smallest nerve fibers, type C (0.5 μm in diameter), convey nerve impulses from sensory endings in the skin that appear to produce sensations of pain when stimulated. Pain impulses are conducted at a velocity of approximately 0.5 M per second.

Classification of Sensory Fibers on the Basis of Fiber Origin

Sensory nerve fibers are classified into four groups based on the type of sensory receptor from which impulses are conducted. The first group (**group I**) is subdivided into subgroups **Ia and Ib.** Group Ia fibers carry impulses from a particular type of sensory receptor, referred to as the **muscle spindle primary receptor**, located in muscles. **Group Ib** fibers carry impulses from sensory receptors located in tendons (the attachment of a muscle to bone) and are referred to as **Golgi tendon organs (GTO).** Diameters of group Ia and Ib fibers are approximately 12 to 20 μm and are considered to be type A α, as classified by axonal diameter. **Group II** fibers are equivalent to type A β in diameter size (4 to 12 μm) and carry impulses from the **secondary receptors** in the muscle spindle (Adal and Barker, 1962). The structure and function of muscle spindles and GTO are described in the section on receptors.

Central Neurons

Nerve fibers are present not only in the peripheral system but also in the CNS, that is, the spinal cord and brain (see Fig. 3–4A). Neurons that carry motor impulses from the brain to motor neurons in the spinal cord are referred to as **upper motor neurons. Lower motor neurons**, in contrast, conduct motor impulses from the spinal cord to activate muscle fibers. Some neurons, termed **interneurons**, reside entirely within the spinal cord and transmit impulses from one neuron to the dendrites or cell body of another neuron nearby. Other neurons extend from a sensory receptor in skin, muscles, tendons, or joints to the spinal cord. After entering the spinal cord, the sensory axon may give off a branch that synapses with interneurons in the spinal cord, but the main fiber usually ascends through the spinal cord to synapse on other neurons in the CNS. A neuron with an uninterrupted axon like this is referred to as a **first-order neuron.** Sensory neurons that receive synaptic input from a peripheral sensory neuron (from a first-order neuron) and conduct action potentials from the spinal cord or brainstem to sensory centers in the CNS may be referred to as **second-order neurons.** Many second-order neurons then transmit the impulse to third-order neurons located in higher centers of the CNS.

Neural Modification of Excitability

Most neurons discharge nerve impulses intermittently; that is, the neurons exhibit a level of firing even while at "rest." The frequency of discharge is modified by the influence of other neurons. Both facilitatory and inhibitory stimuli are constantly being transmitted from motor centers in the brain to interneurons throughout the spinal cord. Similarly, motor neurons receive synaptic connections from thousands of other neurons. Whether a given motor neuron becomes more active or less active depends on the **net effect** of all the facilitatory and inhibitory stimuli that arrive at the motor neuron at any given instant. An inactive motor neuron can be stimulated to discharge nerve impulses by:

- **Increasing** the **facilitatory** stimuli, while the inhibitory stimuli remain constant
- **Decreasing** the **inhibitory** stimuli, while the facilitatory stimuli remain constant
- A **combination** of increasing the facilitatory and decreasing the inhibitory stimuli

The last mechanism is thought to be the most common and reflects the important balance between facilitatory and inhibitory stimuli for effective motor function.

JOINT, TENDON, AND MUSCLE RECEPTORS

Specialized **receptors** are present in joint structures, tendons, and skeletal muscles. The receptors detect **changes** in **tension** and **position** of the structures in which the receptors are situated, and a pattern of nerve impulses is generated in the receptor to convey the information to other parts of the nervous system. As a result, moment-to-moment changes in **joint angle** (position of the joint), **speed** of joint motion, amount of **joint compression** or **distraction**, as well as changes in muscle **length** and **force** of muscle contraction are relayed to centers in the spinal cord and brain. In the CNS, this information is integrated with that coming in from other sensory organs, such as the retina of the eye (vision) and the vestibular apparatus of the inner ear (dealing with balance and position sense). Integrated sensory signals then are used by motor control centers in the brain to automatically adjust the location, type, number, and frequency of motor unit activation so that appropriate muscle tension is developed to perform desired movements.

Joint Receptors

Several different types of sensory receptors are found in joint capsules and ligaments of the joints. The major anatomic features of various sensory receptors are illustrated in Figure 3–9. Most of the receptors emit several action potentials per second as a "resting" output. The receptor is stimulated by being deformed. Depending on the **location** and **magnitude** of deforming forces acting on the joint and the **location** of the receptor, certain receptors are stimulated and discharge a high-frequency burst of nerve impulses when the joint is moved. Receptors typically adapt (frequency of impulses decreases) slightly after movement ceases and then transmit a steady train of nerve impulses thereafter. Further movement of the joint may cause one set of receptors to stop discharging impulses and another set to become active (Fig. 3–10). Thus, information from joint receptors continually provides **feedback** information to the nervous system to apprise the nervous system of momentary **angulation** of joints and of the **rate of movement** of joints.

Golgi Tendon Organs

Golgi tendon organs (GTOs) lie within muscle tendons near the point of attachment of the muscle fiber to the tendon (Fig. 3–11). An average of 10 to 15 muscle fibers is usually connected in direct line (series) with each GTO. The GTO is stimulated by tension produced by the small bundle of muscle fibers. Nerve impulses

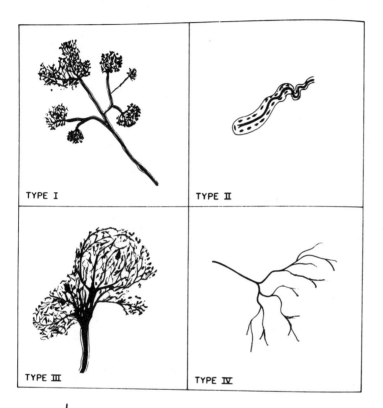

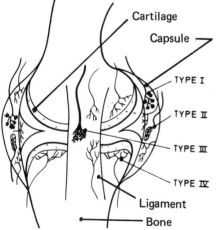

Figure 3–9 *(Top)* Schematic illustration of four receptors that are usually distinguished in joints. *(Bottom)* A diagram of the knee joint, showing the distribution of various receptor types in the capsule and ligaments of the joint. The menisci are free from nerve fibers except at their attachment to the fibrous capsule. (From Brodal, A: *Neurological Anatomy,* ed 3. Oxford University Press, New York, 1981, p 56, with permission.)

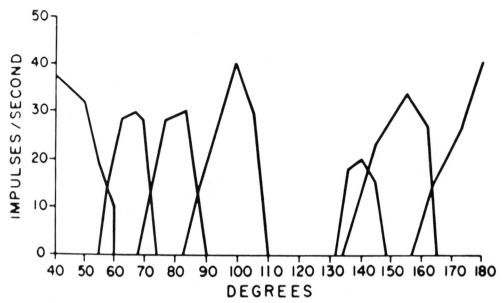

Figure 3–10   Discharge frequency of joint receptors during movement of the joint. Graphs illustrate impulse frequencies for 8 single nerve fibers innervating slowly adapting receptors in the capsule of the knee joint of a cat. The adapted impulse frequency is plotted against the position of the joint in degrees. The figure is not representative for the distribution of endings that are successively activated during full movement, because, in general, activation of endings more often occurs immediately before or at the extremes of joint movement rather than in the intermediate positions of the joint. Joint receptors are sensitive over ranges of 15 to 30 degrees. Ranges are representative of the behavior of most endings. (From Skoglund, S: Anatomical and physiological studies of knee joint innervation in the cat. *Acta Physiol Scand* 36 [Suppl 124]:1, 1956, with permission.)

discharged by the tendon organ are transmitted over large, rapidly conducting afferent axons (**group Ib** fibers) to the spinal cord and cerebellum. Arrival of GTO nerve impulses at the spinal cord excites **inhibitory** interneurons which, in turn, inhibit the neurons (A, α, neurons) of the contracting muscle, thus **limiting** the force developed to that which can be tolerated by the tissues being stressed. Slips of tendon, however, can be torn free from natural points of attachment by the abrupt application of a forceful contraction or by abrupt passive stretch of the tissues. Therefore, to avoid injury, a muscle should be activated or stretched to a moderate degree at first, and then a gradual increase in the force exerted on the points of attachment may occur.

Muscle Spindles

Skeletal muscles are composed of **extrafusal** (L. *extra,* outside of or in addition, plus *fusus,* spindle; in this case, referring to "regular" muscle fibers) **fibers.** Also within muscles lie **muscle spindles,** small but complex organs with multiple functions. A muscle spindle is composed of sets of 3 to 10 small muscle fibers, termed **intrafusal** (L. *intra,* within, plus *fusus,* spindle) **fibers** (Fig. 3–12). Numerous studies have been conducted to gain a better understanding of the structure and functions of the muscle spindle (Taylor and Prochazka, 1981). Although a great deal is known, many questions about muscle spindle functions remain unanswered. The description presented in this chapter is a simplified version that does not consider

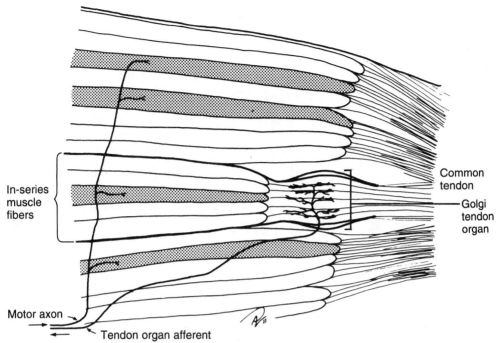

In-series muscle fibers

Common tendon

Golgi tendon organ

Motor axon

Tendon organ afferent

Figure 3–11 A schema to illustrate the anatomic relations among extrafusal muscle fibers, a motor unit (stippled), and a Golgi tendon organ (bracketed area) with the attached afferent projection. The force or tension produced by either contracting or stretching the extrafusal muscle fibers causes the structural fiber network (collagen and elastin) to collapse around the tendon organ. The Golgi tendon organ responds through a force-related neural discharge. Physiologic data indicate that a tendon organ is selectively sensitive to the forces produced by the in-series muscle fibers. A motor unit that activates a given tendon organ typically contributes only one fiber in series with the receptor. (From Houk, JC, Crago, PE, and Rymer, WZ: Functional properties of the Golgi tendon organs. In Desmedt, JE [ed]: *Progress in Clinical Neurophysiology,* Vol 8. Karger, Basel, 1980, p 35, with permission.)

some of the finer distinctions reported regarding structure and functions of muscle spindles (Matthews, 1981).

The lengths of human muscle spindles vary from 0.5 to 13 mm, but the usual length is 2 to 4 mm. Muscle spindles are fusiform in shape (widest in the center and tapering toward each end). Spindles are present in almost all muscles but are most numerous in the muscles of the arms and legs (see Table 3–3). Muscle spindles are especially abundant in the small muscles of the hand and foot. In general, muscle spindles have both afferent and efferent innervation. Muscle spindles function as a **stretch receptor,** sending sensory impulses over afferent axons that "inform" other neurons in the spinal cord and brain of the **length** of the muscle spindle and of the **rate** at which muscle stretch is occurring. Muscle spindles also contain **contractile** fibers that are controlled by nerve impulses reaching them via small-diameter motor axons (**efferent, type A γ motor neurons**) from the spinal cord. **The degree of shortening of the contractile portions of the muscle spindle regulates the sensitivity of the stretch receptor portion of the muscle spindle.** This characteristic is a highly important physiologic property of muscle spindles. In essence, as **α motor neurons** stimulate the contraction of **extrafusal fibers,** γ **motor neuron** discharge causes contraction of the **intrafusal fibers.** The contraction of the intrafusal fibers provides for an adjustable sensitivity range for changing lengths of the muscle.

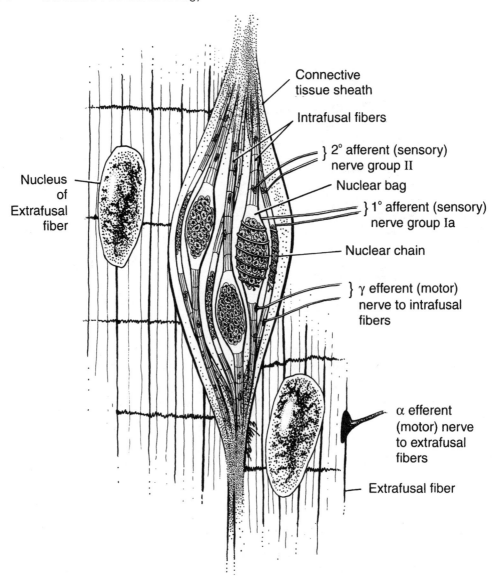

Figure 3–12 The muscle spindle. This diagram shows the anatomic relationships among the major components of a muscle spindle. Although most muscle spindles contain 3 to 10 intrafusal fibers, for simplicity, only 3 are shown. Nuclear bag fibers and nuclear chain fibers also are pictured, as well as the afferent and efferent nerve supplies. Extrafusal muscle fibers alongside the muscle spindle and an α motor neuron to the extrafusal fiber also are shown. **Note:** Fiber diameters are drawn approximately to scale. However, for the lengths of an average muscle spindle and muscle fiber to be illustrated at the magnification pictured here, the figure would extend 8 and 30 pages, respectively. 1^0=primary; 2^0= secondary.

The intrafusal fibers of the muscle spindle are encapsulated within a connective tissue sheath (see Fig. 3–12). The morphologic arrangement of the intrafusal fiber nuclei, along with previously described physiologic properties, distinguishes primary (Ia) from secondary (II) afferent fibers. In general, the primary afferent fibers have nuclei contained in a centralized "bag" region. In contrast, the secondary afferent fibers have nuclei located along the length of the intrafusal fiber in a "chain-like" fashion. The encapsulated systems are attached at their polar ends to the connective tissues of the extrafusal fiber bundles.

As stated previously, intrafusal muscle fibers are controlled by small-diameter motor nerve fibers from the spinal cord, the γ **motor neurons** (termed γ because of the size of their axons). Gamma (γ) motor neurons also are referred to as **fusimotor** neurons because the neurons supply motor impulses to the intrafusal muscle spindle fibers. Thus, the middle, noncontractile part of the muscle spindle can be stretched by two different types of mechanisms. First, when the entire skeletal muscle is stretched, the spindle also is stretched. Second, when the contractile portions at each end of the muscle spindle are activated by impulses arriving over γ motor nerves, the contractile portions shorten, thereby stretching the central "bag" portion of the spindle. In either case, stretch of the nuclear bag portion of the muscle spindle activates one or both of two types of sensory receptors residing there, that is, the primary (Ia) and secondary (II) stretch receptors (see Fig. 3–12).

Activation of the sensory receptors increases the frequency of nerve impulses emitted from the receptors. Afferent nerves (**group Ia**) from the **primary receptor** make synaptic connections with higher **brain centers** and with the **motor neurons** (A, α motor neurons) that control extrafusal muscle fibers in the same muscle. Abrupt stretch of a muscle, therefore, initiates a burst of impulses from the primary stretch receptor in the muscle fiber, which travels to the spinal cord and excites activity in motor units of the same muscle. Shortening of the muscle as a whole relieves stretch on the muscle spindles contained in the muscle, thereby temporarily removing the stimulus from the stretch receptors. Gamma-efferent activity, therefore, adjusts for the new muscle length.

The neural and muscular structures that participate in the stretch reflex are illustrated in Figure 3–13. An abrupt stretch is applied by tapping the patellar tendon with a reflex hammer (a tool specifically designed to test reflex responses). The presence of a reflex contraction in the stretched muscle 100 to 200 msec after tapping the tendon reveals that the circuit is intact. In addition, the briskness and relative amplitude of the reflex contraction reflect the general level of excitability of α motor neurons innervating the stretched muscle.

The stretch reflex circuit is believed to operate in the automatic (reflex) regulation of muscle length when the desired length has been established by voluntary contraction of the muscle. A highly schematic representation of the initial condition is illustrated in Figure 3–14A. Additional sensory impulses are generated when the joint is extended and the muscle spindle is stretched momentarily by an increased load (see Fig. 3–14B). The body part is returned reflexively to the original joint position by the development of increased tension in the extrafusal muscle fibers (see Fig. 3–14C). Clinically speaking, an understanding of the functions of muscle spindles is important when applying stretch to a muscle or group of muscles.

Primary Sensory Endings

The primary sensory endings of muscle spindles detect **velocity** of the stretch as well as the relative **amount** of stretch. As previously described, arrival of impulses from the primary receptor **excites** α motor neurons in the spinal cord, innervating **muscle fibers** in the stretched muscle. In addition, the impulses excite interneurons which, in turn, **inhibit** α motor neurons supplying muscles that perform an

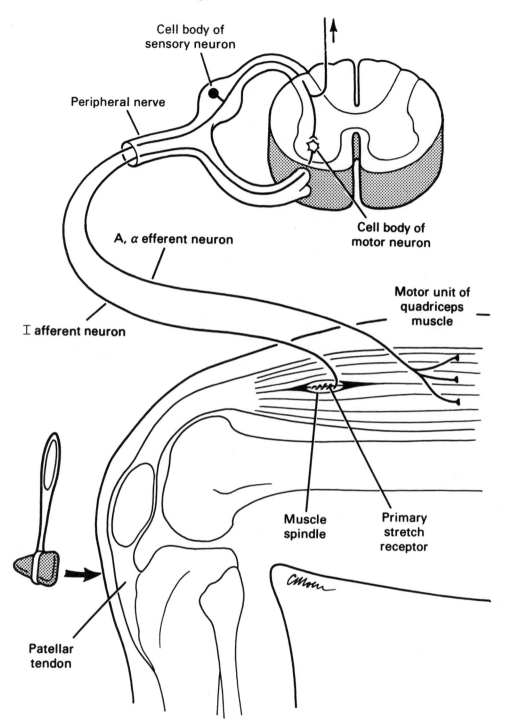

Figure 3–13 The stretch reflex. Four fundamental parts of the simple stretch reflex arc are: (1) A receptor in the muscle generates nerve impulses in proportion to the degree of deformation. (2) An afferent neuron conducts the burst of sensory impulses from the receptor to the spinal cord. (3) An efferent neuron conducts motor impulses from the spinal cord to extrafusal muscle fibers. (4) An effector, the muscle, responds to the motor impulses. Note that the same sensory signals are transmitted to other parts of the central nervous system as well.

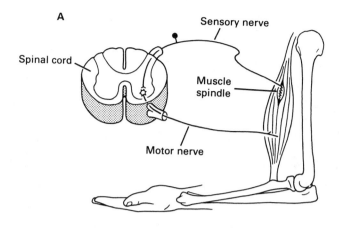

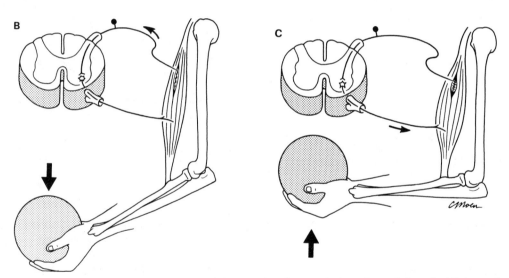

Figure 3–14   Schematic representation of the stretch reflex regulation of muscle length. *(A)* A muscle is under the influence of the stretch reflex when the muscle is engaged in a steady contraction of a voluntary nature, as when a person's elbow is flexed steadily. *(B)* A sudden unexpected increase in the load stretches the muscle, causing the sensory ending on the muscle spindle to send nerve impulses *(small arrow)* to the spinal cord, where the impulses contact a motor nerve cell at the synapse and excite it. *(C)* As a result, motor impulses *(small arrow)* are sent back to the muscle, where the impulses cause the muscle to contract. More complicated nerve pathways than the one shown may also be involved in the stretch reflex. Any actual muscle is, of course, supplied with many motor nerve fibers and spindles. In addition, the synaptic connections to even a single motor neuron are multiple. (Adapted from Merton, PA: How we control the contraction of our muscles. *Sci Am* 228:30, 1972.)

action **opposite** to the action that the stretched muscle performs when it contracts (Fig. 3–15). Such inhibition promotes relaxation of the opposing muscle so that it can be elongated easily while the contracting muscle shortens. As illustrated in Figure 3–15, stretching the elbow toward extension places a stretch on the elbow flexors (ie, the biceps). Impulses from the stretched biceps muscle cause

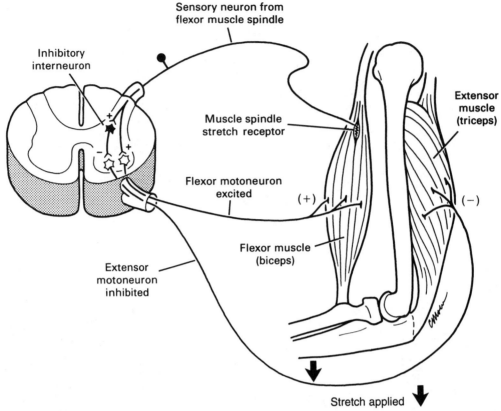

Figure 3–15 Schematic representation of the reciprocal inhibition of motor neurons to the opposing muscle. Impulses from a stretched muscle excite motor units in the same muscle (facilitatory synaptic influence is designated with a plus [+] sign) and inhibit, through an interneuron, motor units in the opposing muscle (inhibitory synaptic influence is designated with a minus [−] sign).

an excitation of motor units in the biceps and an inhibition, through an interneuron, of motor units in the elbow extensor muscle (the triceps muscle) that performs the motion that is the opposite of flexion. Afferent fibers from muscles also send their transduced information of muscle movement to higher centers in the CNS for proprioceptive integration.

Secondary Sensory Endings

Secondary sensory endings appear to detect **amount** of **stretch.** Signals from secondary receptors are transmitted over smaller-diameter afferent neurons (group II fibers), which synapse principally with interneurons and elicit more delayed and more variable patterns of muscle reflexes than the reflex obtained from the output of primary receptors. Signals from secondary sensory endings also are relayed to higher regions of the CNS.

Summary of Muscle Spindle Functions

In essence, muscle spindles function as "comparators," comparing the **length** of the **spindle** with the **length** of **skeletal muscle fibers** that surround the spindle (see Fig. 3–14). If the length of the surrounding extrafusal muscle fibers is **less** than that of the spindle, the **frequency** of nerve impulses discharged from the receptors is **reduced**. When the central portion of the spindle is stretched because of γ-efferent activity, its sensory receptors discharge **more** nerve impulses, which reflexly **excite** α motor neurons to activate the extrafusal muscle fibers. The mechanism is particularly important in the regulation of postural muscle tone.

Patterns of sensory receptor discharge recorded from nerves supplying the primary (Ia) and secondary (II) stretch receptors of the muscle spindle and the GTO (Ib) under various conditions are summarized in Figure 3–16. The major distinctions are that:

- The **primary stretch receptor** signals both the **velocity of stretch** and the **length** of the muscle spindle.
- The **secondary stretch receptor** signals the **length** of the muscle spindle.
- The **GTO** detects the amount of **tension** being exerted by the muscle fibers.

In these roles, the primary stretch receptor exhibits qualities of both phasic (Gr. *phasis,* an appearance, a distinct stage) and tonic (Gr. *tonikos,* continuous tension) activity, while the secondary receptor and tendon organ display tonic activity. A **phasic receptor** signals the **rate of change** of an event, while a **tonic receptor** signals the final **result** of the change. For example, the pattern of discharge from a purely phasic receptor during graded amounts of stretch is shown in Figure 3–17B, and that from a purely tonic receptor is illustrated in Figure 3–17C.

Discharge properties during electrical stimulation of their receptive fields are different for GTOs and muscle spindles. The area of localized sensitivity is approximately 5 mm. A characteristic pause in afferent discharge after electrical stimulation is a positive indicator for muscle spindles. Conversely, an increase in afferent discharge is indicative of GTOs. The properties of the GTO are due to the anatomic arrangement of both receptor types. **Tendon organs,** which exist "in series" with muscular attachments, increase spike activity with linear muscle force. **Muscle spindles** exist in **parallel** with the much larger surrounding skeletal muscle fibers. The contraction of the larger fibers momentarily (35 to 45 msec) unloads the spindle receptor, resulting in a pause in spike discharge. Further testing to distinguish primary from secondary muscle spindles include conduction velocity (primary spindles range from 70 to 100 M per second; secondary spindles range from 40 to 80 M per second in conduction velocity) (Jansen and Rudjord, 1964). Primary and secondary muscle spindles also are distinguished from each other by their discharge characteristics during controlled muscular stretch (primary spindles are more sensitive to the active phase of stretch than are secondary spindles) (Scott, 1990). Other distinguishing discharge properties are found in physiology and neuroscience texts.

SEGMENTAL AND SUPRASEGMENTAL COMPONENTS OF MOTOR CONTROL

Previous portions of the present chapter describe the basic physiologic mechanisms responsible for the development of graded amounts of tension in motor units contained within a **single muscle.** However, to perform skilled motor activities, a highly integrated set of motor commands is required to **activate (or inhibit) appropriate muscles in the proper sequence.** In this text, the term seg-

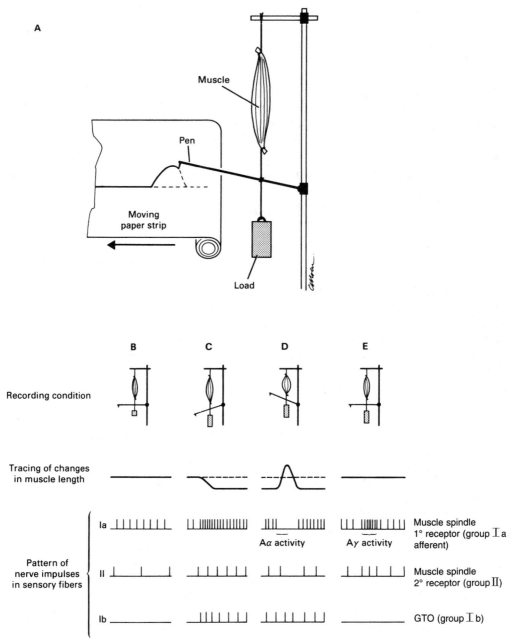

Figure 3–16 Discharge patterns of a muscle spindle's primary receptor (in group Ia sensory nerve fiber), secondary receptor (in group II fiber), and Golgi tendon organ (in group Ib fiber) under various conditions. (*B*) At rest. (*C*) During stretch. (*D*) During transient contraction of the extrafusal muscle fibers produced by activation via alpha motor fibers. (*E*) During contraction of the intrafusal fibers produced by activation via the gamma motor fibers.

mental refers to the neural activity in circuits residing in particular neural segments of the **spinal cord.** The term **suprasegmental** refers to the influence of impulses from the **brain** and **brainstem** on the excitability of neurons within the spinal cord. Further discussion regarding motor control requires that certain ter-

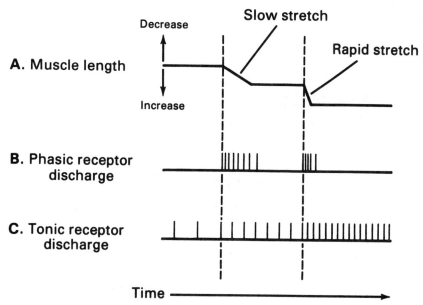

Figure 3–17 Discharge patterns of purely phasic and tonic receptors. The phasic receptor responds to the change in a condition, with the frequency of discharge proportional to the rate of change. The tonic receptor signals the existing status of the condition, such as muscle length.

minology be explained. **Motor control** refers to the regulation of posture and movement. As described previously, the term "tract" is used to describe a bundle of nerve fibers (axons) that connects different regions of the CNS. Because many nerve fibers are covered with a myelin sheath, tracts appear white in unstained histologic sections; hence the term **white matter** is used to describe areas in the CNS that contain predominantly fiber tracts. Within various regions of the CNS, aggregations of anatomically and functionally related neurons (cell bodies) are distinguished from one another, and these aggregations are referred to as **nuclei** or **ganglia.** Regions of the CNS in which nerve cell bodies are concentrated appear gray in color (and are not covered with myelin) and, hence, are referred to as **gray matter.** In the spinal cord, the central region contains nerve cell bodies (gray matter) surrounded by tracts of myelinated axons (white matter) (see Fig. 3–4B). Some of the tracts carry ascending (sensory) impulses, whereas others conduct descending (motor) impulses. In the cerebrum, the situation is reversed, in that the cortex appears gray (because cell bodies of cortical neurons lie in the superficial surface layers). Tissue beneath the gray matter is white (because of the presence of myelinated axons that connect cortical neurons with other regions of the CNS).

The brainstem, located between the cerebrum and the spinal cord, consists of the midbrain, pons, and medulla oblongata (Fig. 3–18). The brainstem contains numerous ascending and descending tracts as well as nuclei and functions as a prespinal integrating system of great complexity. Within the brain, the basal ganglia are comprised of several nuclei, including the caudate, putamen, globus pallidus, and amygdala. Other functionally related areas are included in the basal ganglia complex by some authors (Kandel et al, 1991; Burt, 1993). The following is an overview of several major mechanisms by which the excitability of motor neurons can be altered.

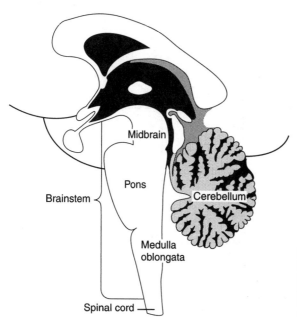

Midbrain

Pons

Brainstem

Cerebellum

Medulla
oblongata

Spinal cord

Figure 3–18 Sagittal view illustrating the positions of the main subdivisions of the brain stem. (From Schmidt, RF [ed]: *Fundamentals of Neurophysiology,* ed 2. Springer-Verlag, New York, 1978, p 187, with permission.)

Motor Centers

Movement cannot be performed effectively unless a **posture** appropriate to the action is assumed by suitable arrangement of the limbs and body as a whole. Thus, the control of posture is an important function of the CNS. Movement is the end product of a number of control systems that interact together extensively. The structures chiefly responsible for the control of posture and movement are the motor centers, which are located in several different parts of the brain. When considering the motor functions of the nervous system, keep in mind that the motor centers can function appropriately only if an uninterrupted stream of afferent (sensory) information about the status of the environment is received from all parts of the body. To emphasize the role of the sense organs in the control of posture and movement, the term **sensorimotor system** is used to denote the combined afferent and efferent processes required to produce coordinated movement. The question of how voluntary movements are initiated is still unanswered, but neuroscientists have established theories regarding the structure and operation of major circuits that execute the "orders" to perform functional activities.

Nerve fibers that descend from the motor cortex collectively form the corticospinal tract (see Figs. 3–4 and 3–19). As the name implies, most of the axons arise from cell bodies in the motor area of the cerebral cortex to the spinal cord, where synaptic contact is made with motor neurons in the gray matter in the anterior horn of the spinal cord. The corticospinal tract also is referred to as the **pyramidal tract** because many of the cell bodies located in the motor cortex are triangular in shape and have the appearance of small pyramids when a section of cortex is stained and viewed under a light microscope. Most of the corticospinal axons cross to the opposite side in the brainstem and descend in the lateral corticospinal tract of the spinal cord (see Figs. 3–4 and 3–19). The crossing fibers from the right and left motor cortex also form a pyramid in the brainstem (the diagrammatic nature of Fig. 3–19 does not depict the pyramid). At the spinal segmental

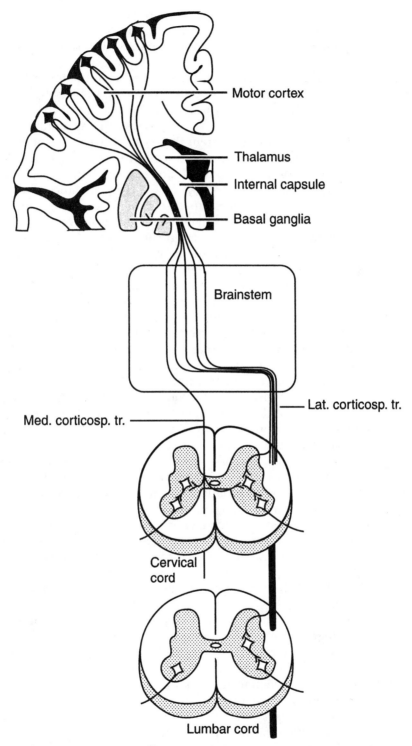

Figure 3–19 Schematic diagram of the course of the lateral and medial corticospinal tracts from the motor cortex to the spinal cord. For simplicity, collaterals to the basal ganglia, the cerebellum, and the motor centers of the brain stem have been omitted. Note that the structures and tracts exist on both the left and right sides; however, only one side is illustrated. For further description, see text. Lat. = lateral; Med. = medial; corticosp. = corticospinal; tr. = tract. (From Schmidt, RF [ed]: *Fundamentals of Neurophysiology,* ed 2. Springer-Verlag. New York, 1978, p 179, with permission.)

level, axons of the corticospinal tract terminate predominantly on interneurons, which in turn, terminate on α motor neurons. The organization of the corticospinal tract suggests that it is designed for precise control of individual muscle groups.

Other cortical neurons originating in the same areas of the motor cortex have shorter axons that synapse with second-order motor neurons lying in the basal ganglia or brainstem, for example, in the reticular formation or in vestibular nuclei. Axons from the second-order neurons do not enter the pyramids. For this reason, axons that descend into the brainstem that synapse there and then continue into the spinal cord frequently are referred to collectively as the **extrapyramidal system.** The distinction of the pyramidal and extrapyramidal systems is an anatomic one, and the descriptions are not totally accurate since the pyramidal and extrapyramidal systems are interconnected (not separate systems). In addition, other areas of the CNS outside the pyramidal and extrapyramidal systems are involved in movement. Furthermore, nuclei in the extrapyramidal system are involved in other functions besides movement (Burt, 1993). For convenience, the term "extrapyramidal" frequently is used (Fig. 3–20).

Bundles of axons that originate from neurons within the reticular formation in the brainstem and terminate within the spinal cord form the reticulospinal tract. Likewise, bundles of axons originating within the vestibular nuclei and terminating within the spinal cord comprise the vestibulospinal tract. The reticulospinal tract and the vestibulospinal tract are examples of two descending tracts that are considered part of the extrapyramidal tract. In general, the reticulospinal tract provides excitatory input to extensor muscles of the arms and flexor muscles of the legs and trunk. In contrast, the vestibulospinal tract carries excitatory input destined for flexor muscles of the arms and extensor muscles of the legs and trunk (Burt, 1993). Clinically, disruptions of the corticospinal tract, the reticulospinal tract, or the vestibulospinal tract result in different clinical symptoms.

A schematic diagram of the spinal and supraspinal motor centers and some of their connections appears in Figure 3–21. Arrows connecting the various centers indicate the **main** direction of information flow underlying muscular activity. On the right in the illustration, a summary indicative of the role each center plays in producing movement is presented. Each center is a site of processing and redirects incoming signals. A conspicuous aspect of the diagram is the key position of the motor cortex. The motor cortex is connected to the spinal cord both directly (by way of the corticospinal tract) and indirectly (by way of the brainstem). In addition, some collateral branches exit the corticospinal tract and pass to the brainstem. Other collateral branches terminate within other high-level motor centers (eg, the cerebellum and the basal ganglia). Centers in the brainstem also are responsible for the integration of incoming sensory information from specific populations of peripheral receptors and, consequently, are responsible for the automatic (reflexive) control of posture and spatial orientation of the body. To accomplish this, centers in the brainstem monitor and evaluate afferent signals of many receptors throughout the body.

The most important sensory receptors for monitoring orientation of the head with respect to the gravitational field are the receptor organs of equilibrium (located within the labyrinth of each inner ear) and the stretch and joint receptors of the neck that monitor the orientation of the head with respect to the trunk. Information in the form of patterns of nerve impulses from these sources enables the brainstem motor centers to provide a continuous regulatory output, so that an upright body posture is adopted and maintained without the need for voluntary con-

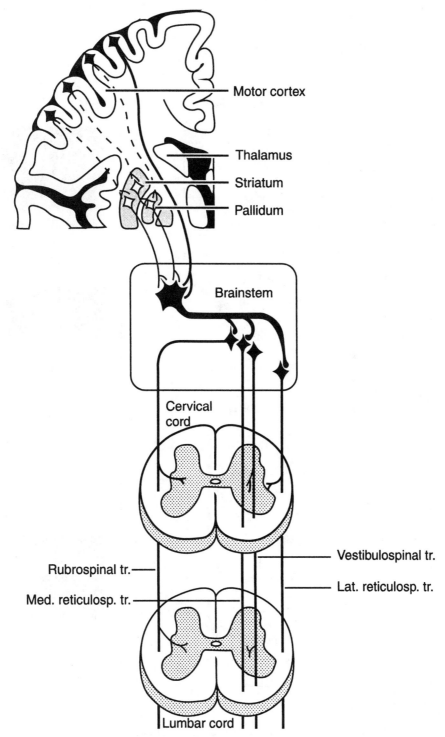

Figure 3–20 Schematic diagram of courses of important extrapyramidal tracts from the supraspinal motor centers to the spinal cord. The neuron with a thick axon in the brainstem symbolizes the crossing of most of the extrapyramidal motor fibers to the opposite side at that level and does not imply convergence. Pathways from the motor cortex to the nuclei in the brainstem are partly collaterals of the corticospinal tract and partly separate efferents. Details of connectivity among the brainstem structures involved in motor activity are extremely complicated; this representation is greatly simplified. Note that the structures and tracts exist on both the left and right sides; however, for simplicity, only one side is illustrated. Lat. = lateral; Med. = medial; reticulosp. = reticulospinal; tr. = tract. (From Schmidt, RF [ed]: *Fundamentals of Neurophysiology*, ed 2. Springer-Verlag, New York, 1978, p 181, with permission.)

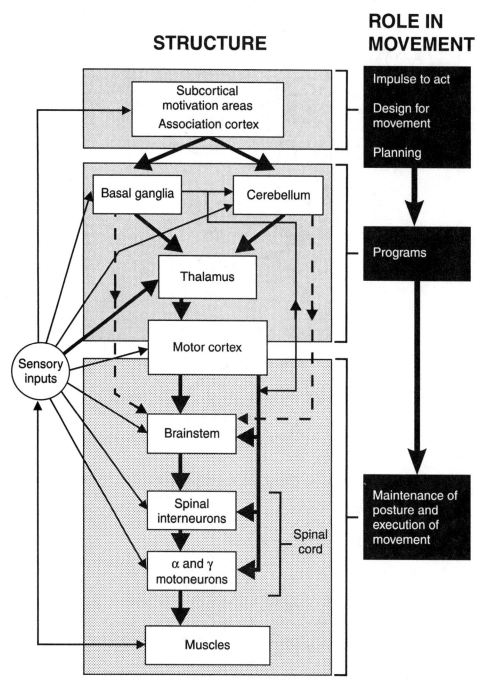

STRUCTURE

ROLE IN MOVEMENT

Subcortical motivation areas
Association cortex

Impulse to act

Design for movement

Planning

Basal ganglia

Cerebellum

Thalamus

Programs

Motor cortex

Sensory inputs

Brainstem

Spinal interneurons

Spinal cord

α and γ motoneurons

Maintenance of posture and execution of movement

Muscles

Figure 3–21 Block diagram of the spinal and supraspinal motor centers and their important connections. Sensory inputs are summarized on the *left,* while the *right column* indicates the chief role played by structures in the middle of the diagram during the performance of movements. Note that motor cortex is assigned to the transition between programs and execution of movement. (From Schmidt, RF [ed]: *Fundamentals of Neurophysiology,* ed 2. Springer-Verlag, New York, 1978, p 176, with permission.)

trol. Note, however, that voluntary motor commands may be superimposed upon the involuntary motor commands to achieve a particular posture or movement.

The **basal ganglia** participate in the conversion of **plans** for movement (which arise in the supplementary motor cortex) into **programs** for movement. Nuclei of the basal ganglia are particularly significant with respect to the **initiation** and **execution** of **slow** movements. The basal ganglia are adjacent to the thalamus, an important sensory relay center in the brain (see Fig. 3–19).

The **cerebellum** is interconnected with all levels of the CNS and functions as an overall "coordinator" of motor activities. The cerebellum is responsible primarily for **programming rapid movements,** correcting the **course** of rapid movements, and **correlating posture and movement** (see Fig. 3–18). Thus, the cerebellum and the basal ganglia serve different but related functions in programming cortically initiated movement patterns.

Sensorimotor Integration

For immediate responses, various suprasegmental motor pathways ultimately converge on a series of simple circuits that link each muscle with the spinal cord. The basic circuit includes:

- Cell bodies of α motor neurons in the spinal cord
- Efferent axons of α motor neurons that extend into the ventral roots of peripheral nerves
- The neuromuscular junctions
- Muscle fibers innervated by the axons
- Sensory receptors
- Afferent axons of sensory receptors that enter the spinal cord (through the dorsal roots)
- Synaptic terminations of the sensory neurons in the spinal cord. (**Note:** The circuit described is the circuit for immediate responses. Sensory input **also** is relayed to **higher centers,** which are not described.)

Sensory neurons that carry impulses from a given muscle are connected with motor neurons that transmit impulses back to that muscle; thus, a loop is formed that regulates the activity of each motor unit in the muscle (Fig. 3–22). The circuit is the basic **segmental** component for control of the motor system.

No movement (reflex or voluntary) can occur except through the operation of the circuit. Some sensory fibers from the muscle establish a direct connection with the motor neurons, whereas other sensory axons connect to the motor neuron indirectly through interneurons. The segmental circuits automatically regulate the length and tension of muscles in accordance with various requirements. The circuits are responsive centrally to neural input from various motor centers and peripherally to mechanical input (such as stretching of the muscle). For example, mechanical deformation of the muscle spindle stimulates the stretch receptors, provoking action potentials that travel to the spinal cord and elicit a reflex response of the muscle (see Figs. 3–13 and 3–14).

Sensory impulses from muscles are not restricted to influencing only their own motor neurons. Afferent input also spreads through collateral branches of primary sensory neurons and through interneuron circuits to reach the motor neurons of closely related muscles and, to some extent, those of more "distant" muscles. Therefore, stretch or contraction of one muscle affects its own motor

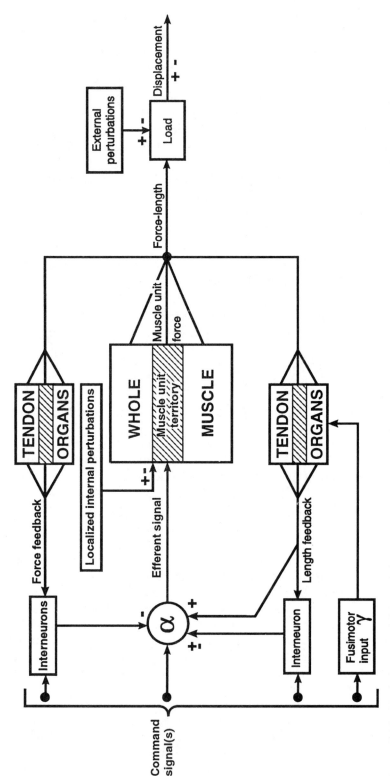

Figure 3–22 Block diagram of the control system that regulates the length of a particular muscle and the force of contraction while performing a motor act. According to the model, the relative amount and strength of muscle contraction are regulated by two feedback pathways, one from the muscle spindle stretch receptors signaling muscle length and velocity of motion, and the other from the Golgi tendon receptors signaling muscle force. The suprasegmental motor centers supply command signals that activate both alpha (α) and gamma (fusimotor) motor neurons as well as interneurons. The degree of further activation is dependent upon the amount the muscle actually shortens in relation to the amount of shortening intended. The influence of any additional forces acting internally or externally that may perturb (disturb) the intended motion is sensed, and corrective motor signals are generated. (From Binder, MD, and Stuart, DC: Motor unit-muscle receptors interactions: Design features of the neuromuscular control system. In Desmedt, JE [ed]: *Progress in Clinical Neurophysiology*, Vol 8. Karger, Basel, 1980, p 74, with permission.)

neurons most strongly and also (to a lesser extent) affects motor neurons of muscles performing an **opposite** action. The effect on the muscles that perform the opposite action is to **inhibit activity** of those muscles (see Fig. 3–15). Motor neurons of other muscles that **assist** in the motion are affected also (but to an even lesser extent). The effect on muscles that assist in the movement is to **facilitate action.** Thus, every primary loop is part of a larger feedback network serving a group of muscles. Transmission in local segmental circuits ("short loop") involves very little delay and ensures rapid responses.

While an immediate response is occurring, the same sensory signals are being transmitted to **higher centers** by way of collaterals, projection tracts, and secondary relays to widely separated parts of the nervous system for more elaborate **analyses** of the information content. The ascending projections permit **integration** of information about the status of the **body** and about the status of the **environment.** Many types of receptors in tendons, joints, and skin, as well as from visual, auditory, and vestibular receptors, provide sensory information regarding the body and the environment. After variable delays, suprasegmental motor signals are relayed back to numerous segmental levels to adjust posture and to perform other motor activities. Thus "long loops," involving higher centers, help regulate the activity of the spinal circuits and of motor units that produce movement.

Kinesthesia and Proprioception

Under most conditions, a person can be consciously aware of the position of the various parts of his or her body relative to all other parts and whether a particular part is moving or still. The awareness is referred to as kinesthesia (Gr. *kinen,* to move, plus *aisthesis,* perception) and position sense. The two terms are often treated as synonyms and are used frequently to cover all aspects of this awareness, whether static or dynamic. Strictly speaking, however, the term **position sense** refers to the awareness of **static** position and the term **kinesthesia** to awareness of dynamic joint **motion.** Kinesthetic signals are generated in various types of **sensory receptors** residing in **muscles, tendons,** and **joints** in response to body **movements** and to **tension** within **tendons.** The impulses produced are transmitted predominantly over group II afferent fibers to the spinal cord, the cerebellum, and sensory nuclei. Thus, other sensorimotor centers in the CNS are "informed" of the exact locations of different parts of the body at each instant to assist in controlling posture and movement.

Proprioception (L. *proprio,* one's own, plus *ceptive,* to receive) is a more inclusive term than kinesthesia and refers to the use of **sensory input** from receptors in **muscle spindles, tendons,** and **joints** to **discriminate joint position** and **joint movement,** including **direction, amplitude,** and **speed,** as well as relative **tension** within tendons. Some neurophysiologists include **vestibular receptors** in each inner ear as part of the proprioceptive system because the output of the vestibular apparatus provides **conscious awareness** of the **orientation** and **movements** of the head. Proprioceptive impulses are transmitted predominantly over group I afferent fibers and are integrated in various sensorimotor centers to automatically regulate adjustments in the contractions of postural muscles, thereby maintaining postural equilibrium.

Several types of **somatosensory** (Gr. *soma,* body, plus L. *sensorius,* pertaining to sensation) **inputs** also are important for the maintenance of equilibrium. For example, **pressure sensations** from the soles of the feet provide information about the distribution of load between the two feet and whether the weight is more forward or backward on the feet. **Visual images** of the location of the body and body parts with respect to reference points in the immediate environment provide complementary information for the maintenance of equilibrium. In fact, visual input sometimes serves as the primary means of maintaining equilibrium when the proprioception system is impaired. The importance of equilibrium is observed not only during daily activities but also when performing various sports or when assessing impairments of equilibrium and suggesting solutions to balance problems.

Muscle Tone

Muscles of individuals with intact neuromusculoskeletal systems exhibit a firmness to palpation, termed **muscle tone.** The firmness present in muscles is observed at rest, even in muscles of well-relaxed subjects. The firmness, however, is impaired if the motor nerve supplying the muscle is not intact. Relaxed muscles exhibit at least a palpable amount of muscle tone, but investigators have failed to detect any muscle action potentials to account for this tone (Clemmeson, 1951; Basmajian, 1952; Ralston and Libet, 1953). Thus, the tone of relaxed muscles in persons with an intact neuromusculoskeletal system appears to be the result of basic physical properties of muscle, such as elasticity, viscosity, and plasticity.

Postural tone is a term used to describe the development of muscular tension in particular muscles that are actively engaged in holding different parts of the skeleton in proper relationships to maintain particular postures. Postural tone is accompanied by recordable electrical activity from the active motor units. Muscles used most often to maintain the body in an erect position are referred to as **antigravity muscles.** In general, muscles of the trunk, flexor muscles of the upper extremities, and extensor muscles of the lower extremities are considered antigravity muscles.

Motor centers supply nerve impulses that influence the excitability of lower motor neurons in the spinal cord segments that supply antigravity muscles. The motor centers include motor areas in the cerebral cortex, the basal ganglia, facilitatory and inhibitory centers in the midbrain, brainstem reticular formation, and the cerebellum (see Fig. 3–21). Postural tone is a reflexive (involuntary) phenomenon that is influenced by both afferent impulses from sensory receptors and by efferent mechanisms from γ motor neurons.

Clinically speaking, normal postural muscle tone has been described as "high enough to hold the head, body and extremities against gravity yet low enough to allow for movement" (DeMauro, 1994). The appropriate amount of muscle tone ensures that the muscle is ready to resist any change in length, thereby helping to maintain posture. In persons with an intact neuromusculoskeletal system, descending motor tracts from the brainstem (particularly from the reticulospinal and vestibulospinal tracts) deliver low-frequency trains of impulses to spinal motor neurons either directly or indirectly through interneurons (see Fig. 3–20). Thus, at any given instant, many local postsynaptic responses (subthreshold depolarizations) occur at widely scattered sites on dendrites and the cell body of the postsynaptic cell. Although local postsynaptic depolarizations may not be dense enough to provoke complete depolarization and firing of the cell, they serve to maintain the neuron in a slightly oscillating state of high excitability, ready to respond to more concentrated presynaptic input. Muscle tone also ensures that the muscle is ready to contract or relax promptly when appropriate control signals reach the motor neurons to produce coordinated movement. Tone may be influenced by disease or injury at various levels of the nervous system and thereby cause symptoms of insufficient muscle tone (low tone, hypotonia) or excessive muscle tone (high tone, hypertonia).

Endurance and Fatigue

Endurance is the ability to perform the same act repeatedly over a period of time. Loss of endurance may be an early sign of cardiopulmonary or neurologic problems. **Fatigue** is defined as a failure to maintain the required or expected force of muscle contraction. Any one of several physiologic mechanisms may be responsible for a state of neuromuscular fatigue at a particular time (Edwards, 1981). For example, fatigue may be of **peripheral** origin because of impairment of excitation-contraction coupling, failure of generating muscle action potentials, or impaired transmission of nerve impulses across the myoneural junction. Similarly, fatigue may be of **central** origin in which failure of neural drive results in a reduction in the number of functioning motor units or in a decrease in the frequency of activation of each functioning motor unit.

Prolonged muscular activity also may lead to fatigue because of metabolic consequences. Examples of metabolic repercussions of extended activity include depletion of ATP supplies for membrane functions (eg, active transport of ions) and accumulation of the products of biochemical reactions, which results in slowing the rate of subsequent reactions. Fatigue becomes important from a clinical standpoint when one or more groups of muscles become unable to continue a given task the individual wants to perform. Furthermore, when disease or injury causes significant weakness of a muscle, endurance of the muscle may be limited. In general, repeated use of a muscle against moderate resistance improves its endurance, but excessive fatigue of an already weak muscle may damage the muscle and produce further weakness (Bennett and Knowlton, 1958; Hickok, 1961; Johnson and Braddom, 1971).

Endurance and **fatigue** also are important clinical considerations in individuals with respiratory diseases. In these persons, an underlying disease process forces the respiratory musculature to perform an excessive amount of work to meet the ventilatory demand. Intramuscular receptors are believed to sense the excessive work, which is compared to the central efferent output (set by ventilatory demand) (Holt and Kelsen, 1993). When the comparison is recognized as a mismatching of input for a given output, the individual may experience dyspnea (shortness of breath) as the perceptual interpretation. If dyspnea and excessive work continue without relief, fatigue and respiratory failure may be the end result. Thus, clinicians and physical educators need to be aware of the effects of resistance and fatigue.

Motor Control

As stated previously, motor control refers to the regulation of posture and movement. The literature is replete with theoretical models of motor control in which investigators attempt to explain how movement and posture are regulated, influenced, learned, or relearned. Models of motor control vary from simple to complex theoretical views, and a few of the models are discussed. The realization that no one theory is all inclusive or totally comprehensive is important.

The simplest theory of motor control, the **reflexive model** (Sherrington, 1906), proposes that the nervous system is similar to a "black box" with sensory input "controlling" motor output. The reflexive model suggests that motor control is provided by a summation of the reflexes affecting an individual and that motor function is directed by sensory receptors (Horak, 1991). However, the reflexive theory is limited in its scope because the human body is capable of substantially more complex movements. Furthermore, the reflexive theory neither considers the importance of interactions between the various systems involved in regulating posture and movement nor the importance of informational feedforward and feedback systems. Motor control, therefore, is more complicated, intricate, and interesting than a simple "stimulus-response" system.

Another theory, the theory of **hierarchy**, proposes that the nervous system has different **levels** of motor control (Jackson, 1884). The hierarchy refers to **higher centers** in the CNS (ie, the motor cortex) that **plan** motor programs and then **relay** the programs to **lower levels** of the nervous system for **execution** of movement and control of posture. The hierarchical theory of motor control is limited, however, because the model proposes that the flow of information occurs in only one direction; no modification of information takes place, and simple motions (reflexes) are controlled by "lower" levels, whereas "higher" centers in the CNS control more complex movements. Motor control, however, is more complicated than the hierarchical theory.

A third model of motor control, the theory of **heterarchy** recognizes that different levels of motor control exist and that portions of the nervous system interact with each other; that is, higher centers interact not only with each other but also with lower centers of the CNS, with the peripheral nervous system, and with ascending and descending pathways (Davis, 1976; Horak, 1991). In the heterarchy:

- Information regarding the environmental milieu both inside and outside the body is provided to "higher centers" of the CNS, that is, the **cerebral cortex, basal ganglia,** and **cerebellum,** which **plan, initiate, execute, coordinate,** and **regulate movement** and **posture.** The higher centers also coordinate the **timing** of specific movements (whether simple or complex), the **sequencing and synchronization** of movements, as well as the amount of **force** generated. Which higher center is considered the "controller" varies depending on the motor task desired and on the information provided to the higher centers at a given time. Therefore, no one center is responsible for the control of all movement and posture (Montgomery and Connolly, 1991).
- "Lower centers" (the **brainstem** and **spinal cord**) generate **patterns** of movement that are often referred to as central or spinal pattern generators (Grillner, 1981; Burt, 1993).
- **Other systems** involved in motor control include **ascending** and **descending pathways** that provide **feedback** and **feedforward** information.
- **Interactions** within and between the various centers provide the most effective and efficient regulation of posture and movement. The model of heterarchy, therefore, considers the importance of interactions of the centers and also the effect of one's ability to **anticipate** movements and **adapt** to changes in the environment.

The heterarchy suggests that the flow of information is in more than one direction; the interaction occurs within and between levels of the neuraxis (the CNS), the interaction is reciprocal, and the information may be modified as a result of feedback and feedforward systems.

When considering motor control, one must realize that movement and posture are exceedingly intricate, complex, and may be affected by an abundance of factors. For example, several systems must be intact for appropriate regulation of posture and movement to occur. The **neuromuscular systems** must be intact (ie, the muscles that experience excitation or inhibition, muscles spindles, GTOs, myoneural junctions, the peripheral nerves that innervate the muscles, the spinal cord ascending and descending pathways, and the higher centers of motor control), as well as the interconnections of these systems. The **skeletal** system (ie, the bones, ligaments, joints, joint capsules, joint receptors, etc) also must be unimpaired. In addition, the **respiratory, cardiovascular,** and **digestive systems** must supply **energy sources** for muscular contractions and for the maintenance of the neuromusculoskeletal systems.

Furthermore, accurate **sensory input** of the internal and external environments must be provided. Examples of essential sensory information include tactile, kinesthetic, proprioceptive, visual, auditory, and vestibular information. Data regarding pressure, temperature, pain, balance, and so forth, also are crucial for appropriate motor control. Not only is the precise functioning of the neuromusculoskeletal systems essential for motor control, but cognition also plays an important role. **Cognitive** factors are necessary to assimilate sensory information, process and integrate the information, and determine appropriate movements and postures at any given instant. Furthermore, **memory** of movement and the ability to **recall** movement information are integral components to the regulation of posture and movement. The execution and efficiency of movement are influenced further by factors such as the ability to **concentrate** (attentional control); the presence or absence of visual, auditory, mental or emotional **distractions;** one's level of **proficiency;** and one's **motivation.** Likewise, **cognitive strategies** and **self-talk** influence motor control (Nideffer, 1985, 1993; Schmidt, 1988; Green, 1994a,b).

Applications of motor control are illustrated in both casual and experimental observations of motor performance. Certainly one can remember the difficulty in beginning a new skill such as learning to read, write, ride a bicycle, play a musical instrument, type on a typewriter, or use a computer. Initially, movements may seem awkward, the task may require a great deal of preparatory thought, and proficiency of performance of the task may be low. The difficulty in performing new tasks may be exaggerated if one's motivation to do the task is low; if visual, auditory, emotional, or mental distractions interfere; or if one's ability to concentrate is low. Additionally, in the beginning, cognitive self-talk may be negative and counterproductive (eg, "I can't do this!" "I'll never get this right!" "This takes too long!" and even, "This is absolutely impossible!").

As one becomes more familiar with a task and has practiced the skill repeatedly, the execution of the skill becomes more "automatic." Execution requires less preparatory thought and seems less awkward, while proficiency improves. Performance may even improve to the point that one becomes highly proficient in the skill and even progress to "elite" status. Furthermore, as one becomes more competent in the performance of the particular task, cognitive strategies change and self-talk becomes less frequent but more positive and productive.

Numerous diseases, injuries, and developmental disabilities may cause disturbances in one or more of the factors involved in the regulation of movement and posture. Knowing that movement of the human body is not simply a stimulus-response system, clinicians can better assess impairments of the neuromuscu-loskeletal systems and suggest possible solutions to clinical problems. In this light, clinicians also become more aware of the effects of impairments on an individ-ual's ability to regulate, learn, or relearn motor control. Numerous rehabilitation strategies have been developed to maximize motor control, including the Rood technique (Rood, 1962), proprioceptive neuromuscular facilitation (PNF) (Voss, 1967), neurodevelopmental treatment (NDT) (Bobath, 1969; 1978), the Brunnstrom technique (Brunnstrom, 1970), and motor relearning approaches (Carr and Shepherd, 1987). Theories supporting these strategies may be found in various rehabilitation textbooks. Most clinicians realize that proper function of the neuromusculoskeletal system is essential for appropriate regulation of movement and posture. Clinicians also recognize the impact of various cognitive factors on motor control. For example, persons with various cognitive deficits (ie, attentional control deficits) have difficulty performing motor tasks even in the **absence** of muscular weakness or paralysis, and without problems with muscle tone, balance, endurance, and so forth.

Exercise and sports scientists, on the other hand, use techniques to enhance motor control in athletes. These techniques are similar to those used by clinicians to properly stretch and strengthen muscles, to increase endurance, to improve bal-ance and muscle tone, and to improve the ability to regulate posture and move-ment. These scientists also realize the importance of practice to enhance skill and recognize that more than just the neuromusculoskeletal system must be enhanced to augment performance in athletes. They acknowledge that cognitive strategies such as mental practice and imagery, as well as positive self-talk, are important for the athlete's success (Feltz and Landers, 1983). In essence, principles of cognition used to enhance athletic performance may be applied clinically so that an individ-ual's mindset for rehabilitation is productive versus counterproductive and that one's self-talk facilitates recovery rather than impairs progress.

CLINICAL CONSIDERATIONS REGARDING MOTOR CONTROL

An understanding of muscle and neural physiology is necessary for appreciating clinical problems associated with disorders of motor control. Impairments of motor control may result from many diseases, injuries, or developmental disabili-ties. The following are some specific "localized" clinical symptoms and conditions intended to introduce the reader to clinical applications. The numerous terms in the literature to describe motor control problems have resulted in some confusion among clinicians. The difficulty is compounded by the fact that actual underlying mechanisms of abnormal tone have not been clearly defined (Craik, 1991). More important, recent theories suggest that rehabilitative strategies do not necessarily need to focus primarily on abnormal tone (Horak, 1991).

Insufficient Muscle Tone

Loss of transmission of motor impulses to muscles may be caused by impaired functioning of either upper motor neurons or lower motor neurons. The loss of motor input may produce a reduction in muscle tone, also referred to as **low tone,** **hypotonia,** or **hypotonicity,** and a state of **flaccid** (L. *flaccidus,* weak, soft, lax) **paralysis.** If the lower motor neuron is intact, the muscle may still respond weakly to segmental reflexes but, without impulses from motor centers in the cortex, cerebellum, and brainstem, the muscle cannot participate in the maintenance of posture or the performance of motor activities. Loss of the lower motor neurons to a muscle may produce profound **flaccidity, loss of reflex responses** of the muscle, and **progressive atrophy** (wasting) of muscle fibers.

Muscular Weakness and Atrophy

When a muscle is not used for long periods of time, the quantity of actin and myosin myofilaments in each muscle fiber actually decreases, leading to atrophy, a reduction in the diameters of individual fibers. A loss of **muscle strength** also may result. **Disuse atrophy** is a term used to describe atrophy that occurs when a person is immobile (eg, on strict bedrest for more than 2 weeks or when a limb is immobilized in a sling or a cast) (Gutmann and Hnik, 1963; Browse, 1965). Atrophy of disuse may be delayed by intermittently contracting the muscle against resistance (Hislop, 1964).

Delivery of action potentials to muscle fibers in a motor unit is accompanied by delivery of trophic (nutrient) substances that prevent atrophy (Guth, 1968; Gutmann, 1976). Lack of use because of disease or injury of the lower motor neurons innervating a muscle removes the source of a continuous supply of trophic substances. The affected fibers may undergo progressive **atrophy of denervation** unless the muscle fibers are reinnervated by sprouts from nearby surviving motor axons or by axons regrowing from the proximal end of the severed peripheral nerve. If reinnervation by the peripheral nerve has not been achieved within about 2 years, the contractile myofibrils may be replaced with fibrous connective tissue and the muscle will not be capable of developing active tension.

Materials are transported in **both** directions through the axon, a process referred to as **axoplasmic flow** (Grafstein and Forman, 1980). A continual supply of trophic substances is needed by both the muscle fiber and the nerve fiber to remain healthy. Activation of the neuromuscular system, therefore, serves as a stimulus for synthesis of trophic substances, and lack of use may lead to functional and structural deterioration. Regardless of the underlying etiology related to these facts, when a muscle is not contracted or exercised voluntarily (or otherwise), weakness, atrophy, or both, of the muscle may occur.

Excessive Muscle Tone

Disease or injury of upper motor neurons may lead to a state of excessive muscle tone. The terms **high tone, hypertonia, hypertonicity,** or **spasticity** (Gr. *spastikos,* pertaining to spasms) are used clinically to indicate excessive muscle tone. **Rigidity** is another term denoting excessive tone in a muscle or group of muscles. Refer to neurophysiologic textbooks for descriptions and etiology of the different types of rigidity.

Excessive tone is indicative of the presence of the following clinical signs: increased **firmness** of the muscle(s) to palpation, increased **resistance** of the muscle(s) to passive elongation (stretch); **impaired voluntary** as well as **reflexive control** of the skeletal muscles (including the sphincters of the bladder and anus); **low threshold** for muscle stretch reflexes and cutaneomuscle reflexes; **spread** of any reflex responses to involve muscles on the **opposite side** of the body; and **irradiation** of any reflex responses to muscles innervated from **higher and lower spinal segments.**

High tone is of great clinical importance because high tone is the end result of many pathologic conditions affecting the CNS. The mechanisms responsible for producing high tone are not well understood. In individuals with an intact neuro-musculoskeletal system, the supply of **facilitatory** impulses maintain motor neurons in a state of high excitability that is balanced by a similar supply of **inhibitory** impulses dispensed to lower motor neurons from inhibitory centers in the brainstem, cerebellum, and cerebral cortex. Inhibition of segmental circuits permits relaxation of muscles. The operation of inhibitory centers in conjunction with excitatory centers during the performance of motor activities causes the excitatory impulses to be channeled only to those motor units needed to produce the desired motions. Disease or injury of upper motor neurons may upset the balance between facilitatory and inhibitory inputs to a portion of the lower motor neurons, especially when damage occurs to motor neurons responsible for conduction of impulses from supraspinal centers that inhibit segmental circuits. Inadequate inhibition of excitatory impulses during attempted movement can cause overflow of excitatory impulses to muscles that should not have been activated, and contraction of those muscles may actually interfere with accomplishment of the desired movement.

Tone of any particular muscle fluctuates from moment to moment, depending on the balance of excitatory and inhibitory influences on the motor neuron pool supplying the muscle. Lesions of the motor cortex or of the lateral corticospinal tract may produce low tone and flaccid paralysis of the muscles innervated by the damaged neurons. In this case, low tone and flaccid paralysis are due to upper motor neuron damage. However, removal of inhibitory influences ordinarily supplied from the reticulospinal region of the brain (located in the pons and medulla) may produce severe high tone. Following traumatic injury to the spinal cord, flaccid paralysis may be present for several weeks, then segmental reflexes below the site of spinal injury return and gradually may become hyperactive. Muscles of the extremities that are innervated by spinal segments located below the level of the lesion in the spinal cord often exhibit the greatest tone, particularly if innervation is lost to the antigravity muscles (flexors of the arms and extensors of the legs). Frequently, characteristics of high tone resulting from injury to the brain differ considerably from high tone following injury to the spinal cord.

If the neural damage occurs at a high level in the CNS, tonic postural and spinal reflexes may be "released" from their inhibited state. The released reflexes may then exert effects on the lower motor neurons and cause stereotyped patterns of increased muscle tone relevant to the reflexes released (Fiorentino, 1973; Brunnstrom, 1970; Bobath, 1985; Haley and Inacio, 1990). For example, asymmetric tonic neck reflex may occur when the head is passively rotated to the side. Tone increases in the extensor muscles of the arm on the same side to which the face is turned and in the flexor muscles of the opposite arm. The hypertonicity appears in opposite muscle groups when the face is turned to the other side. If, however, the head is flexed forward, an increase in tone may occur in the extensor muscles of both arms (tonic labyrinthine reflex). Thus, the pattern of high tone can vary from moment to moment depending on many factors, such as the general position of the person's head and body, the amount and type of damage to the neuraxis, the function of the area of the involved nervous system, the nature of the stimulus applied to the individual, and the amount of effort the individual makes to obtain a voluntary movement. Strong volitional efforts often facilitate an associated reaction. The involuntary reaction may be due to the fact that the threshold of the appropriate motor neuron pools is already low (because of insufficient inhibition), and therefore more sensitive to even minimal incoming stimulus. The arrival of even a few excitatory impulses over preserved corticospinal nerve fibers may trigger the lower motor neurons into action.

If the CNS is damaged so severely that only the spinal reflexes are "released," the individual may demonstrate flexion withdrawal. Reflex withdrawal of a hand or foot is a natural reflex response to noxious (L. *noxious,* injurious) stimuli (eg, touching an extremely hot surface). However, when inhibition is lacking, withdrawal may be the response to almost any stimulus, such as a normal tactile stimulus, noise, or sudden movement. Depending on where a tactile stimulus is applied, flexion or extension responses may occur, but flexion responses are more prevalent. In addition, the presence of noxious stimuli (eg, a bladder infection or a pressure sore) may be the source of a continual supply of afferent impulses that facilitates the motor neuron pool and increases symptoms of high tone.

SELECTED IMPAIRMENTS OF THE NERVOUS SYSTEM

The nervous system may be impaired because of injuries to the spinal cord, brain, peripheral nerve, and so forth. The nervous system also may be impaired as a consequence of numerous diseases (eg, multiple sclerosis, poliomyelitis) or as a result of developmental disabilities. A few specific impairments of the nervous system are described below.

Peripheral Nerve Injury

Peripheral nerves (see Figs. 3–4 and 3–8) may be damaged by disease or trauma, including lacerations, pressure, compression, severance of the nerve, and so forth. If the damage is complete, **flaccid paralysis** of muscle fibers supplied by the motor axons may result (the muscles are no longer stimulated). The muscles may demonstrate low tone and atrophy, and the tendon reflexes may be decreased or absent. **Loss of sensation** in the skin and other structures supplied by the sensory axons also may occur.

Examples of peripheral nerve lesions include the median and ulnar nerves, which are susceptible to damage at the wrist, where the nerves may be severed by glass or knives. Furthermore, the tendons of the long finger flexors pass under the flexor retinaculum (L. *retinaculum,* a rope or cable; in this case, a band of fibrous connective tissue at the wrist). Inflammation of the synovial sheaths of the flexor tendons may lead to compression of the median nerve (which also passes under the flexor retinaculum). Such damage to the median nerve may result in a condition referred to as **carpal tunnel syndrome.** Symptoms associated with the compression of the median nerve include decreased sensation in the area innervated by the nerve, pain and, if the condition progresses, weakness and atrophy of muscles innervated by the median nerve.

Nerves in the arm also may be damaged after a fracture of a bone. For example, a fracture of the humerus may cause a lesion of the radial nerve. Likewise, the nerve may be trapped in calcium deposits formed as the fracture heals. In the lower extremities, the sciatic nerve may be injured by wounds of the pelvis or thigh or by dislocations of the hip. Pressure from tourniquets and improperly applied casts also may lead to interference in nerve conduction.

Peripheral nerve injuries may result in deformities caused by the unopposed action of innervated muscles. For example, following a lesion of the ulnar nerve, the individual is predisposed to developing a clawhand deformity. In this case, the long flexors and extensors of the fingers are not impaired. Their pull, however, is unopposed by intrinsic muscles in the hand, the interossei muscles (innervated by the ulnar nerve). The unopposed positioning may result in a clawing position of the fingers. Another common problem that may develop is a result of no movement by paralyzed muscles. Without occasional movement, adhesions can form between tendons and the sheaths that surround them, as well as between adjacent bundles of muscle fibers. When tissues crossing a joint remain in the same position for several weeks, a contracture may form, whereby the tissues tend to adapt to the shortened position and exhibit a decrease in the range of motion that the tissues would normally allow. Complications may be prevented by maintaining full range of movement and increasing the flow of blood and lymph through the area by physical activity. Splints also may assist in preventing contractures.

Loss of sensation often is a more serious problem than loss of muscle strength for a person with a peripheral nerve lesion. Individuals with impaired sensory function may exhibit a loss of awareness of where certain parts of the body are located and what the body parts are "doing" (loss of proprioception). In addition, the person cannot detect pressure over insensitive areas when blood flow is occluded by external pressure or when the part is in contact with excessively hot or cold objects (loss of touch, pressure, pain, and temperature sensations). Thus the body part is subject to traumatic injuries, ischemia (Gr. *ischein*, to suppress, plus *haima*, blood), burns, pressure sores, and subsequent infections.

Cerebral Palsy

Cerebral palsy (L. *cerebrum*, brain; *palsy*, paralysis) is a general term used to describe a group of motor disorders that generally result from an arrest or retardation of the developing brain. As one of the most common developmental disabilities, cerebral palsy results from a lesion to the brain during prenatal (L. *prae*, before, plus L. *natal*, birth), perinatal, or early postnatal stages of life. The brain lesion, which may be secondary to a wide variety of pathophysiologic events, often results in hypoxia or anoxia of the brain and causes a nonprogressive but permanent damage to an area (or areas) of the brain. Although cerebral palsy is defined as a neurologically static condition, it can be thought of as being orthopedically progressive in nature. The latter is the result of the effects of atypical neuromusculoskeletal symptoms, such as deviations in muscle tone (hypotonus or hypertonus) or movement disorders. In addition, the child's antigravity postural development may be delayed. Therefore, cerebral palsy is the combined result of a delay and a disorder in sensorimotor development.

Depending on the sites of the neurologic lesion, an individual with cerebral palsy may show a variety of motor or other impairments. Because of the close relationship of motor functions with other functions and because of the potential diffuse nature of the lesion, the individual with cerebral palsy also may demonstrate sensory (eg, auditory or visual), communicative, perceptual, and/or cognitive impairments.

A child with cerebral palsy may be unable to acquire some learning experiences if he or she cannot move to explore the environment. The child may be unable to creep, crawl, or walk, or use the hands to discover the meaning of directions, textures, shapes, or temperatures. Furthermore, the child may not be able to look at, reach, or touch different parts of his or her face and body to learn body image and spatial relationships. The paucity of these experiences may disrupt perceptual and conceptual development. Also, the child's delayed motor development may affect speech and language development. A child who is unable to adequately control the muscles that position the head may not be able to observe what makes a specific sound and, thus, may not communicate easily with eye-to-eye contact with another person. Without head control, the child may not observe perceptual aspects, such as the relationships of objects to self and to others that give meaning to words such as "near" and "far" or "up" and "down." Therefore, the contribution of intervention by therapists to the motor development of the child with cerebral palsy has far-reaching effects on the child's total development.

Cerebrovascular Accident (Stroke)

The CNS is very vulnerable to reduction in the blood supply. Cerebrovascular accidents (CVAs), or strokes, occur when the blood supply to an area in the CNS is disrupted. The disruption may be due to atherosclerosis, high blood pressure, malformation of a blood vessel, heart disease, and so forth. Causes of CVA include hemorrhage (bleeding from a blood vessel), thrombosis (a clot that occludes a blood vessel), or embolism (a clot that originates in another area and is transported through the blood stream). Residual problems following a stroke vary greatly depending on numerous factors such as the cause of the CVA, the area of the CNS that incurred the loss of blood supply, the extent of the damage, and the functions of the damaged area(s). The clinical deficits may include weakness or paralysis of the muscles of the face, trunk, and/or extremities; impairment of sensation and proprioception; visual deficits; cognitive difficulties; language impairments; and perceptual problems.

Numerous arteries supply blood and nutrients to the brain and are subject to damage following a CVA. For example, the region of the brain between the thalamus and basal ganglia, through which the bundles of corticospinal fibers pass, is the internal capsule. Rupture or occlusion of an artery supplying nutrients to the region of the internal capsule on one side of the brain may so impair the function of axons passing through the area that impulses are no longer conducted. When this happens, not only the corticospinal tract but other motor tracts from the cortex to the brainstem may be affected (see Fig. 3–20), producing paralysis of muscles whose spinal motor neurons were controlled by those upper motor neurons. After emerging from the internal capsule, 75 to 90 percent of the million or so fibers in the corticospinal tract cross to the opposite side in the brainstem. Thus, impairment of motor impulse conduction through the internal capsule on one side may produce paralysis of muscles on the side opposite the lesion (paralysis of muscles on one side of the body is referred to as hemiplegia).

Basal Ganglia Dysfunction

In general, the basal ganglia convert plans for movement into programs for movement, particularly with respect to the initiation and execution of slow movements. Therefore, impairments of the basal ganglia may result in the individual's exhibiting meaningless intentional movement. The best-known complex of symptoms resulting from disturbance of basal ganglial connections is Parkinson's syndrome. Individuals with Parkinson's disease have symptoms characterized by slowness of movement; rigidity of facial expressions; decreased or absent communicative gestures; a hesitant, shuffling gait with small steps; and trembling of their hands at rest (termed **resting tremor** [L. *tremere,* to shake]).

Athetosis is another movement disorder involving the basal ganglia. Athetosis, however, results in slow, writhing movements that are exhibited especially in the upper extremities. Basal ganglia disorders also include chorea, a complex disorder in which the individual has involuntary, sudden, nonpurposeful movements.

Cerebellar Dysfunction

The cerebellum is primarily responsible for programming rapid movements, correcting the course of rapid movements, and correlating posture and movement. Individuals with impaired functions of the cerebellum perform movements in an uncoordinated, awkward manner. A person with impaired cerebellar function walks with a staggering gait (ataxia) and tends to fall to the same side as the cerebellar lesion. Other motor problems may include general decrease in muscle tone (hypotonia); inability to achieve properly timed and properly graded activation of muscles during attempted movement (may overshoot an object when reaching for it); inability to produce a co-contraction of both flexor and extensor muscles to stabilize a joint; and tremors that appear during attempted purposeful movement and that increase in amplitude as the individual attempts finer control of the movement (referred to as **intention tremor**).

Laboratory Activities |

1. Two-point discrimination

   Two-point discrimination refers to a person's ability to detect two different points on his or her skin when they are touched simultaneously. When the two points are very close together, the individual may perceive only one point. When the two points are farther apart, the person perceives both points.

   The ability to discriminate between two points varies for different areas of the body. For example:
   a. The person can usually discriminate between two points that are close together when the face or palmar surface of the fingers is touched.
   b. The person may, however, perceive only one point when the dorsal surface of the hand or the back of the neck is touched in the same manner (that is, with the two points the same distance apart, as in a).

   Using a compass, test two-point discrimination on your subject's back, neck, dorsal surface of the hand, face, lips, and palmar surface of the index finger. For each area on the body, determine how close together the arms of the compass can be for the subject to perceive two distinct points as opposed to perceiving only one point. Note that you should touch the skin simultaneously with the two arms of the compass.

Compare how close together the compass arms can be on the different areas on the body. Is there a difference?

2. Have an instructor assist you in eliciting stretch reflexes using a reflex hammer to tap the patellar tendons on your partner (see Figure 3–13).

   Have the subject sitting and relaxed, with his or her eyes closed. Test the patellar tendon (at the knee).

   Note the length of time between the tap and the response. Observe the "crispness" of the response. Observe variations among different subjects.

CHAPTER 4

Muscle Activity and Strength

The largest and most frequent source of force generated within the body is by contraction of muscles. Additional passive forces occur from tension on fascia, ligaments, and noncontractile structures of muscle. To simplify problems in mechanics, muscle forces are depicted as acting at a single point on the body. This simplification is helpful in demonstrating principles of biomechanics, but it is important to keep in mind that many complex forces occur in function.

Normally, muscles never contract alone because this would produce a stereotyped nonfunctional motion. For example, the isolated contraction of the biceps brachii would produce elbow flexion, supination, and shoulder flexion. Rather, several muscles in an exquisite combination of forces contribute to produce the desired force and resulting motion or segment position. In addition, soft tissues may transmit active forces of muscles through attachments to fascia, ligaments, cartilage, joint capsules, and tendons of other muscles, as well as to bones. For example, at the knee, the semimembranosus (medial hamstring) attaches to the medial meniscus (a cartilage in the knee joint), the medial collateral ligament, and the posterior capsule of the knee joint as well as to the bony attachment on the medial condyle of the tibia. The purpose of these soft tissue attachments is thought to be movement of these structures to prevent their injury during rapid motions of the knee. An understanding of the active and passive forces in function requires consideration of the behavior of muscle as well as related soft tissues.

MUSCLE ACTIVITY

Recording of Contraction

The role of individual muscles, or a group of muscles, in producing movement or stabilizing body segments may be examined by palpating the muscle to judge when it is active or relaxed. Although palpation of muscles is an important clinical skill to be mastered, the method is of limited usefulness in advancing our knowledge of muscle function. Only one, or perhaps two, superficial muscles can be examined at one time, and there is no record for analyzing the timing or magnitude of muscle contraction. Since activation of a muscle fiber is associated with transient depolarization and repolarization of the muscle fiber membrane (see Fig. 3–5), recording electrodes placed on the skin overlying a muscle (or even introduced into the muscle) can be used to monitor the small changes in electric field produced by the conduction of muscle action potentials over groups of muscle fibers.

Einthoven (1901) used his newly developed string galvanometer to record the action potentials generated by cardiac muscle when the heart of an experimental animal contracted. The technique was further improved by Adrian and Bronk (1929) to study the activity of skeletal muscles. The development of amplifying and recording equipment during World War II made it possible to use improved methods for the study of muscular activity in living human subjects. The gathering of information by this means, with surface, needle, or indwelling wire electrodes, is called **electromyography** (EMG), (L. *elektra,* lit, brilliant, pertaining to electricity; Gr. *myos,* muscle; and L. *graphicus,* to write). Each pair of electrodes is connected to a "channel" of the recording apparatus (Fig. 4–1). The use of multichannel instruments allows the contraction and relaxation patterns of several muscles to be recorded simultaneously during some particular movement or pos-

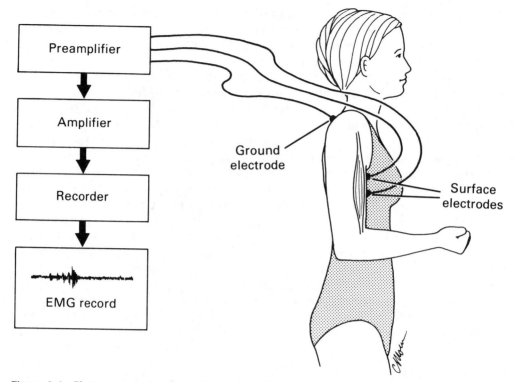

Figure 4–1   Electromyography. Electrodes are placed near the muscle to detect the changes in electric potential associated with activation of muscle fibers. The electric activity "seen" by the electrodes is greatly amplified by electronic equipment and recorded for later analysis of the timing and relative amount of activity exhibited by the muscle(s) being monitored.

tural state of a joint. In this way, the sequence of activation and relaxation, as well as the relative amount of activity of particular muscles, can be studied as they perform various isolated or coordinated functions. Some of the earliest careful studies of kinesiology using EMG were performed by Inman and coworkers (1944) in their analysis of motions of the shoulder. Reports on the uses and limitations of kinesiologic EMG include those by Ralston (1961), Basmajian (1978), and Heckathorne and colleagues (1981). Reports of the use of EMG techniques for kinesiologic studies include those by Basmajian (1978), Smidt (1990), and Perry (1992). A more detailed discussion of the use and limitations of kinesiologic EMG is presented in Chapter 12 under Muscle Activity in the Gait Cycle: Electromyography.

Terminology for Muscle Contractions

Isometric

When a muscle contracts and produces force with no gross change in the joint angle, the contraction is said to be **isometric** (Gr. *isos*, equal; *metron*, measure). Isometric contractions are often called static, or holding, contractions. Functionally these contractions stabilize joints. For example, to reach forward with the hand, the scapula must be stabilized against the thorax.

Concentric

A shortening of the muscle during contraction is called a **concentric** or **shortening contraction**. Examples would be the quadriceps muscle when an individual is rising from a chair or the elbow flexors when an individual is lifting a glass of water to the mouth. Concentric contractions produce acceleration of body segments.

Eccentric

When the muscle lengthens during contraction, it is called an **eccentric** or **lengthening contraction**. Examples for the quadriceps would be when the body is being lowered to sit and for the elbow flexors when the glass of water is lowered to the table. Eccentric contractions decelerate body segments and provide shock absorption as when landing from a jump or in walking.

Isokinetic

An **isokinetic** (Gr. *isos,* equal; *kinetos,* moving) contraction occurs when the rate of movement is constant. In recent years, an electromechanical device (an isokinetic dynamometer) has been developed that limits the rate of movement of a crank-arm or a pulley to some preset angular velocity regardless of the force exerted by the contracting muscles. In 1967, Hislop and Perrine described the concept and principles of isokinetic exercise. The axis of rotation of the crank-arm of the isokinetic device is aligned with the anatomic axis of the moving joint, and the device lever is matched to the skeletal lever (Fig. 4–2). A subject contracts the muscle group being exercised or evaluated, and the device controls the speed of body movement without permitting acceleration to occur. "During isokinetic exercise the resistance accommodates the external force at the skeletal lever so that the muscle maintains maximum output throughout the full range of motion" (Hislop and Perrine, 1967). An experienced therapist can apply a similar accommodating resistance throughout the range of motion by manually resisting the motion. This manually applied, accommodating resistance is still a valuable therapeutic technique. With practice, the therapist can continuously adjust the amount of resistance being offered so that the motion produced is approximately constant throughout the range, thereby approaching an isokinetic condition.

Isotonic

The word **isotonic** is derived from the Greek *isos,* equal, and *tonus,* tension. The term was originally used by muscle physiologists to refer to the **contraction of a muscle detached from the body and lifting a load vertically against gravity** (see Fig. 3–16A). The connotation was that shortening of the muscle occurred and that the load on the muscle was constant throughout the excursion. When the load became great enough to exceed the ability of the muscle to lift it, the contraction became isometric. Truly isotonic contractions seldom, if ever, occur when muscles are acting through the lever systems of the body. Even so, the term is often used, although incorrectly, to refer to a contraction that causes a joint to move through some range of motion, as in flexing the elbow while holding a

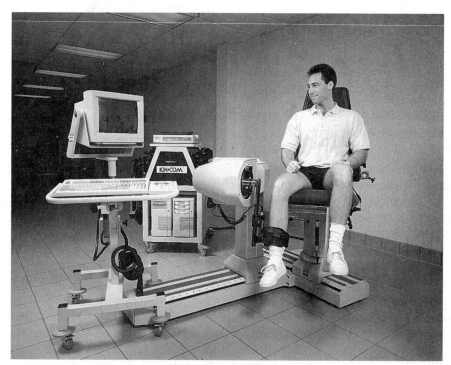

Figure 4–2   One of several types of isokinetic dynamometers, a device for testing and exercising muscle groups during isometric, concentric, and eccentric contractions. Force or torque exerted by the muscle, along with joint angle, is recorded. Calculations are made for average peak torque, work, and power. The subject is seated with his leg coupled to the lever arm to perform motions of extension and flexion of the knee (Courtesy Chattanooga Group, Inc, Hixson, TN).

weight in the hand. Even though the weight remains the same throughout the movement, the tension requirements of the muscle change continuously with changing leverage (see Fig. 2–36), and the torque exerted by the weight changes with changing joint angles (see Fig. 2–14).

Anatomic Actions of Muscles

Anatomically, muscles are described by their **proximal attachments** (origin), **distal attachments** (insertion), and **actions** in producing specific joint motions. Although knowledge of the anatomic attachments and actions is essential to the study of kinesiology, it is important to recognize that these factors can be used to predict muscle function only under the limited circumstances in which all of the following occur: (1) The proximal attachment is stabilized, (2) the distal attachment moves toward the proximal attachment (concentric contraction), (3) the distal segment moves against gravity or resistance, and (4) the muscle acts alone. These circumstances rarely occur in normal function for several reasons: (1) Proximal attachments often move toward fixed distal attachments (closed kinematic chain). (2) Contractions are often eccentric or isometric. (3) Movement of the distal segment is often assisted by the force of gravity. (4) Muscles seldom if ever act alone; they more often act conjointly.

Even though a muscle or muscle group is named after a joint motion (ie, flexor carpi ulnaris, flexor carpi radialis, or wrist flexors), the muscles may or may not be responsible for the motion. For example, when the hand is held with the palm facing the top of the table and the wrist is slowly flexed, the wrist flexors will be inactive, and the motion will be performed by an eccentric contraction of the wrist extensors. Thus, additional terminology is needed to classify muscles as they act in function.

Functional Terminology of Muscle Activity

Many different terms can be found in the literature to classify the function of muscles as they act in joint motion. These terms include agonist, prime mover, antagonist, synergist, true synergist, helping synergist, assistant mover, neutralizer, fixator, and stabilizer. Some of the words are synonymous, and some of the same words have different definitions. Although it is not difficult to determine if a muscle is or is not contracting (by palpation or EMG), it is difficult to ascertain the purpose or reason for which a muscle is contracting. To reduce semantic debate, only three terms or their synonyms are used in this text: agonist, antagonist, and synergist.

Agonist

A contracting muscle (or muscle group) that is considered to be the principal muscle producing a joint motion or maintaining a posture is referred to as an **agonist** (Gr. *agon,* contest), or the prime mover. The agonist always contracts actively to produce a concentric, isometric, or eccentric contraction.

Antagonist

The **antagonist** (Gr. *anti,* against) is a muscle (or muscle group) that possesses the opposite anatomic action of the agonist. Usually the antagonist is a noncontracting muscle that neither assists nor resists the motion but that passively elongates or shortens to permit the motion to occur. Thus, in the example of wrist flexion, when the palm is facing the table top, the wrist extensors are the agonists and the wrist flexors are the antagonists. The classification reverses when the dorsum of the hand is facing the table (forearm supinated) and the wrist is flexed against gravity. Here, the wrist flexors are the agonists, and the wrist extensors are the antagonists.

Synergist

A muscle may be defined as a **synergist** (Gr. *syn,* with, together; *ergon,* work) whenever it contracts at the same time as the agonist. The action of a synergist may be identical, or nearly identical, to that of the agonist—as when the brachioradialis acts with the brachialis during elbow flexion. A synergist may rule out an unwanted action of a prime mover, such as the pronator teres preventing the supination action of the biceps brachii during resisted elbow flexion, or the wrist extensors preventing wrist flexion when the long flexors of the fingers contract to close the hand. Synergists commonly act isometrically at joints far removed from the primary motion to fixate, or stabilize, proximal joints so that motion may occur at distal joints.

Fixating functions are more frequently performed by muscles than the functions of agonists or antagonists. This important function is needed because when the agonist contracts, its force is distributed equally to both its distal and proximal attachments. Thus, both bones (segments) to which the muscle is attached could move. For the desired movement to occur in one segment, the other segment must be fixed. This is accomplished by automatic muscle contractions to stabilize and prevent undesired motion of a segment. This important fixating action of muscles can be demonstrated as one closes the hand and grips forcefully. Even when the forearm is resting on the table, strong isometric contractions can be palpated in muscles of the forearm, arm, shoulder, scapula, and even the trunk.

The relationships of muscles as agonists, antagonists, and synergists are not absolute. They vary with the activity, position of the body, and the direction of the resistance that the muscle must overcome. These changing relationships are illustrated in the EMG records of the triceps brachii and the biceps-brachialis muscles during the motions of elbow flexion and extension (Fig. 4–3). When the seated subject flexes the elbow to lift a load in the hand, the flexors contract concentrically and are classified as the agonists. The antagonistic extensors are relatively relaxed and elongate to permit the motion of elbow flexion. As the elbow is then extended to lower the load, the flexors perform an eccentric contraction and are still classified as agonists (Fig. 4–3A). The extensors remain inactive and are still the antagonists. However, when the subject is placed in the supine position with the shoulder in 90 degrees of flexion and performs the same motions of elbow flexion and extension, the agonist-antagonist relationships are reversed (Fig. 4–3B). Here, the elbow extensors are the agonists for elbow extension (concentric contraction) and for elbow flexion (eccentric contraction), while the flexors are the antagonists for both motions.

Figure 4–3   Electromyographic activity of the triceps brachii (TRI) and the biceps brachialis (B–B) during the motions of elbow flexion and extension, with changes in the position of the body and the direction of the resistive force. (Range of motion of elbow flexion 0° to 120° and extension 120° to 0°.)
(*A*) Subject sitting, shoulder in anatomic position, and 10-lb weight in hand.

Flexion: Agonist = B–B (concentric contraction)
Antagonist = TRI
Extension: Agonist = B–B (eccentric contraction)
Antagonist = TRI

(*B*) Subject backlying, shoulder flexed to 90°, and 10-lb weight in hand.

Flexion: Agonist = TRI (eccentric contraction)
Antagonist = B–B
Extension: Agonist = TRI (concentric contraction)
Antagonist = B–B

(*C*) Subject backlying, shoulder in anatomic position, and 10-lb weight in hand.

Flexion: Agonist 0° to 90° = B–B (concentric contraction)
90° to 120° = TRI (eccentric contraction)
Extension: Agonist 120° to 90° = TRI (concentric contraction)
90° to 0° = B–B (eccentric contraction)

(*D*) Subject sitting, shoulder in anatomic position with manual resistance to elbow flexion and then to elbow extension. (Slight to moderate resistance was applied at the distal forearm.)

Flexion: Agonist = B–B (concentric contraction)
Antagonist = TRI
Extension: Agonist = TRI (concentric contraction)
Antagonist = B–B

Note the decreased frequency and amplitude of electromyographic activity during eccentric contractions as compared with responses during concentric contractions of the same muscle, even though the resistance force and the velocity of motion were approximately the same.

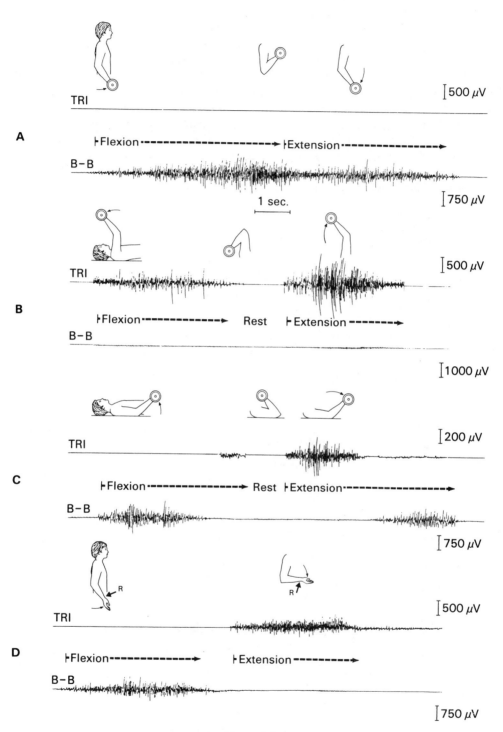

Figure 4–3

An interesting switching of the agonistic-antagonistic classification in the same motions of elbow flexion and extension occurs when the subject is in the back-lying position (Fig. 4–3C). Here, the biceps-brachialis muscles are the agonists for the first part of elbow flexion, but as the elbow passes 90 degrees, the direction of the resistance force changes, and the triceps becomes the agonist. The agonist for elbow extension in this position is the triceps to 90 degrees, but responsibility for controlling the remainder of the motion is assumed by the elbow flexors (eccentric contraction). Application of manual resistance throughout the motion of flexion and then extension (Fig. 4–3D) further illustrates the principle that muscles act according to the resistance they meet rather than the motion of the joint.

Other examples of the varying relationships among these muscles are shown in Figure 4–4. In Figure 4–4A, the biceps is acting as an agonist in the motion of supination (along with the supinator), and the triceps is acting as a synergist to

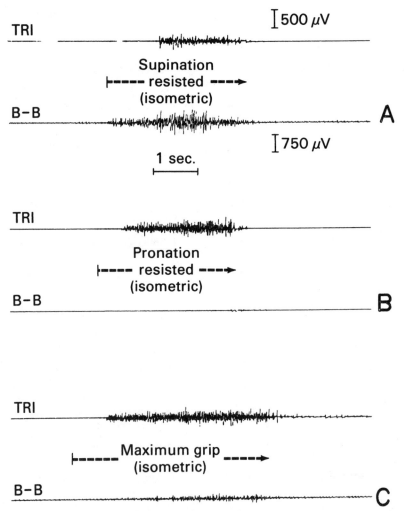

Figure 4–4 Synergistic actions of the triceps brachii (TRI) and biceps brachialis (B–B) muscles. Electromyograph records with the subject sitting, elbow flexed to 90 degrees, and forearm and hand supported. (A) Manual resistance to supination (isometric contraction and moderate resistance). (B) Manual resistance to pronation (isometric contraction and moderate resistance). (C) Maximal isometric grip strength using a hand dynamometer (force recorded = 117 lb or 53 kg).

prevent elbow flexion. The antagonists in this case are the pronator muscles. In the movements of pronation and finger flexion to test grip strength (Fig. 4–4B,C), the elbow extensors are acting as synergists to stabilize the elbow. The elbow flexors are relatively inactive even with a maximal grip effort.

The agonist-antagonist classification is used in simple open-chain motions. In rapid, forceful, or closed-chain motion there may be other terminology used, such as accelerator or decelerator, or there may be co-contraction of muscles. For example, when standing up or sitting down, both the quadriceps femoris and the hamstring muscles contract to produce the movements needed at the knees and the hips. The important concept is that if a muscle is to produce a motion, it cannot be impeded by anatomic antagonistic muscles. Clinically, such impedance occurs with muscle contractures and with hypertonus or spasticity of muscles.

PASSIVE EXCURSION OF MUSCLES

The paired agonist-antagonist relationship of muscles in the lever system requires that each muscle have the ability to accommodate and change length both passively and actively to permit motion. Morrison (1970), for example, measured changes of 3 to 4 inches (8 to 10 cm) in the length of the quadriceps and hamstring muscles during normal walking. The **functional excursion** of a muscle is defined as that distance the muscle is capable of shortening after it has been elongated as far as the joint(s) over which it passes allows. Weber (1851) determined the excursions of a large number of muscles and found that some could shorten to 34 percent of the longest length, and others could shorten to 89 percent, with a mean value of 50 percent. The highest excursions were for those muscles that cross more than one joint, such as the hamstrings. Kaplan (1965) and Boyes (1970) provide specific measurements of the excursion distances for each muscle of the hand and wrist. For example, Boyes (1970) measured an excursion of 3 inches (8 cm) for the flexor digitorum profundus muscle when the middle finger and wrist were moved from full wrist and finger flexion to full extension of these joints.

Passive Insufficiency

When muscles become elongated over two or more joints simultaneously, they may reach the state of passive insufficiency and not allow further motion by the agonist. This antagonistic limitation of motion can be demonstrated with hip flexion in the able-bodied subject. The hip can be flexed to 115 to 125 degrees when the knee is also flexed, but when the knee is kept in extension, hip flexion is limited to 60 to 80 degrees because of passive insufficiency of the hamstrings muscles, which are now stretched over the hip and knee. Certain pathologic conditions may cause muscles and tendons to lose their normal range of excursions. These conditions include muscle tightness, spasticity, shortening from trauma or surgery, and adhesion of tendons to their sheaths. Thus, even though the agonist may contract strongly, motion may be severely limited by the lack of excursion of the antagonist. This restriction is commonly seen in patients with cerebrovascular accidents (hemiplegia) who have spasticity of the finger flexors. Even though these patients may have voluntary control of their finger extensors, they are unable to open the hand because of limitation in lengthening of the finger flexors.

Tendon Action of Muscle

Passive tension may produce movements of joints when the muscle is elongated over two or more joints. This effect is called the tendon or **tenodesis** (Gr. *tenon,* tendon; *desis,* a binding together) action of muscle. In able-bodied subjects, the effect can be seen if the relaxed hand is alternately flexed and extended at the wrist. When the wrist is flexed, the relaxed fingers extend because of the passive tension of the extensor digitorum, which has been elongated over the wrist and fingers. When the wrist is extended, the fingers flex because of the tension of the flexor digitorum profundus and superficialis muscles.

This tenodesis action is sometimes used functionally by quadriplegic patients with spinal cord transection resulting in a C-6 level* of motor functions and by those patients who have the ability to contract wrist extensor muscles but have paralysis of muscles of the fingers. When the wrist is permitted to flex, the fingers extend by passive insufficiency of the extensors and the hand can be placed over an object. As the wrist is voluntarily extended, the passive tension of the finger flexors produces increasing force on the object so that it may be picked up and held. If selective shortening of the long finger flexors has been permitted to occur (or the patient has spasticity in this muscle group), several pounds of grasping force can be generated.

MUSCLE STRENGTH

Muscle strength is a general term without a precise definition. Among the many definitions of strength are the state of being strong, the capacity of a muscle to produce force, and the ability of a muscle to generate active tension. In addition to neurologic, metabolic, endocrine, and psychological factors that affect muscle strength, many other factors determine muscle strength or a maximum voluntary contraction (MVC). These factors include architecture of the muscle fibers, age and gender of the subject, size of the muscles, length of the muscle at the time of contraction, leverage of the muscle, and speed of contraction.

Fiber Architecture

Early investigators have shown a strong correlation between the physiologic cross-sectional area of a detached animal muscle and the maximal force that the muscle can produce when excited by electrical stimuli. The physiologic cross-section transects each fasciculus at a right angle and therefore includes all of the fibers in pennate muscles (L. *penna,* feather; muscle fasciculi attach to the central tendon at angles). The anatomic cross-section transects the muscle as a whole at a right angle and does not include all of the muscle fibers in pennate muscles. Most of the muscles in the body, however, are of pennate structure (eg, interossei, deltoid, and

---

*The designation of the level of a spinal cord injury is based on the lowest normally functioning nerve root segment of the spinal cord. If a patient has complete interruption of upper motor neuron connections to lower motor neurons in the seventh cervical segment and below, the patient is classified as having a C6 level (complete) of motor function. The level of sensory function may also be classified. Incomplete spinal cord injury results in partial preservation of voluntary control of a few muscles or partial preservation of sensation (or both) in regions of the body supplied by nerve roots originating in spinal cord segments below the injury.

hamstrings), designed for increased force at the expense of less shortening distance. The parallel structure of fibers (eg, lumbricales and sartorius) provides greater shortening distance but less force for an equivalent muscle mass.

The term **absolute muscle strength** is used to indicate the maximum tension that can be achieved in the detached muscle. Generally, 3 to 4 kg per square centimeter of physiologic cross-section is accepted as reasonable (Fick, 1911; von Recklinghausen, 1920; Ramsey and Street, 1940; Haxton, 1944). Tables of physiologic cross-sections of muscles measured by Fick can be found in the appendices of the previous editions of this book. Multiplying Fick's value of 175 cm^2 of physiologic cross-section for the quadriceps femoris muscle by 3 to 4 kg per square centimeter gives a theoretical absolute strength of 500 to 700 kg (1100 to 1600 lb). There is, however, considerable variability in the cross-sectional area of a muscle in different people and in the same person over time with exercise or inactivity.

Age and Gender

It is recognized that males are generally stronger than females. In both genders, however, muscle strength is gained from birth through adolescence, peaking between the ages of 20 and 30 years, and gradually declining with advancing age. For example, the grip strength of the dominant hand of males and females between ages 3 and 90 is plotted in Figure 4–5. The muscle strength of young boys is

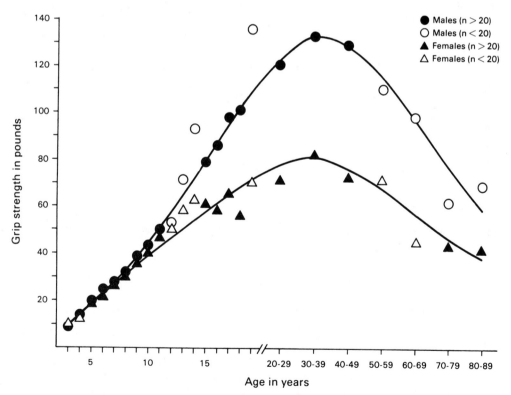

Figure 4–5 Average strength of grip of the dominant hand in able-bodied male and female subjects between 3 and 90 years of age. N = 531 males and 537 females. Data for subjects 20 years of age and older were grouped by decades. Sample sizes greater than or less than 20 are indicated by symbols.

approximately the same as that of young girls up to the age of puberty. Thereafter, males exhibit a significantly greater grip strength than females, with the greatest differences occurring during middle age (between ages 30 and 50). The greater strength of males appears to be related primarily to the greater muscle mass they develop after puberty. Up to about age 16, the ratio of lean body mass to whole body mass is similar in males and females, as indicated by studies of creatinine excretion and potassium counts. After puberty, however, the muscle mass of males becomes as much as 50 percent greater than that of females, and the ratio of lean body mass to whole body mass also becomes greater. On the other hand, muscle strength per cross-sectional area of muscle appears to be similar in males and females, as does the proportion of fast-twitch and slow-twitch muscle fibers in particular muscles (Komi and Karlsson, 1979).

Although muscular strength can be shown to be related to age and gender when considering the population as a whole, many exceptions to the general rule can be found because of the large variation in the rate at which biologic maturation occurs and the large variation in the amount of care that individuals take in keeping themselves in condition through proper diet and exercise.

Muscle Size

It is well known that larger muscles in normal subjects are stronger than smaller ones, and that muscles may increase or decrease in size with exercise or inactivity (hypertrophy and atrophy). Measurement of size and size changes, however, is difficult. Circumferential measurements lack accuracy and reproducibility because they also include skin, fat, fluid, vasculature, and bone and depend on a subjective judgment of the amount of tension on the tape measure. Magnetic resonance imaging provides an anatomic cross-section of the muscle, whereby the area of muscle tissue can be measured and small size changes can be detected (Frontera et al, 1988 and Fiatarone et al, 1990). Muscle biopsy with measurement of fiber areas also can measure small size changes (Leiveseth and Reikeras, 1994). Both of these techniques, however, are expensive, and the biopsy is invasive.

Length-Tension Relationships of Muscle

Detached Muscle

Early investigators working with isolated frog muscle found that muscle force varied with muscle length (Blix, 1895; Ramsey and Street, 1940). Similar studies have been done on humans who have had arm amputations and cineplastic muscle tunnels (Bethe, 1916; Schlesinger, 1920; Inman and Ralston, 1968; Heckathorne and Childress, 1981). This is a surgical procedure that forms a tunnel through the distal end of a muscle tendon that has little function because of the amputation, but can be harnessed to activate parts of the prosthesis, such as the hand or hook. This situation permits study of normal human muscles detached from the skeletal system at one end.

When a detached muscle fiber (or muscle) has no external forces acting on it, the fiber is said to be at **resting length.** At this length, no tension is registered in the muscle. If, starting from resting length, the fiber is slowly elongated by an outside force, tension is produced in the fiber and rises first slowly and then more rapidly until failure occurs (Fig. 4–6). The contractile elements are inactive and,

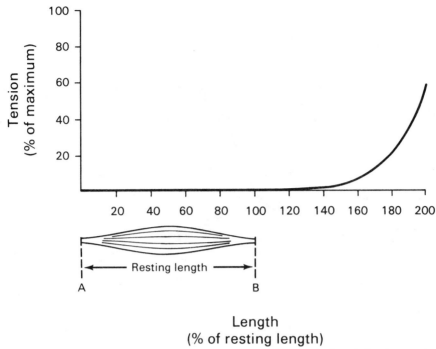

Figure 4-6 Passive tension curve of unstimulated muscle fiber, including fully elongated state of fiber. Length is expressed in percent of resting length; tension, in percent of maximum active tension. Muscle fiber A-B at resting length has been drawn in. (Adapted from Ramsey, RW, and Street, SF: Isometric length-tension diagram of isolated skeletal muscle fibers of frog. *J Cell Comp Physiol* 15:11, 1940.)

therefore, this is passive tension from the sarcolemma of the fiber (and the fascia of the muscle). This curve is known as the **passive tension** or **passive stretch curve.** Tearing of the structural components of the muscle fiber occurred at about 200 percent of resting length in the experiments of Ramsey and Street (1940).

The resting length of a muscle that has been detached from its connections with bones is comparatively easy to determine, whereas the **resting length of a muscle attached to skeletal parts cannot be determined.** Passive tension, however, can be felt in the intact subject. This is most easily found by passively elongating multijoint muscles over their full range of motion. In the upper extremity, passive extension of the wrist, the metacarpophalangeal, and interphalangeal joints through the full range of motion produces tension in the flexor digitorum superficialis and profundus muscles. In the lower extremity, passively flexing the hip and then passively extending the knee produces tension in the hamstring muscles.

LENGTH-TENSION DIAGRAM FOR STIMULATED MUSCLE FIBER The diagram in Figure 4–7 shows the result of an investigation of isometric contraction of frog muscle fibers at lengths shorter and longer than resting length. The muscle fibers were slowly elongated by small increments and electrically stimulated at high frequency to obtain maximal tension. The fibers at lengths less than resting length were not taut before stimulation but rather hung in a loop that had to be taken up by muscle contraction before the fiber could produce tension. Before approximately 50 percent of resting length, the fiber had too much slack for the active tension to be ex-

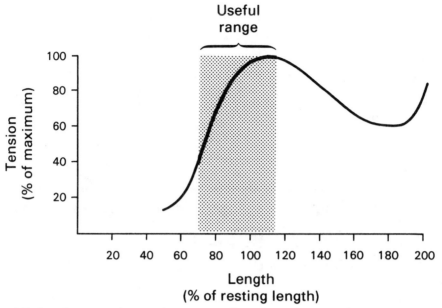

Figure 4–7 Length-tension diagram for isometrically stimulated muscle fiber, including extreme shortened and stretched states of fiber. (Adapted from Ramsey, RW, and Street, SF: Isometric length-tension diagram of isolated skeletal muscle fibers of frog. *J Cell Comp Physiol* 15:11, 1940.)

pressed through the ends of the fiber. From this point, there is a rapid rise in tension to reach a maximum at about 110 percent of resting length. Further lengthening of the fiber produces less tension because the overlap of actin and myosin filaments is reduced, thereby preventing coupling of the full number of cross-bridges (see Fig. 3–3E). The upswing of the tension curve beyond 170 percent of resting length is caused by the rise in passive tension of the fiber (see Fig. 4–6). The tearing point of the fiber occurred at about 200 percent of resting length.

Intact Muscle

In the normal body, the joints do not permit extreme shortening or lengthening of a muscle, so that muscles operate on the ascending portion of the curve and well within safety limits. The physiologically useful portion of the length-tension curve was determined for the gastrocnemius muscle of the frog (Beck, 1921). This portion occurred from about 75 to 105 percent of resting length, a range that is similar to the shaded area in Fig. 4–7. In the intact human, a part of the length-tension curve for the hamstrings can be measured (Fig. 4–8). This is done by placing the subject in a supine position with the knee maintained at 30 degrees of flexion. The subject performs a maximum isometric contraction of the hamstrings against a dynamometer. Then the hamstring muscles are lengthened by elevating the trunk and flexing the hips so that the measurement can be repeated at a shorter muscle length. Recorded forces show the physiologic part of the length-tension curve.

ACTIVE INSUFFICIENCY *Active insufficiency* refers to the weak contractile force of the muscle when its attachments are close together and the muscle is attempting to contract on the lower portion of its length-tension curve (see. Fig. 4–8). The body is designed so that such weak positions are avoided in normal activities requiring

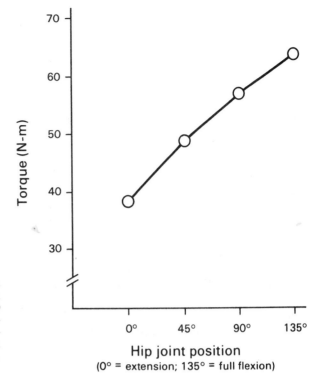

Figure 4–8 Length-tension changes in the hamstring muscles. Maximum isometric torque was measured at 30 degrees of knee flexion in four positions of hip flexion. 135° = full flexion; 0° = extension. (Plotted from data published by Lunnen et al, 1981.)

great force. A large number of muscles, for example, cross more than one joint. Favorable length-tension relationships are maintained by movement combinations whereby the muscle is elongated by motion at one joint while producing motion or force at another joint. Maximum isometric grip strength, for example, is greatest when the wrist is in slight extension (Fig. 4–9), but when the wrist is flexed the grip strength is markedly weakened. The totally ineffectual grip produced when the wrist is held in full flexion is due to the combination of active insufficiency of the long finger flexors (flexor digitorum superficialis and profundus) and passive insufficiency of the antagonistic long finger extensor (extensor digitorum).

Leverage and Length-Tension Interactions

Another unique manner in which the body avoids the weakness of active insufficiency is by changes in the mechanical leverage in the range of joint motion. In the example of the biceps brachii muscle (see Fig. 2–36), the length-tension factor is most favorable when the elbow is in a position of extension, but the maximum tension that can be produced during contraction of the muscle decreases as the elbow approaches and passes 90 degrees of flexion. To compensate for this loss in active muscle tension, the leverage of the muscle (force arm distance) increases to a maximum at 90 degrees. This provides the greatest torque at a point in the range of motion that is important for holding heavy objects. In this instance, the torque that the muscle can produce actually increases, even though the muscle tension may decrease (see Fig. 4-14). The patella serves a similar purpose in the quadriceps muscle group. Not only does the patella increase the force arm distance and, consequently, the torque of the muscle group, but this distance increases as the

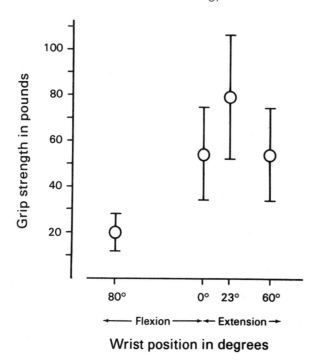

Figure 4–9 Maximum isometric grip strength in four positions of the wrist (mean and standard deviation). The wrist was maintained in 80 degrees of wrist flexion, a neutral position, and 60 degrees of extension while gripping; 23 degrees represents the mean position when subjects gripped without wrist restraint. N = 10 able-bodied adult subjects.

length-tension factor becomes less favorable. Kaufer (1971) measured a 40 percent increase in the force arm distance of the quadriceps from 120 degrees of knee flexion to complete extension (force arm changed from 3.9 cm to 5.8 cm). In the absence of the patella, both the initial force arm distance and the amount of increase with extension were less (force arm changed from 3.5 cm to 4 cm).

Speed of Contraction

Concentric and Isometric Muscle Forces

Speed means rate of motion. Velocity means rate of motion in a particular direction. The rate of muscle shortening or lengthening substantially affects the force a muscle can develop during contraction. The relationship between the maximum force developed by a human muscle with a cineplastic tunnel and the speed of contraction is shown in Figure 4–10 (see Fig. 4–19 for changes in the intact muscle). When the load that the muscle is expected to lift is near zero, the speed of a concentric contraction is the greatest (in this example, nearly 110 cm per second). As the load is increased, the speed of contraction decreases until a load that cannot be lifted is reached (Westing et al, 1988; Lord et al, 1991). At that point (200 N in this example), the speed of shortening is zero. This is a maximum isometric or zero-velocity contraction. The decrease in the contractile force with increasing speed of shortening is explained on the basis of the number of links that can be formed per unit of time between the actin and myosin filaments (see Fig. 3–7). At slow speeds, the maximum number of cross-bridges can be formed. The more rapidly the actin and myosin filaments slide past each other, the smaller the number of links that are formed between the filaments in a unit of time and the less the amount of force is developed.

A

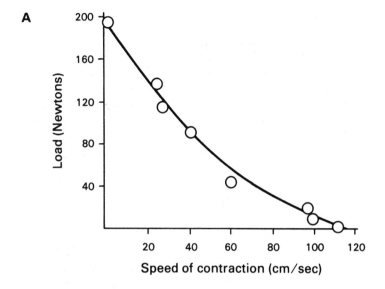

B

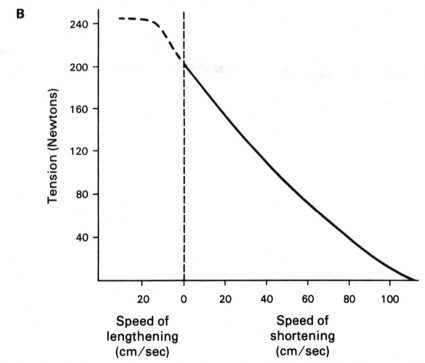

Figure 4–10 Speed of contraction versus load or tension. (*A*) The plotted values were obtained by recording directly from the tendon of the pectoralis major muscle in a subject whose arm had been amputated. Note that the speed of shortening decreased with increasing load. (Adapted from Ralston, HJ, et al: Dynamic features of human isolated voluntary muscle in isometric and free contractions. *J Appl Physiol* 1:526, 1949.) (*B*) Tension developed by the muscle when performing a maximum contraction in which the muscle lifted the load at a particular speed (shortening contraction) or lowered the load at a particular speed (lengthening contraction).

Eccentric Muscle Forces

Submaximal lengthening contractions occur at all the possible velocities in the range of the motion (Fig. 4–10A). However, when the imposed load is increased beyond the force that can be developed by the maximum isometric contraction, the muscle can no longer maintain the position. The load is lowered or decelerated with a maximum eccentric contraction (see Fig. 4–10B and Fig. 4–20). At very slow speeds, the force that the muscle can resist rises rapidly up to 50% greater than the maximum isometric contraction. This rapid increase occurs between ±10 percent of maximum concentric contraction (for the knee joint this is approximately a velocity of 30 degrees per second). The force then remains the same as the velocity increases to maximal levels (Lieber and Bodine-Fowler, 1993). For practical purposes the force of an eccentric contraction is independent of velocity (Westing et al, 1988; Griffin et al, 1993). This ability of muscles to withstand high forces is important in deceleration and shock absorption functions, which occur with high velocities of motion. Examples include throwing, in which deceleration of the forearm by an eccentric contraction of the elbow flexors is essential to prevent elbow joint injury, or running, in which an eccentric contraction of the hamstrings decelerates the swinging leg and the quadriceps femoris absorbs forces of six to seven times the body weight at foot strike (Stanton and Purdam, 1989).

ENERGY EXPENDITURE Higher maximum forces of the lengthening contraction permit lowering heavier loads (negative work) than can be lifted with a maximum shortening contraction (positive work). In the case of submaximal contractions of the same force and velocity, fewer motor units are activated by the lengthening contraction than by the shortening contraction. This phenomenon can be seen in the EMG recordings of the biceps and the triceps brachii in Figure 4–3A,B. Thus, for the same force, energy expenditure (oxygen consumption) is less for the eccentric contraction. The same findings occur with relative metabolic energy measured by P magnetic resonance spectroscopy when the subjects raise, lower, or hold weights with their finger flexor muscles. Metabolic cost with shortening contractions increases proportionally with mechanical power, while the cost of lengthening contractions is not significantly different from resting values (Menard et al, 1991).

Abbott, Bigland, and Ritchie (1952) devised an experiment to measure the relative difference in energy cost of performing positive work (such as that produced by lifting a load a certain distance by means of a concentric contraction) versus the cost of performing so-called negative work (lowering the load the same distance by means of an eccentric contraction). Two bicycle ergometers were placed back to back and coupled by a chain. When one cyclist pedaled in the conventional forward direction, the legs of the other cyclist were driven backward. When the first cyclist pedaled, the muscles shortened and performed positive work; the same muscles of the second cyclist were forcibly stretched as they resisted the motion and work was performed upon them. With practice, the cyclists learned to exert identical force and counterforce so that the pedaling speed remained constant during a given experiment. Experiments were conducted at a variety of pedaling speeds and forces. Oxygen consumption was determined for each cyclist after steady-state conditions had been attained. The results of the experiments showed that the energy cost of forward pedaling was from 2.5 to 6 times greater than the cost of resisting (equal amounts of positive and negative work performed), depending on the rate at which the work was performed. The relative cost of resisting the motion decreased as the rate of motion increased. Thus, less energy is required to lower a given load quickly than to lower it slowly. Most of the energy is used to decelerate the load to prevent it from reaching the velocity it would attain in a free fall.

Dick and Cavanagh (1987) demonstrated that while negative work (running downhill) required less oxygen consumption than positive work (running on the level), there was a gradual increase in oxygen consumption of negative work with time. Oxygen consumption for running at 3.83 M per second at 10 minutes was 33 percent less for running downhill (10 percent grade) than for running on a level surface. There was, however, a 10 percent increase in oxygen consumption in downhill running by 40 minutes, and an increase of only 1.5 percent in level running. The authors also found that EMG activity of the quadriceps femoris muscle during downhill running increased 23 percent between 10 and 40 minutes. The increases in oxygen consumption and EMG activity were proposed to be from muscle fiber and connective tissue damage, which is frequently associated with maximum lengthening contractions and additional motor unit recruitment because of fatigue.

DIFFERENCES IN CROSS-BRIDGE MECHANISMS The ability of the lengthening contraction to exceed the forces of the shortening and isometric contractions, with greater energy efficiency and with independence from velocity of contraction, indicates different mechanisms for the cross-bridges. It is suggested that the attachment, power stroke, and detachment of the cross-bridge may be limited to the shortening contraction and that mechanisms to provide greater force in the isometric and lengthening contractions are different. Differences proposed include strong and weak binding forms of actinomyosin and ATP, multiple active sites on the cross-bridges, different myosin head arrangement, and different states of cross-bridge affinity for attachment or detachment (Huxley, 1990; Sugi and Pollack, 1993). Lombardi and Piazzesi (1990) demonstrated that the tension produced during lengthening contractions of frog muscle fiber was due to a 10 to 20 percent increase in active cross-bridge formation (over that of isometric contraction) and not due to the elastic components of the fiber. The authors present a model of a different type of cross-bridge cycle triggered by steady lengthening (stretch) of the contracted fiber. This cycle produces an early forced detachment of the stretched myosin head in an energized state capable of immediate reattachment to actin. This reattachment occurs 200 times faster than the cycle of the shortening contraction. The stretch stimulus of the contracting muscle occurs below the critical level of 10 percent of the maximum shortening contraction, which can be visualized in Fig. 4–10B (Edman, 1993). The lower EMG activity for comparable loads supports that fewer muscle fibers are activated for a comparable lengthening contraction (Stauber, 1989). Thus, there is a reserve to protect the structures of the muscle fiber if greater forces are needed.

Elastic Forces of Muscle

During activities such as running and jumping, it has been observed since the time of Marey and Demeny (1887) that muscles sometimes behave as if they were capable of storing and transmitting elastic energy. For example, if one performs a maximum vertical jump twice in a row, the second jump is always higher; or if a squat jump is preceded by a quick counterstretch of the contracting hip and knee extensor and plantar flexor muscles, the jump is higher (Komi, 1984; Hakkinen, Komi, and Kauhanen, 1986).

This phenomenon occurs when the muscle is performing negative work (eccentric contraction) and the muscle is contracting while being stretched. The energy absorbed by the muscle is usually dissipated in heat. The contracting muscle, however, can store this energy briefly. If, at this time, a maximum concentric contraction of the muscle is performed, the stored energy can be recovered to increase the force, speed, and power of the contraction beyond that of an isolated maximum concentric contraction (Cavagna, 1977). Activities such as running, in which this type of eccentric-concentric contractions occurs, show a surprising increase in efficiency with increased speed. In the hopping kangaroo, efficiency increases from 0.23 at 10 km per hour to 0.62 at 27.5 km/hour (Cavagna, 1977).

The magnitude of this concentric contraction increases with the intensity of the prestretch (Aura and Komi, 1986). These authors found that EMG activity of the eccentric contraction also increased with the intensity of the prestretch but that there was little change in the EMG of the concentric contraction. Thus, the greater force of the concentric contraction occurs without increased energy expenditure. There is a very short coupling time of the eccentric-concentric contraction. If the stretch is maintained too long (more than one second) or the muscle relaxes, the elastic energy is dissipated in heat. The genesis of this enhancement of the concentric contraction was once thought to be due to elasticity of the connective tissues. Currently the increased force is thought to be due to neural factors including the muscle spindles, Golgi tendon organs, and particularly the force generated by the actin-myosin cross-bridges (Cavagna, 1977; Komi, 1984; Wilk et al, 1993).

This enhancement of the maximum concentric contraction is called the *stretch-shortening cycle* (Komi, 1984). The cycle is used to increase maximum concentric contractions and thereby performance in many sports activities, such as walking, running, jumping, throwing, gymnastics, skiing, and weight lifting. The stretch-shortening cycle also is used in exercise systems such as Proprioceptive Neuromuscular Facilitation (Voss, Ionta, and Myers, 1985) and Plyometrics (Wilk et al, 1993) to obtain stronger concentric muscle contractions. Aspects of the enhancement of the concentric contraction can be seen in the maximum concentric-eccentric contractions in Fig. 4–20. Because of the short time for coupling of the eccentric-concentric contraction, skill and learning are major aspects in achieving maximum performance.

QUANTITATIVE MEASUREMENT OF MUSCLE STRENGTH

Maximum Isometric Muscle Torques

The maximum isometric strength that a muscle group is able to produce can be measured indirectly by having the subject make a maximum effort against a fixed resistance on the bony lever. The force produced is recorded by a transducer, which may be a scale, tensiometer, electronic strain gauge, hand-held dynamometer, or an isokinetic dynamometer that records in torque. When force is recorded, it is multiplied by the distance between the joint axis and the point of attachment of the force transducer to measure the resistance torque ($\tau_R = F \times \perp d$). This value is the same as the muscle torque because at equilibrium the sum of the torques is zero ($\Sigma\tau = 0$; $\tau_M + \tau_R = 0$ or $\tau_M = \tau_R$). Torque is the preferred form of reporting because it is independent of lever arm length and is comparable among individuals when different lever arm lengths are used. Force measurements, on the other hand, change (inversely) with the lever arm length. Rigid control of stabilization and body position are important as well as coupling the force transducer at a right angle to the body segment (Mendler, 1967b). The hand-held dynamometer introduces the added factors of strength and skill of the examiner in meeting the maximum isometric force of the subject and not causing an eccentric contraction or permitting a concentric contraction causing false high or low volumes (Wikholm and Bohannon, 1991).

Early investigators measured maximum isometric force at different points in the range of motion to study the magnitudes and characteristic strength patterns of muscle groups (Figs. 4–11 through 4–18). Although the results of these studies were often labeled "torque curves," it should be noted that the measurements were expressed as pounds force or kilograms. Nevertheless, these studies have made a valuable contribution to the understanding of characteristics of muscle strength. Because the lever arm lengths were constant within each study, the shapes of the curves for force are parallel to those of torque.

Inspection of these curves shows that maximum isometric force changes markedly within the range of motion (40 to 80 percent). Most of the muscles show greater strength when they contract from their elongated position (stretched) than when they contract from their shortened (slack) position. The pronator muscles, for example, show maximum force when the forearm is fully supinated and the least force when the forearm is pronated (see Fig. 4–13). This pattern reflects the length-tension effect. In muscle groups such as the pronators-supinators (see Fig. 4–13), hip flexors (see Fig. 4–15), and the hip abductors-adductors (see Fig. 4–16), a linear decrease in strength shows that the length-tension factor is predominant. Figure 4–17 on the knee flexor muscles shows the effect of increasing the force of the muscles by flexing the hip to increase the stretch on the hamstring muscles. Curves for the elbow flexor muscles (see Fig. 4–14) and the quadriceps femoris muscle (see Fig. 4–18) show peak forces in mid-range of motion. This pattern is one in which the leverage factor is superimposed on the length-tension curve to increase torque in mid-range. In these cases there are marked increases in the muscle lever arm length at mid-range, as can be seen in Figure 2–36 on the elbow flexors. The patella and the shape of the intercondylar groove of the femur increase the lever arm length for the quadriceps femoris muscles at mid-range of knee flexion (Smidt, 1973).

The characteristic patterns of the relationships between joint angle and muscle strength usually can be related to functions that require great force, such as maximum strength of the elbow flexors being available at a joint angle of 90 degrees of flexion, which is a position important for carrying heavy articles. Maximum strength of the knee extensor muscles at 60 degrees of flexion is the position where great force is needed to elevate the body when an individual is rising from a chair or climbing stairs. In Figures 4–12, 4–13, and 4–16, maximum isometric forces of antagonistic muscle groups are recorded. At one point in the range, one muscle is stronger. At another point, the muscles have equal strength. At the other end of the motion, the antagonistic muscle is stronger. Thus, questions of which muscle group is stronger or ratios of strength have little meaning unless referenced to a specific point in the range of motion.

Maximum Isokinetic Torque Curves

The introduction of isokinetic dynamometers that keep speed constant in the range of motion permitted recording of concentric and, later, eccentric muscle

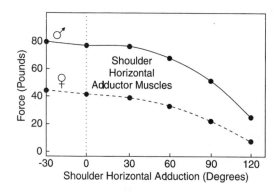

Figure 4–11 Maximum isometric force of the shoulder horizontal adductor muscles (pectoralis major, anterior deltoid, and coracobrachialis muscles) in college men and women. The authors are calling 0 degrees of horizontal adduction the same position as 90 degrees of shoulder abduction. In this illustration, 90 degrees of horizontal adduction is the same as 90 degrees of shoulder flexion. The muscle group demonstrates the greatest force when it is elongated. (Redrawn from Williams and Stutzman, 1959, with permission.)

Figure 4–12 Maximum isometric force of the shoulder flexor muscles (anterior deltoid, coracobrachialis, biceps brachii) and the shoulder extensor muscles (posterior deltoid, teres major, latissimus dorsi, and triceps brachii). Comparison of agonist-antagonist muscle groups in college men. Solid curve = shoulder flexor muscles; dotted curve = shoulder extensor muscles. (Redrawn from Williams and Stutzman, 1959, with permission.)

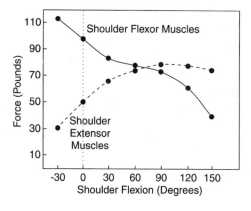

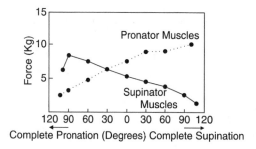

Figure 4–13 Maximum isometric force curves of the pronators (pronator teres and quadratus) and supinators (supinator and biceps brachii) of the right forearm in four male subjects. Solid curve = supinators; dotted curve = pronators. Elbow at 90 degrees of flexion. (Redrawn from Bethe and Franke, 1919.)

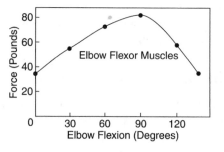

Figure 4–14 Maximum isometric force of elbow flexors (brachialis, biceps brachii, and brachioradialis) in college men. (Redrawn from Williams and Stutzman, 1959, with permission.)

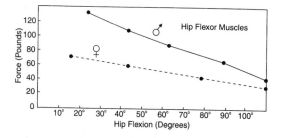

Figure 4–15 Maximum isometric force of the hip flexors (iliopsoas, rectus femoris, sartorius, tensor fasciae latae, pectineus, and adductors) in college men and women. (Redrawn from Williams and Stutzman, 1959, with permission.)

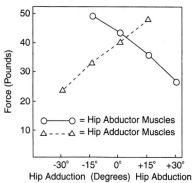

Figure 4–16 Maximum isometric force of the hip abductor (gluteus medius and minimus and tensor fasciae latae and the hip adductor muscles (pectineus; adductors longus, brevis, and magnus; and gracilis) in 25 males aged 20 to 28 years, N = 50. (Plotted from data published by May, WW: Relative isometric force of the hip abductor and adductor muscles. Phys Ther 48:845, 1968.)

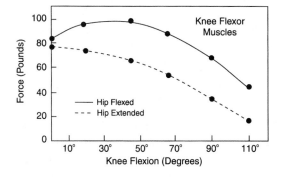

Figure 4–17 Maximum isometric force of the knee flexor muscles (semimembranosis, semitendinosis, biceps femoris, and gastrocnemius). Effect of change of hip position on muscle force. Solid curve = 90 degrees of hip flexion, placing more stretch on the hamstring muscles. Dotted curve = hip in 0 degrees of hip flexion. (Redrawn from Williams and Stutzman, 1959, with permission.)

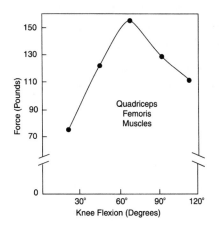

Figure 4–18 Maximum isometric force of the knee extensor muscles (quadriceps femoris) in college men. (Redrawn from Williams and Stutzman, 1959, with permission.)

torques at velocities up to 300 degrees per second (Figs. 4–19 and 4–20). However, people often have difficulty keeping up with the machine at and above 180 degrees per second.

Neither the first nor the last parts of the isokinetic curve are true measures of torque at the stated speed because the segment is either accelerating or decelerating. Acceleration time from 30 to 300 degrees per second was found to vary from 0.03 to 0.08 seconds and to produce errors in work up to 11 percent at the higher velocities and in women (Chen, Su, and Chow, 1994). When the end ranges of isokinetic curves are excluded and corrections are made for the effects of gravity on the weight of the instrument lever arm and the body segment, the shape of the isokinetic concentric curve is similar to the isometric curve (Knapik et al, 1983; Kues, Rothstein, and Lamb, 1994). At less than 30 degrees per second, the magnitude of the concentric isokinetic curves is similar but lower than the isometric contractions. With increasing velocity, the magnitude of these torque curves progressively decreases (see Fig. 4–19).

Recent models of the isokinetic dynamometers are computerized and can display a vast array of derivatives and graphics of torque, work, and power with time, motion, and body weight. Work is torque times angular displacement, and power is work divided by time. These measurements are useful for repetitive and endurance tests. Twenty-five different relationships of isometric, concentric, and eccentric isokinetic torques of the knee extensors were compared and found to be moderately or highly correlated (Kues, Rothstein, and Lamb, 1994). These findings suggest that the many different measurements and derivatives provided by the isokinetic dynamometer are assessing similar aspects of muscle strength. For most clinical orthopedic applications of the knee, peak torque at 60 degrees per second is sufficient unless it is necessary to reduce the joint compression force with a higher velocity (Sapega, 1990).

Reproducibility of Quantitative Muscle Torque Testing

A major use of quantitative force testing is for determining whether there is an increase, decrease, or no change in muscle strength with time, exercise, or treatment. Accurate and reproducible measurements of maximum muscle strength are, however, complex and difficult to achieve. Sapega (1990) well identifies the challenge of quantitative force testing: "It is deceptively easy to measure something other than what one is actually attempting to measure, and it is surprisingly difficult to measure any parameter of muscular performance in reproducible fashion."

Even with the simple measurement of maximum grip strength, there is considerable variability. Grip strength is a familiar activity and not thought to need training or to have a learning effect with repeated testing. Precision of body positions and stabilization are not necessary with grip testing as with measurements of torque in other muscle groups. If the person is permitted postural freedom to perform the grip procedure, the body will select optimum muscle lengths and joint positions to produce a maximum contraction. When free motion is permitted, there are no muscle groups that can provide substitute forces for finger flexion as can happen if the hand dynamometer is stabilized.

An hourly variation of grip strength paralleling body temperature changes occurs. There is a marked drop in strength from midnight to 6 AM and a marked rise from 6 AM to 10 AM (Wright, 1959). Hourly grip strength values during waking hours from 8 AM to 10 PM showed an average coefficient of variation (CV) of ±7

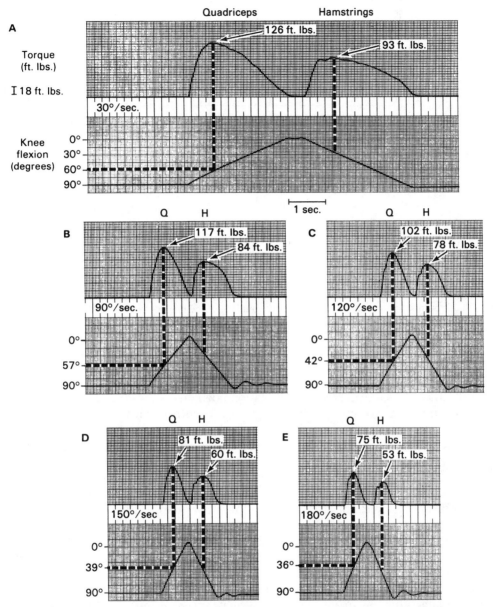

Figure 4–19 Maximum isokinetic concentric torque of the quadriceps (Q) and hamstring (H) muscle groups at 5 velocities of motion *(A–E):* 30, 90, 120, 150, and 180 degrees per sec, respectively. The upper tracing records torque and the lower tracing records knee joint position. Vertical dotted lines have been added to connect the point of peak torque with knee joint position. With corrections for the weight of the leg and lever arm and for acceleration in the early part of the curve, the angle of peak torque is more constant with velocity. (Record adapted from Cybex test results, CYBEX, Ronkonkoma, NY.)

percent in college women (Smith, 1980). CV is one standard deviation from the mean expressed as percent (CV% = SD/X × 100). Thus, with a grip strength of 100 lb, normal hourly variability of two standard deviations would be ±14 lb. The CV for grip-strength measurements taken at the same time of day for 4 weeks was found to be ±6 percent in college men and women (Nilsson, 1978). Weinland

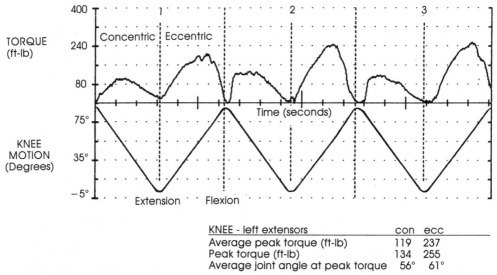

KNEE - left extensors	con	ecc
Average peak torque (ft-lb)	119	237
Peak torque (ft-lb)	134	255
Average joint angle at peak torque	56°	61°

Figure 4–20 Three consecutive maximum isokinetic concentric-eccentric contractions of the quadriceps femoris at 30 degrees per second. The upper record is muscle torque in ft-lb and the lower record is knee range of motion in degrees. Note the rapid coupling of the first eccentric contraction with the second concentric contraction. Note, also, the slower coupling and lower concentric peak torque in the next coupling. Corrections are included for the weight of the lever arm and the leg. (Record adapted from Lido Test Results, Loredan, Sacramento, CA.)

(1947) measured his own grip strength daily for 5 months and found a CV of 5 percent. Both authors found positive correlation coefficients indicating that either neuromuscular learning or increase in strength was occurring with the measurements.

In other muscle groups where torque is measured on the body segment, strong stabilization is needed to prevent motion of proximal muscle attachments and false low forces (Mendler, 1967[b]). For example, the gastrocnemius-soleus muscle group of the calf has been measured with a mean isometric force of 2.4 times body weight at the ball of the foot (Beasley, 1961). For a 150-lb person, the plantar flexion force is 360 lb (SD = +49 lb). Most quantitative force equipment is not able to provide closed-system stabilization to measure this magnitude of force. On the other hand, inadequate stabilization can also permit other muscles to increase the force by substitute actions such as adding a pull or push on the transducer to provide overestimation of the force. Precision in positioning of the joints as well as the total body is essential, for even slight changes in muscle length can produce large changes in muscle force (Bohannon, Gajdosik, and LeVeau, 1986). Some of the additional factors that require attention are instrument calibration, corrections for the effects of gravity, precision in control of velocity of motion, accuracy in the interface of the body part and the instrument, absence of pain or discomfort, subject training and motivation to make a maximum effort, and control of environmental factors.

NEURAL ADAPTATION One of the major factors affecting reproducibility of repeated strength test scores is *neural adaptation* (Sale, 1988). This was previously called motor learning or specificity of exercise. The phenomenon has to do with the tremendous capacity of the body to learn to increase an exercise performance as simple as a maximum isometric contraction performed once a week (Schenck and Forward, 1965). This effect can be seen in the positive correlation coefficients in the daily grip strength recordings (Weinland, 1947; Nilsson, 1978). Other evidence includes the "cross-training effect," in which the unexercised extremity increases performance (Housh and Housh, 1993) when there is no increase in muscle size and when performance gains are maintained 6 to 12 months after the training has stopped. Neural adaptation is specific to a particular task or form of strength testing and does not carry over well into function or other measures of strength. When the test and training are the same, large "apparent strength" gains are made, but when the test is different from the training, strength gains are considerably less. For example, Frontera and coworkers (1988) trained the knee extensors in older men by having them lift the weight equivalent of 80 percent of 1 repetition maximum (1 RM) in 3 sets of 8 repetitions three times a week for 12 weeks. The subjects increased the training load of 1 RM by an average of 112 percent. Peak maximum isometric torque, however, increased only 7 percent, and peak isokinetic torque at 60 degrees per second increased only 9 percent. The area of the quadriceps muscle increased 10 percent as measured from a computed tomography (CT) scan, and the analysis of muscle biopsies showed an increased muscle fiber area of 30 percent. These findings illustrate the large gains that occur from neural adaptation to a specific task and the need for additional measures to assess strength changes, which can be generalized to many exercises and functions.

Studies on the reliability of strength measurements vary with the joint, population, procedure, time elapsed, and technique. Pearson correlation coefficients for the knee and elbow flexors and extensors in people averaging 60 years of age were .58 to .77 at two test sessions (Frontera et al, 1993). The effect of neural adaptation can be reduced with prior practice either before the study starts or before each session. Practice is possible in the research situation using normal subjects but is not usually possible in the clinical situation. With practice sessions, reliability coefficients of .98 were found for concentric-eccentric contractions of the quadriceps (Helgeson and Gajdosik, 1993), .75 to .86 for eccentric contractions of the rotators of the shoulder (Frissello et al, 1994), and .80 to .91 for eccentric quadriceps contractions (Steiner et al, 1993). The latter authors state that clinicians should be aware that variation in measurement of muscle torques from 14 to 30 percent can occur simply from repeated testing.

CLINICAL APPLICATIONS

Exercise-Induced Muscle Injury

Two injuries common in strenuous exercise are attributed to the great forces that occur with maximum eccentric muscle contractions. These can produce up to twice the force of a maximum isometric contraction. One injury is delayed-onset muscle soreness (DOMS), which occurs 8 to 12 hours after the activity and is most severe 48 to 60 hours postexercise. Other functional signs of DOMS are decrease in range of motion because of pain and decrease in maximum concentric and eccentric muscle forces of +50 percent depending on the intensity of the exercise (Clarkson and Tremblay, 1988; Faulkner, Brook, and Opiteck, 1993; Rodenburg, Bar, and DeBoer, 1993). Biochemical signs of injury and destruction of muscle include abnormally high levels of creatine kinase (a muscle enzyme) and myoglobin in venous blood, as well as increased plasma concentrations of myosin heavy-chain fragments from slow-twitch muscle fibers (Golden and Dudley, 1992; Mair et al, 1992). Structural damage to the Z lines with zigzag appearance and sometimes dissolution has been found (Z lines border the ends of the sarcomeres and are a base of attachment of the actin myofilaments; see Fig. 3–1). This alteration of the Z line changes the alignment of the myofilaments, and, in some cases, the myosin filaments are absent (Friden and Lieber, 1992; Faulkner, Brook, and Opiteck, 1993).

Recovery from the functional and structural injuries of DOMS requires from 5 to 30 days depending on the severity of the initial exercise. If, after recovery, the eccentric exercise or activity is repeated, it has been found that muscle soreness does not occur, and the muscle has adapted to the exercise. Even greater eccentric forces can be made; there are minimal signs of muscle damage, but if injury occurs, recovery is more rapid (Clarkson and Tremblay, 1988; Golden and Dudley, 1992).

Prevention of DOMS and the development of the ability to perform high-intensity maximum isometric contractions can occur with training and gradual increases in intensity of activity. In one study, when 24 maximum eccentric contractions were made 2 weeks before performing 70 maximum contractions, the symptoms of DOMS were mild, with recovery occurring within 5 days. With a single 70-maximum contraction bout, symptoms were significantly more severe, and recovery required more than 5 days (Clarkson and Tremblay, 1988).

The second type of exercise-induced muscle injury is the hamstring muscle "pull," which occurs most often in sprinting and jumping activities. This is a sudden and severe injury, frequently causing the athlete to fall to the ground in agony. The injury is a macro–muscle tear of a hamstring with hemorrhage into the muscle. The tear occurs during the late swing phase and early stance phase of running. At this time, the hamstrings are decelerating the forward movement of the thigh and the leg with a maximum eccentric contraction (lengthening) and then instantaneously changing at foot strike to a maximum concentric (shortening) contraction to accelerate the thigh (hip extension) and prevent knee hyperextension.

Stretch-shortening exercises whereby the hamstrings perform a short eccentric contraction immediately followed by a concentric contraction are proposed for rehabilitation of athletes with hamstring muscle pulls and for improvement of the eccentric-concentric coupling to reduce the incidence of the injury (Stanton and Purdam, 1989).

Changes of Muscle Lengths and Lever Arms

Muscle and tendon lengths can be changed by trauma, surgery, or immobilization and thereby alter their length-tension curve and the force that the muscle produces. An example occurs with surgical removal of an inch of the femur to equalize a leg-length discrepancy. All the muscles of the thigh are placed on a slack and are contracting on the lower weak part of the length-tension curve. The quadriceps and the hamstrings lose a significant amount of muscle strength to extend and flex the knee. In time, remodeling of the muscle occurs (loss of sarcomeres), and the contractions become more effective. If, on the other hand, a muscle or tendon such as the flexor carpi radialis (wrist flexor) is abnormally shortened, contraction moves up on the curve and passive tension forces predominate and may prevent wrist extension. In turn, the inability to extend the wrist weakens grip strength because the long finger flexors are on the low part of their length-tension curve.

Surgical alteration of muscle lever arms can alter the torque or strength of muscles. Steindler (1955) developed a method to provide elbow flexion when the biceps brachii and the brachialis were paralyzed and the subject could not flex the elbow. The proximal attachments of the wrist extensors and the pronator teres were moved higher on the humerus to increase their lever arm distances for elbow flexion. This procedure provided satisfactory elbow flexion but also limited elbow extension because of the increased passive tension forces.

Bone loss from fractures can decrease the length of muscle lever arms and muscle strength. Rietveld and coworkers (1988) reported on subjects with extensive fractures of the proximal humerus who were treated with hemiarthroplasty (replacement of the head of the humerus with a metal prosthesis). Some of the subjects failed to gain active abduction of the shoulder even though they had sufficient range of motion and active contraction of the deltoid muscle. These subjects had a decrease in the distance from the center of the humeral head to the lateral surface of the greater tuberosity from 33 mm on the normal shoulder to 12.5 mm on the injured side. This was a 62 percent decrease in the lever arm distance for the deltoid muscle and caused the deltoid force vector to be vertical or at a negative angle. When the muscle contracted, the humerus was directed vertically into the acromion process, and abduction could not occur. Normally, the greater tuberosity directs the force vector of the deltoid laterally at a 10- to 15-degree angle to initiate the motion of abduction (see Fig. 7–20A). The authors recommend that the lever arm principle must be considered in other shoulder conditions and in the design of joint prostheses to allow better function.

Laboratory Activities |

MUSCLE ACTIVITY AND STRENGTH

Demonstrations of the phenomena described in this chapter require force testing, EMG equipment, and an instructor skilled in this type of testing. With attention to detail, however, the following demonstrations can be done using isometric contractions and a hand-held dynamometer. The grip dynamometer in Fig. 6–31 can be modified for use on the extremities by padding with a closed-cell synthetic foam.

1. Part of the length-tension curve for the intact hamstring muscles can be recorded with the subject sitting on a table, the knee in 90 degrees of flexion, and the hip flexion angle changed from 90 degrees (sitting) to 45 degrees (reclining on elbows), and then to 0 degrees (lying down).

   For each position the examiner places the dynamometer at a marked point on the posterior surface of the leg near the ankle and holds the dynamometer still to meet the maximum isometric force produced by the hamstrings in a 4- to 5-second contraction. The subject should provide self-stabilization by holding on with the hands, and the thigh should be stabilized by straps or another person **so that the knee and hip angles do not change during the contraction.**

   The hamstring muscle length can be approximated by measuring the distance between the head of the fibula and the tuberosity of the ischium for each of the three test positions. To make comparisons between subjects, the force measurement should be converted to torque (multiply the force by the distance between the point of dynamometer application and the axis of the knee joint).

Sources of error include inadequate stabilization, failure to obtain maximum isometric contractions, examiner permitting an eccentric or concentric contraction, changing knee-joint angles between tests, subject fatigue from too many contractions or inadequate rest periods, changing placement of dynamometer between tests, and measurements of distances.

2. Using a grip dynamometer, record your partner's maximum grip strength (dynamometers record maximum contractions within 3 to 4 seconds). Allow 30 to 45 seconds of rest, repeat two times, and record each. Then have the subject perform three 75 percent maximum contractions (without knowledge of results and with rest periods). Note that the true maximum contractions are not exactly the same but are very close. This is one way to determine if a person has performed a maximum contraction. The 75 percent contractions are similar to those made by a person who is not motivated or is trying to simulate muscle weakness. There is marked variability to show that this is not a true maximum contraction.

3. Record your partner's maximum grip strength and then repeat the procedure while you hold his or her wrist in 90 degrees of wrist flexion. This requires that the holder be stronger than the one gripping or that other strong stabilization of the forearm and hand be made. Note the marked decrease in the strength of grip because of passive insufficiency of the finger extensors and active insufficiency of the finger flexors.

4. Record your own maximum grip strength 3 to 5 days a week for a month at the same time of day $\pm^{1}/_{2}$ hour. Use the same dynamometer, at the same handspan, and use the same body posture. Note any unusual events on your record. Calculate the mean, standard deviation, and CV of your results (CV% = SD/X × 100).

CHAPTER 5

Elbow and Forearm

The elbow is a structurally stable joint that contains three articulations within a single joint capsule: the ulnohumeral and the radiohumeral joints, which permit flexion and extension, and the proximal radioulnar joint, which permits pronation and supination. The two degrees of freedom serve hand placement by rotating the forearm and lengthening or shortening the distance of the hand to the shoulder. The elbow also is important in elevating the body as in pull-ups and push-ups.

BONES

Palpable Structures

Epicondyles

The epicondyles are bony prominences on the distal enlargements (condyles) of the humerus. Since they are readily identified, they serve as landmarks in this region. When the shoulder is externally rotated, the **medial epicondyle** lies close to the body; the **lateral epicondyle** lies away from the body. When the humerus is internally rotated, however, the medial epicondyle points to the rear; the lateral epicondyle points to the front. The medial epicondyle is known as the **flexor epicondyle** because it serves as the attachment for many flexor muscles of the wrist and digits. For similar reasons, the lateral epicondyle is referred to as the **extensor epicondyle.**

Olecranon Process

When the tip of the elbow is placed on the table with the forearm vertical, the prominent **olecranon process** of the ulna hits the table. This process is quite large, and by following it distally, the dorsal margin of the ulna may be palpated all the way down to the styloid process of the ulna at the wrist. If the palpating fingers move medially from the olecranon process into the groove between it and the medial epicondyle, the ulnar nerve may be felt as a round cord. Friction across the nerve at this point or slightly more proximally produces a prickling sensation in the little finger; hence, the area where the ulnar nerve can be pressed against the bone is popularly known as the "funny bone."

Head of Radius

The **head of the radius** is identified at a point just distal to the lateral epicondyle. When the elbow is fully extended, the circumference of the head of the radius may be felt rolling under the skin as pronation and supination are carried out. Once the head of the radius has been identified with the elbow extended, it should be easy to palpate when the elbow is flexed and the forearm is either supinated or pronated. (The location of the head of the radius with the forearm pronated is seen in Figures 5–5 and 5–10.)

Nonpalpable Structures

Bony structures that lie too deep to be palpated should be studied on the skeleton. Some of these are the **olecranon fossa,** the **trochlea,** and the **capitulum of the** humerus; the **trochlear notch** and the **coronoid process of the ulna**; the **neck of the radius**; and the **radial tuberosity.**

JOINTS

Elbow Joint

The **elbow** is a uniaxial joint of the hinge type (ginglymus), permitting flexion and extension by means of mixed gliding and rolling (one degree of freedom of motion). The trochlea of the humerus articulates with the trochlear notch of the ulna, while the capitulum of the humerus apposes the radius. The joint thus has ulnotrochlear and radiocapitular components that work in unison in flexion and extension. The strong structural stability of the joint is derived from both the bony configuration (corrugated) and the collateral ligaments (see Fig. 5-3).

Axis of Motion

The axis for flexion and extension of the elbow is represented by a line through the centers of the trochlea and the capitulum (Fig. 5–1A). The approximate location of this axis in the living subject may be found by grasping the elbow from side to side slightly distal to the lateral and medial epicondyles of the humerus, which are easily palpated through the skin.

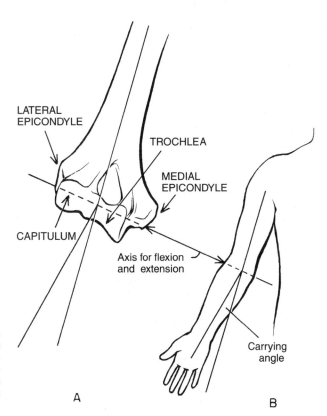

Figure 5–1 (*A*) Axis for flexion and extension of the elbow courses through the trochlea and capitulum (one degree of freedom of motion). (*B*) Carrying angle of the elbow when the forearm is supinated.

Carrying Angle

Since the trochlea extends more distally than the capitulum, the axis for flexion and extension of the elbow is not fully perpendicular to the shaft of the humerus; therefore, when the elbow is extended and the forearm supinated, the forearm deviates laterally in relation to the humerus, which accounts for the **carrying angle**, or cubital angle (Fig. 5–1B). This angle varies somewhat in individuals, the angle usually being more pronounced in women than in men. Reports of studies that measured the carrying angle give mean values from 5 to 19 degrees, with mean differences between men and women of 0 to 6 degrees (Atkinson and Elftman, 1945; Steel and Tomlinson, 1958; Beals, 1976). The variations in these values can be attributed to the different methods of measurement. Excessive lateral angulation of the forearm with respect to the humerus is known as cubitus valgus.

The carrying angle has been suggested to serve the purpose of keeping objects carried in the hand away from the body. However, the natural and common way of carrying an object in the hand is with the forearm pronated, or partly pronated; in these positions in which the radius lies across the ulna, the carrying angle is obliterated. Clearance is gained by abduction or internal rotation of the humerus at the shoulder, or both, or by lateral bending of the trunk. To date, no clear function for the carrying angle has been described.

Radioulnar Articulation

The connections between the radius and the ulna allow the radius to rotate in relation to the ulna so that in one position the two bones lie parallel (supination), and in another position the radius crosses over the ulna (pronation). The hand is attached to the radius at the radiocarpal articulation and follows the movement of the radius so that during supination the palm turns up, and during pronation the palm turns down. The movements of supination and pronation are made possible because there are two separate articulations between the radius and the ulna—one proximal, the other distal. The two joints acting together form a **uniaxial joint** (one degree of freedom) allowing pronation and supination only.

The elbow joint and the radioulnar joints thus both are uniaxial. In the elbow joint, the axis of motion is nearly transverse to the shaft of the bones, whereas in the radioulnar articulation, the axis of motion is almost parallel to the shafts of the participating bony segments (Fig. 5–2).

Axis of Motion

The axis of motion of the radioulnar articulation is represented by a line through the center of the head of the radius proximally and through the center of the head of the ulna distally (see Fig. 5–2). To locate the direction of this line in the human subject, the forearm is held supinated and the circumference of the head of the radius is identified as previously described. The head of the ulna is then palpated near the wrist on the side of the little finger. The location of the center of the heads of the two bones must then be visualized, and an imaginary line passing through these centers must be established.

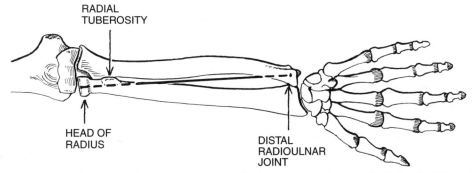

Figure 5–2 Axis for pronation and supination of the forearm courses through the head of the radius proximally and the head of the ulna distally (one degree of freedom of motion). (Redrawn from Grant: *An Atlas of Anatomy*, ed. 7. Williams & Wilkins, Baltimore, 1978.)

Proximal Radioulnar Joint

The **proximal radioulnar joint** lies within the capsule of the elbow joint and may be described as a trochoid or pivot joint. The side of the head of the radius articulates with the radial notch of the ulna. The fibrous **annular ligament** forms a ring around the head of the radius. The annular ligament has firm, fibrous connections with the ulna and is anchored to the neck of the radius by a broad ligament. The radial head thus rotates within a firm ring that permits transverse rotation while preventing movements in other directions. The shallow cup of the radial head pivots on the rounded surface of the capitulum of the humerus.

Distal Radioulnar Joint

The articular surface of the radius (ulnar notch) is concave so that the radius (with wrist and hand) can pivot around the head of the ulna while staying in close proximity to it. An articular disk is interposed between the head of the ulna and the adjacent carpal bones.

Range of Motion

The range of motion of elbow flexion averages 145 degrees, with a normal variation from 120 to 160 degrees. This is among the most variable joint ranges in the body. The motion is usually stopped by contact of the muscles between the forearm and arm with a soft end-feel. In heavily muscled and obese persons, the flexion range can be so reduced that the person may not be able to place the fingers on the shoulder. In lay terminology, this limitation of motion is called being "musclebound." On the other hand, people with little soft tissue have a hard end-feel with bone contact of the coronoid process of the ulna into the coronoid fossa of the humerus.

Elbow extension has a hard end-feel with contact of the olecranon process of the ulna and the olecranon fossa of the humerus. Average motion of extension is 0 degrees with only a few degrees of variation normally found. People who are heavily muscled and with strong ligaments may lack a few degrees of elbow extension, whereas those of lighter structure may have up to 5 degrees or more of normal hyperextension. Clinically, a few degrees of elbow hyperextension is of great functional use to persons with spinal cord severance and quadriplegic involvement with paralysis of their triceps brachii muscles. These individuals cannot hold their elbows extended to push doors or objects or to elevate their bodies in the sitting position. If they have a few degrees of elbow hyperextension, they can learn to use gravity and leverage to lock their elbows and thereby gain some ability to push light objects or perform a sitting push-up to lift their buttocks to permit capillary circulation and prevent pressure sores.

Conventionally, the range of motion of the radioulnar joints is considered to be 90 degrees for supination and 90 degrees for pronation taken from the midposition of the forearm. Most people have only about 80 degrees of pronation.

When range of pronation-supination is observed, the elbow should be held flexed and in contact with the side of the body. This prevents the shoulder from participating in the hand position. The entire range of pronation starting from the fully supinated position is slightly less than 180 degrees (average is 170 degrees). If pronation and supination are carried out with the elbow extended, internal and external rotation of the shoulder occur simultaneously with forearm motions; in this case, the palm of the hand can be turned through almost a full circle or approximately 360 degrees.

Accessory Motions

Accessory motions of the elbow are small compared to the motions possible in the shoulder, wrist, and fingers. The great stability of the joint is due to the corrugated fit of the trochlea and capitulum of the humerus with the matching surfaces of the ulna and radius as well as to the strong medial and lateral collateral ligaments that blend with the joint capsule both anteriorly and posteriorly (Fig. 5–3). When the elbow is flexed, a slight amount of distraction can be felt if the distal end of the humerus is stabilized and posterior force is applied to the anterior surface of the proximal forearm. Mediolateral joint play movements are also present. At the proximal radioulnar joint, dorsoventral gliding of the head of the radius on the capitulum of the humerus can be produced passively.* Determination of normal accessory motions requires that the subject be positioned for and instructed in muscle relaxation, because any muscle contraction causes joint compression, which prevents the evaluation of accessory motions.

The closed-packed position or the most mechanically stable position of the elbow is extension and for the radioulnar joints, 5 degrees of supination.

---

*Students are advised to learn the accessory movements in the metacarpophalangeal joint, the wrist, or even the shoulder before attempting to evaluate the smaller and difficult-to-isolate movements of the elbow.

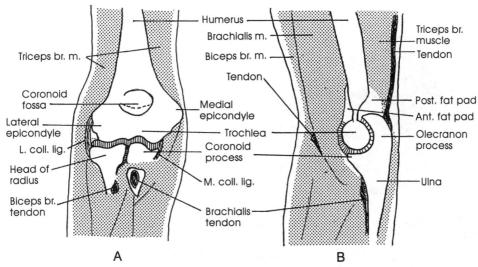

Figure 5–3   (*A*) Coronal plane and (*B*) sagittal plane views of the elbow illustrate the strong bony and ligamentous stability of the joint. Note the corrugated structure of the distal surface of the humerus with the proximal surfaces of the radius and ulna.

MUSCLES

Elbow Flexors

The primary muscles that flex the elbow are the **brachialis, biceps brachii,** and **brachioradialis.** The **pronator teres** and the **extensor carpi radialis longus and brevis** have less leverage and are of smaller size. By manipulating the soft tissue of the arm as seen in Figure 5–4, the biceps brachii, the brachialis, and the flexors of the elbow may be separated from the triceps. Anatomically, these muscle groups are separated both medially and laterally by intermuscular septa of the fasciae. The biceps, originating above the shoulder joint and attaching below the elbow joint, has no direct connection with the humerus and can be moved about easily.

The radial group on the forearm consists of the brachioradialis and extensor carpi radialis longus and brevis. The proximal attachments of all three occur in the region of the lateral epicondyle. When the elbow is flexed, their line of pull is anterior to the axis of the elbow joint. This group is best manipulated when the elbow is flexed and the forearm is in midposition between pronation and supination. In Figure 5–5, a pencil has been placed between the radial and the dorsoulnar group. The bulging shape of the radial groups is seen in Figure 5–6 as the subject grasps around the adjacent dorsoulnar group.

Muscles on the volar-ulnar side of the forearm have their proximal attachments in the region of the medial (flexor) epicondyle of the humerus and are also elbow flexors. They are the pronator teres, flexor carpi radialis and ulnaris, palmaris longus, and the humeral head of the flexor digitorum superficialis. Figure 5–7 illustrates how this group may be identified. The muscles in this group also act in pronation of the forearm or in flexion of the wrist and digits.

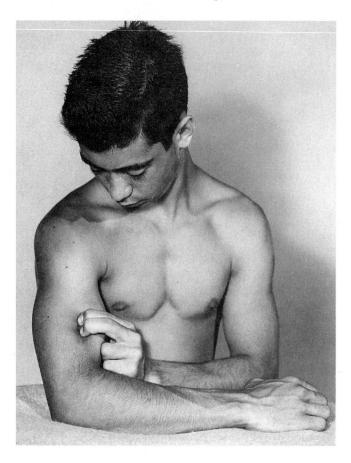

Figure 5–4 Grasp to separate biceps and brachialis from triceps.

Biceps Brachii

The muscular portion of the biceps is located above the elbow. **Proximal attachments:** by two heads from above the glenohumeral joint. The long head is attached by a long tendon from the supraglenoid tubercle of the scapula. The tendon courses within the capsule of the glenohumeral joint and in the intertubercular groove of the humerus. The short head is attached, also by a long tendon, from the coracoid process of the scapula. The two heads have separate bellies in the proximal portion of the arm, and these fuse to form one belly in the middle of the arm. The muscle fibers belonging to the short head make up the medial portion of the common belly, whereas those of the long head make up the lateral portion. **Distal attachment:** tuberosity of the radius and, in part, spreading out to form the bicipital aponeurosis (lacertus fibrosus). **Innervation:** musculocutaneous nerve (C_5-C_6). **Anatomic actions:** shoulder flexion, elbow flexion, and supination of the radioulnar joint.

INSPECTION AND PALPATION The biceps brachii is one of the easiest muscles to identify; to the layman, "making a muscle" means tightening the biceps. The contour of the biceps in a muscular individual is seen in Figure 5–8. The tendon of the biceps is best identified in the "fold" of the elbow when the forearm is supinated. In a muscular subject, the tendon is rather broad, as shown by the examiner's grasp. The examiner's thumb indicates the location of that part of the tendon that dips

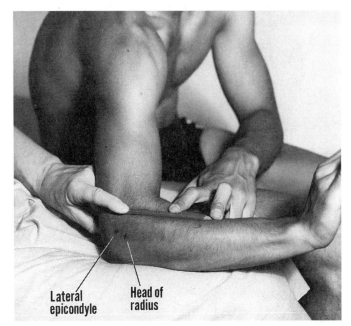

Lateral
epicondyle

Head of
radius

Figure 5–5 Separating the radial group of the forearm (brachioradialis, extensor carpi radialis longus, and extensor carpi radialis brevis) from the dorsoulnar group. Proximal cross-mark is the lateral epicondyle; distal cross-mark, the head of the radius.

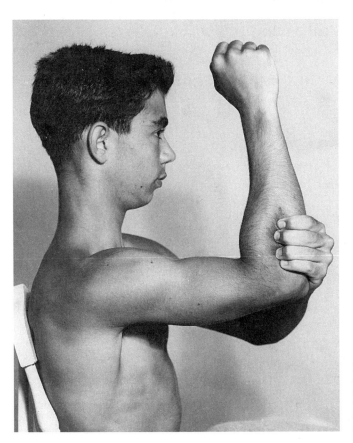

Figure 5–6 Grasp around the dorsoulnar group, simultaneously showing the area of palpation for the supinator. The radial group is being pushed aside.

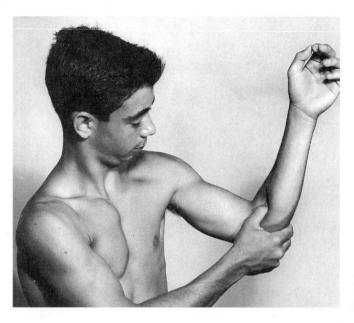

Figure 5–7 Grasping around the volar-ulnar (pronator) group.

into the antecubital fossa on its way to the tuberosity of the radius. The examiner's index finger is seen palpating the bicipital aponeurosis, which spreads out to cover the pronator teres and other muscles of this region.

The biceps and its tendons should next be palpated when the muscle is relaxed, as when the forearm rests on the table or in the lap. It is then possible to

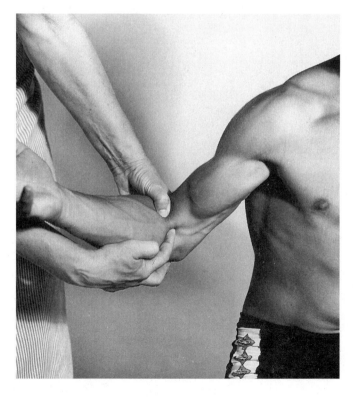

Figure 5–8 The characteristic contour of the biceps is brought out by flexion of the elbow and supination of the forearm. The examiner grasps around the tendon of biceps in the "fold" of the elbow.

grasp around the muscle, lift it from underlying structures, and move it from side to side, a maneuver that is useful in separating it from the more deeply located brachialis muscle (see Fig. 5–4).

When a fist is made, as in squeezing a hand dynamometer, both the elbow flexors and the triceps can be palpated to contract with a tension roughly proportionate to the amount of force recorded on the dynamometer. These contractions are automatic and cannot be inhibited by will. The purpose of synergistic contractions of the elbow muscles in gripping is to stabilize the elbow and thus the proximal attachments of the finger and wrist muscles. Without such stabilization, much of the muscle forces would be dissipated from grip into motions of the elbow. Palpation of the shoulder during the grip-strength maneuver also demonstrates strong contractions to stabilize the proximal attachments of the biceps and triceps.

Brachialis

The **brachialis** muscle has its proximal attachment halfway up the shaft of the humerus and is attached distally to the coronoid process of the ulna and adjacent areas of the ulna. **Innervation:** musculocutaneous nerve (C_5-C_6). **Anatomic action:** elbow flexion.

PALPATION   The muscular portion of the brachialis is located in the lower half of the arm, where it is largely covered by the biceps. The palpating fingers are placed laterally and medially to the biceps, an inch or two higher than the grasp seen in Figure 5–8. The subject's forearm should be pronated and resting in the lap or on a pillow, as seen in Figure 5–4, which ensures relaxation of the biceps. If now the elbow is flexed with as little effort as possible, the contraction of the brachialis may be felt. Under these conditions, the brachialis flexes the elbow with little or no participation by the biceps. Once the palpating fingers are properly placed, a quick flexion in small range may be performed, resulting in stronger contraction of the brachialis.

Brachioradialis

The most prominent and the largest of the three muscles of the radial group of the forearm, the **brachioradialis**, varies considerably in size in individuals. **Proximal attachment:** to a ridge on the humerus above the lateral epicondyle. **Distal attachment:** near the styloid process of the radius. **Innervation:** radial nerve (C_5-C_6). **Anatomic action:** elbow flexion.

INSPECTION AND PALPATION   The brachioradialis is best observed and palpated when resistance is given to flexion of the elbow while the elbow angle is about 90 degrees and the forearm is in midposition between pronation and supination (Fig. 5–9). Figure 5–10 shows the contour of this muscle and its relation to the extensor carpi radialis longus and brevis. The brachioradialis is superficial and can readily be palpated along most of its course. Above the elbow, it lies between the triceps and the brachialis. At and below the elbow, the brachioradialis forms the lateral border of the antecubital fossa. Its muscular part may be followed halfway down the forearm, but its point of distal attachment is less readily palpated because its tendon of attachment is flat and partially covered

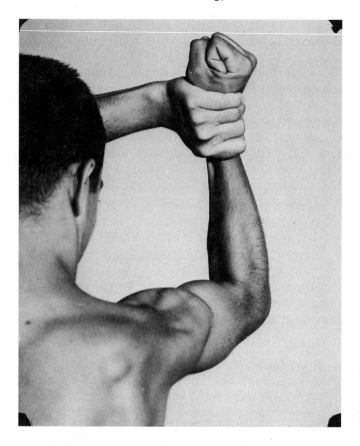

Figure 5–9 Brachioradialis is brought out by resistance to flexion of the elbow with the forearm in midposition between pronation and supination.

by tendons of muscles passing over the wrist to the hand. These tendons are held down by ligamentous structures that cross obliquely from the ulnar to the radial side of the wrist. When the muscle contracts, its upper portion rises from the underlying structures so that its perpendicular distance to the elbow joint increases, which enhances its function.

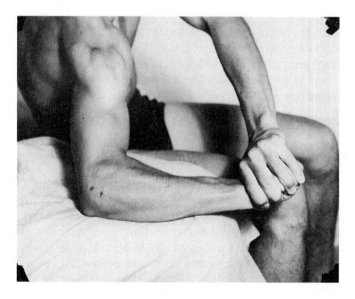

Figure 5–10 Resistance to wrist extension brings out the wrist extensors and also the brachioradialis. Cross-marks identify lateral epicondyle of the humerus *(proximal mark)* and head of radius *(distal mark)*.

Pronator Teres

The bulk of the **pronator teres** muscle is located below the elbow. It courses rather close to the axis of the elbow joint so that it has comparatively poor leverage for elbow flexion. **Proximal attachments:** medial epicondyle of humerus and a smaller portion from the coronoid process of the ulna. The muscle fibers cross obliquely from medial to lateral on the volar aspect of the forearm. **Distal attachment:** lateral side of the radius about halfway down the forearm. **Innervation:** median nerve (C_6-C_7). **Anatomic actions:** radioulnar pronation and elbow flexion.

PALPATION   The muscle is superficial and may be palpated in the fold of the elbow and below. It forms the medial margin of the antecubital fossa, and its fibers are easily identified in this region when the forearm is pronated while the elbow is flexed or semiflexed. Resistance to elbow flexion with the forearm pronated also makes for easy identification.

In Figure 5–7, the subject's thumb grasps around the edge of the pronator teres. If, from the position shown, the forearm is further pronated or resistance is given to pronation or flexion, the muscle hardens markedly.

The pronator teres lies close to the flexor carpi radialis, and both these muscles are covered by the bicipital aponeurosis. More distally, as it crosses over toward the radial side, the pronator teres is covered by the brachioradialis, and if the pronator teres is to be palpated close to its distal attachment, the brachioradialis must be relaxed. This is accomplished by resting the forearm in the lap or on the table. The forearm is then pronated, which activates the pronator while the brachioradialis remains essentially relaxed. The movement of pronation should be performed with little effort, or additional muscles in the region become tense.

Elbow Extensors

The principal extensor of the elbow is the **triceps brachii**, with the small **anconeus** adding only insignificantly to the total strength of elbow extension.

Triceps Brachii

The triceps brachii makes up the entire muscle mass on the posterior aspect of the arm. **Proximal attachments:** by three heads: the long head, the medial head, and the lateral head. The long head is attached to the infraglenoid tubercle of the scapula by a broad tendon that has a close relation to the capsule of the shoulder joint. The medial head is attached to the distal portion of the humerus and has a fleshy origin. The lateral head is attached to the lateral aspect of the humerus, a short distance below the glenohumeral joint. **Distal attachments:** The three heads join a sturdy broad tendon that attaches to the olecranon process of the ulna and that also sends an expansion spreading out over the anconeus muscle into the dorsal fascia of the forearm. **Innervation:** radial (musculospiral) nerve (C_7-C_8). **Anatomic actions:** elbow extension and shoulder extension.

INSPECTION AND PALPATION   The long head is identified in its proximal portion as it emerges from underneath the lowest fibers of the posterior deltoid (Figs. 5–11, 5–12). It may be followed distally halfway down the arm. The muscular portion of the lateral head, which is the strongest of the three heads, is palpated distal to the

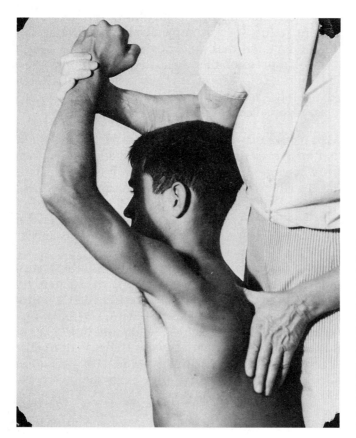

Figure 5–11 Triceps brachii and other muscles are brought out by the examiner's resistance to extension of the elbow. The long head of the triceps is responsible for the contour at the lower margin of the arm. Note its relation to teres major and the latissimus near the axilla. The lateral head appears separated from the deltoid by a groove. The flat area between the lateral and the long heads identifies the broad common tendon of attachment.

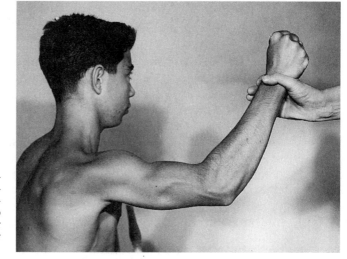

Figure 5–12 Triceps and anconeus. Elbow extension is resisted. The short, triangular-shaped anconeus lies close to the tip of the elbow and near the upper portion of extensor carpi ulnaris.

posterior deltoid. It is well recognizable in Figure 5–11. The long head and the lateral head join the common tendon of insertion from opposite sides, much as the two heads of the gastrocnemius approach the Achilles tendon. Note in the illustration the flat area between the lateral and the long heads. This is the broad superficial portion of the triceps tendon into which the two heads insert, partially from underneath and partially from the sides. The medial head is covered, in part, by the long head and is best palpated in its distal portion, near the medial epicondyle. For palpation of the medial head, it is suggested that the dorsum of the wrist be placed on the edge of a table and pressure be applied in a downward direction, the table supplying resistance to elbow extension. The medial head may then be felt contracting.

Anconeus

Proximal attachment: the region of the lateral epicondyle of the humerus. **Distal attachment:** the ulna, partly into the olecranon process, partly below this process. **Innervation:** radial nerve (C_7-C_8). **Anatomic action:** elbow extension.

PALPATION If one fingertip is placed on the lateral epicondyle and one on the olecranon process, the muscular portion of the anconeus is palpated distally at a point that forms a triangle with the other two points. The anconeus may be identified in Figure 5–11 but should not be confused with the extensor carpi ulnaris that lies close to it. In the illustration, the two muscles appear almost as one; but each muscle may be identified by keeping in mind that the direction of the two muscles differs and that the anconeus lies more proximally and is very short, whereas the extensor carpi ulnaris runs down the forearm.

Muscles Performing Supination

The muscles in a position that enables them to supinate the forearm are the **biceps brachii, supinator, abductor pollicis longus, extensor pollicis brevis,** and **extensor indicis proprius.** The first two muscles are the most important supinators. The last three are mechanically capable of aiding in supination but are small in size and have poor leverage for supination.

Location of the proximal and distal attachments and palpation of the biceps brachii have already been discussed.

Supinator

The supinator is a deep muscle located on the dorsal side of the interosseous membrane between the two bones of the forearm. It is covered by the anconeus, the extensor carpi radialis longus, and the brachioradialis. **Proximal attachments:** lateral epicondyle of the humerus and adjacent areas of the ulna. It is a fairly short and rather flat muscle, triangular in shape, which winds around the proximal portion of the radius close to the bone. **Distal attachments:** volar and lateral surfaces of the proximal part of the radius. **Innervation:** a branch of the radial nerve (C_5-C_7). **Anatomic action:** Radioulnar supination.

PALPATION The area where the supinator, although deeply located, may be palpated is shown in Figure 5–6. The fingertips are pushing the muscles of the radial group in a radial direction so that there is no interference with palpation. The best position for palpation is perhaps to sit with the pronated forearm resting in the lap and to grasp the radial muscle group from the radial side, pulling it out of the way as much as possible. As the forearm is supinated slowly through short range to avoid activating the biceps, the supinator may be felt under the palpating fingers.

Muscles Performing Pronation

The muscles that are capable of pronating the forearm are the **pronator teres, pronator quadratus, flexor carpi radialis, palmaris longus,** and **extensor carpi radialis longus.** The last three muscles have poor leverage for pronation and contribute little force. The pronator teres has been discussed previously in this chapter.

Pronator Quadratus

The **pronator quadratus** crosses transversely over the ulna and the radius in the distal region of the forearm near the wrist. It is deeply situated on the palmar side, lying directly over the bones and the interosseous membrane, and is covered by the flexors of wrist and digits. **Attachments:** the distal one fourth of the ulna and radius on the volar surfaces. **Innervation:** a branch of the median nerve (C_8-T_1). **Anatomic action:** radioulnar pronation. **Palpation** is impossible because the muscle is covered by tendons of the fingers and the wrist. The approximate length and direction of the muscle fibers are indicated in Figure 5–13.

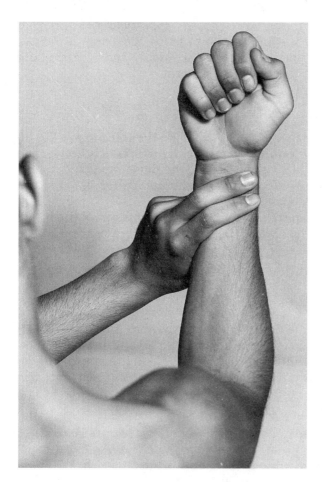

Figure 5–13 Demonstrating the line of action of the deeply situated pronator quadratus.

Selection of Muscles in Movement: Synergistic Contractions

In general, it may be stated that those muscles that best serve a particular purpose with the least amount of expenditure of energy are the ones selected by the nervous system to perform the task. For any movement combination, however, a perfect selection of muscles is achieved only by highly skilled individuals. Unskilled movements are wasteful of energy because muscles not necessarily needed for the movement contract along with those needed. As skill increases, the selection improves and gradation of contraction becomes more refined, resulting in smoother movements that are less fatiguing and, from the aesthetic standpoint, more pleasing to the eye.

The number of muscles involved in movements also is determined by the effort needed for a particular task. Thus, if great resistance is encountered, more muscles are recruited, not only at the joint or joints where the movements take place but also at joints far away from the scene of action. A typical example is that of making a fist, which involves primarily the flexors of the digits and the extensors of the wrist. When the effort increases, as in testing grip strength on a dynamometer, not only do the finger flexors and the wrist extensors increase their tension, but there is a successive recruitment of muscles at the elbow, the shoulder, and even the trunk until with greatest effort practically all muscles of the body appear to participate.

Many muscles act over more than one joint, and they are the ones usually selected for a task involving these joints. For example, the biceps brachii is a flexor of the elbow and a supinator of the forearm; when both these movements are wanted simultaneously, the biceps is the logical selection. This movement combination, of course, could also be performed by the brachioradialis and the supinator, as is indeed the case in musculocutaneous nerve injuries when the biceps and the brachialis are paralyzed. Ordinarily, for light tasks, the nervous system prefers to have one muscle perform the job of two when such a muscle is available.

The brachialis, a one-joint muscle, is the perfect selection for flexion of the elbow if neither supination nor pronation is willed. For such motion, it is wasteful to use the biceps because supination has to be neutralized by the pronators, and it is equally wasteful to use the pronator teres, because pronation has to be prevented by the supinators.

Often, it becomes economical to use a two-joint muscle to produce movement over one joint only, in which case synergic muscle action (or gravitational force) stabilizes the other joint or moves that joint in the opposite direction. This latter arrangement enables a muscle to perform work in a relatively elongated state through a large range of motion, thus using a favorable portion of the length-tension diagram (see Chapter 4).

The foregoing discussion emphasizes that muscles may team up in many different ways and that synergism among muscles is always changing depending on requirements. Consequently, it can never be stated that two specific muscles are always synergists or antagonists; the muscles may be so labeled for specific movement combinations only.

Elbow Flexion

The manner in which the individual muscles team up to flex the elbow has been the subject of much discussion and a considerable amount of dissension, mainly because the variety of requirements and individual variations in skill have not been sufficiently appreciated. Recent EMG studies indicate that, as would be expected, there are considerable variations of muscle action among individuals, both in the selection of muscles and in the sequence of recruitment of the muscles.

BRACHIALIS The brachialis is the least controversial of the flexors of the elbow. It is uninfluenced by the position of the forearm, being as effective when the forearm is pronated as when it is supinated. Studies by Basmajian and Latif (1957) show that the brachialis is always active as an elbow flexor with or without a load and whether the motion is rapid or slow.

BRACHIORADIALIS This muscle is clearly a flexor of the elbow, but actions of supination and pronation have also been ascribed to it. Early anatomists called it the **supinator longus.** Fick states that, mechanically, the brachioradialis is capable of performing a limited range of supination from the fully pronated position. Beevor (1903) considered it to be a pure flexor of the elbow. His observations have been substantiated by EMG studies (Basmajian and Latif, 1957). Persons with paralysis of the biceps, supinator, and pronators and with a strong brachioradialis cannot generate force in supination or pronation. Functionally, they have difficulty holding a glass of water and keeping it from turning over and spilling. For practical purposes, the brachioradialis may be considered a pure flexor of the elbow when the forearm is in midposition.

BICEPS BRACHII An isolated, unopposed contraction of the biceps would produce simultaneous flexion of the shoulder and elbow and supination of the forearm. In function, undesired motions are prevented by synergistic contraction of other muscles or gravity.

The EMG studies cited previously show that the biceps takes little or no part in slow flexion of the elbow when the forearm is pronated, even when a load of 2 lb, held loosely in the hand, is lifted or lowered. When the forearm is supinated, however, the biceps acts in flexion of the elbow both with and without a load, in slow as well as in fast movements, and regardless of whether it acts in a concentric or eccentric contraction. With increasing speed and increasing load, however, the biceps acts also when the forearm is pronated.

COMPARISON OF ACTIONS OF THE BICEPS BRACHII AND THE SUPINATOR The biceps acts most effectively as a supinator when the elbow is flexed at an angle of about 90 degrees, a conclusion gained from observing the angle of approach of its tendon to the long axis of the radius. As the elbow extends, the effectiveness of the muscle as a supinator lessens; the effectiveness of the supinator muscle is not influenced by the elbow angle. Fick (1911) calculated that, at an angle of 90 degrees, the biceps is almost four times as effective as the supinator in performing supination. When the elbow is extended and supinated, however, the effectiveness of the biceps is only twice that of the supinator.

Because the supinator's sole action is supination, whereas the biceps is also a flexor of the elbow, it is logical to conclude that the supinator would be called upon to contract when supination without elbow flexion is willed, provided that the movement is performed slowly and without resistance. Clinically, this assumption may be confirmed as follows: The subject is seated with the forearm resting in the lap. The palpating fingers are placed on the tendon of the biceps in the fold of the elbow. If supination is performed slowly and the forearm remains in the lap, the tendon of the biceps remains relaxed, and one may conclude that the movement is performed by the supinator. But, if a quick supination is performed, the biceps immediately springs into action and its tendon stands out markedly.

This procedure is employed for isolated testing of the supinator, although in normal individuals no information about the strength of the supinator is obtained. The test is also useful in patients with radial nerve injuries to determine when regeneration of the nerve has progressed to the supinator. As long as the supinator is denervated, a slow supination of the forearm in the position described causes the biceps tendon to become prominent. When the supinator has been reinnervated, this is no longer the case.

The ability of the supinator to perform supination without the aid of the biceps has been verified by Basmajian and Latif (1957). In most subjects, no electrical activity was registered in either head of the biceps when the forearm was supinated while the elbow was in extension. But if resistance was applied to supination, the biceps became active.

COMPARISON OF ACTIONS OF THE PRONATOR TERES AND THE PRONATOR QUADRATUS   The pronator teres is the strongest of the pronators, and because it is superficial, its contraction can be ascertained by palpation. The role played by the pronator quadratus is difficult to assess because it cannot be palpated readily. Its cross-section is almost two-thirds of that of the pronator teres and compares favorably with that of the supinator. The shortening distance of the pronator quadratus, however, is small. One may assume that the pronator quadratus pronates the forearm unaided by other muscles if pronation is performed slowly without resistance and without active elbow flexion. These conditions are met if the subject lies prone with the forearm hanging vertically over the edge of the table and if little effort is used in pronation.

COMPARISON OF ACTION OF THE TRICEPS AND THE ANCONEUS   Both the triceps and the anconeus are extensors of the elbow, the triceps being by far the more powerful of the two. The triceps has a cross-section about five times, and a shortening range about twice that of the anconeus (Fick, 1911, p 131, cited in Lehmkuhl and Smith, 1983). The fascia over the triceps tendon continues over the anconeus, which has a close relation to the elbow joint and the proximal radioulnar joint. Both muscles, therefore, contribute to the protection of these joints.

Multijoint Muscles

When a muscle crosses more than one joint, the muscle not only has an effect on each joint but is in turn influenced by the position of the joints. The biceps brachii is a three-joint muscle crossing the glenohumeral, the elbow, and the radioulnar joints. The long head of the triceps brachii and the pronator teres are two-joint muscles, with the long head of the triceps crossing the glenohumeral joint and the elbow and the pronator crossing the elbow and the radioulnar joints.

Minimum Muscle Length: Active Insufficiency

The shortest length of a muscle is in a position of full motion of all of its anatomic actions. When a muscle contracts at this length, the contraction force is weak because the muscle is at its lowest point on its length-tension curve. The muscle is stated to be in **active insufficiency.** For the biceps, this is full shoulder flexion, elbow flexion, and supination with the palm touching the back of the shoulder. Testing the maximum force of supination in this position compared with when the arm is at the side and the elbow is in 90 degrees of flexion demonstrates the marked loss of force of the biceps (the biceps also loses some leverage in the shortened position). The position of active insufficiency for the long head of the triceps is shoulder and elbow extension, and for the pronator teres it is elbow flexion and pronation.

The body in movement seeks to avoid active insufficiency and maintains muscle lengths at more optimal positions on the length-tension curve. The biceps muscle is elongated when the shoulder is extended or hyperextended. Therefore, elbow flexion combined with shoulder hyperextension maintains a favorable tension while flexing the elbow through a large range of motion. The brachialis, on the other hand, produces its greatest force when the elbow is extended, and the force decreases as the elbow is flexed. This combination—elbow flexion and shoulder hyperextension—is used in "pulling" activities and contributes materially to the strength of elbow flexion.

The long head of the triceps, because of its attachment to the infraglenoid tuberosity of the scapula, is elongated when the shoulder is flexed. Therefore, elbow extension combined with shoulder flexion enhances the force of the long head of the triceps. This two-joint mechanism is the reverse of the flexion combination and is used to advantage in "pushing" activities. The flexion and extension combinations are used alternately in scores of functional activities, such as sanding, polishing, pulling the beater of a loom, using a carpet sweeper, sawing wood, throwing a ball, and so forth. Examples of such multijoint mechanisms are numerous throughout the body.

Maximum Length of Multijoint Muscles

The maximum length of a multijoint muscle is the full range of all of its antagonistic anatomic actions. For the biceps brachii, this is shoulder hyperextension, elbow extension, and pronation. This position is necessary to determine if a multijoint muscle is abnormally shortened or if the muscle or its attachments have been injured. In such cases, individual passive joint motions are usually within normal ranges. The problem is not identified until the multijoint muscles are passively elongated toward their full range. If the muscle has a contracture or is shortened, the last motion attempted will be abnormally limited with a firm end-feel. If the muscle has been injured, pain occurs before the last joint motion is completed and the end-feel is called "empty."

The long head of the triceps brachii is stretched to maximum length by simultaneous shoulder flexion and elbow flexion, and the pronator teres is placed at maximum length by elbow extension and supination.

Agonistic, Antagonistic, and Synergistic Actions

The anatomic classification of muscle actions occurs when the muscle acts alone, its proximal attachment is stabilized (by other muscles or body weight), and the distal attachment moves in open-chain motion with a concentric contraction against gravity or very light resistance (see Fig. 4–3). Thus it is not surprising that the definitions agonist, antagonist, and synergist are not constant for muscles but rather vary with motion and imposed forces that occur in function. While the biceps and triceps may act antagonistically in the motions described earlier, they are more likely to contract simultaneously as synergists, as when a forceful grip is made (see Fig. 4–4C). These muscles do so to stabilize the elbow from being moved by the strong contractions of the wrist and finger flexors and extensors. Turning a doorknob or using a screwdriver also illustrates synergistic actions of the biceps and triceps. The triceps stabilize the elbow and prevent elbow flexion by the biceps or the pronator teres as they participate in supination or pronation (see Fig. 4–4A,B).

Closed-Chain Motion of the Elbow

Closed-chain motion at the elbow occurs when the hand is fixed and the shoulder is moving as in pull-ups or push-ups. In the case of pull-ups, the elbow flexors provide the muscle force to raise and lower the body by concentric and eccentric muscle contractions. In this instance, the elbow flexors are both flexing and extending the elbow. The opposite occurs with push-ups, where the triceps extend the elbow with a concentric contraction to raise the body and then with an eccentric contraction to lower the body, thus flexing the elbow. In both instances, the shoulder-elbow combinations to maintain optimal length-tension relationships of the multijoint muscles are in operation.

Even though the pectoralis major does not cross the elbow, the muscle is able to cause elbow extension in closed-chain motion as the muscle acts to adduct the shoulder. This action can be observed and palpated in subjects performing prone push-ups and is extremely useful to persons with spinal cord lesions who have paralysis of the triceps brachii (C_7–C_8) but innervation of the pectoralis major (C_5–C_7). Light objects can be pushed, drawers shut, and doors closed. This is done by placing the hand on the object with the elbow flexed and then contracting the pectoralis major to extend the elbow.

CLINICAL APPLICATIONS

Effect of Nerve Lesions on Function

Paralysis of the triceps brachii can occur with a **radial nerve injury** or a **spinal cord severance at the sixth cervical segment.** When the person is sitting upright, elbow flexion and extension are performed easily by concentric and eccentric contractions of the biceps and brachialis muscles. The person, however, does not have an effective push and cannot press down with the hand as is necessary in cutting food. When the person is supine, he or she can flex the elbow to 90 degrees with the elbow flexors, but then the hand suddenly falls into the person's face and the elbow cannot be extended to return the hand to the side.

If the biceps brachii and the brachialis are paralyzed, as can occur in a **musculocutaneous nerve lesion** and some types of **muscular dystrophy,** only weak elbow flexion can be achieved. This is accomplished by the brachioradialis, pronator teres, and the extensor carpi radialis longus and brevis. Because the leverage of these muscles is poor for elbow flexion when the elbow is in a position of extension, these individuals frequently swing the whole upper extremity, using momentum to start the motion. Then the forearm muscles can hold the elbow flexed at 90 degrees, where leverage is better. This compensation is useful for hand placement and lifting very light objects.

A **median nerve injury** above the elbow causes paralysis of the pronator teres and quadratus with profound loss of pronation force. Subjects are unable to produce sufficient force to turn a key or hold a glass and keep it from tipping.

Laboratory Activities

ELBOW AND FOREARM

1. On disarticulated bones or the skeleton, identify these bones and bony landmarks:

Humerus	*Ulna*	*Radius*
shaft	shaft	head
capitulum	olecranon process	neck
coronoid fossa	coronoid process	shaft
trochlea	trochlear notch	tuberosity of radius
olecranon fossa	head	radioulnar
medial epicondyle	radial notch	articulations
lateral epicondyle	styloid process	Lister's tubercle

2. Which of these bony landmarks can you palpate? Locate these on yourself and then on a partner.

3. Identify and examine bony surfaces where the movements of elbow flexion, elbow extension, pronation, and supination take place. Move the radius on the ulna by turning the palm of the hand up (supinate) and then by turning it down (pronate). Note that when the palm turns up (supination), radius and ulna are parallel; when the palm turns down (pronation), these bones are crossed—that is, the radius rotates and crosses over the ulna.

4. Perform elbow and forearm movements on yourself and then observe as a subject performs them:
   a. Flex and extend the elbow first with the forearm supinated, then with the forearm pronated.
   b. Pronate and supinate the forearm while palpating the head of the radius. As you do this, hold your upper arm against the side of your body, maintain your wrist in one position, and maintain your elbow flexed at a right angle. Note that isolated forearm movement occurs for approximately 180 degrees of total motion.
   c. Pronate both forearms as described. Now extend your elbows, lift your arms to shoulder height, and continue to turn the palms of your hands in the direction of pronation and then supination as far as they will move. Note the increased movement that results from shoulder rotation (approximately 360 degrees). Now isolate the forearm movement by again flexing the elbow and holding the upper arm against the side of the body.
      Which forearm and shoulder movements occur synchronously?

5. On the skeleton, on yourself, and on a partner, identify and visualize the axes for elbow flexion and extension and for forearm pronation and supination. Identify and palpate bony landmarks to locate these axes.

6. Using anatomy text and skeleton, determine points of attachment for:

biceps brachii	triceps brachii	anconeus
brachialis	pronator teres	pronator quadratus
brachioradialis	supinator	wrist extensors

Note particularly the action line of each muscle and the axes each one crosses; from these observations, determine the movements each can perform. A helpful method to facilitate such observations is to cut lengths of adhesive tape to reach from one attachment of the muscle to the other and then to tape these pieces on the skeleton from the point of proximal attachment to point of distal attachment.

7. Determine muscles that:
   a. Flex the elbow
   b. Extend the elbow
   c. Pronate the forearm
   d. Supinate the forearm

8. Select a partner. Following the descriptions in Chapter 5, palpate the biceps brachii, brachialis, brachioradialis, pronator teres, triceps brachii, supinator, and anconeus. Identify these muscles and tendons first on yourself and then on your partner. How can you determine whether:
   a. The motion of supination is being produced by the biceps brachii or the supinator?
   b. The motion of elbow flexion is being produced by the biceps brachii, the brachialis, or brachioradialis?

9. End-feels: Perform slow passive motion to the end of the range of motion of elbow flexion, extension, pronation, and supination. Describe the end-feels and the tissues that limit the motion.

10. Muscle excursion: Measure the excursion of the biceps brachii from its shortest length (full shoulder flexion, elbow flexion and supination) to its longest length (shoulder hyperextension, elbow extension, and pronation) on an articulated skeleton or on your partner. In the human subject, consider the acromion as the approximate proximal attachment of the muscle. How many inches of excursion does the muscle have? What is the percent excursion of the shortened length?

11. Active insufficiency of the biceps brachii: Test the strength of supination with the arm at the side and the elbow in 90 degrees of flexion and then when the biceps brachii is in its shortest position of shoulder flexion, elbow flexion, and supination.

CHAPTER 6

Wrist and Hand

The hand is a complex, multipurpose organ. As a prehensile organ (L. *prehensus,* to seize), the hand can grasp with forces exceeding 100 lb (445 N or 45 kg) as well as hold and manipulate a delicate thread. In addition, the hand is used for pushing, striking blows, and even locomoting with crutches or wheelchairs. As a sense organ for touch, the hand is an extension of the brain to provide information to the visual system about the environment. The hand is also an important organ for expression and nonverbal communication.

Placement and stabilization of the hand depend on the trunk, shoulder, elbow, and wrist. With the multiple degrees of freedom allowed by the upper extremity, the versatility of hand placement is high. For example, the palm or surface of the hand can be rotated in a full circle (360 degrees) and placed on any surface of the body with the exception of the ipsilateral arm and forearm.

BONES

Palpable Structures of the Wrist

Head of the Ulna

If the wrist is grasped from side to side at its narrowest portion, as seen in Figure 6–1, the bony eminence proximal to the examiner's index finger on the dorsum of the wrist is identified as the **head of the ulna.** In the pronated position of the forearm, this eminence is seen beneath the skin. If one fingertip is placed on the highest part of this bony eminence and the forearm is slowly supinated, this portion of the bone recedes and can no longer be palpated, because during supination the distal portion of the radius rotates around the head of the ulna, thus partially hiding the ulnar head from palpation.

Styloid Process of the Ulna

The position of the examiner's index finger in Figure 6–1 indicates the approximate location of the **styloid process of the ulna.** The tendon of the extensor carpi ulnaris, however, courses in this region and interferes with palpation. By sliding the index finger over this tendon in a palmar direction, the styloid process becomes more accessible for palpation. This process is smaller and feels sharper than the head of the ulna, and it may be palpated both in the pronated and in the supinated position of the forearm.

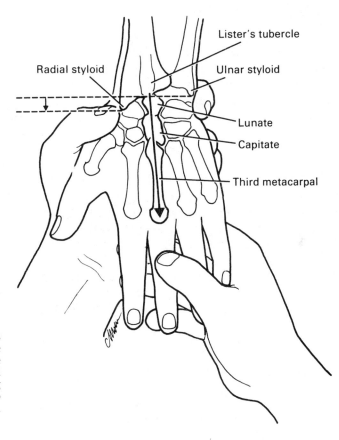

Lister's tubercle

Radial styloid

Ulnar styloid

Lunate

Capitate

Third metacarpal

Figure 6–1 Bony landmarks on the dorsum of the wrist. The approximate location of the axis for radiocarpal flexion and extension is a line connecting the tips of the palpating thumb and forefinger of the proximal hand.

Styloid Process of the Radius

The position of the examiner's thumb in Figure 6–1 indicates the point where the **styloid process of the radius** may be palpated. This process extends somewhat more distally than the corresponding process of the ulna. The styloid processes serve as attachments for the ulnar and radial carpal collateral ligaments, respectively.

Grooves and Prominences on the Distal End of the Radius

On the dorsal aspect of the broad distal end of the radius are found a number of grooves for tendons passing to the hand, these grooves being separated by prominences. The **tubercle of the radius**, sometimes referred to as **Lister's tubercle**, may be palpated about level with the head of the ulna (see Fig. 6–1). The tendon of the extensor pollicis longus lies in a groove on the ulnar side of this tubercle and, on palpation, appears to be hooked around it. The tubercle serves as a landmark for locating several other tendons in this region: the deeply situated tendon of the extensor carpi radialis brevis; the tendon of the extensor indicis proprius, which crosses over the tendon of the extensor carpi radialis brevis; and the tendon of the extensor digitorum to the index finger, which is superficial and visible under the skin. The deep tendons, however, are difficult to identify with certainty by palpation.

Carpal Bones

There are eight cuboid-shaped carpal bones in the wrist. They have articulating surfaces proximally, distally, medially, and laterally with roughened surfaces for attachments of ligaments on their volar and dorsal sides. The exception is the pisiform bone, which has only one articulating surface. The **proximal row** of carpal bones contains the **scaphoid, lunate, triquetrum,** and **pisiform.** The **distal row** contains the **trapezium, trapezoid, capitate,** and **hamate** (Fig. 6–2).

Occupying a central position at the wrist (in line with the middle finger), the **capitate bone** (os magnum) is best approached from the dorsum, where a slight depression indicates its location (see Fig. 6–2). The axis of motion for ulnar and radial abduction goes through this bone in a dorsopalmar direction.

The **scaphoid (navicular) bone** is palpated distally to the styloid process of the radius (see Fig. 6–2). Ulnar deviation of the wrist causes the bone to become prominent to the palpating fingers, while radial deviation causes the bone to recede. The scaphoid is the most commonly fractured of the carpal bones. The scaphoid bone and the trapezium make up the floor of the "anatomic snuff box" (fovea radialis), the depression seen between the tendons of the thumb extensor muscles (extensor pollicis longus and brevis) when these muscles are tensed. It should be remembered that the scaphoid belongs to the proximal row and the trapezium to the distal row of carpal bones.

The **trapezium** (greater multangular) can be palpated proximally to the first carpometacarpal (CMC) joint of the thumb (passively flex and extend the thumb) and distal to the identified scaphoid (see Fig. 6–2).

The **lunate** is palpated distally to Lister's tubercle and proximally to the capitate (see Fig. 6–1). In normal subjects, the lunate becomes prominent to the palpating finger as the wrist is passively flexed and recedes as the wrist is passively ex-

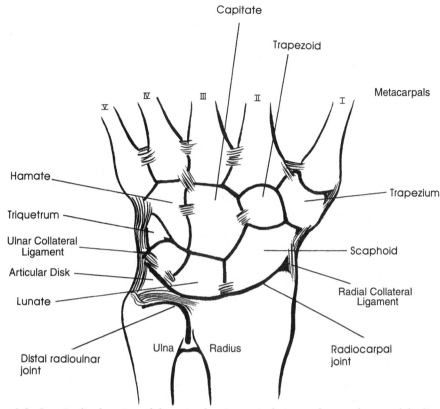

Figure 6–2 Longitudinal section of the wrist showing articulating surfaces and some of the ligaments. The midcarpal joint is formed by the distal articulating surfaces of the proximal row of carpals and the proximal articulating surfaces of the distal row.

tended. The lunate is the most frequently dislocated bone in the wrist (Hoppenfeld, 1976).

The pea-shaped bone palpated on the palmar side of the wrist near the ulnar border is the **pisiform** bone, which can be grasped and moved from side to side. It serves as the point of attachment for the tendon of the flexor carpi ulnaris.

The **trapezoid** (lesser multangular), the **triquetrum** (triangular), and the **hamate** (unciform) **bones** seen in Figure 6–2 are more difficult to identify directly by palpation. They can, however, be precisely palpated using their relationships to carpal bones and bony structures that are more easily palpated.

Palpable Structures of the Digits

Five Metacarpals

Each metacarpal has a base that articulates proximally with one or more carpal bones and with adjacent metacarpals (see Fig. 6–2), a shaft that is slightly curved, and a head that articulates with the base of a proximal phalanx. Each metacarpal can be palpated throughout its length on the dorsum of the hand. **Note the tubercle at the base of the fifth metacarpal**, which is located just distal to the examiner's finger in Figure 6–1, and which serves as the distal attachment for the extensor carpi ulnaris. At the base of the second metacarpal bone (dorsally), an eminence may be felt that serves as the distal attachment for the extensor carpi radialis longus. The palmar surface of the base of the second metacarpal also presents a rough area, which serves as the attachment for the flexor carpi radialis, but this lies in a position that is too deep for palpation. The head of each metacarpal bone presents a biconvex articular surface that becomes part of the metacarpophalangeal (MCP) joint, and that may, in part, be palpated when the joint is flexed.

Phalanges

The two phalanges of the thumb and the three phalanges of each of the other digits may be palpated without difficulty. To differentiate the phalanges of the thumb, the terms **proximal** and **distal** are used; for the other digits, **proximal, middle**, and **distal**. The base of the proximal phalanges is biconcave and has a smaller articular surface than the metacarpal head. The distal heads are bicondylar with an intercondylar depression. This can be palpated at the distal end of the phalanges when the proximal interphalangeal joints are flexed. The middle phalanges and the base of the distal phalanges have articulating surfaces similar to the proximal phalanges.

JOINTS

Wrist

The wrist provides wide mobility of the hand along with great structural stability. Although the wrist is often classified as a condyloid joint with two degrees of freedom, it is in reality a highly complex area of 15 bones, 17 joints, and an extensive ligament system.

Radiocarpal Joint

The **radiocarpal joint** is formed by the biconcave distal end of the radius and the biconvex proximal articulating surfaces of the scaphoid and lunate bones. A triangular fibrocartilaginous disk attaches to the distal end of the radius, the styloid process of the ulna with the apex of the disk attached to the triquetrum (see Fig. 6–2). The disk binds the radius and ulna together and separates the distal radioulnar joint and the ulna from the radiocarpal joint. Part of the wrist motions of flexion (volar flexion), extension (hyperextension), radial abduction (radial deviation), and ulnar abduction (ulnar deviation) occurs at the radiocarpal joint.

Midcarpal Joint

The **midcarpal joint** is formed by the proximal and distal carpal rows. The scaphoid articulates with the trapezium, trapezoid, and capitate; the lunate articulates with the capitate; and the triquetrum with the hamate (see Fig. 6–2). The wrist motions of flexion, extension, and radial and ulnar abduction also take place at this joint.

Carpometacarpal Joints

The bases of the second to the fourth metacarpals articulate with each other and with the distal row of carpal bones in an irregular manner to form mortices

(Gr. *murtazza,* joined or fixed in). A common joint cavity occurs between the four carpals, the CMC articulations, and into the intermetacarpal joints. The motion in the second and third CMC joints may be one or two degrees or less, the fourth has 10 to 15 degrees of dorsovolar movement, and the fifth is more flexible with 25 to 30 degrees of motion (Razemon and Fisk, 1988). While movements at each individual joint are small, the motions are important for hand function and provide for a large change in the shape of the transverse arch of the hand from the closed fist to the open hand (Fig. 6–3).

The **CMC joint of the thumb** is formed by the trapezium and the base of the first metacarpal, the surfaces of which are both convex and concave and form the sellar or saddle joint (see Fig. 1–7). The joint capsule is thick but loose, and the metacarpal can be distracted up to 3 mm from the trapezium. Motions are abduction and adduction (in a plane at a right angle to the palm); flexion and extension (in a plane parallel to the palm); and **opposition**, which is a rotation of the first metacarpal on the trapezium to place the pad of the thumb opposite the pads of the fingers (see Fig. 6–21). If there were close congruence of the sellar joint, only two degrees of freedom would exist, but the laxity of the joint capsule allows 15 to 20 degrees of rotation (Spinner, 1984). Kapandji (1982), however, states that the joint acts by axial compression like a pivot. **Reposition** or retroposition is the reverse of opposition.

Ligaments of the Wrist

Ligaments cover the volar, dorsal, radial, and ulnar areas of the wrist. These ligaments function to stabilize joints, to permit and guide motion of bones, to limit joint motion, to transmit forces from the hand to the forearm, and to prevent dislocation of carpal bones with movement.

The complexity of these ligaments is illustrated in Table 6–1. In this classification, extrinsic ligaments connect the radius, ulna, or metacarpals to the carpal bones, and intrinsic ligaments run between the carpal bones only. Short, strong ligaments bind the distal row of carpal bones to each other (intrinsic, short, interossei) and to the bases of the metacarpals (extrinsic, distal, CMC ligaments) (see Fig. 6–2). The distal row of the carpal bones and the second to fourth metacarpals form a fixed unit or block without appreciable motion. Intrinsic, intermediate-length ligaments permitting more motion connect the carpal bones, where most of individual carpal movements occur—the triquetrum, lunate, scaphoid, and trapezium.

The two rows of carpals are articulated to each other and to the radius and the

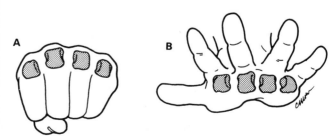

Figure 6–3 The flexible transverse arch of the hand showing the position of the metacarpal heads when (*A*) making a fist and (*B*) opening the hand. The third carpometacarpal joint is stable while the second, fourth, and fifth joints provide increasing mobility. Thus, as the extended hand is opened, the span of the fingers increases to surround objects, and as the hand is closed, the fingers are approximated to increase the force of the grip.

Table 6–1 Classification of Ligaments of the Wrist*

Extrinsic ligaments	Proximal (radiocarpal)	Radial collateral	Superficial / Deep	Radio-scaphoid-capitate / Radiolunate / Radio-scaphoid-lunate
		Volar radiocarpal		
		Ulnocarpal ligamentous complex		Meniscus (radio-triquetral) / Triangular fibrocartilage
	Distal (carpo-metacarpal)	Radiocarpal dorsal		Ulno lunate ligament / Medial collateral ligament
Intrinsic ligaments	Short	Volar / Dorsal / Interosseous		
	Intermediate	Lunate-triquetral / Scaphoid-lunate / Scaphoid-trapezial		
	Long	Volar intercarpal (deltoid, V, radiate or arcuate) / Dorsal intercarpal		

*Extrinsic ligaments are those that connect carpal bones to the radius, ulna, or metacarpals. Intrinsic ligaments attach between the carpal bones only.
SOURCE: Adapted from Taleisnik, J: Ligaments of the carpus. In: Razemon, JP and Fisk, GR (Eds.): The Wrist. Churchill Livingstone, Edinburgh, 1988, p. 17, with permission.

ulnar fibrocartilaginous disk by medial and lateral collateral ligaments and strong oblique V-shaped ligaments. The extrinsic ligaments extend from the radius and ulna to converge on the capitate and the lunate (Fig. 6–4). The intrinsic V ligament attaches to the triquetrum and the scaphoid and converges on the capitate. There are no ligamentous connections between the capitate and lunate. Thus, considerable movement is allowed, including 2 to 3 mm of distraction.

The extra-articular ligamentous structures of the wrist are the flexor and extensor retinacula (L. *halter*), which contain the tendons going to the fingers. Part of the flexor retinaculum includes the transverse carpal ligament. The ligament is 1 to 2 mm thick and 2 to 3 cm wide, attaching to the hook of the hamate and pisiform bones and coursing to the radial side, where it attaches to the trapezium and the scaphoid. These attachments maintain the transverse carpal arch and form a tunnel through which the median nerve and the tendons of the flexor pollicis longus, flexor digitorum superficialis, and flexor digitorum profundus travel to the hand. Trauma or swelling in this area can cause carpal tunnel syndrome, producing compression of the median nerve, which may result in pain, loss of sensation, and paralysis of the thenar muscles.

Some muscle tendons have attachments on the retinacula. When the muscles contract, they pull on the retinacula and stabilize it (dynamic stabilization). These muscles include the flexor and extensor carpi ulnaris, abductor pollicis longus, extensor pollicis brevis, palmaris longus, and thenar and hypothenar muscles. The actions of these muscles are discussed later.

Motions and Axes of the Wrist

Planar motions of the wrist occur at the radiocarpal and the midcarpal joints. According to Kapandji (1982), the midcarpal joint is responsible for one-half of the

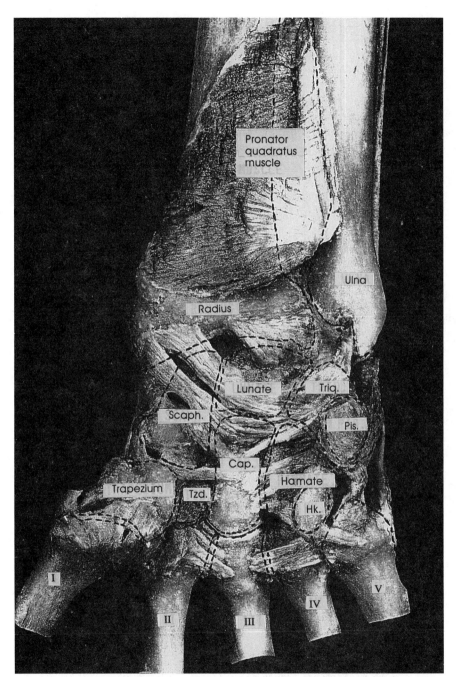

Figure 6–4 Cadaver dissection showing some of the ligaments on the volar surface of the wrist. Note the V-shaped ligaments converging on the lunate and the capitate bones. Underlying bones have been identified with dotted lines as follows: scaphoid (Scaph.); lunate; triquetrum (Triq.); pisiform (Pis.); trapezium; trapezoid (Tzd.); capitate (Cap.); and hamate hook (Hk.). I–V = first-fifth metacarpals. (Adapted from Guyot, J. *Atlas of Human Limb Joints*. Springer-Verlag, New York, 1981, p 168, with permission.)

motion of radial abduction and for one-third of the range of ulnar abduction with the remaining motion occurring at the radiocarpal joint. These motions occur around an axis through the head of the capitate. The normal end-feel for radial abduction is usually hard from contact of the scaphoid on the styloid process of the radius. Ulnar abduction provides more motion and has a firm end-feel from tension on the radial collateral ligament.

In wrist flexion, Kapandji (1982) states there are 50 degrees of motion at the radiocarpal joint and 35 degrees at the midcarpal joint. In full extension, these values reverse with 35 degrees occurring at the radiocarpal and 50 degrees at the midcarpal joint. The axis of motion again goes through the capitate. This axis, however, migrates distally from full flexion to extension (Fig. 6–5). The migration is caused by complex movements of the lunate and scaphoid, which include rotational and translatory motions with change in their effective height. These complex motions are compensatory in order to maintain tension of the ligaments at all times (Kuhlmann and Tubiana, 1988).

Full wrist extension requires slight spreading of the distal radius and ulna. If these bones are grasped and held together firmly, the subject is unable to completely extend the wrist.

ACCESSORY MOTIONS   When the forearm and hand are relaxed, the wrist is unstable and permits a considerable amount of passive joint play movements. If the examiner stabilizes the distal radius and ulna with one hand and places the other hand around the proximal carpal row, the carpals can be moved with ease in dorsal, volar, medial, and lateral translatory glides and distracted several millimeters. Similar movements with less motion occur with hand placement on either side of the midcarpal joint. In addition, each metacarpal bone can be passively moved relative to its neighbors. For example, the capitate can be stabilized on its dorsal and

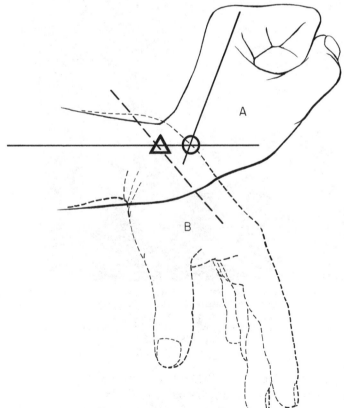

Figure 6–5 For maximum range of motion at wrist, the fist should be (*A*) closed in extension and (*B*) open in flexion. The axis for extension (o) is distal to axis for flexion (Δ).

volar surfaces by the examiner's left thumb and forefinger, and the individual carpals (trapezoid, scaphoid, lunate, and hamate) can be grasped between the examiner's right thumb and forefinger and moved one at a time on the capitate. The most stable (close-packed) position of the wrist is in full extension.

Fingers and Thumb

Metacarpophalangeal Joints

The MCP joints of the fingers are of the condyloid type with two degrees of freedom. The rounded surfaces of the heads of the metacarpals articulate with the shallow concave surfaces on the bases of the proximal phalanges. Approximately three-quarters of the circumference of the heads of the metacarpals are covered with articular cartilage, which extends onto the volar surface. The articular surfaces of the base of the phalanges are extended by fibrocartilaginous volar plates (Fig. 6–6). As the joint is flexed the volar plate slides proximally under the metacarpal with a folding of the membranous part. This mechanism permits a large range of motion for the small articulating surface of the phalanx. Accessory collateral ligaments control movement of the volar plate, and the metacarpal pulley for the long flexor tendons blends with these structures.

Medial and lateral collateral ligaments attach from the heads of the metacarpals to the bases of the phalanges (Fig. 6–6). There is a longer distance between the points of attachment of these ligaments when the joints are flexed than when they are extended. Thus abduction and adduction can occur when the

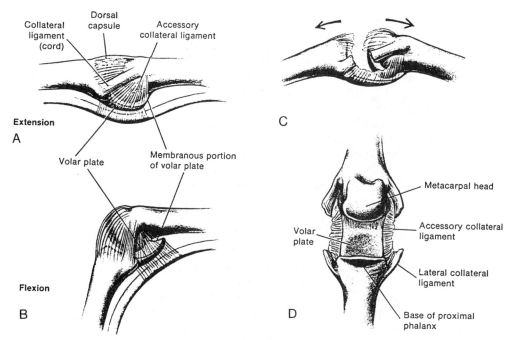

Figure 6–6 (*A,B*) Lateral views of the capsular and ligamentous structures of the metacarpophalangeal joint. Note the relationships of the volar plate, articulating surfaces, capsule, and collateral ligaments (*A*) in extension and (*B*) in flexion. In (*C*) and (*D*), the capsule and ligaments have been cut to show the volar plate. (Adapted from Spinner, M: *Kaplan's Functional and Surgical Anatomy of the Hand.* JB Lippincott, Philadelphia, 1984, p 42, with permission.)

joints are extended. When the MCP joints are flexed to 90 degrees, the collateral ligaments become taut and abduction cannot be performed. The MCP joints are then mechanically stabilized for gripping.

The deep transverse metacarpal ligament is attached to the volar plate and runs between the metacarpal heads to connect adjacent sides of metacarpals II to V. The ligament permits a flexible metacarpal arch and limits the spread of the bones (see Fig. 6–3).

In the thumb, two sesamoid bones are attached to the volar plate on its palmar surface. They are in the tendons of attachment of the adductor pollicis and the first dorsal interosseous ulnarly and the flexor pollicis brevis and the abductor pollicis brevis radially. The sesamoid bones have medial and lateral ligaments at the metacarpals as well as several ligaments joining the structure to the base of the phalanx (Kapandji, 1982). The sesamoid mechanism produces a dynamic rotation of the thumb segment for precision of the pinch.

Interphalangeal Joints

Each of the digits II to V has two interphalangeal (IP) joints, referred to as the proximal interphalangeal (PIP) and distal interphalangeal (DIP) joints. The thumb has only two phalanges and therefore only one IP joint. IP joints are classified as hinge joints with one degree of freedom. The IP joints possess volar plate mechanisms similar to the MCP joints with the addition of check rein ligaments, which prevent hyperextension. These ligaments cross the joints on the volar surface on either side of the flexor tendon sheath.

Motions of the Fingers

Metacarpophalangeal joints of the fingers have approximately 90 degrees of flexion, with the index finger having slightly less and the middle, ring, and little fingers having successively more range. The end-feel may be hard with contact of the phalanx on the metacarpal or firm from capsular limitation. Hyperextension is variable depending on ligamentous structure. Some people may be able to extend the MCP joints to only 0 degrees whereas others with ligamentous laxity may be able to actively hyperextend up to 45 degrees. Passively, some can hyperextend to 90 degrees. The normal end-feel is firm from limitation by the volar plate and capsule.

When the MCP joint is extended, the collateral ligaments are slack and permit about 20 degrees of abduction and, if adjacent fingers are moved away, about 20 degrees of adduction. In 90 degrees of flexion, the collateral ligaments are taut and abduction or adduction are limited to a few degrees at best. This is the close-packed position of the joint.

The MCP joint of the thumb is usually described as a hinge joint. It has less motion than the MCP joints of the fingers. Flexion occurs to 45 to 60 degrees and hyperextension from 0 to 20 degrees. In full flexion and extension, ligaments tighten and there is little abduction or adduction. In semiflexion, 5 to 10 degrees of side-to-side motion can occur plus a dynamic rotation of the phalanx produced by contraction of the muscles to the medial or the lateral sesamoid bone. These small motions precisely fit the thumb around objects for grasping.

Proximal and distal IP joints are hinge joints with one degree of freedom. The bicondylar heads of the phalanges and the greater tension of the collateral ligaments prohibit motions of abduction and adduction. Flexion of the PIP joints is about 120 degrees and of the DIP and the IP joints, slightly less than 90 degrees. Extension of the PIP and DIP joints is to 0 degrees except in individuals with ligamentous laxity, in which some hyperextension is seen. Hyperextension of the thumb IP joint may be 5 to 10 degrees and can be considerably more passive, as when pressing down with the thumb pad.

ACCESSORY MOTIONS Large joint play movements are possible when a person is relaxed and the capsules of the MCP joints are loose. If the examiner stabilizes the metacarpal with one hand and holds the proximal phalanx with the other hand, translatory motions of dorsal, volar, and lateral glides; rotation; and distraction can be made with the base of the phalanx (see Fig. 1–10).

Similar motions but with smaller movements are found in the IP joints.

MUSCLES

Function of the hand is complex and difficult to understand for many reasons. One, the hand is a compact multipurpose organ with interdependency of structures in which injury to one may affect many others. Two, the hand possesses both great mobility and great stability and can shift from one to the other in a fraction of a second. Three, almost all of the muscles are pluriarticular and therefore can have an effect on each joint crossed. Some cross as many as seven joints, and to prevent an undesired motion by the muscle, other muscles must contract. Four, the hand has many automatic neurophysiologic synergies that are so strongly linked that a person cannot willfully separate them. For example, when making a fist, the wrist extensors contract forcefully and cannot be voluntarily inhibited.

Basic to the understanding of muscle function is knowledge of the anatomic actions of each muscle. This information is used to determine the effect of a muscle if it were to shorten completely, to elongate a muscle passively to its normal length, and to isolate muscles (as possible) to test for their presence or strength. Muscles should be studied on the skeleton, the cadaver, and the living subject, considering: (1) over which joints each muscle passes; (2) the line of action of the muscle and its tendon; (3) the distance of the muscle to the axis of joint motion at various positions of the joint; and (4) the relative length of the muscle.

Muscles Acting on the Wrist (and Elbow)

Extensor carpi radialis longus
Extensor carpi radialis brevis
Extensor carpi ulnaris
Flexor carpi radialis
Palmaris longus
Flexor carpi ulnaris

Palpation of Muscles Acting in Extension of the Wrist

If the wrist is extended with the fist closed, the tendon of the **extensor carpi radialis longus** becomes prominent and is palpated as seen in Figure 6–7. The tendon

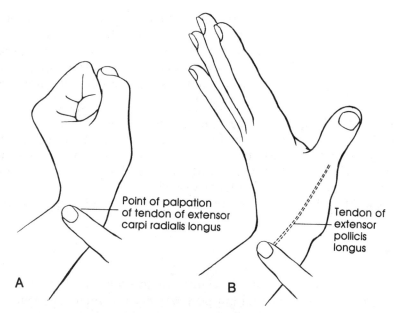

Point of palpation
of tendon of extensor
carpi radialis longus

Tendon of
extensor
pollicis
longus

A

B

Figure 6–7 (A) Palpation of the tendon of extensor carpi radialis longus at the base of the second metacarpal when the fist is closed. (B) When the fingers are extended, extensor digitorum takes over the task of extending the wrist. Note that the tendon of extensor pollicis longus also courses on the extensor side of the wrist, not far from the tendon of extensor carpi radialis longus.

lies on the radial side of the capitate bone but on the ulnar side of the tubercle of the radius and courses toward the base of the metacarpal bone of the index finger, to which it is attached. The distal attachment of the **extensor carpi radialis brevis** is the base of the metacarpal bone of the middle finger. The tendon of the extensor of the index finger crosses over the extensor carpi radialis brevis, making identification of the muscle by palpation somewhat difficult. Its tendon can usually be felt rising if the thumb is moved in a palmar direction, in a plane perpendicular to the palm of the hand.

The muscular parts of the two radial wrist extensors, together with the brachioradialis, make up the radial muscle group at the elbow. By manipulating the muscle tissue, this group may be separated from the other extensors on the dorsum of the forearm and from the flexor group on the palmar side of the forearm. To locate the radial extensors of the wrist, the brachioradialis is first identified by resistance to elbow flexion with the forearm halfway between pronation and supination (see Fig. 5–9). The muscular portion of the extensor carpi radialis longus is then located close to the brachioradialis, toward the dorsal side of the forearm. It is a superficial muscle and may be readily identified when resistance is given to extension of the wrist (see Fig. 5–10). The extensor carpi radialis brevis is found somewhat more distally.

The **extensor digitorum** participates in extension of the wrist only when the fingers are simultaneously extended; in fact, the finger extensors then appear to take over the task of wrist extension altogether. To feel the shift from wrist extensors to finger extensors, the wrist should first be extended with the fist closed, and the prominent tendon of extensor carpi radialis longus palpated at the base of the second metacarpal (see Fig. 6–7A). While maintaining the wrist in this position, the fingers are extended (see Fig. 6–7B). It is then noted that the prominent tendon being palpated "disappears," a sign that the muscle "lets go" or diminishes its contraction. At the same time, the tendons of the extensor digitorum can be seen and palpated on the dorsum of the hand. This shift is regulated automatically. If, however, the wrist is held in the extreme of hyperextension, both tendons are found to be prominent.

The tendon of the **extensor carpi ulnaris** is palpated between the head of the ulna and a prominent tubercle on the base of the fifth metacarpal bone, the latter serving as its point of distal attachment. The tendon becomes prominent if the wrist is extended with the fist closed and even more prominent if the wrist is simultaneously abducted ulnarward (Fig. 6–8). The tendon is also easily palpable when the thumb is extended and abducted (see Fig. 6–22).

The muscular portion of the **extensor carpi ulnaris** is best palpated about 2 inches (5 cm) below the lateral epicondyle of the humerus, where it lies between the anconeus and the extensor digitorum (see Fig. 5–12). From this point on, it may be followed distally along the dorsoulnar aspect of the forearm in a direction toward the head of the ulna.

The proximal attachments of the wrist extensors have a common tendon attachment from the lateral epicondyle of the humerus with the extensor carpi radialis longus also attaching higher onto the lateral supracondylar ridge. When the elbow is extended, the line of action of these muscles crosses on or slightly posterior to the axis of the elbow. After 15 degrees of elbow flexion, their line of pull is anterior to the axis, and the wrist extensors are elbow flexors. The higher attachment of the extensor carpi radialis longus provides good lever arm distance from the elbow axis when the elbow is flexed to 90 degrees. This muscle is often used to flex the elbow if the brachialis and biceps are paralyzed.

Palpation of Muscles Acting in Flexion of the Wrist

The three tendons of the wrist flexors become prominent if resistance is given to flexion of the wrist (Fig. 6–9). The most centrally located tendon is that of the **palmaris longus**; it varies in size in different individuals, or it may be missing altogether. Radial to it, the strong tendon of the **flexor carpi radialis** is identified.

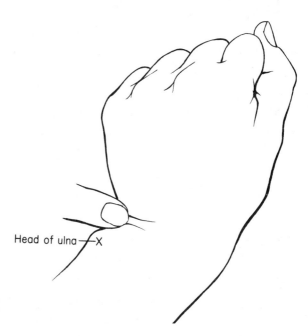

Head of ulna—X

Figure 6–8 Palpation of extensor carpi ulnaris at the base of the fifth metacarpal in power grip.

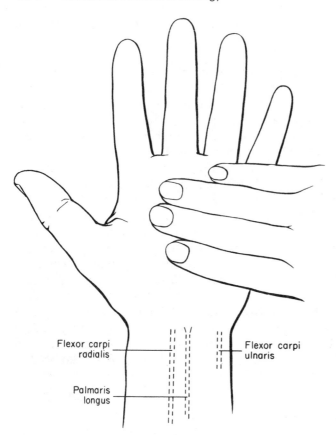

Flexor carpi
radialis

Flexor carpi
ulnaris

Palmaris
longus

Figure 6–9   Resistance to wrist flexion applied in the palm of the hand brings out tendons of wrist flexors.

This tendon lies in a superficial position in the lower part of the forearm, is held down by the transverse carpal ligament at the wrist, and disappears into a groove in the trapezium bone. It cannot be followed to its distal attachment on the base of the second metacarpal bone. The tendon of the **flexor carpi ulnaris** lies close to the ulnar border of the forearm and may be palpated between the styloid process of the ulna and the pisiform bone, to which it is attached.

If the fist is tightly closed and wrist flexion is simultaneously resisted, one or more tendons of the **flexor digitorum superficialis** become prominent in the space between the palmaris longus and the flexor carpi ulnaris (Fig. 6–10). The tendon of the fourth digit appears to rise to the surface. In individuals lacking the palmaris longus, a more complete display of the tendons of the long finger flexors may be observed if flexion of the wrist is resisted and the subject then flexes one finger after the other or flexes all fingers simultaneously.

Part of the proximal attachment of the wrist flexors is the common flexor tendon from the medial epicondyle of the humerus. When the elbow is flexed, these muscles lie on the anterior side of the elbow axis. Their leverage for elbow flexion is not as good as the wrist extensors, but their maximum elongation occurs when the wrist and elbow are extended.

Muscles Acting in Radial and Ulnar Abduction of the Wrist

The palmaris longus and the extensor carpi radialis brevis have a central location at the wrist; the other wrist flexors and extensors are situated either toward the ra-

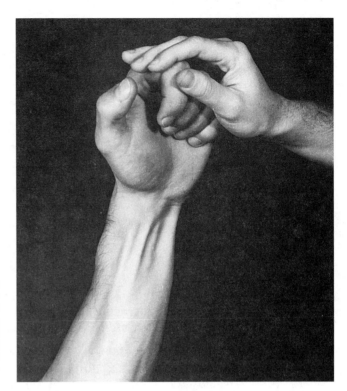

Figure 6–10 When a tight fist is made and wrist flexion is resisted, four tendons are visible: on the ulnar side of the wrist, the flexor carpi ulnaris; next, the flexor digitorum superficialis; then, the prominent palmaris longus; and, on the radial side, the flexor carpi radialis.

dial or toward the ulnar side of the wrist. They are therefore capable of producing movements from side to side as well as flexion and extension.

When the extensor carpi ulnaris and flexor carpi ulnaris combine their actions, ulnar abduction of the wrist results. The extensor carpi radialis longus and the flexor carpi radialis, aided by the abductor pollicis longus and the extensor pollicis brevis, produce radial abduction. The latter two muscles have a favorable line of action for performing radial abduction, and they do so regardless of the position of the thumb, whether flexed, extended, abducted, or adducted.

The wrist furnishes typical examples of how muscles may act as either synergists or antagonists. For instance, in flexion and extension of the wrist, the flexor carpi ulnaris and the extensor carpi ulnaris are antagonists, but in ulnar abduction of the wrist these two muscles act as synergists.

ROLE OF THE WRIST EXTENSORS IN GRASPING   When the fist closes, the fingers fold into the palm of the hand or close around an object by the action of the long finger flexors (profundus and superficialis), probably aided by some of the intrinsic muscles of the hand. Because these long finger flexors have proximal attachments in the forearm and their tendons pass on the flexor side of the wrist, these muscles, if unopposed, would cause the wrist to flex during grasp. Such action is prevented by the stabilizing action of the wrist extensors. The strength of contraction of the wrist extensors is in direct proportion to the effort of the grip—the harder the grip, the stronger the contraction of the wrist extensors.

If the wrist is allowed to flex during finger flexion, the grip is markedly weakened (see Fig. 4–9); in fact, it then becomes almost impossible to close the fist completely (Fig. 6–11). This difficulty arises partly because the finger extension apparatus may not permit further elongation (passive insufficiency) and partly be-

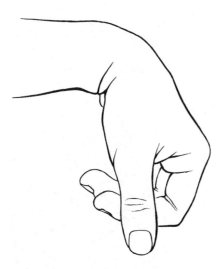

Figure 6–11   Weakness of grasp when the wrist is fully flexed. In this position, it becomes difficult or impossible to close the fist completely.

cause of the marked approximation of the proximal and distal attachments of the finger flexors, which weakens their contraction so that they may attain a length at which they are unable to produce effective tension (active insufficiency).

PALPATION OF THE WRIST EXTENSORS IN GRASPING   For palpation of the **extensor carpi radialis longus,** the subject places the lightly closed fist on the table or in the lap, forearm pronated, and the examiner palpates on the radiodorsal aspect of the wrist, as explained previously. By having the subject alternately close the fist firmly and relax the grip, the rise and fall of the tendon of the extensor carpi radialis longus may be felt and its contracting muscle belly identified in the forearm close to the brachioradialis. To eliminate the possibility of palpating the wrong tendon, the tendon of the extensor pollicis longus should first be identified. This poses no difficulty because the tendon is visible under the skin when the thumb is held in extension.

The **extensor carpi radialis brevis** also participates in wrist fixation for grasp, but its tendon protrudes less than that of the extensor carpi radialis longus and is therefore somewhat more difficult to identify. Its tendon may be palpated on the dorsum of the wrist, in line with the third metacarpal bone, when the fist is firmly closed.

The **extensor carpi ulnaris** also participates in wrist fixation for grasp. When a fist is made, its tendon and muscle belly may be palpated in the location previously described (see Fig. 6–8).

ROLE OF THE WRIST FLEXORS IN EXTENSION OF THE FINGERS   The long extensor muscles of the fingers are attached in the forearm and pass over the wrist and then over the MCP joints. If these muscles were to contract in an isolated fashion, they would extend not only the joints of the fingers but also the wrist. To prevent them from moving the wrist, the wrist flexors contract synergically, keeping the wrist in a neutral position or flexing it. The association between finger extensors and wrist flexors is strong, and it takes concentrated effort to interrupt the linkage.

If complete finger extension is alternated with grasp in rapid succession, it can be observed that the wrist as well as the fingers are in constant motion: flexion of the wrist accompanies finger extension; extension of the wrist occurs when the fist is closed. These combinations are automatic, and the less attention the performer pays to the details of the performance, the more obvious they will be. Note that the wrist movements are in a direction opposite to the finger motions, so that an alternate elongation of the finger extensors and the finger flexors over the wrist is obtained. Such elongation adds to the efficiency of these muscles in extending and flexing the fingers.

PALPATION OF THE WRIST FLEXORS IN EXTENSION OF THE FINGERS When the fingers are extended, the tendons of the wrist flexors are palpated on the palmar side of the wrist: the flexor carpi radialis and the palmaris longus in the center, the flexor carpi ulnaris near the pisiform bone—all three muscles spring into action. With increased forcefulness of finger extension, increased tension can be felt in the wrist flexors.

Muscles Acting on the Digits

Functions of the hand depend on the teamwork of the many muscles of the wrist and digits. The muscles of the digits have been classified as (1) extrinsic muscles, which have proximal attachments in the forearm or humerus; and (2) intrinsic muscles, which have both proximal and distal attachments within the hand:

Extrinsic Muscles	**Intrinsic Muscles**
Extensor digitorum	Four lumbricals
Extensor indicis proprius	Three palmar interossei
Extensor digiti minimi	Four dorsal interossei
Extensor pollicis longus	Thenar muscles
Extensor pollicis brevis	Opponens pollicis
Abductor pollicis longus	Abductor pollicis brevis
Flexor digitorum superficialis	Adductor pollicis
Flexor digitorum profundus	Flexor pollicis brevis
Flexor pollicis longus	Hypothenar muscles
	Opponens digiti minimi
	Abductor digiti minimi
	Flexor digiti minimi brevis
	Palmaris brevis

Proximal Attachments

Because extrinsic muscles have their proximal attachments in the forearm or on the humerus, they all have an effect on the wrist as flexors or extensors when the muscles contract. If the muscles lack normal length, they may affect the range of motion of the digits and the wrist. The extensor digitorum and the extensor digiti minimi have their proximal attachments on the lateral epicondyle of the humerus in the common extensor tendon, and the flexor digitorum superficialis has a proximal attachment on the medial epicondyle in the common flexor tendon. In addition to their effects on the digits and the wrist, these muscles can contribute to elbow flexion.

The proximal attachments of the lumbricals are on the tendons of the flexor digitorum profundus in the palm. Thus, if the profundus is relaxed, the lumbricals can pull these tendons distally. The dorsal and palmar interossei have their proximal attachments on the side of the shafts of the metacarpals. Most of the thenar and hypothenar muscles have attachments on the flexor retinaculum and on the carpal bones. The flexor retinaculum is in turn stabilized by the contraction of the palmaris longus and the flexor carpi ulnaris through attachment on the pisiform and its radiating fascia.

Extensor Assembly

The digital tendons of the extensor muscles and almost all of the intrinsic muscles terminate in the extensor assembly (exceptions: palmaris brevis, opponens pollicis, and the opponens, abductor, and flexor digiti minimi muscles) (Fig. 6–12). Among its other names are the extensor expansion, apparatus, aponeurosis, retinaculum, or hood. The extensor assembly is made up of a tendinous system composed of the distal tendons of attachment of the extensor muscles, lumbricals, interossei, and thenar and hypothenar muscles and a retinacular system of fasciae and ligaments to retain and stabilize the tendons and the skin. The purpose of the assembly is to extend the digits in different positions of finger flexion. Another purpose is to provide shortcuts for the extensor tendon across the joints and to permit the digits full flexion (see Fig. 6–12, finger flexed). The extensor tendons must cover a longer distance from full hyperextension to full flexion. This distance is about 25 mm and can be approximated in the normal subject by placing a string over the dorsum of a finger and marking the change in length from extension to flexion.

TENDINOUS SYSTEM The long extensor tendon (ie, extensor digitorum) crosses the MCP joint and from the undersurface extends a lax tendon, which inserts into the MCP joint capsule and the base of the proximal phalanx (Zancolli, 1979). Over the proximal phalanx the extensor tendon divides into three bands: the central band, which inserts into the base of the middle phalanx, and two lateral bands that course on either side to the PIP joint and continue on to rejoin over the middle phalanx and insert into the base of the distal phalanx.

Interossei muscles have several terminal tendons on the sides of each finger (see Fig. 6–12). These include bony insertions into the base of the proximal phalanges, attachments to the volar plate, tendons that contribute to the lateral bands, and tendons that contribute to the base of the middle phalanx. The terminal attachments of the lumbricals pass on the radial side of the MCP joints and volar to the tendons of the interossei. The distal lumbrical tendon inserts into and helps form the lateral band. Thus, for each finger, the motor input into the lateral bands, which extend the PIP and DIP joints, is provided by at least four muscles: the extrinsic extensor(s), two interossei, and a lumbrical.

The tendon of the extensor indicis proprius parallels the extensor digitorum on the ulnar side of the finger. The indicis has a separate muscle belly in the forearm and provides independent movement of the index finger even when the other fingers are flexed. The extensor digiti minimi usually divides into two tendons in the area of the hood and is the primary long extensor of the little finger. According to Brand (1985), the extensor digitorum tendon to the fifth digit is usually small and inadequate to extend the finger. The abductor digiti minimi inserts into the hood and the lateral bands of the extensor assembly, as do the interossei.

The thumb has a similar extensor assembly with tendinous insertions from the adductor pollicis, flexor pollicis brevis, and abductor pollicis brevis.

RETINACULAR SYSTEM The complex fascial and ligamentous parts of the retinacular system enclose, compartmentalize, and restrain the joints and tendons as well as the nerves, blood vessels, and skin. A fibrous hood or dorsal expansion encircles the MCP joints and retains the tendons crossing the joint.

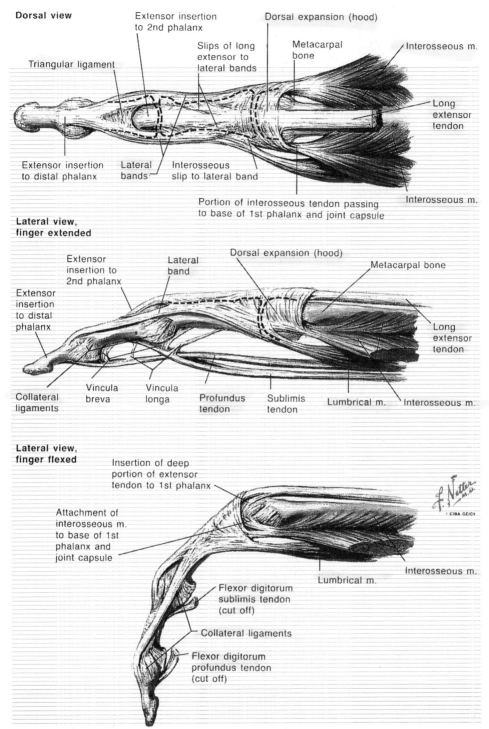

Dorsal view

Extensor insertion to 2nd phalanx

Dorsal expansion (hood)

Slips of long extensor to lateral bands

Metacarpal bone

Interosseous m.

Triangular ligament

Long extensor tendon

Extensor insertion to distal phalanx

Lateral bands

Interosseous slip to lateral band

Portion of interosseous tendon passing to base of 1st phalanx and joint capsule

Interosseous m.

Lateral view, finger extended

Extensor insertion to 2nd phalanx

Lateral band

Dorsal expansion (hood)

Metacarpal bone

Extensor insertion to distal phalanx

Long extensor tendon

Collateral ligaments

Vincula breva

Vincula longa

Profundus tendon

Sublimis tendon

Lumbrical m.

Interosseous m.

Lateral view, finger flexed

Insertion of deep portion of extensor tendon to 1st phalanx

Attachment of interosseous m. to base of 1st phalanx and joint capsule

Lumbrical m.

Interosseous m.

Flexor digitorum sublimis tendon (cut off)

Collateral ligaments

Flexor digitorum profundus tendon (cut off)

Figure 6–12 Dorsal and lateral views of the anatomic structures of the extensor assembly of a finger. (© Copyright 1969, CIBA Pharmaceutical Company, Division of CIBA-GEIGY Corporation. Reprinted with permission. Adapted from CLINICAL SYMPOSIA illustrated by Frank H. Netter, MD. All rights reserved.)

Attachments of the hood are on the palmar sides at the junction of the volar plate and the transverse intermetacarpal ligament (see Fig. 6–6). Distally, the hood and tendons are difficult to distinguish. When the fingers are flexed, the extensor hood is pulled distally so that the hood lies over the proximal phalange rather than over the MCP joint (see Fig. 6–12). At the level of the PIP joint, the retinacular system joins and restrains the tendinous system, capsular structures, and skin. During finger flexion, for example, the lateral bands must move volarly on the PIP joint to permit the motion, but to be effective in extension of the IP joints, the tendons must move dorsally. It is the purpose of the fascia and ligaments of the retinacular system to control and to limit these motions.

Flexor Pulleys

The retinacular system is also connected to the flexor compartment. The flexor digitorum superficialis and profundus tendons are enclosed in synovial-lined tunnels, which are maintained against the palmar surfaces of the phalanges by pulleys. Annular (L., ring) pulleys attach to the shafts of the proximal and distal phalanges and to the sides of the volar plates of the MCP, PIP, and DIP joints at the junctions with the extensor hood and the retinaculum. Cruciate pulleys attach on the shafts of the phalanges and cross to form distal attachments on the volar plates of the PIP and DIP joints (Amadio, Lin, and An, 1989). These pulleys prevent bowstringing of the long flexor tendons. Severance of a pulley causes loss of finger motion (Lin et al, 1989). Some of these pulleys can be seen supporting the flexor digitorum profundus tendon in Figure 6–20 views. Removal of the pulleys has occurred in Figure 6–12, lateral views.

Thus the retinacular system can be compared to an interconnecting structure that encircles the digit and creates balanced forces. Destruction of a ligament by injury or disease such as rheumatoid arthritis can cause disruption of the balanced forces and movement of tendons to abnormal positions, which create further deforming forces. For example, destruction of an accessory collateral ligament (see Fig. 6–6) can cause the extensor digitorum tendon to slide off the dorsum of the MCP joint into the intercarpal gutter as well as loss of restraint and bowstringing of the flexor tendons.

Role of the Long Finger Flexors in Grasping

Flexor digitorum superficialis and profundus serve the second to fifth digits for flexion at the IP joints. Because the tendons of these muscles pass on the palmar side of the wrist and the MCP joints, they also tend to produce flexion of these joints. In using the hand for grasping, flexion of the MCP joints is necessary for proper shape of the hand, while flexion at the wrist is undesirable because it decreases the force exerted by the flexors by shortening them. Fortunately, wrist flexion is prevented by synergic contraction of the wrist extensors.

The flexor digitorum superficialis, attaching to the base of the middle phalanx, flexes the proximal IP joint. The flexor digitorum profundus tendon, after perforating the superficialis tendon, attaches to the base of the distal phalanx and acts as a flexor of the distal as well as the proximal IP joint. The profundus is the only muscle capable of flexing the distal joint.

In the motion of closing the hand, flexion of the finger is almost simultaneous at the digital joints. The IP joints initiate the motion and the PIP has the greatest amount of motion. This mechanism permits the pads of the fingers to contact and feel the object to be grasped. The only muscle that shows EMG activity during easy unresisted motion is the flexor digitorum profundus (Backhouse and Catton, 1954; Long and Brown, 1964). MCP flexion is attributed to passive tension of the lateral bands and the tendons of the intrinsic muscles (Landsmeer and Long, 1965; Long, 1968; Zancolli, 1979). Contraction of the flexor digitorum profundus exerts traction on the proximal attachment of the lumbrical, and the simultaneous flexion of the IP joints places the intrinsic muscles on a stretch distally, thus producing MCP flexion. The existence of passive tension can be seen in the semiflexed position of the fingers in the resting hand. This same position is seen in astronauts sleeping in space, where no gravitational force acts on the hand.

When the wrist is extended, length-tension relationships of the flexor digitorum profundus are favorable for producing tensions, and sufficient tension is developed to close the fist. With progressive flexion of the wrist, however, length-tension relationships of the profundus become less favorable, and the flexor digitorum superficialis is recruited to aid in fist closure. Forceful closure of the hand or power grip elicits high-level activity of the flexor digitorum superficialis, the interossei, and the flexor digitorum profundus.

Subjects with long-standing paralysis of the intrinsic muscles, even though the flexor digitorum profundus and superficialis are intact, have an ineffective grasp. Such a subject is still capable of making a fist, but the IP joints flex first and the MCP joints flex a fraction of a second later (Fig. 6–13). Without the intrinsic muscles, some difficulty arises when the subject attempts an activity that requires quick closure of the hand, as in catching a ball. Disturbance of the extrinsic-intrinsic muscle balance eventually results in a "claw" posture of the hand. Changes in capsules and ligaments and atrophy and loss of elastic properties of the intrinsic muscles are part of the reason for this problem.

Palpation and Testing of the Long Finger Flexors

The **flexor digitorum superficialis** is located underneath the flexor carpi radialis and the palmaris longus, and the general direction of the muscle is from the flexor

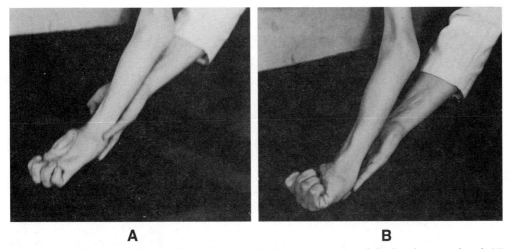

A   **B**

Figure 6–13 Manner of closure of the fist when the intrinsic muscles of the hand are paralyzed. (*A*) The interphalangeal joints are first flexed by the long finger flexors. (*B*) In continued action, these muscles also flex the metacarpophalangeal joints, so that the fingers "roll" into the palm. Simultaneous flexion of all finger joints, such as is needed in catching a ball, cannot be accomplished.

(medial) epicondyle to the center of the palmar side of the wrist. It is difficult or impossible to palpate the muscle at its proximal attachment because this is widespread and in part tendinous, and impossible to distinguish the separate muscle bellies serving the four fingers. However, movement of the tendons of the superficialis may be observed in the forearm and at the wrist beneath the tendons of the flexor carpi radialis and palmaris longus, and particularly in the space between the two tendons. In this region, as previously mentioned, the tendon serving the fourth digit usually stands out prominently if a firm fist is made while the wrist is somewhat flexed. In subjects lacking the palmaris longus, observation is considerably easier.

Isolated action of the flexor digitorum superficialis is obtained if the proximal IP joint is flexed while the distal joint remains inactive, a movement that is best performed with one finger at a time (Fig. 6–14A). The coordination needed for this movement can be mastered by most individuals; if some difficulty arises, the examiner should stabilize the proximal phalanx.

Another way in which the superficialis of one digit may be tested without participation by the profundus is for the examiner to maintain the other digits in full extension at all joints (Fig. 6–14B). This inactivates the profundus so that the subject is unable to flex the distal joint.

The **flexor digitorum profundus** is deeply located, being covered by the flexor digitorum superficialis, flexor carpi ulnaris, palmaris longus, flexor carpi radialis, and pronator teres. It is muscular only in the upper half of the forearm. The muscle bellies serving the individual fingers are not nearly as well separated as those of the superficialis.

In spite of the deep location of the profundus, its contracting muscle belly may be palpated, provided that tension is minimal in the more superficial muscles. To achieve relative relaxation of the overlying muscles, the subject is seated with the forearm supinated and resting in the lap while the wrist is extended by the weight of the hand (protruding over the lap). When the arm is in this position and the subject closes the fist fully but with moderate effort, the profundus may

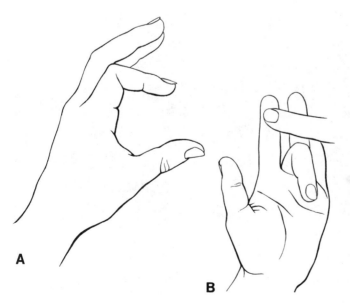

A

B

Figure 6–14 (*A*) Isolated action of the flexor digitorum superficialis of the index finger. (*B*) Method for testing individual flexor digitorum superficialis muscles by holding all other fingers in extension. Light pressure on the pulp of the finger will show the relaxation of the flexor digitorum profundus.

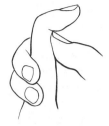

Figure 6–15 Testing flexor digitorum profundus of the index finger by stabilizing the proximal interphalangeal joint. Strength of the muscle can be felt by resisting distal interphalangeal joint flexion.

be felt rising under the examiner's fingers, which are placed in the region between the pronator teres and the flexor carpi ulnaris, about 2 inches (5 cm) below the medial epicondyle of the humerus.

In testing the profundus, one finger at a time is stabilized over the middle phalanx, as seen in Figure 6–15. During this test, it may be observed that the index finger is able to move well without drawing the other fingers into action, and the middle finger can be moved alone comparatively well, while isolated flexion of the fourth and the fifth fingers is difficult or impossible.

Ordinarily, a subject is unable to move the distal IP joint separately when no fixation of the middle phalanx is given. This is understandable, because the tendon of the profundus acts on the two IP joints simultaneously. Under normal circumstances, there is no extensor mechanism capable of extending the proximal joint separately. There are subjects, however, whose proximal IP joints allow hyperextension, and these persons will succeed in flexing the distal joints in an isolated fashion (Fig. 6–16). The middle band of the extensor mechanism then "locks" the proximal joint in hyperextension, preventing the profundus from flexing it. When the proximal joint is hyperextended, the lateral band becomes slack and therefore can exert no action on the distal joint.

Role of the Intrinsic Muscles in Grasping

The location of the dorsal interosseous muscles with the MCP joints extended would indicate that these muscles are essentially neutral with respect to flexion and extension of the MCP joints. But the palmar interossei and the lumbrical muscles course definitely on the palmar side of the axis for flexion and extension

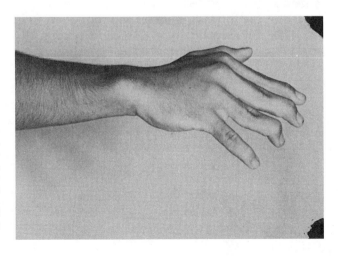

Figure 6–16 A subject who is capable of stabilizing the proximal interphalangeal joint in hyperextension can flex the distal joint in an isolated fashion by flexor digitorum profundus. Ordinarily, the profundus acts on both joints. Note the dorsal medial position of the lateral bands to the axis of the PIP joints.

of these joints and are therefore mechanically capable of producing flexion. The leverage of the lumbrical muscles for flexion is more favorable than that of the palmar interossei—the former course on the palmar, the latter on the dorsal side of the transverse metacarpal ligament (see Fig. 6–12). As mentioned previously, none of the intrinsic muscles show EMG activity with easy or light-resisted closure of the fingers. Their role in MCP flexion is thought to be from passive stretch.

When a lumbrical is stimulated by a high-intensity electric current, the result is strong extension of the IP joints and flexion of the MCP joint to about 80 degrees. However, when a low current is used (minimal to produce response) the IP joints extend, but the MCP joint flexes very little or not at all (Backhouse and Catton, 1954). This suggests that the leverage of a lumbrical muscle for extension of the IP joints is far better than its leverage for flexion of the MCP joint. The high-current experiment also demonstrates that a lumbrical muscle when contracting maximally is capable of shortening effectively through a long range. Such long effective excursion is remarkable when one considers that, under such experimental conditions, the proximal attachment of the lumbrical muscle must be poorly stabilized because the flexor digitorum profundus muscle is inactive.

Flexion of the finger pulls the extensor hood distally over the proximal phalange, and the tendons of the interossei cross the MCP joint on the volar side with considerable distance from the joint center. In pinching, grasping, and power grip, the interossei are found to have high levels of activity (Long et al, 1970). This muscle contraction serves to rotate the finger to fit the surface of the object, strengthen the grip, stabilize the proximal phalanges against the metacarpal head, and stabilize the extensor tendons on the dorsum of the MCP joints through attachments to the extensor hood.

Although the lumbricals cross the MCP joint at a farther distance from the joint center than do the interossei, the lumbricals are electrically silent in MCP flexion unless the IP joints are extended. The lumbricals do not participate in grip and rarely contract synchronously with the flexor digitorum profundus.

INTRINSIC-PLUS AND INTRINSIC-MINUS POSITIONS The motion of MCP flexion with IP extension produces major EMG activity in the intrinsic muscles and slight variable activity in the extrinsic muscles (Fig. 6–17). This position of the digits is called the "intrinsic-plus" hand position. It is also the position in which interossei and the lumbricals assume their shortest length. The hand assumes this position with contracture of the intrinsic muscles as is often found in rheumatoid arthritis. Normal length of the intrinsic muscles should permit full passive flexion of the DIPs and the PIPs followed by hyperextension of the MCP joints. An "intrinsic-minus" hand has paralysis of the interossei and lumbrical muscles. The resting posture of

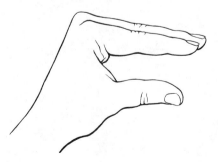

Figure 6–17 Flexion of the metacarpophalangeal joints, extension of the interphalangeal joints ("intrinsic-plus" hand position).

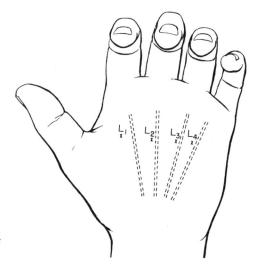

Figure 6–18 The muscular portions of the lumbricals are located on the radial side of the tendons of
the long finger flexors.

this hand is referred to as a "clawhand," with the MCP joints in slight hyperextension and the IP joints in partial flexion.

As mentioned previously, none of the intrinsic muscles show EMG activity
with easy or lightly resisted closure of the fingers. Their role in MCP flexion is
thought to be from passive stretch.

Palpation of the Intrinsic Muscles

The muscular portions of the lumbricals are located on the radial side of the tendons of the long finger flexors. In most hands, these tendons are best visible in the
clawhand position, that is, when the MCP joints are hyperextended and the IP
joints are flexed (Fig. 6–18). Identification of the lumbrical muscles by palpation is
difficult because these muscles are small and covered with fascia and skin.

The palmar interossei are located deep in the palm of the hand beneath the
lumbricals and between the metacarpal bones. They are even less accessible to palpation than the lumbricals.

The muscular portion of the first interosseus is easily observed and palpated in
the space between the metacarpal bones of the thumb and the index finger when
resistance is applied to abduction of the index finger, by manual resistance or by
using a rubber band, as seen in Figure 6–19A. The second, third, and fourth dorsal
interossei are more difficult to palpate in the narrow spaces between the
metacarpal bones, but their attachments at the base of the proximal phalanges
may be felt, although some practice is needed to do so. By applying a rubber band
around the fingers in various combinations, the action of each finger abductor, including the abductor of the fifth finger, may be brought out.

The abductor digiti minimi may be palpated on the ulnar border of the hand.

Extension of the Fingers

The extensor digitorum through its attachments on the bases of the proximal,
middle, and distal phalanges is mechanically capable of extending the MCP, PIP,
and DIP joints but not at the same time. When the extensor digitorum contracts

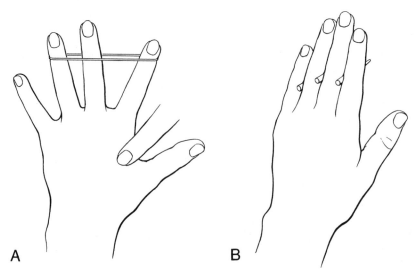

Figure 6–19 (*A*) Palpation of the muscular portion of the first dorsal interosseus. A rubber band offers resistance to the first and fourth dorsal interossei. (*B*) Adduction of the fingers to compress dowel (or card) activates the palmar interossei.

alone, as with intrinsic muscle paralysis or electrical stimulation, the MCP joints extend but the IP joints remain semiflexed in a clawhand position. This flexion is due to the passive resistance of the flexor digitorum profundus and active insufficiency of the extensor digitorum. If, however, the MCP joint is blocked at 0 degrees of extension, the force of the long extensor is transmitted to the IP joints and they extend. This phenomenon (ie, blocking hyperextension at the MCP joint) is used in splinting the hand that has intrinsic muscle paralysis and permits functional opening of the hand.

The line of pull of the interossei and the lumbricals through the lateral bands and the retinaculum is dorsal to the joint centers of the PIP and DIP joints, making them mechanically capable of extending these joints. Physiologically, the muscles demonstrate this ability with strong electrical stimulation as previously described. Thus the intrinsic muscles have been called the primary extensors of the IP joints. In function, however, this does not always hold true.

During unresisted opening of the hand, synchronous EMG activity takes place in the long extensors and the lumbricals only. The interossei are electrically silent. The lumbricals could be considered acting to extend the IP joints, but they have very poor proximal fixation because of the inactivity of the flexor digitorum profundus. Several authors have suggested that the function of the lumbrical is to pull the profundus tendon distally to decrease the passive tension and thus facilitate digital extension by the extensor digitorum (Sunderland, 1945; Backhouse and Catton, 1954; Long, 1968; Spinner, 1984). That such passive resistance exists may be concluded from the semiflexed position of the fingers when the arm hangs relaxed at the side of the body. Ranney and Wells (1988) propose that the lumbrical pulls the profundus tendon distally and also extends the IP joints but that its direct contribution is small compared to its indirect contribution of release of tension. The authors consider that the lumbrical also prevents MCP joint hyperextension by the extensor digitorum. An additional function of the lumbrical contraction during digital extension may be to stretch the profundus into a more favorable length-tension position before its subsequent contraction.

Forceful or resisted extension of the digits produces electrical activity in the interossei muscles.

THE LUMBRICALS   The lumbricals have a number of unusual characteristics and their function is puzzling. Both their proximal and distal attachments are movable unless fixed by other muscles. The lumbricals and the flexor digitorum profundus, however, seldom contract at the same time (Long and Brown, 1964; Citron and Foster, 1988). Anatomically, the size and proximal attachments of the lumbricals have a high rate of variability. The muscles are richly innervated. They have a low number of muscle fibers per motor unit and a high number of muscle spindles even compared to the first dorsal interosseous (see Table 3–3). Rabischong (1962) found a wide variety of muscle and tendon receptors and suggested that the lumbrical may have a highly specialized proprioceptive function such as a tensiometer. The lumbrical is in an unusual position as a neuromuscular connection between the flexor and extensor mechanisms of the finger.

Abduction and Adduction of Digits II to V

NOMENCLATURE   Movements away from the midline of the hand are called **abduction**; movements toward the midline are called **adduction.** The midline is a longitudinal line through the center of the forearm and hand and through the middle finger; thus, when the fingers spread apart they are abducted, and when they lie close together they are adducted. The third finger, being in the midline, has both radial and ulnar abduction.

RELATIONSHIP OF ABDUCTION AND ADDUCTION TO FLEXION AND EXTENSION   Abduction and adduction movements are free when the MCP joints are extended (collateral ligaments are loose); when these joints flex, the fingers automatically adduct, and the range of abduction becomes extremely limited or is absent (collateral ligaments tight). The natural tendency is to abduct the fingers as they extend; it may be said that extension and abduction belong together, as do flexion and adduction. If the fist is closed and opened in rapid succession, this pattern becomes obvious: The fingers abduct as they extend and adduct as they flex. In slower motions, and with some concentration, it is entirely possible to keep the fingers adducted as they extend. The extension-abduction combination appears to be part of a mass movement that is considerably easier to execute than other combinations.

When the fingers are flexed one at a time, they point toward the base of the thumb. The literature often states that the point of convergence is on the scaphoid. Fess (1989), however, found more variability among hands and even some variation between dominant and nondominant hands. Knowledge of this motion is of particular importance in applying stretching techniques to fingers that have limited range of motion.

MUSCLES ACTING IN ABDUCTION OF THE FINGERS   The four dorsal interossei are responsible for abduction of the second and fourth fingers and for radial and ulnar abduction of the third finger. The fifth finger has its own abductor, the abductor digiti minimi, located on the ulnar border of the hand and being part of the hypothenar muscle group.

The dorsal interosseous muscles are located between the metacarpal bones, each muscle having double proximal attachments; that is, each is attached to two adjacent bones. The action of the dorsal interosseous muscles as abductors of the fingers may be concluded from knowing the location of their distal attachments:

First dorsal interosseus—radial side of base of index finger
Second dorsal interosseus—radial side of base of middle finger
Third dorsal interosseus—ulnar side of base of middle finger
Fourth dorsal interosseus–ulnar side of base of ring finger

The extensor digiti minimi, with its proximal attachment above the wrist, has its distal attachment at the base of the proximal phalanx in such a manner that it is able to both extend and abduct the little finger. This muscle receives its innervation from the radial nerve. The ability of this muscle to abduct the little finger (in small range) is clearly seen in cases of ulnar nerve paralysis when the hypothenar muscle group is paralyzed. The little finger then tends to maintain a somewhat abducted position, and the subject is unable to adduct it.

MUSCLES ACTING IN ADDUCTION OF THE FINGERS   The palmar interossei are responsible for adduction of the index, ring, and little fingers. These muscles, unlike the dorsal interossei, have only a single proximal attachment to the metacarpal bone of the digits that they serve. The palmar interossei may be tested by manual resistance to adduction of each finger separately or by squeezing three small objects between the fingers (see Fig. 6–19B). If a piece of paper is slipped between two adjacent fingers and the subject is asked to hold on to it, one palmar and one dorsal interosseous muscle are tested simultaneously.

Some anatomists speak of the deep portion of the flexor pollicis brevis (innervated by the ulnar nerve), or of a division of the adductor pollicis, as the first palmar interosseous muscle. In that case, the index finger is served by the second, the ring finger by the third, and the little finger by the fourth palmar interosseus.

OPPOSITION OF THE LITTLE FINGER   The opponens digiti minimi, aided by the flexor digiti minimi and by the palmaris longus and brevis, is responsible for the motion referred to as opposition of the fifth finger. The movement is not nearly as well developed as is opposition of the thumb. When both thumb and little finger move toward each other in opposition, "cupping" of the hand results; that is, the hand narrows considerably from side to side.

Balanced Forces

A way of beginning to appreciate the vast complexity of muscle function of the hand is through biomechanical analysis of a force applied to the finger. Figure 6–20 depicts a 2-kg* force applied to the tip of the finger as may occur when pressing down on a table. If the torques created by the applied force are not balanced by equal muscle torques at the DIP, PIP, MCP, and wrist joints, the joints extend. Conversely, if the muscle torque at a joint exceeds the applied torque, the joint flexes.

The torque created at each joint by the resistance force can be found by multiplying the force by the resistance arm distance ($\tau = F \times \perp d$):

Joint	F_R	R_A	τ_R	
DIP	2 kg $\times$	2.0 cm =	4 kg-cm*	τ_R = Resistance torque
PIP	2 kg $\times$	5.5 cm =	11 kg-cm	F_R = Resistive force
MCP	2 kg $\times$	10.5 cm =	21 kg-cm	
Wrist	2 kg $\times$	20.0 cm =	40 kg-cm	R_A = Resistance arm

---

*Some authors use kilograms instead of newtons for force units and kg-cm for torque.

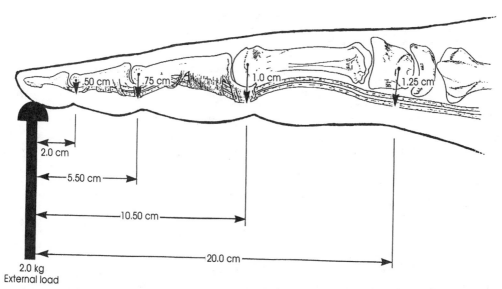

Figure 6–20 Vector representation of a 2-kg force applied to the distal phalanx. The *horizontal arrows* are the resistance arms of the force to the joints of the finger and wrist (perpendicular distance from the action line to the joint axis). The *vertical arrows* are the force arm distances of the flexor digitorum profundus tendon (FDP) to each joint axis. (Adapted from Brand, P, and Hollister, A: *Clinical Mechanics of the Hand* (2nd ed.). Mosby Year Book: St. Louis, 1992, p 83, with permission.)

Using the measured resistance and force arm distances for the DIP joint, the force in the flexor digitorum tendon and muscle can be calculated using the formulas for torque ($\tau = F \times \perp d$ and $\Sigma\tau = 0$):

$$\Sigma\tau = 0$$
$$\tau_R - \tau_M = 0$$
$$(2 \text{ kg} \times 2 \text{ cm}) - (F_M \times 0.5 \text{ cm}) = 0$$
$$F_M = \frac{2 \text{ kg} \times 2 \text{ cm}}{0.5 \text{ cm}}$$
$$F_M = 8 \text{ kg}$$

τ_M = Muscle torque
F_M = Muscle force

The 8 kg of muscle force exists throughout the length of the tendon. The torque created at each joint can be found by multiplying by the force arm distance:

Joint	F_M	F_A	τ_M	τ_R	
DIP	8 kg × 0.5 cm =		4 kg-cm	(4 kg-cm)	
PIP	8 kg × 0.75 cm =		6 kg-cm	(11 kg-cm)	F_A = Muscle
MCP	8 kg × 1.0 cm =		8 kg-cm	(21 kg-cm)	force arm
Wrist	8 kg × 1.25 cm =		10 kg-cm	(40 kg-cm)	

Comparison of the muscle torques with the resistance torques (as calculated) shows balance only at the DIP joint and illustrates that the resistance torques exceed those of the profundus at the other joints. The PIP, MCP, and wrist joints will extend or hyperextend. To maintain the position, additional muscles must participate. Table 6–2 shows the contribution of the superficialis with a contraction force of 6.66 kg to achieve equilibrium at the PIP joint and the further but insufficient contribution to the MCP and wrist joints. The intrinsic muscles are added to balance the MCP joints, and the wrist flexors are added to balance the torques at the wrist. The intrinsic muscles must be balanced to avoid lateral motions of abduc-

Table 6-2 Tabulation of Muscle Torques Necessary in the Joints of the Finger and Wrist to Balance a 2-kg Force Applied to the Tip of the Distal Phalange*

Tensions	Moment or Torque (kg·cm)			
	DIP	PIP	MCP	Wrist
Profundus—8 kg	4	6	8	10
Superficialis—6.66 kg	—	5	6.66	8.33
Intrinsics	—	—	6.33	—
Wrist flexors—10.66 kg	—	—	—	21.66
Totals	4	11	21	40

*The muscle force calculated for the flexor digitorum profundus is 8 kg; the flexor digitorum superficialis (sublimus), 6.66 kg; and the wrist flexors, 10.66 kg.
SOURCE: Brand, P and Hollister, A: Clinical Mechanics of the Hand, ed 2. Mosby Year Book, St Louis, 1992, p 82, with permission.

tion or adduction and cannot exceed the flexor torques of the IP joints. Similarly, the wrist flexors must be balanced to avoid radial or ulnar torques at the wrist and must be counteracted at the elbow to prevent flexion. This simplified example of maintaining balanced forces in the extended finger does not include the more complex passive and dynamic forces occurring in the extensor mechanism, the flexor pulleys, and the retinacular system of the finger.

Thumb Movements

The marked mobility that the thumb possesses as compared with the other fingers is made possible **first,** because the saddle-shaped CMC joint of the thumb has two degrees of freedom of motion and the capsule is loose, permitting rotation and a third degree of freedom; **second,** because the metacarpal bone of the thumb is not bound to the other metacarpals by ligaments, so that a wide separation between index finger and thumb can take place; **third,** because the movements that occur at the MCP and IP joints of the thumb add substantially to the versatility of thumb movements; and **fourth,** because the nine muscles that move the thumb can combine their actions in numerous ways in finely graded movement combinations.

Nomenclature

A considerable difference in terminology exists, which leads to potential confusion in the description of thumb movements, especially for those of the CMC joint. Movements at this joint have been labeled variously as flexion, extension, abduction, adduction, palmar abduction, opposition, reposition, pronation and supination, and have been described as taking place either in the plane of the palm or in a plane perpendicular to the palm. To add to the confusion, movements are sometimes defined as related to the entire thumb rather than to movements of separate joints. Clinically, for example, opposition of the thumb means the ability to bring the palmar surface of the tip of the thumb in contact with the palmar surfaces of the other digits. Functionally, this is justifiable, but anatomically, each joint has to be dealt with separately.

The **CMC** joint of the thumb is a saddle joint (see Fig. 1–7) with two degrees of freedom of motion. If this conception is adhered to, movements at this joint may be defined as **opposition-reposition** and as **abduction-adduction** (which occurs in a plane perpendicular to the palm of the hand). The term **flexion-extension** is then reserved for the two distal thumb joints but is frequently used in reference to the carpometacarpal joint.

The axes of the **CMC joint** are determined by the shape of the "saddle" of the trapezium; the "rider" is the metacarpal bone. One axis passes longitudinally, the other transversely through the saddle, so that the "rider" may slide from side to side or tip forward and backward in the "saddle."

The **MCP** joint of the thumb is more stable than the MCP joints of the other digits. Approximately 50 to 60 degrees of flexion can occur, whereas hyperextension and abduction-adduction are negligible.

The thumb contains only two phalanges and therefore has only one IP joint. Flexion is 90 degrees or less. Passive hyperextension, as in pressing down on the thumb, may have a large range.

It is important to recognize that a wide range of terminology exists for thumb motions. In this text, the terminology used in **Gray's Anatomy** (Goss, 1973) and by Kendall and associates (1971) is followed (Fig. 6–21).

Muscles of the Thumb

The **extrinsic muscles** of the thumb are the **flexor pollicis longus, extensor pollicis longus** and **brevis,** and **abductor pollicis longus.** The **intrinsic muscles** are the **adductor pollicis, flexor pollicis brevis, abductor pollicis brevis,** and **opponens pollicis.** In addition, the **lateral head of the first dorsal interosseous** attaches to the shaft of the first metacarpal. The muscles have been named after motions they produce. Because of the large range of motion of the thumb as well as multiple attachments of the intrinsic muscles, additional motions occur.

The flexor pollicis longus is the only flexor of the IP joint and also contributes to MCP, CMC, and wrist joint flexion as well as adduction from the abducted position. The flexor pollicis brevis, abductor pollicis brevis, and opponens pollicis all participate in movements of unresisted opposition, MCP flexion, and CMC abduction. The abductor and flexor brevis have attachments into the dorsal hood and also can extend the IP joint. The adductor pollicis is an extensor of the IP joint via its attachment to the hood and can flex the MCP and CMC joints from a position of extension. The extensor pollicis longus and brevis extend the thumb and from this position can act as adductors.

The thumb seldom acts alone except to press or play instruments. The thumb is mostly used against the fingers in gripping, pinching, or precision handling. Muscle function can be categorized for positioning the thumb and for stabilizing the thumb. In the positioning category are the extensors and the abductor pollicis longus to reposition the thumb around objects and the thenar muscles to oppose the object (opponens and flexor and abductor pollicis brevis). Muscles used primarily for applying force are the flexor pollicis longus, adductor pollicis, and the first dorsal interosseous. In most functional movements of the thumb all of the muscles participate in varying degrees. All of the muscles of the thumb have an effect on first CMC joint movements and provide strong stabilization of the joint in forceful opposition and grasp. All of the muscles except the opponens and the abductor pollicis longus also cross the MCP joint.

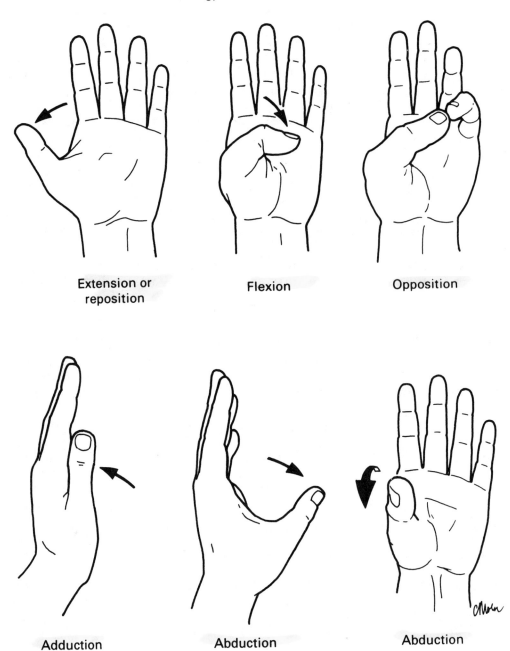

Figure 6–21 Terminology used in this text for motions of the thumb. Extension and flexion occur in the plane of the palm, whereas abduction and adduction occur in a plane perpendicular to the palm. Opposition requires rotation of the metacarpal at the carpometacarpal joint and contains elements of abduction and flexion.

Synergic Action of Wrist Muscles in Movements of the Thumb and Little Finger

Synergic actions of the wrist muscles should be noted in the following movements:

1. When the little finger is abducted (by abductor digiti minimi), the flexor carpi ulnaris contracts to furnish countertraction on the pisiform bone (Fig.

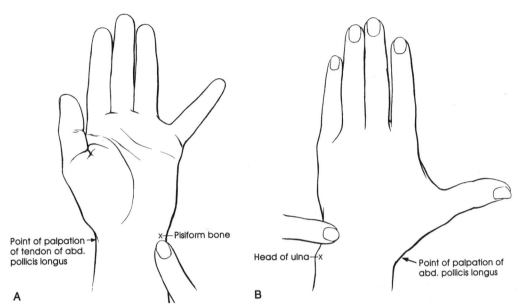

Figure 6–22 (*A*) Palpation of flexor carpi ulnaris proximal to the pisiform bone in abduction of the little finger. Abductor pollicis longus contracts synergically. (*B*) Palpation of extensor carpi ulnaris distal to the head of the ulna in extension of the thumb. Abductor pollicis longus may be palpated as indicated by the *arrow*. (Forearm and hand should be relaxed on table.)

6–22A). To prevent the flexor carpi ulnaris from abducting the wrist ulnarward, the abductor pollicis longus contracts. Its tendon may be palpated as indicated in the illustration.

2. When the thumb is extended to the position seen in Figure 6–22B, the tensed tendon of the extensor carpi ulnaris is palpated on the opposite side of the wrist. This muscle springs into action to prevent radial abduction of the wrist by the abductor pollicis longus. The points of palpation of the tendons of both muscles are indicated. The tendon of the abductor pollicis longus lies close to, and is partially covered by, the tendon of the extensor pollicis brevis.

3. When the entire thumb is brought in a palmar direction (flexion) by the thenar muscles, the palmaris longus aids the movement by tensing the fascia of the palm. To prevent the palmaris longus from flexing the wrist, the extensor carpi radialis brevis contracts.

Motor Innervation of the Hand

The innervation of muscles acting on the wrist and digits is as follows:

Radial Nerve

Extensor carpi radialis longus (C_6-C_7)
Extensor carpi radialis brevis (C_6-C_7)
Extensor carpi ulnaris (C_7-C_8)
Extensor digitorum (C_6-C_8)
Extensor indicis proprius (C_7-C_8)
Extensor digiti minimi proprius (C_7-C_8)
Extensor pollicis longus (C_7-C_8)

Extensor pollicis brevis (C_7-C_8)
Abductor pollicis longus (C_7-C_8)

Median Nerve

Flexor carpi radialis (C_6-C_7)
Palmaris longus (C_7-C_8)
Flexor digitorum superficialis (C_7-T_1)
Radial half of flexor digitorum profundus (C_8-T_1) and the two radial lumbricals (C_8-T_1)
Flexor pollicis longus (C_8-T_1)
Superficial portion of flexor pollicis brevis (C_8-T_1)
Opponens pollicis (C_7-T_1)
Abductor pollicis brevis (may have ulnar innervation; Belson, Smith, and Puentes, 1976) (C_5-T_1)

Ulnar Nerve

Flexor carpi ulnaris (C_8)
Ulnar half of flexor digitorum profundus (C_8-T_1) and the two ulnar lumbricals (C_8-T_1)
All interossei muscles (C_8-T_1)
All hypothenar muscles (C_8-T_1)
Palmaris brevis (C_8-T_1)
Deep portion of flexor pollicis brevis (C_8-T_1)
Adductor pollicis (C_8-T_1)

The muscles may be thought of in groups, innervated as follows: The **radial nerve** supplies all the extensors of wrist and digits with proximal attachments on the forearm and in the region of the lateral epicondyle. The **median nerve** supplies most of the flexors of the wrist and digits with proximal attachments on the forearm and in the region of the medial epicondyle. The **ulnar nerve** supplies most of the small muscles in the hand. Exceptions are "half-half" supply of flexor digitorum profundus and lumbricals (median and ulnar), ulnar nerve supply to flexor carpi ulnaris, and median nerve supply to thenar muscles.

Peripheral Nerve Injuries Affecting Wrist and Hand

In **radial nerve paralysis**, the extensors of the wrist and the long extensors of the digits are paralyzed. A wrist-drop develops causing a hand position much like the one seen in Figure 6–5B. The wrist can be neither actively extended nor stabilized for effective grasp. In the drop-wrist position, the digits are partially extended, but such extension is due to tendon action, not to active contraction. The grasp becomes awkward and weak (see Fig. 6–11), but if the wrist is supported in extension by means of a splint (see Fig. 2–13B), the strength of the grip is good because the flexor muscles are intact.

In **ulnar nerve paralysis**, the habitual position of the hand is a characteristic one (Fig. 6–23). The fourth and the fifth digits are the ones mostly affected because the flexor digitorum profundus, the lumbricals, and the interossei belonging to these fingers are paralyzed and the hypothenar group is also out of function. The extensor digitorum tends to keep the MCP joints of digits IV and V hyperextended. If the examiner holds the MCP joints in a flexed position, however, the subject is capable of extending the IP joints by using the extensor digitorum. Al-

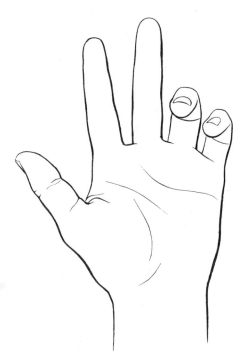

Figure 6–23 Characteristic hand posture in ulnar nerve paralysis. The fourth and fifth fingers cannot be extended because the long extensors of these digits, in the absence of the intrinsic muscles, cause hyperextension of the metacarpophalangeal joints but are incapable of extending the interphalangeal joints.

though the abductor of the little finger is paralyzed, this finger is maintained somewhat abducted (by the extensor digiti minimi proprius), but it cannot be adducted because the action of the palmar interosseus cannot be taken over by any other muscle. Abduction and adduction movements of all digits served by the interosseous muscles are affected. Occasionally, however, there is some median nerve supply to the more radially located interossei, in which case some movements may be preserved.

A **median nerve paralysis** causes most of the flexors of the digits to lose action and therefore seriously affects the grasp. The digits on the radial side, having only median nerve supply, are affected to a greater extent than those on the ulnar side. Flexion and opposition of the thumb are lost, the thenar muscles atrophy, and the entire thumb is pulled in a dorsal direction by the extensor muscles so that it remains in the plane of the palm or is taken even farther back toward the dorsum of the hand. The adductor is the only useful thenar muscle and, with the first dorsal interosseous muscle, may enable the subject to hold a small object between the thumb and the index finger. Because the flexor digitorum superficialis and profundus, and also the lumbricals of the index and middle fingers, have median nerve supply, these two fingers lose their ability to flex. The index finger tends to remain in an extended position while the middle finger may be drawn into some flexion when the two ulnar fingers flex. However, if the subject extends the wrist as far as possible, both index and middle fingers may flex by tendon action, but this is not an active grasp.

Deficits in hand function are additionally influenced by sensory loss resulting from peripheral nerve injury. Hand rehabilitation programs have always included motor retraining; in recent years, these programs have been emphasizing the importance of sensory retraining as well. The effect of sensory loss resulting from peripheral nerve injuries is that of diminishing power and precision of hand function (Wynn-Parry, 1981). Wynn-Parry divides re-education into stereognosis and localization of touch. He states that his experience has shown that patients can be trained to improve their sensory function remarkably and in too short a time to be explained by reinnervation.

Types of Prehension Patterns

The hand may be used in a multitude of postures and movements that in most cases involve both the thumb and the other digits. Napier (1956) describes two basic postures of the human hand: the "power grip" and the "precision grip." The power grip, used when full strength is needed, involves holding an object between the partially flexed fingers and the palm while the thumb applies counterpressure (Fig. 6–24A). In the precision grip, the object is pinched between the flexor surfaces of one or more fingers and the opposing thumb (Fig. 6–24B). It is used when accuracy and refinement of touch are needed. The thumb postures differ in the two grips. In power grip, the thumb is adducted, and it reinforces the pressure of the fingers. In precision grip, the thumb is abducted, and it is positioned to oppose the pulp of the fingers. Napier (1956) states that the nature of the task to be performed determines the working posture to be used and that these two postures incorporate the whole range of prehensile activity in the human hand.

Other graphic terms have been used to describe hand prehension patterns. Their names imply that hand posture is conditioned by the shape of the object being held. These terms should be noted, too, because they continue to be used in rehabilitation even though the terms power grip and precision grip are quite universally accepted.

Schlesinger (1919), in investigating designs for terminal devices for artificial arms, studied the versatility of the human hand in grasping and holding objects of various sizes and shapes. He distinguished among 12 different types of prehension; 7 are described below:

HOOK GRASP   Digits II to V are used as a hook, as in carrying a briefcase. The thumb is not necessarily active (Fig. 6–25).

CYLINDRIC GRASP   The entire palmar surface of the hand grasps around a cylindric object, such as a glass jar. The thumb closes in over the object (Fig. 6–26).

FIST GRASP   The fist closes over a comparatively narrow object, and the grip is secured by the thumb over the other digits, as in grasping a golf club or a hammer (see Fig. 6–24A).

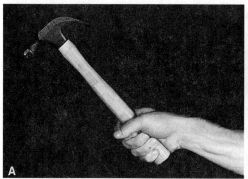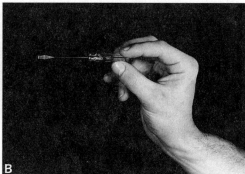

Figure 6–24   (A) Power grip. (B) Precision grip.

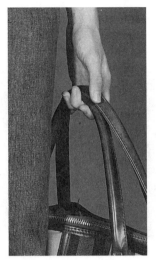

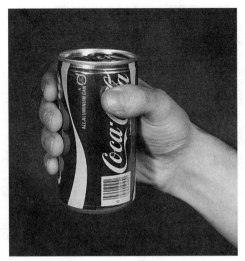

Figure 6–25   Hook grasp.   Figure 6–26   Cylindric grasp.

SPHERIC GRASP   The grasp is adjusted to a spheric object, such as a ball or an apple (Fig. 6–27).

TIP PREHENSION   The tip of the thumb is used against the tip of another digit to pick up a small object, such as a bead, a pin, or a coin (Fig. 6–28).

PALMAR PREHENSION   The thumb opposes one or more of the other digits; contact is made by the palmar surfaces of the distal phalanges of the digits. This grip is used to pick up and hold small objects, such as an eraser or a pen. Larger objects may also be held in this manner by widening the grip (Fig. 6–29).

LATERAL PREHENSION   A thin object, such as a card or a key, is grasped between the thumb and the lateral side of the index finger (Fig. 6–30).

Schlesinger also points out that some of these prehension types may be compared to simple tools, such as a hook (hook grasp), pincers (tip prehension), and

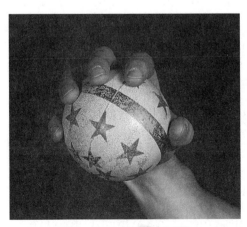

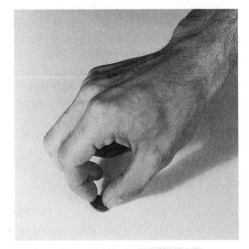

Figure 6–27   Spheric grasp.   Figure 6–28   Tip prehension.

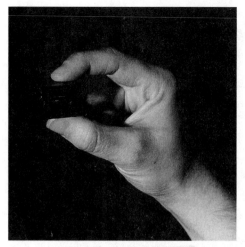

Figure 6–29   Palmar prehension.

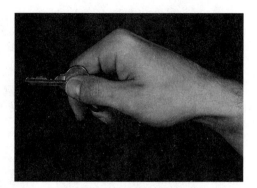

Figure 6–30   Lateral prehension.

pliers (palmar prehension). Current terminology applies the mechanical analogue "three-jaw chuck" to the palmar prehension pattern of the thumb pad opposing the index and middle digits.

Keller, Taylor, and Zahm (cited by Taylor and Schwartz [1955]) investigated the frequency of three types of common prehension patterns in picking up objects and holding them for use. Their findings were as follows:

	Palmar	Tip	Lateral
Pick up	50%	17%	33%
Hold for use	88%	2%	10%

This study showed that palmar prehension is by far the most commonly used type for both picking up and holding small objects. An adaptation of this grasp was subsequently used in the design of terminal devices for artificial arms.

Palmar and tip prehension require that the thumb and fingers be opposed to each other, and their frequent use in daily activities points to the importance of opposition of the thumb in the human hand.

Patients who have lost their ability to oppose the thumb but who are capable of adducting it, however, may use lateral prehension for grasping and holding small objects. Lateral prehension makes use of pressure of the thumb against the radial side of the index finger, which is held semiflexed. It is the prehension pattern of choice for patients with upper motor neuron lesions, in whom contact on the palmar surface of the fingers causes spasticity of the finger flexors, which is frequently the case. Such patients may be able to release an object held with lateral prehension, while an object that touches the palm of the hand may be very difficult to release.

Strength of Grip

Swanson, Matev, and deGroot (1970) studied normal grip and pinch strength to establish a baseline for evaluation of the disabled hand. Strength measurements were taken on 50 normal males and 50 females ranging in age from 17 to 60 years. Some of the mean values expressed in pounds are as follows:

	Age	Male	Female
Grip (major hand)	20	100	53
	20–30	107	54
	30–40	109	68
	40–50	108	52
	50–60	101	49
Chuck pinch (major hand)	17–60	17	11
Lateral pinch (major hand)	17–60	17	11

In addition to providing some normal values useful for making comparisons, this study found only a 4 to 9 percent decrease between the major and minor hands, which substantiates the 6 percent difference found by Toews (1964). This small differential does not necessarily hold true for individuals. Swanson and associates (1970) found that 29 percent of the subjects had the same or greater grip strength in the minor hand. Jarit (1991) found no significant difference between dominant and nondominant grip in college baseball players or in the control group. If a noticeable difference exists in the grip strength of the two hands, it is important to suspect pathology. Mean values for grip strength from ages 3 to 90 are found in Figure 4–5.

To determine forces of grip and pinch that should be provided in artificial hands, Keller and associates (cited in Klopsteg and Wilson [1968]) measured the minimum prehension forces required in the manipulation of common objects and other activities of everyday life. They found, for example, that pulling on a sock required a 7.7-lb force, whereas manipulation of a screw cap like that found on a toothpaste tube required a 2.5-lb force, and holding a soup spoon, a 1.6-lb force. It is estimated that adults with arm amputations, using prostheses, use 3 to 10 or 15 lb prehension force in their activities (New York University, 1971). Prehension forces available in the natural hand as shown by the Swanson and associates' study (1970) are considerably higher than forces required for most everyday activities.

CLINICAL APPLICATIONS

Knowledge of muscle attachments, actions, and functional behaviors is frequently the basis for locating the source of injuries. An example is tennis elbow or lateral epicondylitis, which is a repetitive stress injury actually found more commonly in the workplace than in tennis. The individual complains of pain on the lateral side of the elbow, particularly when picking up objects or reaching with the forearm pronated. There is usually pain to palpation distal to the lateral epicondyle, but range of motion of elbow flexion and extension as well as supination and pronation are normal and pain-free. In addition, strength testing of these motions is usually pain-free. Performing a maximum grip-strength test, however, usually reproduces the pain. To determine the possible injured structures, the following questions should be answered: What structures lie in the area of the lateral epicondyle? What muscles contract when performing maximum grip strength or picking up an object with the forearm pronated?

Answers should lead the student to the four wrist extensors and specific testing of their maximum lengths and contraction against resistance. Limitation of full muscle excursion and reproduction of the pain occurs when attempting to gain passive elbow extension along with wrist flexion (and finger flexion in the case of the extensor digitorum). Resisting isolated contractions of the injured muscle also causes pain. An immediate kinesiologic solution toward preventing further pain and injury, yet maintaining function, is to teach the person to hold objects or to lift with the forearm supinated.

The muscles most frequently affected in tennis elbow are the proximal attachments of the extensor carpi radialis brevis, the extensor carpi radialis longus, and the extensor digitorum (Powell and Burke, 1991). The authors state that elite tennis players and athletes who throw are more likely to get medial epicondylitis from injury to the proximal attachments of the wrist and finger flexors from the forehand strokes or the throwing motion. Lateral epicondylitis is more likely to occur in typists and others who perform repetitive wrist motions, such as needlepoint work, and in tennis players with poor backhand mechanics.

Laboratory Activities

WRIST AND HAND

1. On disarticulated bones or the skeleton, identify the following bones and bony landmarks of the wrist and hand. Determine which of these are palpable and palpate them on yourself and on a partner.

head of the ulna	eight individual carpal bones
styloid process of the ulna	shafts of metacarpal bones
styloid process of the radius	heads of metacarpal bones
dorsal radial tubercle	phalanges

2. Examine and identify the following joint surfaces:

radiocarpal	metacarpophalangeal (MCP)
midcarpal	interphalangeal (IP)
intercarpals	carpometacarpal joint of the thumb (CMC)
carpometacarpal; II–V	

3. Analyze wrist and finger movements (excluding thumb) on yourself and on a partner. Identify and palpate bony landmarks that locate axes of these movements.

4. Analyze all thumb movements (CMC, MCP, IP) on yourself and on a partner. Palpate in your own hand and in several subjects' hands the location of the "saddle" joint of the thumb.

5. Passively move the joints of your partner's wrist, fingers, and thumb through their ranges of motion in flexion, extension, and lateral motions (if present) and:
   a. State the approximate range of motion in degrees
   b. Describe the end-feel

6. Place your forearm and hand on a table, palm down. Extend and hyperextend your fingers actively (keeping the palm on the table), then passively perform the same motions. Notice that there is always slightly greater range of motion passively. If you observe a number of female and male subjects, you will find that the females usually have more flexibility in these joints.

7. Perform gentle passive accessory motions for the carpal bones and the joints of the fingers. Points to remember are that the subject's forearm and hand

must be relaxed and the examiner must stabilize one bone and move the joint surface of the other bone in glides, rotation, and distraction.

8. On the skeleton, locate the points of attachment for these muscles:

extensor carpi radialis longus
extensor carpi radialis brevis
extensor carpi ulnaris
extensor digitorum
flexor pollicis longus
abductor pollicis longus

extensor pollicis longus
extensor pollicis brevis
flexor carpi ulnaris
flexor carpi radialis
flexor digitorum profundus
flexor digitorum superficialis

Analyze the:
a. Joints these muscles cross
b. Motions that these muscles can produce.

9. Palpate tendons and muscle bellies of wrist and finger flexors and extensors, tracing their action line to their proximal bony attachments in the region of the elbow. Palpate tendons about the wrist and analyze their relationships so that you can identify them accurately irrespective of forearm or hand position.

10. Using skin pencils, sketch on your own hand the extrinsic tendons, including those of the thumb. Next add the "short" (ie, intrinsic) muscles and analyze their relationships to the extrinsic muscles. Determine hand, finger, and thumb movements performed by the intrinsics. Analyze integrated action of intrinsic and extrinsic hand muscles.

11. Pick up or manipulate these objects: thumb tacks, straight pins, paper clips, cards, coins, keys, glass, weights, pencil or pen, briefcase, handbag, cup, doorknob, scissors, magazine, newspaper, screwdriver, book, ball. Analyze prehension patterns, noting particularly the wrist positions, the specific finger movements and the continuous transition from pattern to pattern. (See Figs. 6–24—power grip and precision grip, 6–29—palmar prehension, 6–30—lateral prehension, 6–28—tip prehension, 6–26—cylindric grasp, 6–27—spheric grasp, 6–25—hook grasp.)

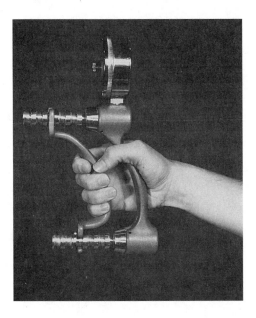

Figure 6–31 Adjustable hand dynamometer for measuring grip strength.

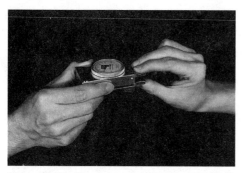

Figure 6–32 Pinch meter. The examiner *(left)* holds the meter, and the subject performs a chuck pinch.

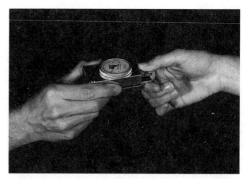

Figure 6–33 Pinch meter. The subject *(right)* performs a lateral pinch.

12. With a hand dynamometer and a pinch meter, test the strength of your grip, chuck pinch, and lateral pinch (Figs. 6–31—grip, 6–32—chuck pinch, 6–33—lateral pinch). Test your major and your minor hand. Compile and compare results among all class members and determine average scores. Ensure standardization of the test procedure with respect to the number of repetitions and to the position and support (or nonsupport) of the forearm.

13. Predict dysfunction of the elbow, wrist, and hand that could occur when:
    a. Radial nerve is severed in the region of the spinal groove in the humerus
    b. Median nerve is cut at the wrist joint
    c. Ulnar nerve is crushed at the elbow between the medial epicondyle of the humerus and the olecranon process
    d. The lateral cord of the brachial plexus is damaged
    In your analysis, determine functions that will be lost, functions decreased, and functions remaining.

CHAPTER 7

Shoulder Complex

The shoulder region is a complex of 20 muscles, 3 bony articulations, and 3 soft tissue moving surfaces (functional joints) that permit the greatest mobility of any joint area found in the body (approximately 180 degrees of flexion, abduction, and rotation and 60 degrees of hyperextension). The shoulder complex not only provides a wide range for hand placement but also carries out the important functions of stabilization for hand use, lifting and pushing, elevation of the body, forced inspiration and expiration, and even weight bearing as in crutch-walking or handstands. The extensive mobility is provided by the six moving areas:

1. Bony articulations
   a. Sternoclavicular
   b. Acromioclavicular
   c. Glenohumeral
2. Functional joints
   a. Scapulothoracic
   b. Suprahumeral (or subacromial)
   c. Bicipital groove

Mobility, however, is at the expense of structural stability. The only attachment of the upper extremity to the trunk is at the sternoclavicular joint, and the head of the humerus hangs loosely on the inclined plane of the glenoid fossa. Thus, support and stabilization of the shoulder primarily depend on muscles and ligaments.

BONES

The osseous parts participating in movements of the upper extremity in relation to the trunk are:

Sternum (breast bone)	(Gr. *sternon*, chest)
Costae (ribs)	(L. *costa*, rib)
Clavicle (collar bone)	(L. *clavicula*, diminutive of *clavus*, key)
Scapula (shoulder blade)	(L. *scapula*, shoulder blade)
Humerus (bone of upper arm)	(L. *humerus*, shoulder)

Palpation

Sternum

The sternum may be palpated anteriorly on the thorax from the **xiphoid process** at its lower end to the **manubrium sterni** at its upper end (Gr. *xiphos*, sword, and *eidos*, appearance; L. *manubrium,* handle).

Clavicle

The sternal portion of the clavicle is prominent where it articulates with the manubrium sterni (sternoclavicular joint). From this point, the clavicle may be followed laterally to its acromial end. The curved shape of this bone should be noted—it is convex forward medially and concave forward laterally (Fig. 7–1). The acromial end, like the sternal end, is enlarged and may be palpated as a protuberance.

Standing and running animals, such as horses and dogs, do not have clavicles, and their scapulae are on the lateral surfaces of the thorax. Humans have a strong, well-developed clavicle that acts as a lateral strut to the scapula and the humerus. This increases glenohumeral mobility to permit reaching and climbing activities (O'Brien et al, 1990).

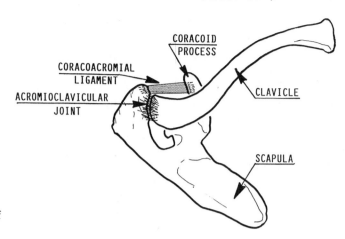

Figure 7–1 Superior view of the left clavicle and scapula.

Scapula

At the tip of the shoulder, the broad **acromion process**, which extends like a shelf over the shoulder joint, is palpated (Gr. *acron*, tip; *omox*, shoulder). Anteriorly, its free edge may be felt. Its junction with the clavicle (acromioclavicular joint) lies somewhat protected, being covered by the acromioclavicular ligament; hence, it is difficult to palpate with accuracy. In most individuals, two bony enlargements may be felt in this region, one on the acromion, the other on the clavicle. The acromioclavicular joint is found in the area between these two prominences (see Fig. 7–1).

By following the acromion process posteriorly, the **spine of the scapula** is palpated; it is continuous with the acromion process. The spine of the scapula may be followed transversely across the scapula to the medial (vertebral) border of the scapula where it flattens out to form a smooth triangular-shaped area. The **supraspinous fossa** of the scapula, above the spine, and **infraspinous fossa**, below the spine, should be identified; because both are filled with muscles, their depths cannot be appreciated. This applies particularly to the supraspinous fossa, which is not accessible to palpation in its deeper parts. The **medial (vertebral) border** of the scapula and its **lateral (axillary) border** are easily palpable if the scapular muscles are relaxed. The **inferior angle** of the scapula is the lowest part of the scapula where the medial and lateral borders join. The **superior angle** of the scapula is well covered by muscles and therefore more difficult to palpate. Anteriorly, below the clavicle, where the roundness of the shoulder begins, the **coracoid process** is palpated (Gr. *korax*, raven, curved door handle; *eidos*, appearance).

The **glenoid cavity** of the scapula (Gr. *glene*, a socket), which receives the head of the humerus, cannot be palpated. This also applies to the **supraglenoid tubercle**, which serves as proximal attachment for the long head of the biceps, and to the **infraglenoid tubercle**, where the long head of the triceps attaches.

Humerus

If the humerus is internally rotated while the arm is at the side of the body, the **greater tubercle** of the humerus may be palpated just distal to the acromion process. Once this tubercle has been identified, the palpating fingers may follow its changing position as the shoulder is rotated externally. In full external rotation, this tubercle is no longer palpable because it disappears under the heavy portion of the deltoid muscle. The greater tubercle has three facets, serving as points of attachment for muscles, but these facets cannot be distinguished easily by palpation. The lesser tubercle is best felt when the shoulder is externally rotated and may be followed during internal rotation. The proximal portion of the humerus also may be approached from the axilla, but palpation must be done gently because of the many nerves and vessels in this area. The name **anatomic neck** is applied to a narrow area distal to the articular surface of the humeral head. Fractures in this region tend to occur at the surgical neck, below the tubercles.

On the proximal portion of the shaft of the humerus, the **crest of the greater tubercle** and the **crest of the lesser tubercle** should be noted. Between the two crests is the **intertubercular** (bicipital) **groove**. These structures should be studied on a skeleton, as they are difficult to palpate through the muscles. Note the changing position of the intertubercular groove during humeral rotation; in complete external rotation, the groove is in line with the acromion process.

JOINTS

The bones of the shoulder complex are joined at three articulations: the clavicle articulates with the manubrium sterni at the **sternoclavicular joint;** the clavicle and the scapula join at the **acromioclavicular joint;** and the humerus articulates with the scapula at the **glenohumeral joint**. During movements of the upper extremity, the scapula also slides freely on the thorax (scapulothoracic "joint"). In motions of flexion and abduction, the head of the humerus slides beneath the acromion (suprahumeral "joint"), and the tendon of the long head of the biceps brachii slides in the bicipital groove. Pain or limitation of motion in any of these true or functional joints will lead to shoulder dysfunction.

Scapulothoracic Joint

The **serratus anterior** muscle attaches to the medial border of the scapula and passes under the scapula to attach on the anterolateral border of the first nine ribs. A large amount of motion occurs between the fascia of the muscle and the fascia of the thorax. Because there are no bony articulations, the moving surfaces are called **false** or **functional joints**. Normal function of the scapulothoracic joint is essential for the mobility and stability of the upper extremity. Motion of the scapulothoracic joint provides a movable base for the humerus and thereby increases the range of motion of the arm, maintains favorable length-tension relationships for the deltoid muscle to function above 90 degrees of arm elevation, provides glenohumeral stability for work in the overhead position or for handstands, provides shock absorption for forces applied to the outstretched arm, and permits elevation of the body in crutch-walking or sitting push-ups for transfers by persons with paraplegia.

Definition of Shoulder Girdle Movements

Special terms used to describe the motions of the scapula (scapulothoracic joint) and also the clavicle (sternoclavicular joint) are illustrated in Figure 7–2:

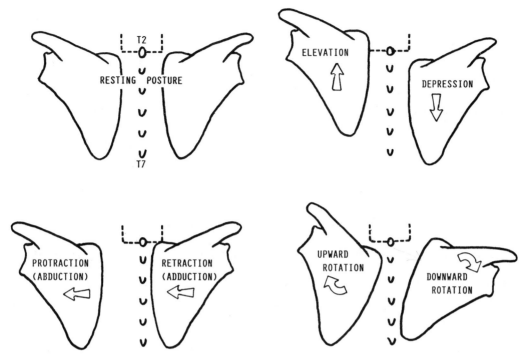

Figure 7–2 Motions of the scapula occur at the sternoclavicular, acromioclavicular, and scapulothoracic joints. The dotted lines at the second thoracic vertebra (T-2) provide a reference for the location of the superior and medial borders of the scapula in the resting posture.

Elevation—The distal end of the clavicle and the acromion process of the scapula (acromioclavicular joint) move superiorly (toward the ear) approximately 60 degrees (Kapandji, 1982).

Depression—Motion of the acromioclavicular area inferiorly. From a sitting resting position, only 5 to 10 degrees of depression can be achieved. The importance of the movement, however, is in stabilization of the scapula and elevation of the body as in crutch-walking or wheelchair transfers for patients with paraplegia. From a position of maximum elevation, the movement of shoulder depression can elevate the trunk 4 to 6 inches (10 to 15 cm).

Protraction—The distal end of the clavicle and the scapula move anteriorly around the rib cage, with the medial borders of the scapula moving away from the midline 5 to 6 inches (13 to 15 cm). This motion is also referred to as **abduction of the scapula.**

Retraction—The distal end of the clavicle and the scapula move posteriorly, and the medial borders of the scapula approach the midline. This motion is also called **adduction of the scapula.** At the sternoclavicular joint, the total range for protraction and retraction is approximately 25 degrees (Kapandji, 1982).

A circling movement may be performed by moving the shoulder girdle upward-forward-downward-backward (involving a combination of elevation, protraction, depression, and retraction) or in the opposite direction. During these movements, the sternoclavicular joint is the pivot point, and the tip of the shoulder moves in a circular path. The scapula, because it articulates with the clavicle at the acromioclavicular joints, adjusts its position and stays close to the thorax.

Scapular motions are further described by the rotations that occur at the acromioclavicular joint:

Upward rotation is a movement of the scapula in which the glenoid fossa faces superiorly and the inferior angle of the scapula slides laterally and anteriorly on the thorax. Maximum range of upward rotation is seen with the full shoulder flexion.

Downward rotation of the scapula is a movement of the glenoid fossa to face inferiorly. Complete range of downward rotation occurs when the hand is placed in the small of the back. The total range of upward and downward rotation is approximately 60 degrees.

Shoulder abduction in the plane of the scapula occurs 30 to 40 degrees anterior to the frontal plane. This motion is advocated for evaluation of elevation of the arm because the capsule remains in a loose-packed position, and there is less likelihood of impingement on the coracoacromial structures (Perry, 1988). Thus, it is important to identify the plane of abduction that is used because the ranges of motion vary slightly and the torque of the external rotators is greater in the plane of the scapula than in the frontal plane (Greenfield et al, 1990).

Sternoclavicular Joint

The sternoclavicular joint is the only joint that connects the upper extremity directly with the thorax. The shoulder girdle, together with the entire upper extremity, is suspended from the skull and the cervical spine by muscles, ligaments, and fascia. The position of this hanging structure is determined partly by the action of gravity and partly by the clavicle, which restricts shoulder girdle movements in all directions, particularly in a forward direction. Cases of the clavicle's being absent have been reported in the medical literature—these individuals were able to move their shoulders so far forward that the tips of the shoulders almost met in front of the body. With complete surgical removal of the clavicle, Lewis and associates (1985) found shoulder ranges of motion to be the same as those on the uninvolved side. The maximum isokinetic torques for shoulder extension, as well as internal and external rotation, were also the same. The shoulder flexors, abductors, and adductors on the involved side, however, had a 50 percent loss of isokinetic torque.

Type of Joint

The sternoclavicular joint is a sellar joint with three degrees of freedom. The enlarged sternal end of the clavicle and the articular notch of the sternum are separated by an articular disk. Motions thus take place both between the clavicle and the disk and between the disk and the sternum. The disk serves as a hinge for motion and for shock absorption of forces delivered through the arm. Although the bony articulations appear small, the ligamentous attachments are strong, and the clavicle usually fractures before the joint dislocates. The clavicles are connected to each other by the interclavicular ligaments, to the sternum by the anterior and posterior sternoclavicular ligaments, and to the first ribs by the costoclavicular ligaments. These ligaments support the weight of the upper extremities, limit clavicular motions, and prevent dislocation of the joint. The joint capsule and ligaments are further reinforced by the proximal tendinous attachments of the sternocleidomastoid muscles.

Axes of Motion and Movements

The axis for elevation and depression of the shoulder girdle is an oblique one that pierces the sternal end of the clavicle and takes a backward-downward course. Movement about this axis takes place between the sternal end of the clavicle and the articular disk. Because of the obliquity of this axis, shoulder girdle elevation occurs in an upward-backward direction, and depression, in a forward-downward direction. Elevation of the sternoclavicular joint is 30 to 45 degrees (Inman et al, 1944; Moseley, 1968), with most of the motion occurring in the first 90 degrees of arm elevation. The joint motion is limited by the costoclavicular and interclavicular ligaments and the subclavius muscle. From the resting position, the joint can be depressed 5 to 10 degrees until the clavicle is stopped by the first rib.

The joint between the articular cartilage and the sternum is involved mainly in retraction-protraction of the shoulder girdle. These motions take place about a nearly vertical axis, which pierces the manubrium sterni close to the joint. From the resting position, protraction of the sternoclavicular joint is 15 degrees and retraction is 15 degrees (Moseley, 1968). The posterior sternoclavicular ligament and the costoclavicular ligament limit protraction, and the anterior sternoclavicular ligament limits retraction (Peat, 1986). Scapular excursion accompanies retraction and protraction of the clavicle.

Transverse Rotation of the Clavicle

In addition to elevation-depression and protraction-retraction, the clavicle also rotates at the sternoclavicular joint approximately 40 degrees around its long axis (Inman et al, 1944). This transverse rotation occurs after the shoulder has been abducted or flexed to 90 degrees and is essential for complete upward rotation of the scapula and shoulder flexion or abduction. If rotation of the clavicle is prevented, elevation of the arm is limited to 110 degrees (Inman et al, 1944).

This axial rotation occurs as the arm is elevated above 90 degrees where the sternoclavicular joint starts to reach maximum elevation. The upward rotation of the clavicle is caused by the tightening of the acromioclavicular ligaments—the trapezoid and the conoid (Fig. 7–3)—which are attached to the inferior surface of the clavicle and at right angles to each other. As the conoid ligament becomes taut, the attachment on the clavicle becomes an axis for upward rotation occurring at the sternoclavicular joint. Because of the S shape of the bone, the acromial end becomes higher to further elevate and upwardly rotate the scapula. These two ligaments also function to limit separation of the clavicle from the scapula.

Acromioclavicular Joint

The acromioclavicular joint is a single arthrodial joint involving the medial margin of the acromion and the acromial end of the clavicle (see Fig. 7–1). This joint binds the scapula and clavicle in similar motions and at the same time accommodates individual motions of the bones. The joint has three axes and three degrees

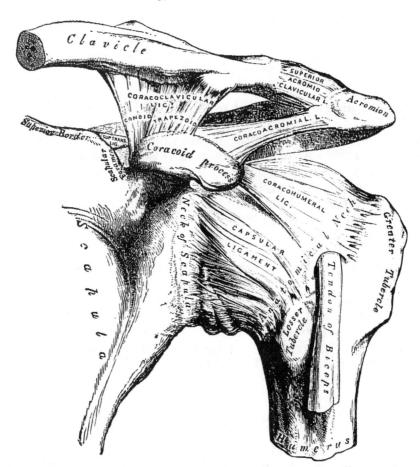

Figure 7–3 Anterior view of the left shoulder showing the acromioclavicular and glenohumeral joints, the coracoid process, ligaments, and capsular structures. Note the folds in the inferior part of the glenohumeral capsule. (From Gray, H: In Goss, C [ed]: *Anatomy of the Human Body*. Lea & Febiger, Philadelphia, 1966, p 327, with permission.)

of freedom, and the motions are reflected in scapular movements of elevation, abduction, and rotation. During full arm elevation, the acromioclavicular joint contributes 20 degrees of scapular elevation and about 20 degrees of upward rotation (Inman et al, 1944). Neer and Rockwood (1984), however, measured a maximum of 8 degrees of acromioclavicular motion and stated that no loss of scapular rotation was apparent with acromioclavicular joint fixation. Small anterior and posterior movements of the acromion (scapular abduction and adduction) keep the glenoid fossa aligned with the humeral head during motions of shoulder flexion or abduction. These motions are permitted and limited by two strong ligamentous pairs: the anterior and posterior ligaments of the joint and the more proximally located coracoclavicular ligaments, the conoid and the trapezoid (see Fig. 7–3).

The combined effect of acromioclavicular and sternoclavicular motions is to permit scapular movement so that the glenoid fossa may face forward, upward, or downward, as the need may be, while the costal surface remains close to the thorax. The sum of the ranges of motion at the sternoclavicular and acromioclavicular joints equals the range of motion of the scapula.

Glenohumeral Joint

Type of Joint

Although the glenohumeral joint is called a ball-and-socket, spheroidal, or universal joint and has three degrees of freedom, the joint has little bony stability. The hemispheric-shaped head of the humerus rests on the small, shallow, inclined plane of the glenoid cavity (see Fig. 1–6A). Surrounding the rim of the glenoid is a cartilaginous labrum, or lip. The loose and thin joint capsule covers the joint from the neck of the glenoid to the anatomic neck of the humerus. This capsule has a surface area twice that of the humeral head and, in the normal subject, permits injection of 10 to 15 mL of fluid (O'Brien et al, 1990).

Capsular Reinforcement

Ligaments and tendons provide capsular reinforcement. The coracohumeral ligament crosses from the coracoid process of the scapula to the greater and lesser tuberosities of the humerus, where it forms a tunnel for the tendon of the long head of the biceps brachii (see Fig. 7–3). The superior, middle, and inferior glenohumeral ligaments (called capsular ligaments in Fig. 7–3) arise from the glenoid and its labrum, form capsular thickenings, and attach to the humeral neck and lesser tuberosity. The coracohumeral, superior, and middle glenohumeral ligaments support the dependent (hanging down) arm and limit external rotation in the lower ranges of abduction (Ferrari, 1990). The inferior glenohumeral ligament forms a hammock-like sling with anterior and posterior bands around the head of the humerus. O'Brien and associates (1990) consider this ligament the main stabilizer of the abducted shoulder. In this position, different parts of the ligament tighten to limit internal and external rotation.

The deep muscles of the shoulder provide intimate reinforcement of the joint capsule by their tendons of attachment. Anteriorly, the tendon of the long head of the biceps brachii arises from the supraglenoid tuberosity and the glenoid labrum. The tendon arches over the head of the humerus under the joint capsule to exit and descend in the intertubercular groove of the humerus (see Fig. 7–3). While the bicipital tendon is within the joint capsule, the tendon is covered by reflection of the synovial membrane; therefore, the tendon is not exposed to the synovial fluid of the joint cavity. Thus, the tendon is considered to be intra-articular but extrasynovial. Strong contraction of the biceps brachii muscle, as when the elbow is flexed and a weight is held in the hand, produces depression force on the head of the humerus (Neer, 1990). The forces causing that effect are similar in action to forces that restrain the pull on a rope by "snubbing" the rope around a pole or tree. Such depression of the head of the humerus prevents elevation of the head, which might otherwise cause impingement injuries to suprahumeral tissues stressed between the humeral head and the rigid acromial structures.

Posteriorly, the long head of the triceps brachii has a broad proximal attachment on the infraglenoid tubercle of the scapula. This tendon blends with and becomes a part of the posterior capsule.

The Rotator Cuff

The tendons of four short scapulohumeral muscles that produce internal and external rotation of the glenohumeral joint blend with the capsule and form their distal attachments on the tuberosities of the humerus. Anteriorly, the subscapularis attaches by a broad tendon to the lesser tubercle of the humerus. This tendon covers the head of the humerus below 90 degrees of abduction and is considered by Jobe (1990) to be a passive stabilizer to prevent anterior subluxation of the humerus. The lower part of the capsule and the subscapularis are the primary structures limiting external rotation (Ovesen and Nielsen, 1985). Superiorly, the supraspinatus muscle attaches to the lesser tubercle of the humerus, and posteriorly, the infraspinatus and the teres minor blend with the capsule to attach lower on the greater tuberosity. These tendons were found by Ovesen and Nielsen (1985) to be the major structures limiting internal rotation in the first half of abduction. The rotator cuff structures can be injured when striking against the acromion or coracoid processes or against the strong connecting coracoacromial ligament (see Fig. 7–3). This injury occurs with activities requiring elevation of the arm, such as working overhead or sports activities requiring throwing.

Axes of Motion and Movements Permitted

The following ranges of motion can be attributed to the glenohumeral joint **only when the scapula is stabilized** to prevent movement at the sternoclavicular, acromioclavicular, or scapulothoracic joints. **Flexion** takes place in the sagittal plane about a transverse axis through the head of the humerus. Approximately 90 degrees of flexion are permitted. The inferior glenohumeral ligaments become taut and limit further motion (Morrey and An, 1990). **Extension** is the reverse of flexion. When the arm passes behind the body, the motion is termed **hyperextension**. The range of hyperextension is 40 to 60 degrees and is limited by the superior and middle glenohumeral ligaments. **Abduction** occurs in the frontal plane around a horizontal axis directed dorsoventrally. The amount of abduction that is permitted depends on the rotation at the glenohumeral joint. When the joint is in full internal rotation, active abduction is limited to approximately 60 degrees, because the greater tubercle strikes the acromion process and the acromioclavicular ligament. With 90 degrees of external rotation, the greater tubercle goes behind and under the acromion and active abduction increases to approximately 90 degrees, where it becomes limited by active insufficiency of the deltoid muscle. Abduction can be continued passively to 120 degrees, where it is then limited by the inferior glenohumeral ligament. In full shoulder abduction, Murray (1985) measured an average of 124 degrees of glenohumeral motion (Table 7–1).

Rotation takes place about an axis longitudinally through the head and shaft of the humerus in the horizontal plane. Rotation at the glenohumeral joint is isolated from supination and pronation of the forearm by flexion of the elbow to 90 degrees. If the arm is at the side of the body, **external (lateral) rotation** causes the medial epicondyle of the humerus to move anteriorly, and internal (medial) rotation causes the condyle to move posteriorly. The amount of rotation changes with elevation of the arm. Approximately 180 degrees of total rotation are present when the arm is at the side (Bechtol, 1980) and are reduced to about 90 degrees because of the twisting and tightening of the coracohumeral and glenohumeral ligaments when the arm is fully elevated. When the glenohumeral joint is placed in the standard goniometric position of 90 degrees of shoulder abduction and 90 degrees of elbow flexion (Norkin and White, 1995), the normal range of motion for external rotation is approximately 90 degrees and for internal rotation, approximately 70 degrees (see Table 7–1). Brown and associates (1988) found 141 de-

Table 7-1 Average Shoulder Range of Motion in Normal Subjects
(Degrees)

Author	Boone and Azen (1979)		Murray et al (1985)		Brown et al (1988)	Chang, Buschbacher, and Edlich (1988)	
Subjects	109 M		20 M 20 F		41 M*	10 M 10 M†	
Age (yrs)	2–19	19–54	25–66		27 ± 4.2	21–35	
Flexion	168	165	167	171	163	171	157
Abduction	185	183	178	179	168	—	—
Extension	67	57	56	59	76	55	42
External rotation	108	100	88	97	136	82	78
Internal rotation	71	67	54‡	54‡	84	83	56
Glenohumeral abduction	—	—	122	126	99	—	—

NOTE: Notice the tendency for more flexibility in the younger males (Boone and Azen) and in the females versus the males (Murray et al), the decreased flexibility of the power lifters versus normal controls (Chang, Buschbacher, and Edlich), and the marked amount of external rotation in the baseball players (Brown et al).
*Major league baseball players.
†Power lifters.
‡The goniometric positions were described as standard, except that the scapula was stabilized.

grees of external rotation in major league baseball pitchers, and Chang, Busch-bacher, and Edlich (1988) found 78 degrees in power lifters.

Two other terms are frequently used to describe glenohumeral joint motion. They are **horizontal abduction** and **horizontal adduction**. These motions occur from a starting position of 90 degrees of abduction. Horizontal abduction is a posterior motion from this position, and horizontal adduction is an anterior motion across the body.

All the normal limitations of motion on the glenohumeral joint are due to ligamentous and passive muscle tightening. Thus, the end-feels are all firm. Even when the greater tuberosity of the humerus strikes on the acromion process, the end-feel is firm because of the intervening soft tissues.

Accessory Motions

Passively small gliding motions of the sternoclavicular and acromioclavicular joints can occur (Kaltenborn, 1980). The shallow bony structure and the loose capsule of the glenohumeral joint normally permits 1 to 2 cm of joint play motions in distal and lateral distraction of the humeral head on the glenoid as well as anterior and posterior translatory glides.

The close-packed position of the glenohumeral joint occurs in abduction and external rotation where the capsular structures are twisted tightly. This is a common position of the shoulder in people who sleep on their abdomen and is frequently a source of shoulder pain and injury. The close-packed position of the sternoclavicular joint occurs when the arm is fully elevated and the close-packed position of the acromioclavicular joint occurs when the arm is abducted to 90 degrees (Kaltenborn, 1980).

Suprahumeral or Subacromial Joint

Motions of the glenohumeral joint require large movements between the head of the humerus and the arch formed by the neck of the scapula, the acromion process, the rigid coracoacromial ligament, and the coracoid process. This area has also been named the **supraspinatus outlet** by Neer and Poppen (1987). The clinical importance of this area is the propensity for compression and injury of the soft tissues that lie between the rigid structures: the tendons of the rotator cuff (especially the supraspinatus), the tendon of the long head of the biceps brachii, the capsule, the capsular ligaments, and the subdeltoid and subacromial bursae. Shoulder impingement injuries occur because the line of pull of the deltoid muscle for elevation of the arm is directly superior and causes the humerus to move vertically and strike the acromion. Normally, this vertical movement is prevented by the downward line of pull of the rotator cuff muscles and depression of the head of the humerus by the tendons of the supraspinatus and the long head of the biceps brachii. Unfortunately, there is no space for error in the supraspinatus outlet, and impingement injuries occur with muscle weakness, fatigue, or uncontrollable forces. Microtrauma and repetitive stress injuries are common, for example, causing 50 to 60 percent of all problems in competitive swimmers (Reid, Saboe, and Burham, 1987). People with poliomyelitis and paraplegia who have been crutch-walking, propelling manual wheelchairs, or performing sitting push-ups to transfer the body have an extraordinarily high incidence of shoulder pain and rotator cuff tears (Bayley, Cochran, and Sledge, 1987; Smith, 1990). Neer (1990) considers the most frequent cause of injuries to be narrowing of the supraspinatus outlet, which may be congenital or caused by inflammation, scarring, or the development of bone spurs. Attrition (wearing down) of the capsular structures has a high incidence in cadaver dissections and has been documented with aging by Brewer (1979) and Ferrari (1990).

The Bicipital Groove

The tendon of the long head of the biceps brachii attaches to the supraglenoid tubercle of the scapula and arches over the head of the humerus to descend in the intertubercular groove of the humerus (see Fig. 7–3). The tendon is retained in the groove by the coracohumeral ligament and by the transverse humeral ligament (not shown in Fig. 7–3), which covers the groove from the lesser to the greater tuberosity. During motions of the shoulder, the head of the humerus slides on the undersurface of the tendon. A fixed point on the groove moves along $1^1/2$ inches of tendon with full elevation of the arm (Burkhead, 1990). When the glenohumeral joint is in full external rotation, the proximal and distal attachments of the tendon are in line, but in all other positions of rotation, the bicipital tendon is bent around the medial wall of the groove (Perry, 1988). Thus, the bicipital tendon is subject to wear and injury with time as well as impingement injuries on the coracoacromial arch.

Scapulohumeral Rhythm

Normally, shoulder elevation occurs in a precisely coordinated series of synchronous motions termed **scapulohumeral rhythm**. The classic work by Inman and associates (1944) demonstrated that both the scapular and humeral segments participate throughout the motion. The early phase of abduction was individually variable, but after 30 degrees of abduction, a 2:1 ratio occurred: For every 15 degrees of motion between 30 and 170 degrees of abduction, 10 degrees occurred at the glenohumeral joint and 5 degrees occurred at the scapulothoracic joint

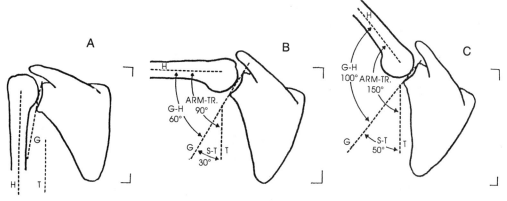

Figure 7–4 Scapulohumeral rhythm. Schematic illustration of the motions of the glenohumeral joint and the scapula during abduction of the shoulder. *(A)* Arm at side with zero degrees of shoulder abduction. *(B)* Shoulder in 90 degrees of abduction. *(C)* Shoulder in 150 degrees of abduction. H = long axis of the humerus; G = plane of the glenoid fossa; T = line parallel to the long axis of the trunk; ARM-TR. = arm-trunk angle; G-H = glenohumeral joint angle; S-T = scapulothoracic joint angle.

(Fig. 7–4). Other investigations have found that the motions are not as linear as the 2:1 ratio implies and that there is variation in patterns. The most common pattern, found by Bagg and Forrest (1988), showed greater glenohumeral motion at the beginning and end of the range and more scapular motion between 80 and 140 degrees of abduction. The average ratio of glenohumeral to scapulothoracic joint motions was 1.25:1, which is the same as the mean values obtained by Poppen and Walker (1976). Both of these investigators used the plane of the scapula for the motion of abduction, while Inman used the frontal plane.

The motions that occur at the scapulothoracic joint in elevation of the arm are elevation, abduction, and upward rotation, with the inferior angle of the scapula moving to the lateral side of the thorax and the glenoid fossa directed upward. The axis of rotation of the scapula migrates from the medial root of the spine of the scapula to the region of the acromioclavicular joint during the motion (Bagg, 1988). This large movement of the axis causes marked changes in the force arms of the trapezius and the serratus anterior, which will be considered later.

Elevation of the Arm

Normal range of shoulder flexion or abduction is conventionally reported as 180 degrees, but when carefully measured to eliminate trunk motions, the mean angle is close to 170 degrees (Freedman and Munro, 1966; Doody et al, 1970; Boone and Azen, 1979; see Table 7–1). This is a measurement of an angle between the arm and the trunk. The motion occurs at both the glenohumeral and scapulothoracic joints, with the scapular movements accompanied by motions at the sternoclavicular and acromioclavicular joints. Ninety to 110 degrees of motion occur at the glenohumeral joint and an additional 60 to 70 degrees occur at the sternoclavicular and acromioclavicular joints. The remainder of the motion needed to achieve 180 degrees occurs in the trunk with lateral flexion for shoulder abduction or with trunk extension for shoulder flexion. Achievement of the glenohumeral range requires external rotation of the shoulder in abduction and internal rotation for flexion (Blakely and Palmer, 1984).

Clinical treatment of shoulder problems requires a careful assessment of all the motions permitted at each of the three synovial and the three moving surfaces to determine if and where limitation of motion or pain occurs.

MUSCLES OF THE SHOULDER REGION

The muscles of the shoulder region give fixation to and produce movements of the shoulder girdle and control scapulohumeral relationships. All joints previously discussed, to a variable extent, participate in such movements. The resulting mobility of the shoulder is largely responsible for the ability of using the hand in all desired positions—in front of the body, overhead, behind the body, and so forth. The muscles of the shoulder girdle also participate significantly in skilled movements of the upper extremity, such as writing, and are essential in activities requiring pulling, pushing, and throwing, to mention only a few of the important activities of the upper extremity.

The shoulder region muscles are divided into three groups for study:

- Muscles connecting the shoulder girdle with the trunk, the neck, and the skull.
- Muscles connecting the scapula and the humerus.
- Muscles connecting the trunk and the humerus, having little or no attachment to the scapula.

Muscles From Trunk to Shoulder Girdle

Serratus Anterior

Serratus anterior (L. *serra*, saw) is one of the most important muscles of the shoulder girdle. Without it, the arm cannot be raised overhead. **Proximal attachments**: By nine muscular slips from the anterolateral aspect of the thorax, from the first to the ninth ribs—hence its name, the "saw muscle." The lowest four or five slips interdigitate with the external oblique abdominal muscle. Lying close to the thorax, the muscle passes underneath the scapula with the **distal attachment** occurring along the medial border of the scapula. The lowest five digitations converge on the inferior angle of the scapula, attaching to its costal surface. This is the strongest portion of the muscle. **Innervation**: Long thoracic nerve (C_5-C_7). **Anatomic actions**: Abduction and upward rotation of the scapula.

INSPECTION AND PALPATION On well-developed individuals, the lower digitations may be seen and palpated near their proximal attachment on the ribs when the arm is overhead (Fig. 7–5). The middle and upper portions of the muscle are largely covered by pectoral muscles but may be palpated in the axilla close to the ribs, posterior to the pectoralis major. For palpation of the muscle in the axilla, the subject first elevates the arm to a horizontal position halfway between flexion and abduction, then reaches forward so that the scapula slides forward on the thorax. This isolated action of the serratus occurs at approximately 135 degrees of shoulder flexion and abduction. When the serratus is paralyzed and forward reaching is attempted (Fig. 7–6A), a typical "winging" of the medial border of the scapula is seen, and the scapula fails to slide forward on the rib cage (Brunnstrom, 1941).

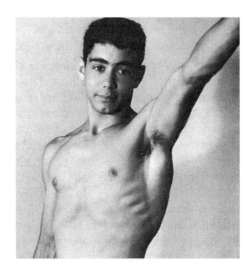

Figure 7–5 Lower digitations of the serratus anterior near their origins on the ribs. The upper portion of the muscle is covered by the pectoralis major.

Trapezius

The **trapezius** is a superficial muscle of the neck and upper back and is accessible for observation and palpation in its entirety. Because of its shape, it has been called the "shawl" muscle. Early anatomists named it "musculus cucullaris" (shaped like a monk's hood). The present name refers to a geometric figure. **Proximal attachments**: Occipital bone, ligamentum nuchae, and spinous processes from C_7–T_{12}. From this widespread origin, the muscle fibers converge to their **distal attachments** on the acromial end of the clavicle, the acromion, and the spine

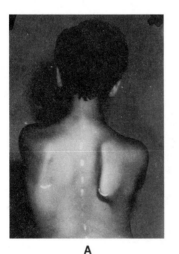
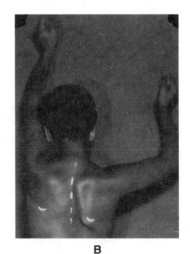

A **B**

Figure 7–6 Isolated paralysis of the serratus anterior. *(A)* Forward reach is poor. The scapula fails to slide forward on the rib cage, and there is a typical winging of its medial border. *(B)* In retraction of the shoulder girdle, the medial border of the scapula does not stay close to the rib cage. The right arm cannot be raised overhead because the trapezius does not provide sufficient upward rotation of the scapula. (From Brunnstrom, S: Muscle testing around the shoulder girdle. *J Bone Joint Surg [Am]* 23:263, 1941, with permission.)

of the scapula. The fibers of the upper portion course downward and laterally, those of the middle portion more horizontally, and those of the lower portion obliquely upward. **Innervation**: Spinal accessory nerve (C_3-C_4 and spinal portion of cranial nerve XI). **Anatomic actions**: The upper trapezius performs elevation and upward rotation of the scapula, as well as extension, lateral flexion, and contralateral rotation of the neck; the lower trapezius performs upward rotation, adduction, and depression of the scapula; the middle trapezius performs upward rotation and adduction of the scapula. Upward rotation occurs with abduction of the scapula during elevation of the arm. As the axis for rotation moves from the root of the scapular spine to the acromion process, the force arm for the lower trapezius becomes larger for upward rotation (Bagg and Forrest, 1988).

INSPECTION AND PALPATION   For observation of the entire muscle in action bilaterally, the subject abducts the shoulders and retracts the shoulder girdles, as seen in Figure 7–7. This position requires the action of all parts of the trapezius, retraction of the shoulder girdle by the entire muscle, and upward rotation of the scapula by the upper and lower portions of the muscle. If the trunk is simultaneously inclined forward or the subject lies prone, the muscle has to act against the force of gravity to hold the shoulders back, and the intensity of the contraction increases. The upper portion of the trapezius should also be observed and palpated as it performs its function of shoulder elevation, as well as the lower portion, as it carries out its function of shoulder depression.

Rhomboid Major and Minor

The **rhomboids** (Gr. *rhombos*, a lozenge-shaped figure), which connect the scapula with the vertebral column, lie underneath the trapezius. The upper portion is known as **rhomboid minor**; the lower (larger) portion, as **rhomboid major**. **Proximal attachments**: Ligamentum nuchae and spinous processes of the lowest two cervical and the upper four thoracic vertebrae. **Distal attachment**: Medial border of scapula. The oblique direction of the muscles indicates that they serve to ele-

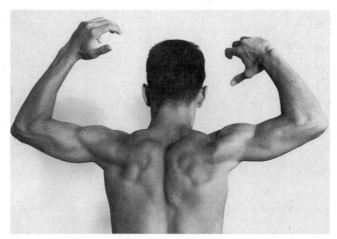

Figure 7–7   All portions of the trapezius in contraction. For strong action of this muscle, the subject inclines trunk forward. Note also the contraction of the posterior deltoid, infraspinatus, and teres minor.

vate as well as to retract the scapula. The rhomboid major also has the important function of downward rotation of the scapula since it attaches to the inferior angle of the scapula. The rhomboids are made up of parallel fibers, the direction of which is almost perpendicular to those of the lower trapezius. **Innervation**: Dorsal scapular nerve ("the nerve to the rhomboids," C_4-C_5). **Anatomic actions**: Downward rotation, adduction, and elevation of the scapula.

INSPECTION AND PALPATION   Because the rhomboids are covered by the trapezius, they are best palpated when the trapezius is relaxed. The subject's hand is placed in the small of the back. The investigator places the palpating fingers underneath the medial border of the scapula, which can be done without causing discomfort to the subject, provided that the muscles in this region are relaxed (Fig. 7–8). If the subject raises the hand just off the small of the back, the rhomboid major contracts vigorously as a downward rotator of the scapula and pushes the palpating fingers out from underneath the medial border of the scapula (Fig. 7–9). If the lower trapezius is not too bulky, the direction of the contracting fibers of the rhomboids may be seen under the skin. In the case of trapezius paralysis, the course of the rhomboids is easier to observe (Fig. 7–10).

Pectoralis Minor

The **pectoralis minor** (L. *pectus*, breast bone, chest) is located anteriorly on the upper chest, being entirely covered by the pectoralis major. **Proximal attachments**: By four tendomuscular slips from the second to the fifth ribs. These mus-

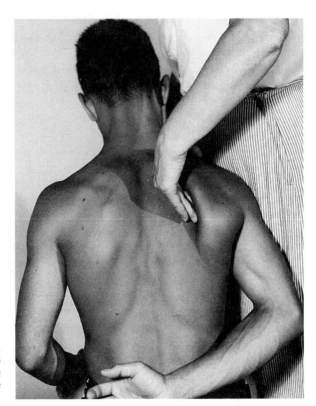

Figure 7–8 Palpation of rhomboids. When the trapezius and rhomboids are relaxed, the examiner's finger may be placed under the medial border of the scapula.

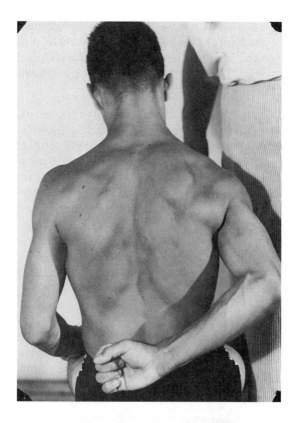

Figure 7–9   The rhomboids. As the subject raises the hand off the back, contraction of the rhomboideus major is observed. Note also the contraction of the teres major.

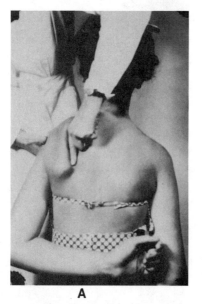

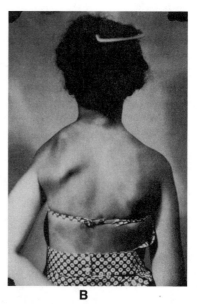

| **A** | **B** |

Figure 7–10   Testing the rhomboids in a subject with trapezius paralysis. *(A)* The examiner's finger lies along the medial border of the scapula. *(B)* When the subject raises the hand off the back, the lower border of the rhomboid major is easily seen. (From Brunnstrom, S: Muscle testing around the shoulder girdle. *J Bone Joint Surg [Am]* 23:263, 1941, with permission.)

cular slips converge with their **distal attachment** into the coracoid process of the scapula. This gives the muscle a triangular shape. **Innervation**: Medial pectoral nerve (C_7-T_1). **Anatomic actions**: Depression and ventral tilt of the scapula as well as elevation of ribs 2 to 5.

INSPECTION AND PALPATION The forearm is placed in the small of the back. In this position, the pectoralis major is relaxed, a prerequisite for palpation of the pectoralis minor. The examiner places one finger just below the coracoid process of the scapula, as seen in Figure 7–11, pressing down gently to let the finger sink in as far as possible.

In this position, the finger lies across the tendon of the pectoralis minor, the muscle of which is relaxed as long as the forearm rests in the small of the back. When the subject raises the forearm off the back, the pectoralis minor contracts, and its tendon becomes tense under the palpating fingers. The muscle can also be palpated in its important function of shoulder depression (trunk elevation). The palpating fingers should be placed distal to the coracoid process, and the subject (sitting on a table) should be asked to push down on the table with the hands as if to elevate the body (actual trunk elevation or sitting push-up will cause other muscles to contract and obscure palpation of the muscle).

Levator Scapulae

The **levator scapulae**, as its name indicates, is an elevator of the scapula, an action it shares with the upper portion of the trapezius and with the rhomboids. **Proximal attachments**: Transverse processes of the upper cervical vertebrae. **Distal attachment**: Medial border of the scapula, above the spine, near the superior

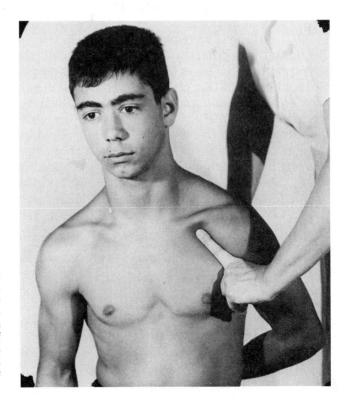

Figure 7–11 Palpation of the pectoralis minor. With the subject's hand resting in the lumbar region of the back, both the pectoralis major and the pectoralis minor are relaxed. The tendon of pectoralis minor is palpated below the coracoid process when the subject raises the hand off the back.

angle. **Innervation**: Dorsal scapular nerve (C_3-C_5). **Anatomic actions**: Elevation and downward rotation of the scapula as well as lateral flexion and ipsilateral rotation of the cervical spine.

INSPECTION AND PALPATION   The levator is covered by the upper trapezius and in its upper portion also by the sternocleidomastoid muscle. Posteriorly, its border extends to the rhomboid minor and the splenius muscle of the neck. Ordinarily, in elevation of the shoulder girdle, the upper trapezius and the levator contract together. The levator is difficult to isolate and palpate. To bring out levator action with a minimum of trapezius participation, the subject places the forearm in the small of the back, then shrugs the shoulder. The levator may then be palpated in the neck region, anterior to the trapezius but posterior to the sternocleidomastoid muscle.

Note that the line of action of the upper trapezius produces elevation and upward rotation of the scapula, whereas the levator, at least in a certain range, has a downward rotary action on the scapula. Therefore, the levator muscle will more likely be used as an elevator when elevation is carried out with the scapula in a downward rotation position, as in shrugging the shoulder when the hand is behind the body. A comparatively isolated action of the levator may be obtained if the shrug is made briefly and quickly and in short range. If much effort is exerted in raising the shoulder and if the elevated position is maintained, the trapezius will contract in spite of above precautions.

Inspection and palpation of the sternocleidomastoid muscle are discussed in Chapter 11.

Muscles From Shoulder Girdle to Humerus

Deltoid

The **deltoid** (Gr. *delta*, the letter Δ; *eidos*, resemblance) is a large superficial muscle consisting of three parts: anterior, middle, and posterior. The muscle covers the glenohumeral joint on all sides except the axilla and comprises 40 percent of the mass of the scapulohumeral muscles (O'Brien et al, 1990). **Proximal attachments**: The acromial end of the clavicle, the acromion process, and the spine of the scapula. From this widespread origin, the three portions of the muscle converge to have their **distal attachment** onto the deltoid tuberosity, a rather rough area about halfway down the shaft of the humerus. **Innervation**: Axillary nerve (C_5-C_6). **Anatomic actions**: Abduction of the glenohumeral joint. Anterior deltoid performs flexion and horizontal adduction of the glenohumeral joint. Posterior deltoid performs extension and horizontal abduction of the glenohumeral joint.

INSPECTION AND PALPATION   The muscle is covered by skin only and may therefore be observed and palpated in its entirety. The characteristic roundness of the normal shoulder is due to the deltoid muscle. All parts of the deltoid are easily identified in Figures 5–9 and 5–10.

The **anterior deltoid** may be observed and palpated when the arm is held in a horizontal position (Fig. 7–12). Note that its inferior border lies close to the upper portion of the pectoralis major. The anterior deltoid contracts strongly when horizontal adduction is resisted.

The **middle deltoid** has the best anatomic position for abduction and is seen

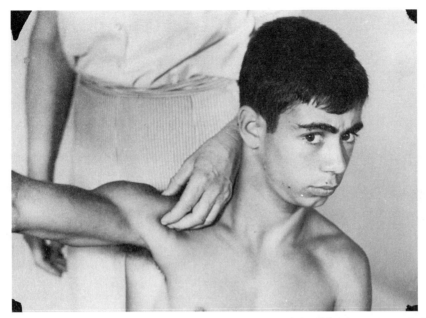

Figure 7–12 The examiner grasps around the anterior portion of the deltoid, separating it from the middle deltoid and from the pectoralis major.

contracting whenever this movement is carried out or the abducted position is maintained.

The **posterior deltoid** contracts strongly when the shoulder is hyperextended against resistance, or resistance is given to horizontal abduction. The inferior border of the posterior portion of the deltoid has a close relation to the long head of the triceps and to the teres muscles (see Figs. 5–11 and 7–14). Isolated action of the posterior deltoid may be seen in Figure 7–13. The patient (postpoliomyelitis) had extensive paralysis of the shoulder muscles, including the middle and anterior portions of the deltoid, while the posterior portion was more or less preserved.

The three portions of the deltoid should be observed in action while horizontal abduction and adduction are performed and in pulling and pushing activities. It will then be seen that the anterior and posterior portions often act antagonistically—the anterior portion exerting traction forward, the posterior portion backward—on the arm.

Early anatomists thought that the supraspinatus initiated abduction. It has been shown, however, in persons with supraspinatus paralysis from nerve blocks or from poliomyelitis, that the deltoid alone is capable of abducting the humerus throughout the range of motion but with less than normal strength. Howell and associates (1986) found an approximately 50 percent reduction in maximum isokinetic abduction torque with nerve blocks to the suprascapular nerve. After recovery from surgical removal of the deltoid muscle (because of soft tissue tumors), Markhede, Monastyrski, and Stener (1985) documented a loss of 5 to 15 degrees of active abduction and a decrease in maximum isometric torques of only 30 to 40 percent. The authors propose that the reduction in isometric torques does not reflect the true loss of the deltoid muscle. Compensatory hypertrophy and increased activity of the rotator cuff muscles may have made a greater relative contribution to the recorded torques.

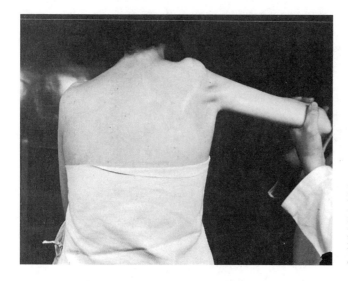

Figure 7-13 Isolated action of the posterior deltoid in a postpoliomyelitis patient. The examiner holds the arm abducted while the patient pushes back against resistance. Note atrophy of the middle deltoid.

Supraspinatus

As its name indicates, the **supraspinatus** muscle is located above the spine of the scapula. It is hidden by the trapezius and the deltoid, the trapezius covering its muscular portion, the deltoid, its tendon. **Proximal attachment**: Supraspinous fossa of the scapula, which it completely fills. The muscle fibers converge toward the tip of the shoulder to form a short tendon that passes underneath the acromion and that adheres to the capsule of the shoulder joint. **Distal attachment**: Uppermost facet of the greater tubercle of the humerus. **Innervation**: Suprascapular nerve (C_5-C_6). **Anatomic action**: Abduction of the glenohumeral joint.

PALPATION The deepest portion of the supraspinatus lies too deep in the supraspinous fossa to be palpated, but its more superficial fibers may be felt through the trapezius. The spine of the scapula is first identified, and the palpating fingers are placed above the spine (they should be moved to various positions so that the best spot for palpation is located). A quick abduction movement in short range is carried out and a momentary contraction of the muscle is felt. In wider range of abduction, the supraspinatus is more difficult to palpate because the trapezius becomes increasingly tense and it is then not easy to distinguish one muscle from the other.

Palpation of the supraspinatus also may be done with the subject prone and the arm hanging over the edge of the table. In this position, the scapula has moved forward on the rib cage by the weight of the arm and is already partially upwardly rotated. When abduction is carried out in this position, a contraction of the supraspinatus may be felt with little or no interference by the trapezius. The supraspinatus also may be palpated when the subject lifts a heavy briefcase or the like, preferably with the trunk inclined forward. As the weight of the object exerts its downward traction, the supraspinatus becomes tense, apparently for the purpose of preventing excessive separation of the glenohumeral joint.

The supraspinatus is capable of performing the total motion of abduction without the assistance of the deltoid. This has been demonstrated in persons with paralysis of the deltoid muscle in both poliomyelitis and axillary nerve block.

Howell and associates (1986) found the supraspinatus to be able to abduct the humerus against resistance and to contribute approximately 50 percent of normal maximum isokinetic torque.

Infraspinatus and Teres Minor

Although the **infraspinatus** and **teres minor** are supplied by two different nerves, they are described together because they are closely related in location and action and are sometimes inseparable. **Proximal attachments**: Infraspinous fossa and lateral border of the scapula. The infraspinatus lies closest to the spine of the scapula and occupies most of the infraspinous fossa. The teres minor (L. *teretis*, round and long) is attached mainly to the lateral border of the scapula. **Distal attachments**: Greater tubercle of the humerus, infraspinatus into its middle facet, and teres minor into its lower (posterior) facet. The tendons of both muscles are adherent to the capsule. **Innervation**: Infraspinatus by the suprascapular nerve and teres minor by the axillary nerve (C_5-C_6). **Anatomic actions**: External rotation and adduction of the glenohumeral joint.

INSPECTION AND PALPATION   The largest parts of the infraspinatus and the teres minor are superficial and may be palpated; some portions are covered by the trapezius and the posterior deltoid. To have as large parts of the muscle as possible available for palpation, the arm must be away from the body and the posterior deltoid must be relaxed. This is accomplished if the subject lies prone or stands with the trunk inclined forward and if the arm hangs vertically (Fig. 7–14). The margin of the posterior deltoid is first identified. The palpating fingers are placed below the deltoid on the scapula, near its lateral margin. While the subject maintains the arm in a vertical position, the subject externally rotates the shoulder by turning the palm forward. The two muscles then rise under the palpating fingers, the teres minor being felt next to the infraspinatus, but farther away from the spine of the scapula than the infraspinatus. External rotation in this position requires only a mild contraction of these muscles, and consequently they do not show beneath the skin in the illustration. A more vigorous contraction is seen in Figure 7–7, where a large number of other muscles are also activated.

The distal attachments of these muscles (as well as the supraspinatus) as they blend into the joint capsule are a frequent site of injury and cause of shoulder pain. These attachments can be palpated on the head of the humerus if the glenohumeral joint is passively hyperextended and the deltoid muscle is relaxed.

Subscapularis

The **subscapularis** is located underneath the scapula, close to the rib cage, but it is not attached to the rib cage. The smooth connective-tissue covering of the subscapularis provides a sliding surface for the scapular on the rib cage. **Proximal attachment**: Costal surface of scapula. Fiber bundles converge toward the axilla to form a broad tendon, which passes over the anterior aspect of the capsule of the glenohumeral joint. **Distal attachments**: Lesser tubercle of the humerus and shaft below the tubercle. **Innervation**: Subscapular nerves (C_5-C_6). **Anatomic action**: Inward rotation of the glenohumeral joint. Depending on the arm position, the subscapularis can flex, extend, adduct, or abduct the gleno-

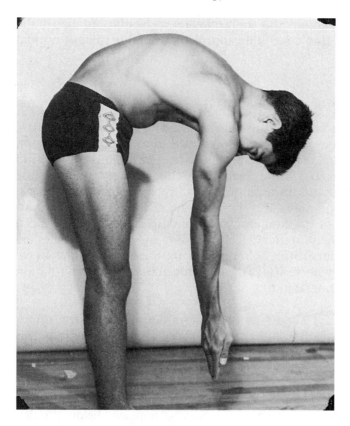

Figure 7–14 The infraspinatus and the teres minor may be felt contracting near the lateral border of the scapula when the shoulder is externally rotated. Vertical position of the arm allows activation of these two muscles in a rather isolated fashion.

humeral joint. Howell and associates (1986) proposed that the supraspinatus may contribute to 12 percent of abduction torque at and above 120 degrees of motion.

PALPATION   With the subject in the erect standing position, the muscle cannot be reached very well for palpation, but if the trunk is inclined forward so that the scapula slides forward on the rib cage by the weight of the hanging arm, a portion of this muscle may be palpated. The fingers are placed in the axilla anterior to the latissimus dorsi and, with gentle pressure, are moved in the direction of the costal surface of the scapula. With the arm hanging vertically, the subject internally rotates the shoulder by turning the palm backward and laterally (Fig. 7–15). The firm, round belly of the subscapularis can then be felt rising under the palpating fingers. If a person wishes to feel the muscle on himself or herself, the thumb is used for palpation. As far as can be ascertained by palpation, the size of the muscle varies considerably from person to person. The subscapularis has a cross section approximately equal to that of the middle deltoid, which indicates that it is a muscle of considerable size (Lehmkuhl and Smith, 1983, p. 397).

Teres Major

The **teres major** is located at the axillary border of the scapula distal to the teres minor. It is round like the minor, but larger. **Proximal attachment**: Inferior angle

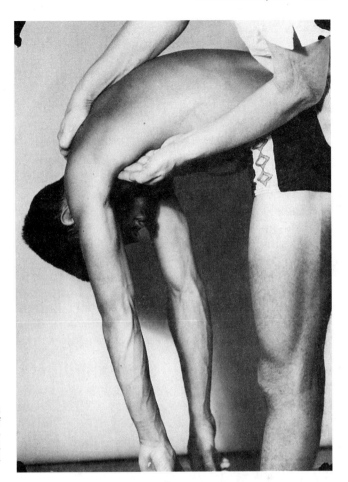

Figure 7–15 The subscapularis is palpated in internal rotation of the shoulder. The palpating fingers are placed in the axilla and are moved in a direction toward the costal surface of the scapula.

of the scapula. The muscle fibers course upward and laterally and have their **distal attachments** to the crest of the lesser tubercle of the humerus by means of a strong broad tendon. **Innervation:** Subscapular nerves (C_5-C_6). **Anatomic actions:** Internal rotation, adduction, and extension of the glenohumeral joint.

INSPECTION AND PALPATION The muscular portion of the teres major is well accessible to palpation, but the tendon of its distal attachment is not. The belly of the muscle can be palpated on the inferior aspect of the axillary border of the scapula when the subject is prone on a table with the arm hanging over the side or in the positions in Figures 7–14 and 7–15. If the relaxed subject inwardly rotates the glenohumeral joint, the teres major rises under the palpating fingers. If at the same time other fingers are placed higher on the axillary border and the subject is asked to externally rotate, the teres minor is felt to contract as the teres major relaxes.

The teres major acts in most pulling activities when the shoulder is extended or adducted against resistance. If the examiner gives manual resistance to adduction, as seen in Figure 5–11, the muscle may be palpated lateral to the inferior angle of the scapula. In this illustration, resistance is given simultaneously to extension of the elbow and adduction of the shoulder so that the triceps as well as the teres major contracts. (The teres major is also seen in Figure 7–17.) In most subjects, it is difficult to isolate the teres major from the adjacent latissimus dorsi muscle.

Coracobrachialis

Proximal attachment: Coracoid process of scapula. **Distal attachment**: Medial surface of humerus, about halfway down the shaft of the humerus. **Innervation**: Musculocutaneous nerve (C_6-C_7). **Anatomic actions**: Flexion and adduction of the glenohumeral joint.

INSPECTION AND PALPATION   Part of this muscle is covered by the deltoid and the pectoralis major. The coracobrachialis may be palpated in the distal portion of the axillary region if the arm is elevated above the horizontal, as seen in Figure 7–16. It emerges from underneath the inferior border of the pectoralis major where it lies medial to, and parallel with, the tendon of the short head of the biceps. The biceps is first identified by supination of the forearm; the palpating fingers then follow the short head of the biceps proximally until the muscle tapers off, and this is the height best suited for palpation of the coracobrachialis. In the illustration, the subject is bringing the arm in a direction toward the head.

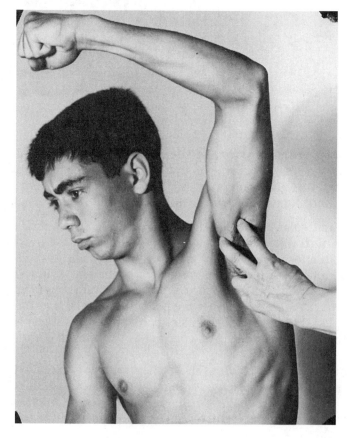

Figure 7–16 Identification of the coracobrachialis. This muscle emerges from underneath the inferior border of the pectoralis major, where it lies close to the tendon of the short head of the biceps.

Biceps Brachii and Triceps Brachii

The **biceps** and **triceps** muscles do not belong to the scapulohumeral group because they do not have their distal attachments on the humerus; however, the two heads of the biceps and the long head of the triceps cross the shoulder joint and therefore act on it. It should be recalled that the heads of the biceps attach to the supraglenoid tubercle and to the coracoid process, and that the triceps attaches to the infraglenoid tubercle.

The biceps is a flexor and an abductor, and the triceps is an extensor and an adductor of the glenohumeral joint. The long head of the biceps is capable of elevating the arm when the deltoid and the supraspinatus are paralyzed. The motion occurs in a position of external rotation of the glenohumeral joint, slightly anterior to the frontal plane and without resistance or a tool in the hand. This motion is useful for placement of the hand over the head, but the long head of the biceps is not strong enough to lift objects or to perform work in this position.

Muscles From Trunk to Humerus

These muscles have their proximal attachments on the trunk and their distal attachments on the humerus, having little or no attachment to the scapula. They act primarily on the humerus but also indirectly affect the position of the shoulder girdle. There are only two muscles in this group, the latissimus dorsi and the pectoralis major, which perform multiple actions at the shoulder including adduction, extension, internal rotation, and depression.

Latissimus Dorsi

The name **latissimus dorsi** is derived from the Latin *latus*, meaning broad. This muscle is the broadest muscle of the back and the lateral thoracic region. It lies superficially, except for a small part that is covered by the lower trapezius. **Proximal attachments**: Spinous processes of the thoracic vertebrae from T-6 downward, dorsolumbar fascia, crest of ilium (posterior portion), and the lowest ribs, here interdigitating with the external oblique abdominal muscle. The fibers converge toward the axilla, some fibers passing over or near the inferior angle of the scapula, often adhering to it. The **distal attachment** is by a tendon that courses in the axilla and attaches to the crest of the lesser tubercle of the humerus, proximal to that of the teres major. **Innervation**: Thoracodorsal nerve (C_6-C_8). **Anatomic actions**: Internal rotation, extension and adduction of the glenohumeral joint, scapular depression, elevation of pelvis.

INSPECTION AND PALPATION   The largest part of this muscle is thin and sheet-like, which makes it difficult to distinguish from the fascia and from the deeper muscles of the back. Laterally, in the axillary line and where the fibers converge, the muscle has considerable bulk, and here it is easy to observe and palpate (Fig. 7–17). The latissimus and the teres major contract when adduction or extension of the shoulder is resisted, as seen in the illustration, in which the subject is pressing down on the examiner's shoulder. The latissimus forms the posterior fold of the axilla. Its relation to the teres major and the long head of the triceps in this region should be noted.

The latissimus dorsi is attached, in part, to the crest of the ilium. When the arms are stabilized as in pushing down on crutch handles (closed-chain motion),

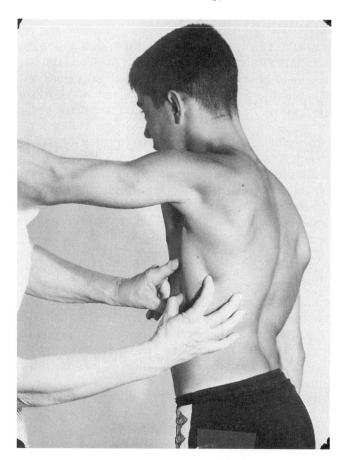

Figure 7–17 Palpation of the lower portion of the latissimus dorsi. The subject presses downward on the examiner's shoulder. The teres major may also be seen contracting strongly.

the distal attachment can aid in lifting the pelvis so that the foot clears the ground in walking. This function is of particular importance to someone with paraplegia; whose lower extremity muscles, including the hip-hikers (quadratus lumborum and lateral abdominals), are paralyzed because of an injury of the spinal cord. By placing the hands on the armrests of the wheelchair, the person can perform a sitting push-up and decrease pressure from sitting on the buttocks and the likelihood of pressure sores. The latissimus dorsi is innervated by the thoracodorsal nerve, derived from C_6, C_7, and C_8, and therefore is not involved in injuries to the spinal cord below C_8.

Pectoralis Major

Its name (L. *pectus*, breast bone, chest) indicates that the **pectoralis major** is a large muscle of the chest. It has an extensive origin but does not cover nearly as large an area as the latissimus dorsi. **Proximal attachments**: Clavicle (sternal half), sternum, and costal cartilages of the second to seventh ribs, and the aponeurosis over the abdominal muscles. The muscle is described as consisting of three parts: the clavicular, sternocostal, and abdominal. From the standpoint of action, the muscle has an upper portion (clavicular) and a lower portion (sternocostal and abdominal). Because of its wide origin and the convergence of its fibers toward the axilla, the muscle takes the shape of a fan. **Distal attachment**: Crest of the greater tuberosity of the humerus, on an area several inches long. Before reaching its attachment, the tendon bridges the intertubercular (bicipital) groove. The manner in which the muscle fibers approach their distal attachment should be noted—the tendon appears to be twisted around itself, so that the uppermost fibers attach lowest on the crest and the lower fibers attach more proximally. **Innervation**: Medial and lateral pectoral nerves (C_5-T_1). **Anatomic actions**: Adduction and internal rotation of the glenohumeral joint. Clavicular head performs flexion of the glenohumeral joint.

INSPECTION AND PALPATION   Being superficial and of considerable bulk, the muscle is easily observed and palpated. It is best palpated where the fibers converge toward the axilla. The entire muscle contracts when horizontal adduction is resisted, as in pressing the palms together in front of the body.

The upper portion acts separately if the arm is brought obliquely upward toward the head against resistance, as seen in Figure 7–18. A pencil has been placed across the lower portion of the muscle to show that it is not contracting. The lower portion contracts separately when the arm is adducted in a lower position (Fig. 7–19). The examiner's fingers are placed across the upper portion to show that it is relatively relaxed. The external oblique abdominal muscle is also seen contracting (note its interdigitations with the serratus anterior).

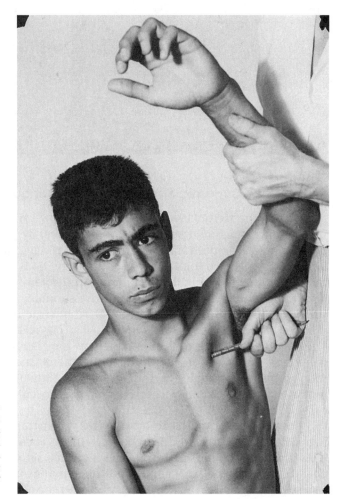

Figure 7–18 The upper portion of the pectoralis major is seen contracting as the subject pulls the arm in the direction toward the head against resistance. A pencil has been placed across the lower portion of pectoralis major to show that it is relaxed.

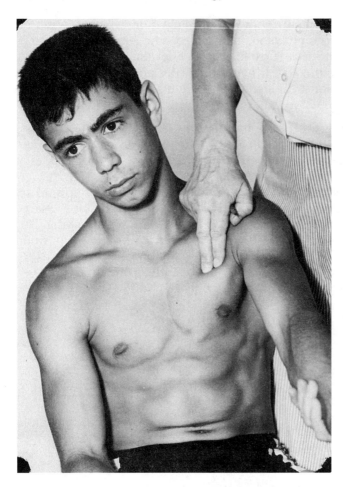

Figure 7–19 The lower portion of the pectoralis major contracts as the subject adducts the arm against resistance. The examiner's fingers are separating the lower portion from the upper.

Support and Dynamic Stabilization of the Shoulder

Motions at the sternoclavicular and acromioclavicular joints are limited by strong ligamentous attachments and, to a lesser degree, by bony configuration. The glenohumeral and scapulothoracic joints, however, have little ligamentous or bony stability. The latter two joints are attached to the body by muscles and, in the case of the glenohumeral joint, by the joint capsule reinforced by ligaments. Normally, there is no contraction of muscles of the shoulder girdle during relaxed sitting or standing, giving rise to the question of what structures prevent the humerus from subluxating when the person is upright. The clavicle and scapula rest on the thorax. The head of the humerus is maintained on the glenoid fossa by the horizontal coracohumeral and superior glenohumeral ligaments and by negative atmospheric pressure within the capsule. In fresh cadavers, Kumar and Balasubramaniam (1985) found that subluxation of the humeral head occurred only after puncture of the capsule.

Low-level continuous activity of the upper trapezius is frequently found during sitting and standing, but when attention is called to this activity, most subjects can relax the muscle easily. The trapezius activity is probably related to head posture because the upper fibers are neck extensors as well as scapula elevators, and such continuous muscle activity is a common source of tension and neck pain in people who work at a desk. Nevertheless, it has long been noted that paralysis of the trapezius is accompanied by dropping and downward rotation of the scapula (Brunnstrom, 1941; Sakellarides, 1986). Maintenance of the normal resting position of the scapula may be from passive fascial forces produced by the 15 muscles that make attachments on the scapula as well as from the support of the rib cage.

Rotator Cuff Stabilization

It was once thought that, when a person is carrying a heavy load such as a briefcase in the hand, contraction of the deltoid, biceps, or triceps brachii muscles with their vertical action lines kept the humeral head apposed to the glenoid cavity. These muscles, however, have been found to be electromyographically silent even with loads of 25 lb in the hand (Bearn, 1961; Basmajian, 1978). Instead, EMG activity has been found in the horizontally directed rotator cuff muscles—the supraspinatus, infraspinatus, and teres minor (Fig. 7–20A). Contraction of these

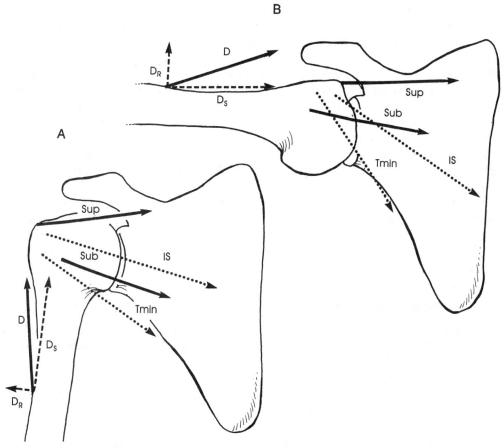

Figure 7–20 Shearing, stabilizing, and rotary effects of the forces of the deltoid and rotator cuff muscles at the glenohumeral joint. The vectors depict the direction of the muscle action lines in *(A)* initiation of abduction and *(B)* at 90 degrees of glenohumeral abduction. The solid lines represent the medial or anterior lines of action of the middle deltoid (D), supraspinatus (Sup), and the subscapularis (Sub); the dotted lines represent the posterior lines of action of the infraspinatus (IS) and the teres minor (Tmin). The vector of the deltoid has been resolved into a rotary component (D_R) and a stabilizing component (D_S). Vector lengths are not related to force but are of equal length in *(A)* and *(B)* to visualize decreases in muscle length (and therefore force) with increased abduction.

muscles holds the humeral head tightly against the glenoid to prevent subluxation when carrying a weight in the hand.

Biceps Brachii

The tendon of the long head of the biceps brachii courses over the humeral head and descends in the intertubercular groove. When the muscle contracts, tension occurs in the tendon to produce a downward and inward force on the head of the humerus, compressing it against the glenoid cavity. This force is similar to pulling a rope around a post. Thus, when the elbow is flexed with a weight in the hand, the biceps aids in preventing subluxation of the glenohumeral joint.

The Deltoid

In the evolution of primate and human development, the deltoid muscle increases its relative size markedly with the upright position (O'Brien et al, 1990). In humans, the muscle is prominent and surrounds the glenohumeral joint on three sides. Attention has been focused on the deltoid in its function as an abductor of the glenohumeral joint. The deltoid, however, has a small rotary component to its muscle force vector (see Fig. 7–20). In the early part of elevation, the major force of the deltoid is directed vertically, producing a shear on the glenoid and causing the humeral head to strike the coracoacromial arch. This movement is prevented by the horizontal and downward lines of action of the rotator cuff muscles. Some consider the posterior deltoid itself to be an adductor or to cause joint compression in the early part of the motion and have found lines of force inferior or very close to the axis of motion (Duca and Forrest, 1973; Poppen and Walker, 1978). As elevation progresses, the lever arms for abduction increase, but **most of the force generated by the deltoid is directed into the stabilizing component**, which compresses the head of the humerus against the glenoid. In the position of arm elevation, the deltoid and the horizontal forces of the rotator cuff muscles provide stability for the glenohumeral joint. In full shoulder elevation, as in pressing upward or standing on the hands, the abducted and upwardly rotated scapula forms a platform for the head of the humerus. The scapula, in turn, is stabilized by the serratus anterior and the trapezius muscles.

Synergistic Muscle Actions

Classification of shoulder muscles in function as prime movers and antagonists is of limited value in the shoulder except for a specific motion. Individual muscles and parts of the same muscle in the shoulder girdle have multiple anatomic actions because of the number of joints, the large range of motion, and the absence of structural stability. The majority of the shoulder muscles contract during any motion of the arm. For example, elevation of the arm can activate 11 of the 17 major muscles of the shoulder girdle, and it is of little value to attempt to identify a single prime mover. In the many motion combinations, muscles or their parts can be classified as synergists or antagonists for a particular movement only. Examples are the trapezius and the serratus anterior as they act together to produce upward rotation of the scapula but act as antagonists in retraction and protraction of the scapula. Even the parts of the same muscle may act as synergists or antagonists as occurs with the trapezius. The upper and lower trapezius act synchronously in upward rotation of the scapula but are antagonists in elevation and depression of the scapula.

Several important synergies, or force couples, occur in the shoulder. In mechanics, a **force couple** is defined as two forces whose points of application occur on opposite sides of an axis and in opposite directions to produce rotation of the body. This situation occurs during elevation of the arm. The trapezius and the serratus anterior combine forces to produce abduction and upward rotation of the scapula. The deltoid and the supraspinatus contract together to produce abduction (or flexion) at the glenohumeral joint.

Muscle Forces and Torques

Large forces occur in the shoulder with hand use because the resistance arm can be 2 ft, or longer with a tool, while the muscle force arms are measured in inches. Determination of the magnitude of the forces is difficult because of the number of muscles participating in the motions (see Fig. 7–20). Biomechanical equations become indeterminant because of the number of unknown forces. Thus, all estimates of the forces require assumptions. In Figure 7–21, the forces occurring in 90 degrees of abduction are diagrammed with the assumption that the deltoid is the only active glenohumeral abductor and using average distances and angles for a 150-lb person. The magnitude of the deltoid muscle force (D) can be found using the equilibrium equation for torques (see Fig. 7–21 for known values):

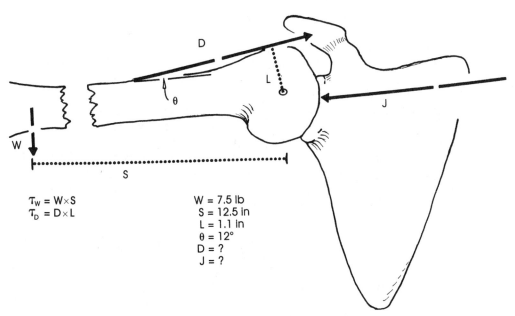

$$T_W = W \times S$$
$$T_D = D \times L$$

W = 7.5 lb
S = 12.5 in
L = 1.1 in
θ = 12°
D = ?
J = ?

Figure 7–21 Diagram of the forces on the humerus when the arm/trunk angle is in 90 degrees of abduction. D = deltoid muscle; W = weight of the arm, forearm, and hand acting at the center of gravity; J = joint compression force; L = force arm distance for the middle deltoid (Poppen and Walker, 1977); S = distance of the center of gravity of the upper extremity to the axis of motion (weight arm distance); θ = angle of the action line of the deltoid with the long axis of the arm. It is assumed that only the deltoid is acting to maintain the position of abduction. The weight of the upper extremity was calculated as 5% of 150 lb of body weight. See the text for equations to solve for unknown forces.

$$\Sigma\tau = 0$$
$$-\tau_W + \tau_D = 0$$
$$(-W \times S) + (D \times L) = 0$$
$$-(7.5 \text{ lb} \times 12.5 \text{ in}) + (D \times 1.1 \text{ in}) = 0$$
$$D = \frac{7.5 \text{ lb} \times 12.5 \text{ in}}{1.1 \text{ in}}$$
$$\boxed{D = 85 \text{ lb}}$$

The magnitude and direction of the joint force (J) can be found using the equilibrium equations for forces:

$$\Sigma F_x = 0$$
$$D_x - J_x = 0$$
$$D \cos \theta - J_x = 0$$
$$85 \text{ lb} \times \cos 12° - J_x = 0$$
$$-J_x = -85 \text{ lb} \times .978$$
$$J_x = 83 \text{ lb}$$
$$\Sigma F_y = 0$$
$$-W_y + D_y + J_y = 0$$
$$-W_y + D \sin \theta + J_y = 0$$
$$-7.5 \text{ lb} + 85 \text{ lb} \times \sin 12° + J_y = 0$$
$$+J_y = +7.5 \text{ lb} - (85 \text{ lb} \times .2079)$$
$$+J_y = -10 \text{ lb}$$

The joint compression force (J) can be found using the Pythagorean theorem:

$$J = \sqrt{J_x^2 + J_y^2}$$
$$J = \sqrt{6889 + 100}$$
$$\boxed{J = 84 \text{ lb}}$$

This estimation of a joint compression force of 84 lb is similar to that of Inman, Saunders, and Abbott (1944), who calculated the joint force to be 10.2 times the weight of the arm, which would be 75.5 lb in a 150-lb person (with weight of arm equal to 5 percent of body weight). Poppen and Walker (1978) calculated the joint reaction force to be 0.89 times body weight, which would be 134 lb in the 150-lb person. These authors' assumptions, however, were that the relative force in a given muscle is proportional to its cross-sectional area times its integrated EMG signal. The forces become even larger with resistance applied to the arm or tools held in the hand. In the equation above, adding a 5-lb weight in the hand (2 ft from the axis of motion) increases the joint compression force from 84 to 190 lb.

Maximum isometric torque measurements in the shoulder demonstrate that the greatest strength occurs when the muscles contract in the elongated position and that torque decreases as the muscles shorten (see Figs. 4–11 and 4–12; Murray et al, 1985; Otis et al, 1990). Maintenance of favorable length-tension relationships over such a large range of motion (ie, up to 180 degrees) is accomplished by movement of the base of support of the humerus by the scapula and by changes in muscle lever arms. Lever arm lengths for the deltoid increase with the motion of abduction. Poppen and Walker (1978) found that the middle deltoid almost doubled its leverage from 17 to 30 mm, the anterior deltoid increased eightfold from 5 to 40 mm, and the posterior deltoid increased from −5 mm (an adduction or joint compression force) to +20 mm. The supraspinatus maintained a relatively constant lever arm of about 20 mm throughout the motion of abduction. In the first 30 to 60 degrees of abduction, the leverage for the supraspinatus was greater than that of the deltoid, which indicates that the supraspinatus provides a major force in the initiation of shoulder abduction.

Small changes in lever arm lengths can have great effects on strength and function of shoulder motions. In persons who had complex fractures of the proximal humerus treated surgically by hemiarthroplasty, Rietveld and associates (1988) found that functional outcomes (ie, ability to actively elevate the arm) were related to the loss of lever arm lengths of the supraspinatus and the deltoid. Failures increased as the distance from the joint center to the lateral margin of the head of the humerus progressively decreased.

Maximum Isometric and Isokinetic Torque Measurements

Table 7–2 shows maximum isometric torques in normal subjects taken from two investigations (Murray et al, 1985; Otis et al, 1990). Where more than one position was tested, it can be seen that the torques are higher when the muscle is contracted in the elongated position. Differences between men and women and between younger and older persons also are represented.

Table 7-2 Average Maximum Isometric Torque in Normal Subjects (ft-lb)*

	Shoulder Abduction			Shoulder Flexion		
Joint position	0°	45°	90°	0°	45°	90°
Subjects and age						
36 Males † ($\bar{X}$ = 25.8 yr)	53	43	42	69	59	55
20 Males ‡ ($\bar{X}$ = 31 yr)	—	45	—	76	41	—
20 Males ‡ ($\bar{X}$ = 62 yr)	—	31	—	62	35	—
20 Females ‡ ($\bar{X}$ = 29 yr)	—	20	—	37	24	—
20 Females ‡ ($\bar{X}$ = 62 yr)	—	16	—	28	16	—

* Maximum isometric torques from two studies that used similar methods have been converted from newtonmeters and kilograms-centimeters to foot-pounds. One foot-pound of resistance is the application of 1-lb force just above the elbow.
† Otis et al (1990).
‡ Murray et al (1985).

Peak isokinetic torque decreases when the velocity of the motion increases as can be seen in the values for shoulder flexion in baseball pitchers (Alderink and Kuck, 1986):

Velocity (degrees/sec)	Peak Torque (ft-lb)
90	43
120	41
210	35
300	28

Ivey et al (1985) measured isokinetic torques in normal subjects at 60 and 180 degrees per second. Peak torque ratios were found to be 3:2 between the internal and external rotators, 2:1 for the adductors and abductors, and 5:4 for the extensors and flexors. There was no significant difference between dominant and nondominant sides. The angle at which the peak torque occurred was constant for the same person but had a wide variation among individuals. Isokinetic studies on athletes in throwing sports show slightly different ratios, particularly at high speeds, and some significant differences between dominant and nondominant sides (Brown et al, 1988; Hinton, 1988).

Motions and Muscular Activity in Function

Functionally, muscles participate in postures and movements according to limb and body position in relation to gravity, applied resistance, and velocity of motion rather than by anatomic actions. For example, reaching overhead (a flexion-abduction-upward rotation movement) requires concentric contraction of the anterior deltoid, pectoralis major (clavicular head), coracobrachialis, biceps brachii, and the rotator cuff muscles at the glenohumeral joint as well as the trapezius and serratus anterior muscles at the scapulothoracic joint. Returning the arm to the side is an antagonistic motion (extension-adduction-downward rotation). The active muscles, however, do not become the antagonists. Rather, the flexors, abductors, and upward rotators perform eccentric contractions to lower the arm. Therefore, knowledge of muscle actions is essential in the analysis of muscular activity in function as well as in isolation of individual muscles for evaluation of length or strength. A summary classification of muscles according to their anatomic actions at the shoulder joints is presented in Table 7–3.

In forceful movements, all muscles in the upper extremity may contract, making it difficult to analyze the muscle activity. They may be contracting to produce or restrain the motion, to hold the desired position, to counteract an undesired motion of another active muscle, or to stabilize the glenohumeral joint. The rotator cuff muscles are almost always active in shoulder motions to provide gleno-

Table 7–3 Classification of Muscles According to Anatomic Actions at Joints

Scapulothoracic	Glenohumeral

Elevation
  Upper trapezius
  Levator scapulae
  Rhomboids
Depression
  Pectoralis minor
  Lower trapezius
  (pectoralis major and latissimus dorsi
    acting on humerus)
Protraction
  Serratus anterior
  Pectoralis major
  Pectoralis minor
Abduction
  Serratus anterior
Retraction-Adduction
  Trapezius
  Rhomboids
Upward rotation
  Trapezius
  Serratus anterior
Downward rotation
  Levator scapulae
  Rhomboids
	Flexion
	  Pectoralis major (clavicular head)
	  Anterior deltoid
	  Coracobrachialis
	  Biceps brachii
	Extension
	  Latissimus dorsi
	  Teres major
	  Triceps brachii (long head)
	  Posterior deltoid
	Abduction
	  Deltoid
	  Supraspinatus
	  Biceps brachii (long head)
	Adduction
	  Pectoralis major
	  Latissimus dorsi
	  Teres major
	  Triceps brachii (long head)
	  Posterior deltoid
	External rotation
	  Infraspinatus
	  Teres minor
	  Posterior deltoid
	Internal rotation
	  Subscapularis
	  Teres major
	  Pectoralis major
	  Latissimus dorsi
	  Anterior deltoid

humeral stabilization even if the muscles are not called upon for their actions in rotation. In the following analysis of muscle activity, it is helpful to have a subject perform the activity with a minimum of resistance so that the prime movers can more easily be identified visually and by palpation.

Placing the Hand Behind the Head

Placing the hand behind the head, as in combing one's hair, requires motions of elbow flexion; sternoclavicular joint elevation and upward rotation; scapular elevation, upward rotation, and abduction; and glenohumeral joint abduction and full external rotation. Shoulder muscles producing these motions in the standing position are the biceps brachii at the elbow; the trapezius and serratus anterior force-couple at the scapula; the deltoid and supraspinatus couple at the glenohumeral joint; and the infraspinatus and teres minor. When the arm is overhead, the triceps brachii contracts to control elbow flexion for hand placement. The contractions of the muscles are concentric except for the eccentric contraction of the trapezius during scapular abduction and the posterior parts of the deltoid, which lengthen during movement from 0 to 60 degrees and then shorten (Jiang et al, 1988). When the extremity is returned to the side, the motions reverse to sternoclavicular depression and downward rotation; scapular depression, downward rotation, and adduction with glenohumeral adduction, extension, and internal rotation. However, the primary muscles controlling this motion are the same as with elevation. The type of contraction changes to eccentric to control the lowering of the arm.

Pulling

If a similar adduction-extension motion is performed against external resistance, muscle activity reverses. This occurs with a motion such as pulling down on a window or exercise pulley. With the hands in place on the overhead pulley, the pulling motion is open chain: elbow flexion; sternoclavicular depression and derotation; scapular adduction, downward rotation, and depression; and glenohumeral adduction and extension with rotational changes relative to initial hand placement close together in internal rotation or widely separated in external rotation. Concentric muscle activity is required of the elbow flexors; the glenohumeral adductors and extensors (latissimus dorsi, pectoralis major, long head of the triceps brachii, and posterior deltoid); and the scapular downward rotators and depressors (pectoralis minor and rhomboids).

When the overhead bar is fixed and the person performs a chin-up to lift the body weight, closed-chain motion occurs. The elbows flex; the glenohumeral joint moves toward adduction, extension, and internal rotation; and the scapula is adducted, downwardly rotated, and depressed. Concentric muscle activity occurs in the same muscles used in pulling down on the overhead bar. Both the motions and the muscle activity are the same except that in the first instance the bar moves down and in the second the body moves up. When the person lowers the body from the chin-up position, eccentric contractions of the same muscle groups occur (elbow flexors, glenohumeral extensors and adductors, and the scapular downward rotators and depressors) to extend the elbows; flex and abduct the glenohumeral joint, and upwardly rotate, abduct, and elevate the scapula. Motions and muscle activity in the chin-up are similar to those needed in a pull-up when patients grasp overhead bed trapezes to lift their body weight for transfers and bedpan use.

Pushing

Another method used by persons with paraplegia to lift and move their bodies is to perform wheelchair or sitting push-ups. After the hands have been placed on the armrests of the chair, the motion is closed chain with elbow extension, glenohumeral adduction, scapular retraction, and depression. These motions require concentric contractions of the corresponding muscle groups. Lowering of the body then requires elbow flexion, glenohumeral abduction, scapular elevation, and abduction with eccentric contractions of the same muscles (triceps brachii, pectoralis major, latissimus dorsi, teres major, posterior deltoid, pectoralis minor, rhomboids, and trapezius). Persons with quadriplegia resulting from severance of the spinal cord at the sixth cervical segment lose the triceps brachii (C-7 to C-8) and the ability to extend the elbows against gravity or resistance. They can lift and shift their body weight using the scapular depressors. This is done by pushing down on the chair armrests with flexed elbows or getting the elbow into an extended and locked or braced position in the wheelchair and pushing down on the wheelchair seat. Able-bodied subjects can lift the body weight up to 5 to 7 inches using scapular depression alone. In the weight-bearing phases of crutch-walking, the muscle activity is similar to the sitting push-up: triceps brachii, pectoralis major, latissimus dorsi, teres major, posterior deltoid, pectoralis minor, rhomboids, and lower trapezius.

Throwing

The overhead throwing motion is found in many types of athletics (baseball, football, racquet sports, gymnastics, javelin, and swimming). Both the acceleration and deceleration phases frequently lead to injuries of the glenoid labrum and the rotator cuff. In the baseball throw, the peak internal rotation torque has been calculated at 220 ft-lb occurring within a time period of 0.01 seconds. Analysis of such rapid motion requires use of dynamics rather than statics, and the reader is referred to LeVeau (1977).

In general terms, the great force imparted to the ball is gained by elevation and rotation of the body and by transmitting this potential energy along with the kinetic energy of the large muscles of the legs and trunk through the shoulder and elbow into kinetic energy of the hand. The ball leaves the hand in a 90-mile-an-hour pitch with 88 Joules (J) of energy (65 ft-lb) and there remains 217 (155 ft-lb) of energy to be dissipated (Jobe et al, 1990).

The motion can be divided into phases of cocking (wind-up), acceleration, and deceleration (follow through). In the shoulder and arm during the cocking-phase motions of elbow flexion and supination, glenohumeral abduction, horizontal abduction, and maximal external rotation as well as scapular retraction occur. These motions place the muscles to be used in the acceleration phase on a stretch and increase their force: pronators, triceps brachii, pectoralis major, subscapularis, anterior deltoid, and serratus anterior. In deceleration, the same muscles are active but with eccentric contractions. Werner and coworkers (1993) found insufficient force in the triceps muscle to account for the magnitude of the acceleration. They believed that acceleration of the elbow from the cocked position of 85 degrees of elbow flexion to extension in less that 0.07 seconds occurs from the centrifugal force generated by trunk rotation, sudden decrease in elbow flexor contraction, and then triceps muscle activity. Detailed analyses of throwing are found in publications by Jobe and coworkers (1983, 1990b), Perry (1983), and Werner and coworkers (1993).

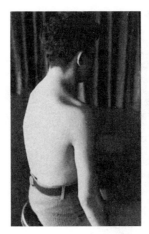
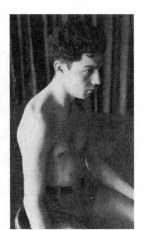

Figure 7–22 The emptiness in the supraspinous region is easily observed in this boy, who had involvement of the trapezius and the supraspinatus following poliomyelitis. The subject experienced no difficulty in raising his arm over his head.

CLINICAL APPLICATIONS

At the glenohumeral joint, there are 3 to 5 muscles that can perform each motion (see Table 7–3). For example, either the deltoid or the supraspinatus is capable of performing glenohumeral abduction (Figs. 7–22 and 7–23). Thus, paralysis of individual muscles will cause functional deficits from loss of strength, but through substitution, the arm and hand often can be placed in desired positions.

The scapular muscles, however, do not have as much redundancy, and paralysis of single muscles can seriously compromise use of the hand and arm. In normal subjects standing in the erect position with the arms at the sides, the medial border of the scapula is more or less parallel to the vertebral column. When the arm is raised overhead, the scapula rotates upward while simultaneously sliding forward on the rib cage, so that the medial border of the scapula assumes an oblique position and its inferior angle comes to lie approximately in the axillary line. The serratus anterior and the trapezius work together to bring about this movement and to give fixation to the scapula in any partially upward rotated position. With paralysis of the serratus, the scapula is not held against the rib cage and the medial border is winged (see Fig. 7–6). Scapulohumeral rhythm is abnormal and the subject is unable to fully elevate the arm. The scapula fails to abduct and upwardly rotate. In some people, the trapezius combined with a lateral trunk shift can produce sufficient upward rotation to gain an overhead position of the hand. In addition to the inability to elevate the shoulder for hand placement, the

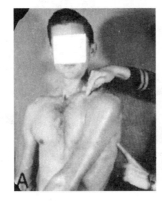
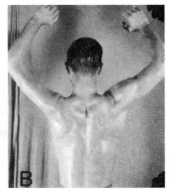

Figure 7–23 Deltoid and teres minor paralysis caused by a gunshot injury to the axillary nerve. *(A)* The examiner is indicating points of entry and exit of projectile. Note flaccidity of the left deltoid. *(B)* The subject was able to abduct arm full range. (From Brunnstrom, S: Muscle testing around the shoulder girdle. *J Bone Joint Surg [Am]* 23:263, 1941, with permission.)

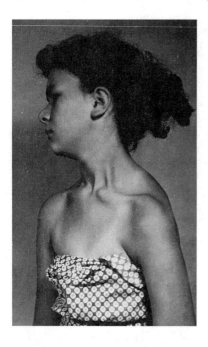

Figure 7–24 Paralysis of the trapezius. Note the subluxation of the sternoclavicular joint and the sharp outline of the posterior border of the clavicle; also note the skin fold in the anterior axillary region, characteristic of trapezius paralysis. (From Brunnstrom, S: Muscle testing around the shoulder girdle. *J Bone Joint Surg [Am]* 23:263, 1941, with permission.)

person with serratus paralysis has an ineffective ability to push on doors or drawers because without stabilization of the scapula by the serratus, pressure on the extended hand causes the scapula to move posteriorly.

Isolated paralysis of the trapezius muscle occurs if the spinal accessory nerve is severed during radial neck dissection surgery for complete removal of lymph nodes in people with cancer of the head and neck. Although the trapezius is electromyographically inactive in the erect posture, clinicians have long noted that the resting posture of the scapula in the presence of paralysis of the trapezius is that of downward rotation, abduction, and depression (Brunnstrom, 1941; Herring et al, 1987). This dropped position is best attributed to loss of passive tension of the trapezius. The downward rotation position of the scapula in turn places the glenohumeral joint in a position of abduction, with forces on the humeral head promoting subluxation and pain in the sternoclavicular joint (Fig. 7–24). Functionally, people with trapezius paralysis cannot retract the scapula (Fig. 7–25), but

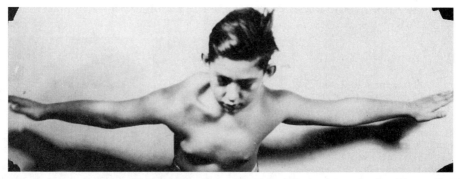

Figure 7–25 Paralysis of the right trapezius. The subject is unable to retract the shoulder girdle when the trunk is inclined forward. (From Brunnstrom, S: Muscle testing around the shoulder girdle. *J Bone Joint Surg [Am]* 23:263, 1941, with permission.)

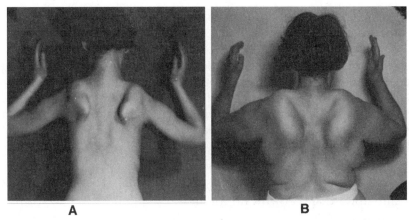

A   **B**

Figure 7–26   Bilateral paralysis of the trapezius and serratus. Maximum arm elevation of which these subjects are capable is demonstrated. Note the downward-rotated position of the scapulae. (*[A]* From Brunnstrom, S: Muscle testing around the shoulder girdle. *J Bone Joint Surg [Am]* 23:263, 1941, with permission.)

usually they can partially elevate the arm by using the levator scapulae, the serratus anterior, the deltoid, and the pectoralis major.

Paralysis of both the trapezius and the serratus destroys scapular stability, and the arm cannot be elevated (Fig. 7–26). Absence of scapular fixation causes the forces of the contracting scapulohumeral muscles to downwardly rotate and abduct the scapula, making the 90 degrees of glenohumeral abduction that can be performed by the deltoid less effective in elevating the arm.

Laboratory Activities

SHOULDER COMPLEX

1. On the bones, identify the following parts and bony landmarks. Determine which ones are palpable, and identify these on a partner. (Wear appropriate attire for this unit to permit exposure of the shoulder and shoulder girdle.)

Scapula	*Humerus*	*Sternum*	*Clavicle*
acromion process	head	manubrium	trapezoid line
spine	neck	body	conoid tubercle
coracoid process	greater tubercle	xiphoid process	articulating
supraspinous fossa	lesser tubercle	jugular (sternal)	surfaces of
infraspinous fossa	bicipital	notch	sternal and
glenoid cavity	(intertubercular)	facet for clavicle	acromial ends
superior angle	groove		
inferior angle	deltoid tuberosity		
medial border			
axillary border			
supraglenoid tubercle			
infraglenoid tubercle			

2. Locate the sternoclavicular, acromioclavicular, and glenohumeral joints on the bones or skeleton, and perform all movements that are possible at these joints. Identify axes about which these movements occur.

3. Passively move your partner's shoulder through its range of flexion and hyper-extension; internal and external rotation (shoulder abducted to 90 degrees and elbow flexed to 90 degrees to rule out supination and pronation); and ab-duction (externally rotate at 90 degrees of abduction) to reach maximum range of motion. State the approximate range of motion and the end-feels for each.

4. With your partner in a face-lying position, passively move the scapula through its normal ranges of elevation and depression, protraction and retrac-tion, and upward and downward rotation.

5. With a skin pen, mark the following landmarks on your partner (in a sitting position):
   a. The two angles of the scapula
   b. The three borders of the scapula
   c. The spine, acromion process, and glenoid fossa
   d. Spinous processes of C-7 and T-12
   e. Outline the clavicle

6. Use the marked side for reference and have your partner perform motions of abduction, flexion, internal rotation (place hand behind back), and external rotation (place hand behind neck). Observe the motions from the back and the front and palpate the motions of both the scapula and the humerus when the shoulder is at the side (0 degrees) and when the shoulder is at 45, 90, 135, and 180 degrees of abduction.

7. On the bones, determine attachments for the muscles connecting:
   a. Shoulder girdle with trunk
   b. Scapula and humerus
   c. Trunk and humerus
   Note particularly the:
   a. Lines of action
   b. Muscles with extensive proximal attachments and, hence, the multiple ac-tions
   c. Movements these muscles can perform

8. Determine muscles that:
   a. Flex the shoulder
   b. Extend the shoulder
   c. Abduct the shoulder
   d. Adduct the shoulder
   e. Internally and externally rotate the shoulder
   f. Elevate the shoulder girdle
   g. Depress the shoulder girdle
   h. Protract the shoulder girdle
   i. Retract the shoulder girdle
   j. Upwardly rotate the scapula
   k. Downwardly rotate the scapula

9. Palpate and obtain isolated contractions of muscles as described in the text:

Shoulder girdle to trunk	*Scapula to humerus*	*Trunk to humerus*
serratus anterior	deltoid	pectoralis major
trapezius	supraspinatus	latissimus dorsi
rhomboids	infraspinatus	
pectoralis minor	teres minor	
levator scapulae	subscapularis	
	teres major	
	biceps brachii	
	triceps brachii	
	coracobrachialis	

10. Functional analysis of the shoulder, elbow, wrist, and hand in activities: Perform the analysis by palpating muscles at rest and in activity and observing motions and muscles on a partner or a member of a small group. The analysis should include the name of the motion at each joint area, the primary muscle group(s) responsible for the motion or for maintaining a position, and the type of contraction that occurs (eccentric, concentric, or isometric). Difficult activities should be modified so that injury or exhaustion does not occur with the repetitions required; for example, push-ups should be done from the knees instead of the toes, and chin-ups should be done with partial support of the feet on the floor.

    a. Sitting push-up in a wheelchair (or arm chair) or standing push-up in parallel bars.

    b. Have the person perform a sitting or standing push-up; when in the highest position keep the elbows straight and lower the body by permitting the scapula to elevate. Measure how many inches the body can be elevated by scapular elevation and depression alone.

    c. Prone push-ups (modify). How do they differ in muscle activity from push-ups in the erect position?

    d. Chin-ups from the erect position (modify).

    e. Pull-ups from a supine position.

    f. Push forward on an object such as a table or door.

    g. Pull back.

    h. Reach over head to grasp a pulley or a window shade. Then pull down.

    i. Lift a briefcase or a purse from the floor. Then lower it back to the floor.

    j. Crutch-walking, non–weight-bearing one leg.

    k. Propelling a manual wheelchair.

    l. Sports activities such as swimming, throwing, or tennis or playing musical instruments such as violin, cello, flute, and so on. All of these activities can lead to injuries of the upper extremities.

CHAPTER 8

Hip and Pelvic Region

The pelvis (L., a basin) consists of the **sacrum, coccyx,** and the **two innominate bones,** which are formed by a fusion of the ilium, ischium, and pubis. The pelvic basin, or pelvic girdle, provides support and protection to the abdominal organs and transmits forces from the head, arms, and trunk to the lower extremities. Seven joints are formed by the pelvic bones: **lumbosacral, sacroiliac** (two), **sacrococcygeal, symphysis pubis,** and the **hip** (two). Although motions at the sacroiliac, symphysis pubis, and sacrococcygeal joints are small, the ability to have movement at these joints is very important. These joints are subject to injury, and they may become hypomobile or hypermobile with resulting pain and dysfunction. These joints also play an important role in permitting childbirth.

The hip joint (acetabulofemoral) is the most structurally stable, yet mobile, single joint in the body. In addition to transmitting large forces between the trunk and the ground, the hip region is a major component of the locomotor system. It participates in elevating and lowering the body, as in climbing or rising from a chair, and it is important in bringing the foot toward the body or hands, as in putting on a shoe. With every step, the hip abductor muscles (on the stance leg) must create a force to balance about 85 percent of the body weight (head, arms, trunk, and opposite leg). The hip joint serves as the fulcrum in this system and therefore sustains more than twice the body weight with each step.

BONES

Palpable Structures

Palpation may conveniently begin by placing the thumbs laterally on the **crests of the ilia,** one on the right and one on the left side. Under normal conditions, these two points are level in the standing position. Clinically, a lateral tilt of the pelvis is discovered by checking the height of the crests of the ilia. The symmetry of the pelvis also may be checked from the front by placing the thumbs on the **anterior superior spines of the ilia,** which, in most individuals, are easily located, often being visible under the skin. In obese individuals, it may be best to start palpation on the crests of the ilia laterally, and to follow the downward curve of the crests anteriorly until the anterior superior iliac spines are located.

If the crests are followed in a posterior direction, the **posterior superior spines of the ilia** are located. The subject in Figure 8–1 is palpating them with the thumbs. These prominences are broader and sturdier than the anterior spines and feel rough under the palpating fingers. Below each posterior spine is a depression, which is the posterior landmark for the sacroiliac joint.

To locate the greater **trochanter of the femur,** the subject places the thumb on the crest of the ilium laterally and reaches down on the thigh as far as possible with the middle finger. The greater trochanter is a large bony prominence, over which the fingers may slide from side to side and upward and downward. If the subject stands on the opposite leg and the examiner passively rotates the femur, the greater trochanter can be palpated with more certainty. In the standing position, the height of the greater trochanter should be the same for both legs.

The **tuberosities of the ischia** (the "sit bones") are easy to locate when the subject is sitting on a hard chair or is lying on the side with hips and knees flexed. Once located in these positions, the tuberosities also should be palpated in the standing position. They are then approached below the gluteal fold and are best

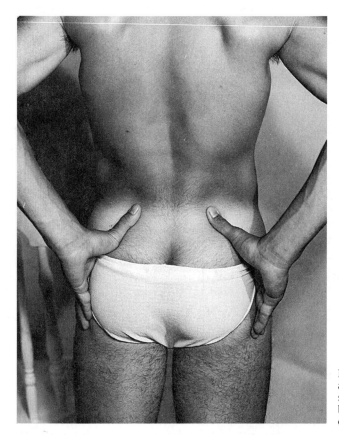

Figure 8–1 The subject's thumbs are palpating the posterior superior spines of the ilia. The spines are best located by following the crests of the ilia in a posterior direction.

palpated when the gluteus maximus and the hamstrings are relaxed. Such relaxation is achieved by having the subject stand in front of a table or in parallel bars. The subject bends forward at the waist and flexes the hips while supporting the weight of the trunk on the hands. The ischial tuberosities can be palpated when the hips are flexed and then can be followed as the subject returns to the erect posture by pushing the trunk up with the arms. This technique of palpation is used clinically to determine the relationship of the ischial tuberosities to the posterior brim of a prosthesis or the thigh cuff of an orthosis.

The **rami of the pubic bones** and the **superior aspect of the symphysis** can be palpated in the supine position with relaxation of the abdominal muscles. First, ask the subject to identify the top of the pubic bone with his thumbs. Then, place the extended hand on the abdomen with the fingers pointing toward the pubis. Slide the hand down so that the middle finger contacts the symphysis and the adjacent fingers contact the rami. The rami can take considerable pressure and should be smooth and without pain.

Nonpalpable Structures

A disarticulated set of bones and anatomic atlases should be used to identify the articulating surfaces of the sacrum; the **acetabulum** (L., a shallow vinegar vessel or cup), the socket of the hip joint, into which the head of the femur fits; the **posterior, anterior, and inferior gluteal lines** on the outer surface of the ilium, which separate the areas of attachment of the three gluteal muscles; the **anterior inferior iliac spine**, located below the superior spine and separated from it by a notch; the **posterior inferior iliac spine;** the **greater sciatic notch;** the **spine of the ischium;** the **head and neck of the femur;** and the **lesser trochanter of the femur.**

The sacrum (L., sacred) is a complex bone formed by the parts of the sacral vertebrae: body, vertebral arches (two), and costal elements (two) called ala (L., wing). These parts fuse by the 8th year, and then after the 20th year, the five sacral vertebrae fuse to form the sacral bone (Lee, 1989). The sacrum has six articulating surfaces: superiorly with the body and the two articular processes of the fifth lumbar vertebra to form the lumbosacral junction, bilaterally with the two ilia at the sacroiliac joints, and inferiorly with the coccyx. The articular surfaces with the ilium are found on the lateral surfaces of the sacrum. These surfaces are L-shaped and are usually irregular and roughened in skeletal bones because of sclerosis and degeneration of the joint with aging.

The **head of the femur** is connected to the shaft by the neck. This lateral projection increases the lever arm distance of the femur from the axis of motion and therefore increases the torque produced by the muscles with distal attachments in the area of the greater trochanter (gluteus medius, minimus, and maximus; piriformis, obturator internus and externus, quadratus femoris, and the gemelli). The shaft of the femur angles medially in adduction to place the knee under the weight-bearing line of the head of the femur (see Fig. 8–9). The neck-shaft angle averages 125 degrees (Kapandji, 1987). If the neck-shaft angle is smaller (ie, approaches 90 degrees), the deviation is called **coxa vara**, and there is a decrease in leg length. An increase in the neck-shaft angle is called **coxa valga** and results in an increase of limb length. Both of these structural changes also lead to decreased muscle strength because of changes in torque from alterations in muscle lever arms and length-tension relationships.

A second angle occurring in the femur is called the angle of anteversion (Fig. 8–2). When the femur is viewed from above with the axis of the femoral condyles in the frontal plane, the neck of the femur is seen to have an anterior angle with the frontal plane of 13 to 15 degrees (Yoshioka, Siu, and Cooke, 1987). An increase in this angle is called **anteversion** and is one factor that is considered to cause intoeing, or pigeon toes. A decrease in the angle is called **retroversion**, which may lead to out-toeing (external rotation) during standing and walking. The angle of anteversion normally decreases with growth and development of the child, causing orthopedists to be conservative in treatment of children who walk with intoeing.

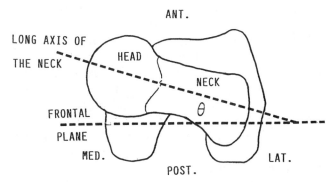

Figure 8–2 Superior view of the right femur showing the angle of anteversion (θ). This angle is visualized by aligning the femoral condyles in the frontal plane and projecting a line through the long axis of the neck of the femur. The average normal angle is 15 degrees.

JOINTS

Sacroiliac Joint

The sacroiliac joint (SIJ) was thought by ancient practitioners to be immobile except for slight motions occurring during pregnancy. In the 20th century, it has been established that small motions in these joints occur in both men and women (Sashin, 1930; Mennell, 1947; Weisl, 1955; Colachis et al, 1963; Ro, 1990). Because SIJ motions are small (1 to 3 mm) and difficult to measure, there is a tendency to consider the motions insignificant and unimportant. Many practitioners, however, consider injuries to the ligaments, hypermobility or hypomobility, and inflammatory conditions of the SIJ to be primary sources of low back pain (Mennell, 1947; Grieve, 1986; DonTigny, 1990), with the most frequent problems occurring following childbirth (Ro, 1990).

Type of Joint

Most authors classify the SIJ as a freely movable diarthrodial joint. The sacral surface is covered in hyalin cartilage, and the iliac surface is covered in fibrocartilage. Synovial fluid is found in the joint cavity and the joint is covered with a capsule. With aging, the incidence of osteophytes and ankylosis of the SIJs is high, especially in men. Sashin (1930) found gliding and anterior-posterior motion in the cadavers of men up to 30 years of age at their deaths, slight motion in the cadavers of men up to 40 years, and ankylosis in most cases after that. Slight motion was also found in the cadavers of women up to 50 and 60 years of age, and none showed advanced ankylosis at any age.

Motions

Movements of the SIJ are small. In 32 fresh cadavers of persons who were under 29 years of age at their deaths, Sashin (1930) found up-and-down gliding and slight anterior-posterior movement of sacrum on the ilia or the ilia on the fixed sacrum. The average motion of the SIJs was 4 degrees, with a range from 2 to 8 degrees. Weisl (1955) measured the movement of the sacral promontory radiographically in living people. He found that the greatest movement in the sacral promontory was 5.6 mm (±1.4) in the ventral direction when the subjects moved from the supine to the standing position. Steel pins were imbedded in the posterior superior iliac spines of medical students by Colachis and coworkers (1963). The greatest change between the right and left sides was 4 mm near the skin with full forward flexion in the standing position. Trigonometrically, the measurements indicate approximately 2 to 3.5 degrees of movement per SI joint.

Kapandji (1987) described the motions of nutation (L. *nutare*, to nod) and counternutation. In nutation, the promontory of the sacrum moves inferiorly and anteriorly while the distal aspect of the sacrum and the coccyx move posteriorly. In addition, the iliac crests are approximated and the ischial tuberosities move apart. Nutation causes the pelvic outlet to become larger. Counternutation is the opposite movement with the sacral promontory moving upward and posteriorly. The coccyx moves anteriorly, the iliac crests move apart, and the ischial tuberosities are approximated. These motions enlarge the pelvic inlet. Secretion of the hormone relaxin during pregnancy causes ligamentous laxity and permits increase in the magnitude of the motions of the SIJs and the symphysis pubis. Thus, the pelvic inlet can become larger to accommodate the fetus, and the pelvic outlet can become larger at birth. This excessive ligamentous laxity, however, can produce severe pain and sometimes spontaneous dislocation of the SIJs and the symphysis pubis. Following lactation, the secretion of relaxin ceases and the ligaments tighten up again. It is not uncommon to find that the reapproximation has occurred with an asymmetric alignment of the SIJs and the symphysis pubis with resulting chronic low back and hip pain.

In standing and walking, the superincumbent weight of the head, arms, and trunk is distributed from the fifth lumbar vertebra to the sacrum and through the pelvis to the pubic symphysis and the heads of the femurs, and then down to the floor (the floor reaction force would be of the same magnitude but in the opposite direction). In the sitting position, the weight is distributed to the pubic symphysis and the ischial tuberosities and then to the seat of the chair. These forces cause the sacrum to be driven distally and anteriorly between the ilia (or the ilia to be driven proximally and posteriorly on the sacrum). An extensive, strong ligamentous system limits these motions.

Ligaments

Posteriorly, interosseus ligaments fill the space between the lateral sacral crest and the inner side of the iliac tuberosity (Fig. 8–3B). These ligaments have multidirectional fibers and cover about one half of the length of the joint. Several layers of short and long posterior sacroiliac ligaments cover the interosseus ligaments and

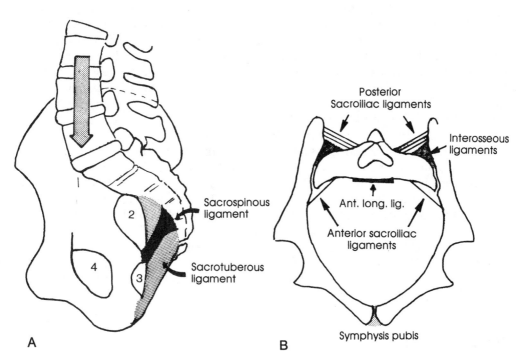

Figure 8–3 Ligaments stabilizing the sacroiliac joint. (*A*) Sagittal view of the pelvic bones showing the direction of the force of the head, arms, and trunk through the lumbar vertebrae to the sacrum. The strong sacrospinous and sacrotuberous ligaments with their long lever arms prevent anterior and distal motion of the base and promontory of the sacrum. 1 = sacral promontory, 2 = greater sciatic foramen, 3 = lesser sciatic foramen, and 4 = obturator foramen. (*B*) Transverse view of the sacrum and the ilia illustrates the ligaments surrounding the sacrum. These ligaments serve as a sling to limit the distal and anterior motion of the sacrum between the ilia. The anterior and posterior sacroiliac ligaments cover the entire length of the sacrum.

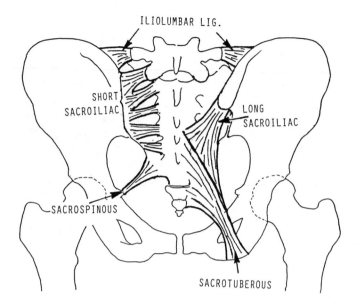

ILIOLUMBAR LIG.

SHORT SACROILIAC

LONG SACROILIAC

SACROSPINOUS

SACROTUBEROUS

Figure 8–4 Posterior view of the arrangement of the pelvic ligaments. The deeper short sacroiliac and sacrospinous ligaments are outlined on the *left* and the more superficial long sacroiliac and sacrotuberous ligaments are on the *right*.

the posterior aspect of the sacrum (Fig. 8–4). These attach on the tuberosity of the ilia (to the posterior gluteal line) and are directed medially and distally to attach on the sacrum. On the ventral side are the anterior sacroiliac ligaments, which are thin and not as extensive as the posterior ligaments. The anterior and posterior sacroiliac ligaments suspend the sacrum from the ilia and, as weight bearing drives the sacrum distally on the ilia, these ligaments act as shock absorbers. This suspensory mechanism has caused some authors to describe the SIJs as non–weight-bearing joints (DonTigny, 1985). In addition, the length of these ligaments places limits on the motion of counternutation. The strong anterior longitudinal ligament, which covers the lumbar vertebrae and attaches to the sacrum and the iliolumbar ligaments, is discussed with the vertebrae.

The sacrotuberous and the sacrospinous ligaments are broad, long ligaments connecting the lower aspect of the sacrum to the spine and the tuberosity of the ischium (see Figs. 8–3 and 8–4). These ligaments have excellent leverage to hold the distal aspect of the sacrum in place against the anterior weight-bearing forces that tend to cause the sacral promontory to tilt anteriorly and distally. The length of these ligaments controls the amount of nutation that is possible.

The combined bony architecture and the strong and extensive ligamentous system of the SIJ produces a self-locking mechanism. As forces increase to cause downward movement of the sacrum on the ilia, the posterior ligaments tighten and pull the ilia closer together like a clamp.

Symphysis Pubis

Articulating surfaces of the pubic bones are covered by hyaline cartilage and separated by fibrocartilaginous disks. The joint is protected by strong ligaments on all sides, and the fibrocartilage is reinforced by the attachments of the rectus abdominus, pyramidalis, and internal abdominal oblique muscles. The symphysis pubis completes the closure of the ring of the pelvic articulations of the sacrum and the innominate bones. Thus, even small motions occurring at the SIJs must be accompanied by motion at the symphysis pubis. Generally, there is little motion at this joint. Excessive forces, however, may occur to produce injury or dislocation of the SIJ and the symphysis pubis. These forces can occur with landing on the feet from a jump, hitting the knees on the dashboard in an auto accident, walking with a leg-length discrepancy, or having a forceful motion of hip flexion suddenly obstructed as with a blocked football kick.

Coccygeal Joints

The sacrococcygeal and the intercoccygeal joints are classified as symphyses. Slight anterior-posterior motion occurs and is limited by ventral, dorsal, and lateral ligaments. Motion increases during pregnancy and ossification of the joints occurs with aging.

Pelvic Balance

The rigid sacral portion of the vertebral column, firmly connected with the ilia, is part of the pelvis. The pelvis, interposed between the lower extremities and the flexible portions of the vertebral column, possesses movements of its own. Because of the firmness of the sacroiliac and lumbosacral junctions, however, every pelvic movement is accompanied by a realignment of the spine, most markedly in the lumbar region.

Pelvic Inclination

In erect standing, when the hip is flexed by a pelvic movement while the upper part of the body remains erect, the **inclination** of the pelvis is said to be **increased**—a **forward tilt** of the pelvis has occurred. When this movement takes place, the anterior superior spines of the ilia come to lie anterior to the foremost part of the symphysis pubis, whereas these spines are normally in vertical alignment with, or lie slightly posterior to, the symphysis (Fig. 8–5A). The opposite

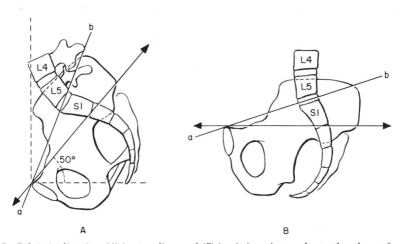

A   B

Figure 8–5   Pelvic inclination (*A*) in standing and (*B*) in sitting. Arrow shows the plane of pelvic inclination. Line a-b represents "plane of the inlet." (Redrawn from Fick, 1911, pp 438 and 439.)

movement of the pelvis (in direction of extension) is referred to as a **backward tilt** of the pelvis, and the resulting position is referred to as a **decreased pelvic inclination**.

A determination of the pelvic inclination in degrees can be made by laying an oblique plane through the posterior superior spines of the ilia and the foremost portion of the symphysis pubis. The angle of this plane with the horizontal plane is said to be the **angle of pelvic inclination** (see Fig. 8–5A). This method of measuring the pelvic inclination was advocated by Fick (1911), who considered an angle of 50 to 60 degrees to be normal for adult men and a somewhat larger angle to be normal for women.

Fick's method of measuring the angle of pelvic inclination has been used by many investigators but has not been adopted universally. Sometimes, the "plane of the inlet" (inlet to the lesser pelvis) is used as a reference plane. This plane, indicated by the line a-b in the illustration, passes through the lumbosacral junction and through the foremost portion of the symphysis pubis. If this plane is used, the angle of pelvic inclination is greater than when determined by Fick's method.

The range of backward tilt of the pelvis in the erect standing position is determined by the tension of the capsule of the hip joints and the reinforcing ligaments, noticeably, the iliofemoral or Y ligament (see Fig. 8–7B). If further backward tilt is attempted, this can be accomplished only by flexing the knees simultaneously with the pelvic movement, which also causes hip flexion and slackening of the ligaments.

In the sitting position, these ligaments no longer restrict pelvic movement, and the pelvis tilts backward so that the plane through the posterior superior spine of the ilia and the symphysis pubis becomes horizontal (Fig. 8–5B). A backward tilt of the pelvis is accompanied by a decrease in, or obliteration of, the physiologic lumbar curve. Such flattening of the lumbar spine is particularly marked in sitting. A forward inclination of the pelvis is accompanied by an increase in the physiologic lumbar curve.

Clinical Evaluation of Pelvic Inclination

It is difficult to measure the angle of pelvic inclination in the living subject. Clinically, therefore, a more practical method to determine normal or abnormal inclination of the pelvis is needed. Because the anterior superior spines of the ilia and the front part of the symphysis pubis are superficial and easily located, the alignment of these points may be observed. When the subject is viewed from the side, the pelvic inclination may be considered normal if these two points are approximately in vertical alignment, as seen in Figure 8–5A. Walker and associates (1987) measured the angle of pelvic tilt by placing a caliper on the anterior superior iliac spine and the posterior superior iliac spine. An inclinometer was attached to the caliper to measure the angle formed with the horizontal plane.

Hip Joint

Type of Joint

The hip joint is the best example of a ball-and-socket joint in the human body. The joint surfaces of the head of the femur and the acetabulum correspond better to each other and have firmer connections than the joint surfaces of the glenohumeral joint. This promotes stability but limits range of motion. The hip joint has three degrees of freedom of motion: flexion-extension, abduction-adduction, and internal-external rotation. In most activities, combinations of these three types of movements occur, and hip motions are accompanied by movements of the lumbar spine for total mobility.

Despite being called a ball-and-socket joint, the articulating surface of the acetabulum covers only the anterior, superior, and posterior sides. The area medial to the horseshoe-shaped articular cartilage is called the **acetabular fossa** and contains the ligamentum teres, a mobile fat pad and synovial membrane (Fig. 8–6). While the ligamentum teres is strong, its primary function is to carry the vascular supply to the head of the femur. Tension on this structure does not occur until extreme positions of adduction, flexion, and external rotation or adduction, extension, and internal rotation are achieved (Kapandji, 1987). The acetabular fossa permits the necessary movement of the ligamentum teres and importantly serves as a reservoir for synovial fluid when the hip is heavily loaded (Palastanga, Field, and Soames, 1989). When the forces on the joint decrease, synovial fluid again returns to the joint space to provide lubrication and nutrition to the articular cartilages.

The femoral head is two thirds of a sphere, and the acetabulum is a hemisphere with three notches bridged by ligaments. A triangular fibrocartilaginous labrum encircles the rim of the acetabulum and substantially encloses the head of the femur (see Fig. 8–6). In the quadrupled position in which the hips are flexed, slightly abducted, and externally rotated, the surfaces of the femoral head are completely covered by the acetabulum.

The joint capsule is a strong structure attaching to the outer rim of the acetabulum, enclosing the neck of the femur like a tube, and with distal attachments along the trochanteric line anteriorly and just above the trochanteric crest posteriorly (see Fig. 8–6).

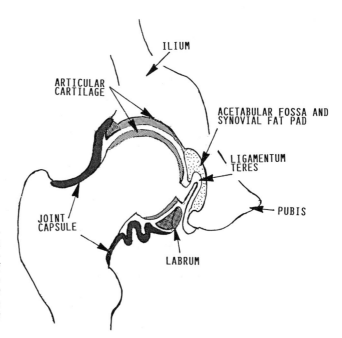

Figure 8–6 Schematic longitudinal section of the acetabulum and the head of the femur, illustrating the relationships of the ligamentum teres, which attaches to the head of the femur (fovea), the acetabular fossa, the acetabular labrum, the articular cartilage, and the joint capsule.

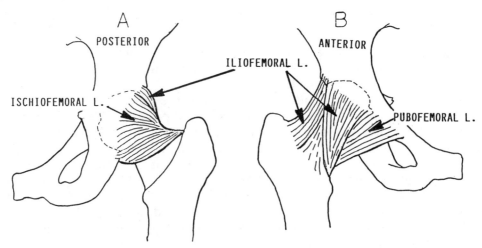

Figure 8–7 Ligaments of the right hip joint. (*A*) Posterior view illustrates the ischiofemoral ligament. (*B*) Anterior view demonstrates the iliofemoral or Y ligament and the pubofemoral ligament.

Ligaments

Strong ligaments reinforce the capsule on all sides (Fig. 8–7). The iliofemoral ligament covers the hip joint anteriorly and superiorly. This ligament is also called the **Y ligament** because it resembles an inverted letter Y. The pubofemoral ligament is anterior and inferior to the hip joint and the ischiofemoral ligament is posterior and inferior. All of these ligaments become slack when the hip is flexed and become taut when the hip is extended. Thus in the standing position, the iliofemoral ligament, particularly the inferior band, prevents posterior motion of the pelvis on the femur (hyperextension of the hip) (Fig. 8–8). The anterior ligaments, especially the pubofemoral ligament, limit the motion of external rotation, and the ischiofemoral ligament limits internal rotation. Abduction of the hip is limited by tension on the pubofemoral and ischiofemoral ligaments. Adduction is limited by tension of the superior or iliotrochanteric portion of the Y ligament.

Axes of Motion and Movements

At the hip joint, movement may take place about any number of axes, all passing through the center of the femoral head; but for descriptive purposes, three axes perpendicular to each other are usually chosen.

In standing, the axis for flexion and extension is transverse (horizontal, in a side-to-side direction). A line connecting the centers of the two femoral heads is called the **common hip axis**. Movement about the common hip axis takes place when, for example, the pelvis rocks forward and backward in standing or when, in a back-lying position, both knees are pulled up toward the chest. Unilateral hip flexion with the knee flexed can be carried out until the thigh contacts the anterior surface of the trunk. When the knee is extended, the muscle length of the hamstrings limits hip flexion to 70 to 90 degrees. Hyperextension of the hip is limited to 0 to 10 degrees by the iliofemoral ligament. As further motion is attempted, the lumbar vertebrae extend (lordosis) and may give a misleading impression of the amount of true hip extension present.

The axis for abduction and adduction (in standing) is horizontal, in a front-to-back direction. The limb may move in relation to the pelvis, as in lifting the

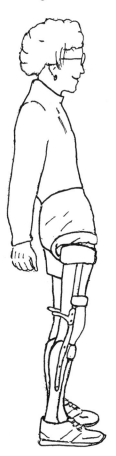

Figure 8–8   This lady has paralysis of muscles from the waist down. She is wearing bilateral knee-ankle-foot orthoses (KAFOs), which stabilize the knees and ankles. Standing balance is achieved by placing the center of gravity of the head, arms, and trunk (HAT) posterior to the hip joint axis and hanging on the iliofemoral ligaments.

limb laterally, or the pelvis may move in relation to the limb, as in inclining the trunk to the side of the stance leg (see Fig. 1–3). In each instance, whether the limb or the pelvis moves, the correct term to use is abduction or adduction of the hip. Hip abduction is approximately 45 degrees and is usually accompanied by elevation of the pelvis (hip hiking). Hip adduction is frequently given as contact of the two thighs or 0 degrees. The legs may be crossed, however, to adducted positions of 30 to 40 degrees. While this is not pure planar motion (since one hip must be in flexion and the other in extension), it is an important motion in running and turning and crossing the thighs.

The axis for internal and external rotation (in standing) is vertical, and this axis is identical to the mechanical axis of the femur (Fig. 8–9). In internal rotation, the greater trochanter moves forward in relation to the front part of the pelvis or, conversely, the front part of the pelvis moves toward the greater trochanter. External rotation is a movement in the opposite direction. When the knee is flexed to 90 degrees, hip rotation can be observed by the motion of the tibia from the neutral position.

ANATOMIC AND MECHANICAL AXES OF FEMUR   The anatomic axis of the femur is represented by a line through the femoral shaft (see Fig. 8–9). However, the mechanical axis is represented by a line connecting the centers of the hip and knee joints. In the erect position, the mechanical axis is usually vertical. The neck of the femur forms an angle of approximately 125 degrees with the anatomic axis of the femur.

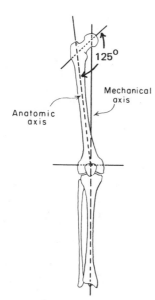

Figure 8–9 The anatomic and mechanical axes of the femur.

NORMAL RANGES OF MOTION End-feels of hip ranges of motion in normal subjects usually are firm because of ligamentous limitations. The exception is hip flexion with simultaneous knee flexion, which may be limited by abdominal adipose tissue. In severe obesity, this limitation can limit functions such as tying shoes or driving a car, as well as the ability to reach and carry objects. Hip flexion with simultaneous knee extension is limited by the length of the hamstring muscles.

Normal range of hip joint motions vary considerably with age and may deviate markedly from the average values found in Table 1–1. For example, the normal hip posture of infants is flexion, and hip extension is markedly limited. In newborns, Haas, Epps, and Adams (1973) measured hip extension of −28 degrees (SD = 8.2). Over the next 5 to 6 years, the limitation of hip extension decreases. Coon and coworkers (1975) found −19 degrees at 6 weeks and −7 degrees at 6 months. Inability to extend the hip and assume the zero starting position of hip flexion persists in subjects under 6 years of age (Boone and Azen, 1979).

Flexibility of other hip joint motions decreases gradually throughout childhood, adolescence, and maturity (Table 8–1). Hip ranges of motion in active, healthy people 60 years and older show decreases from the averages as found in Table 1–1 (Walker et al, 1984). James and Parker (1989) found significant decreases in all hip motions from ages 70 to 92, with the largest loss of 33 percent occurring in abduction (see Table 8–1).

In normal subjects, no significant difference in motion between the right and left hips has been found (Haas, Epps, and Adams, 1973; Boone and Azen, 1979; Svenningsen et al, 1989). This finding permits measurement of the uninvolved side as a guide for normal motion of the involved side. Because of measurement error, Ellison, Rose, and Sahrmann (1990) state that there should be more than a 10-degree difference between rotation measurements of the two sides in an individual before a difference can be considered clinically significant.

ACCESSORY MOTIONS The accessory motions of the hip are distal traction and lateral, dorsal, and ventral glides. Normally, a relatively negative atmospheric pressure prevents distraction and dislocation of the joint. A force of 45 lb was required in adult

Table 8–1 Normal Range of Hip Rotation and Abduction with Growth and Aging*

Author	Age	No.	Internal Rotation X̄	(SD)	External Rotation X̄	(SD)	Abduction X̄	(SD)
Coon et al (1975)	6 wk	40	24°		48°		—	—
				(±5)		(±11)		
	6 mo	40	21°		46°		—	—
				(±4)		(±5)		
Svenningsen et al (1989; males)	4 yr	52	51°		48°		53°	
				(±15)		(±14)		(±8)
	11 yr	65	46°		42°		44°	
				(±14)		(±15)		(±11)
	15 yr	57	41°		43°		42°	
				(±15)		(±14)		(±8)
	23 yr (±3)	102	38°		43°		40°	
				(±15)		(±13)		(±7)
Ellison et al (1990)	26 yr (±5)	100	38°		35°		—	—
				(±11)		(±8)		
Boone and Azen (1979; males)	35 yr (±3)	56	44°		44°		41°	
				(±4)		(±5)		(±6)
James and Parker (1989; males)	73 yr (±2)	10	34°		33°		34°	
				(±2)†		(±2)†		(±2)†
	87 yr (±2)	10	22°		26°		21°	
				(±2)†		(±2)†		(±2)†

*Normal ranges of motion of hip rotation and abduction in healthy, active persons show variations that may occur with growth and aging. These motions were selected because there is some similarity in positions and measurements. Hip extension, flexion, and adduction were not tabulated because there are more differences in measurement procedures. In the studies presented in this table, hip abduction was measured in the supine position, and rotation was measured in the prone position with the knees flexed, except for James and Parker (1989), who measured rotation in the sitting position. Ellison, Rose, and Sahrmann (1990) established that there was no significant difference between measurements in the two positions in adults. Svenningsen and associates (1989) and James and Parker (1989) also presented data on females. In the majority of the motions, they found that females had a greater range of motion than males in all age groups.
†Standard error of the mean.

cadavers to laterally distract the joint 3 mm, but when the joint capsule was incised to release the vacuum, the femur could be distracted about 8 mm without significant traction force (Wingstrand, Wingstrand, and Krantz, 1990). In adults, Arvidsson (1990) found that traction forces above 90 lb were required to produce a significant joint separation in the loose-packed position. When the hip is in the closed-packed positions of hyperextension, internal rotation, and abduction, however, the capsule and ligaments are taut and produce additional resistance to accessory motions and dislocations. Because of the large forces needed, the ability to perform normal accessory motions at the hip usually requires additional mechanical stabilization and straps to support body parts (Kaltenborn, 1980).

MUSCLES

Posterior Muscles

The posterior muscles are the **gluteus maximus**; the **biceps femoris**, the **semitendinosus**, and the **semimembranosus** (collectively called the **hamstrings**); and the posterior portion of the adductor magnus. In addition, there is a deeply located group consisting of six small muscles, all **external rotators** of the hip.

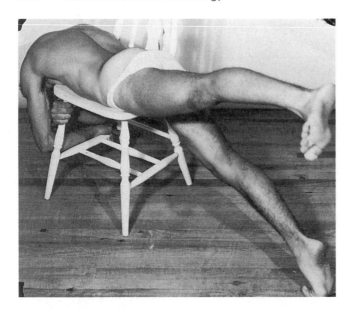

Figure 8–10 The gluteus maximus is strongly activated when the hip is extended and externally rotated.

Gluteus Maximus

The **gluteus maximus** (Gr. *gloutos*, buttock) is the large, superficial muscle that is responsible for the roundness of the buttock region. **Proximal attachments:** Posterior portion of the crest of the ilium, lumbodorsal fascia, parts of the sacrum and coccyx, and sacrotuberous ligament. The fibers take a downward and lateral course and have their **distal attachments** (1) into the iliotibial tract and (2) into the gluteal tuberosity of the shaft of the femur, on the posterior aspect of the femur. **Innervation:** Inferior gluteal nerve (L_5, S_1-S_2). **Anatomic actions:** Extension and external rotation of the hip.

INSPECTION AND PALPATION The gluteus maximus may be observed when the subject is prone or standing erect. Like the quadriceps, it can be tightened by simply "setting" it without any joint motion being carried out. For stronger activation of the muscle, the hip is extended and externally rotated (Fig. 8–10), in which case the muscle acts in two functions simultaneously. If palpated when the limb is in this position, the muscle feels very firm. Strong contraction of the gluteus maximus also may be observed in climbing stairs and in running and jumping.

Hamstrings

The **hamstrings** have their **proximal attachments** on the ischial tuberosity and their **distal attachments** on the proximal shaft of the tibia (see Chapter 9 for more details). They should now be observed and palpated in their function as hip extensors.

PALPATION IN PRONE POSITION If the hip is extended and simultaneously internally rotated (Fig. 8–11), the hamstrings and part of the adductor magnus, all with attachments on the tuberosity of the ischium, may be felt contracting while the gluteus maximus, at least in part, ceases contracting. Note that this inner extensor group of muscles cannot extend the hip as high as when the gluteus maximus participates in the movement. The shift from one muscle group to the other should be

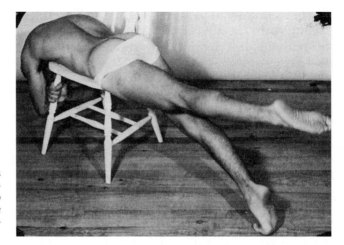

Figure 8–11 When the hip is extended and internally rotated, the inner extensor group of muscles contracts while the gluteus maximus markedly decreases its contraction.

observed by maintaining the hip extended while alternating internal rotation with external rotation.

PALPATION IN STANDING ERECT   In standing, the hamstrings may be palpated close to their proximal attachments on the ischial tuberosity. First, the subject inclines the trunk somewhat backward so that the center-of-gravity line of the upper part of the body falls well behind the axis of the hip joint. This secures relaxation of the hip extensors, and the ischial tuberosities may then be palpated more easily. The fingertips are placed below the tuberosities, but close to them, and as deeply as the tissue will allow. The subject now reverses the trunk movement, that is, inclines the trunk slightly forward. The instant the center-of-gravity line passes anterior to the common hip axis, a contraction of the hamstrings, acting as hip extensors, is felt. By swaying the trunk slightly forward and backward, alternating contraction and relaxation of these muscles are brought about.

When the same trunk movements are repeated while the buttocks are being palpated, very little, if any, contraction of the gluteus maximus can be detected. The hamstrings, rather than the gluteus maximus, appear to be used in small-range anteroposterior balance of the pelvis. On the other hand, if a large range of hip flexion is performed by inclining the trunk forward and then quickly returning the trunk to the erect position, a strong contraction of the gluteus maximus may be felt. These clinical observations have been substantiated by EMG (Joseph, 1960).

External Rotators

The **six small external rotators** are located in the posterior gluteal region and covered by the gluteus maximus. They have **proximal attachments** both inside and outside the pelvis, have a more or less horizontal direction, and have **distal attachments** in the region of the greater trochanter in such a fashion that they have an external rotary action at the hip.

The uppermost of the six external rotators is the **piriformis;** the lowermost is the **quadratus femoris.** These two muscles can be palpated with fair accuracy. Palpation of the piriformis is described with that of the lateral group with which this muscle is closely associated. The quadratus femoris is palpated in the area between the tuberosity of the ischium and the greater trochanter, and it may be felt contracting when the hip is externally rotated. The other four, the **gemellus superior**, the **gemellus inferior**, the **obturator internus**, and the **obturator externus**, are located between the piriformis and the quadratus femoris. They can be palpated as a group but not very well individually.

Anterior Muscles

This group of muscles includes the **rectus femoris**, the **sartorius**, the **tensor fasciae latae**, the **iliopsoas**, and the **pectineus**. The tensor has an anterolateral location, and the pectineus has an anteromedial location.

Rectus Femoris and Sartorius

The **proximal attachment** of the **rectus femoris** on the anterior inferior spine of the ilium and above the acetabulum and its **distal attachment** on the patella is described in Chapter 9. Palpation of its proximal attachment as the muscle acts in flexion of the hip is described under the tensor fasciae latae.

The **sartorius** (L. *sartor*, a tailor) is a superficial, band-like muscle extending obliquely down the thigh from the anterior to the medial side of the thigh. **Proximal attachment**: Anterior superior spine of the ilium. **Distal attachment**: Medial surface of the tibia close to the crest of the tibia (anterior to the distal attachments of the gracilis and semitendinosus tendons). **Innervation**: Femoral nerve (L_2-L_3). **Anatomic actions**: Flexion, external rotation, and abduction of the hip as well as flexion and medial rotation of the knee.

INSPECTION AND PALPATION   When the hip is flexed and externally rotated, the sartorius may be observed and palpated from its proximal attachment down almost to its distal attachment (Fig. 8–12). In many subjects, the lower portion of the muscle cannot be observed well but may be followed by palpation if the subject alternately contracts and relaxes the muscle. This is best accomplished if the examiner carries the weight of the limb with the hip flexed and externally rotated and the knee flexed (muscle relaxed), and then asks the subject to hold the limb in position actively (muscle contracts).

The perpendicular distance from the axis for flexion and extension of the hip to the line of action of the sartorius is considerable. Therefore, even though the muscle's cross-section is relatively small, it can exert a comparatively large torque. Note that, as the muscle contracts, it rises from the underlying structures, and this mechanically enhances its action. Because of its great length, the sartorius muscle can shorten a long distance.

The sartorius is a two-joint muscle, passing on the flexor side of the knee, where it is in close relation to the tendons of the gracilis and the semitendinosus muscles.

Tensor Fasciae Latae

The **tensor fasciae latae**, like the sartorius, has effects on both the hip and the knee. **Proximal attachment**: Crest of the ilium and adjacent structures, lateral to the proximal attachment of the sartorius. **Distal attachment**: Iliotibial tract, about one third of the way down the thigh. **Innervation**: Branch of the superior

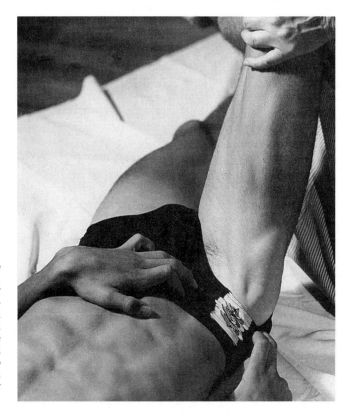

Figure 8–12 Near the hip (flexed and externally rotated), the sartorius and the tensor muscles form a V, with the sartorius taking a medial direction and the tensor taking a lateral direction. The tendon of the rectus femoris may be palpated in the V between the other two muscles. The muscular portion of the rectus is seen farther down the thigh.

gluteal nerve (L_4-S_5, S_1). **Anatomic actions**: Flexion, abduction, and internal rotation of the hip.

INSPECTION AND PALPATION   The tensor fasciae latae is palpated near the hip, but more laterally than the upper portion of the sartorius. A strong contraction is brought out by resisting flexion of the internally rotated hip (Fig. 8–13). The relation of the tensor to the sartorius and the rectus femoris is seen in Figure 8–12. The tensor forms the lateral border of the V-shaped area where the tendon of the rectus femoris is palpated. The relation of the tensor to the anterior portion of the gluteus medius should be noted—the two muscles lie side by side in the anterolateral hip region. In closed-chain motion with the foot on the floor, both the gluteus maximus and the tensor fasciae latae can extend and stabilize the knee.

Iliopsoas

The **iliopsoas** consists of two parts, the **iliacus** and the **psoas major**, which have separate proximal attachments but a common distal attachment. That portion of the iliopsoas that lies below the hip joint is located medial to, and is partially covered by, the upper portion of the sartorius.

The **iliacus** has **proximal attachments** on the iliac fossa and the inner sides of the anterior spines of the ilium. The muscle covers the anterior side of the hip joint and the femoral neck. It winds around the neck in a medial and posterior direction and has its **distal attachment** on the lesser trochanter of the femur. **Innervation**: Branches of the femoral nerve (L_1-L_4).

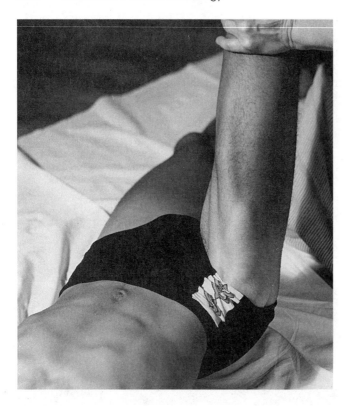

Figure 8–13 The tensor fasciae latae are seen contracting as resistance is given to flexion of the internally rotated hip. The rectus femoris and the sartorius are also seen.

The **psoas major** (Gr. *psoa*, the loins) is located in the posterior wall of the abdominal cavity, close to the lumbar vertebrae and the ilium. **Proximal attachments**: Vertebral bodies, intervertebral disks, and transverse processes of T_{12}-L_5. The muscle fibers form a round, rather long belly that lies medial to the iliacus. **Distal attachment**: Lesser trochanter of the femur. **Innervation**: By branches directly from the lumbar plexus (L_1-L_4). **Anatomic actions of the iliopsoas**: Flexion and external rotation of the hip. When the legs are fixed in the supine position, the combined action of muscles on both sides elevates the trunk and flexes the pelvis on the femur as in a sit-up.

PALPATION OF THE ILIACUS AND PSOAS MAJOR   The iliacus is difficult to palpate because it lies behind the abdominal viscera and is rather flat. It follows, and partly fills out, the iliac fossa.

The psoas major, in spite of its deep location, may be palpated as follows: In the sitting position, the subject inclines the trunk slightly forward to secure relaxation of the abdominal muscles. The palpating fingers are placed at the waist, between the lower ribs and the crest of the ilium, and with gentle pressure, are made to sink in as deeply as possible toward the posterior wall of the abdominal cavity, near the vertebral column. In some subjects, this meets with no difficulty. The subject now flexes the hip, raising the foot just off the floor (Fig. 8–14), and the round, firm belly of the psoas major may be felt as the muscle contracts.

It is suggested that the student first palpate the psoas major on himself or herself before attempting to do so on another person. Palpation is best done if the bowels are fairly empty, and it should not be attempted if it causes discomfort.

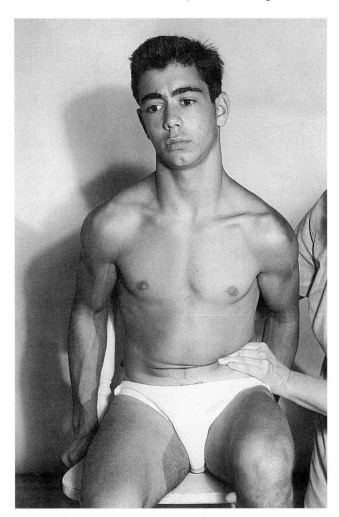

Figure 8–14 Palpation of the psoas major. If the subject's abdominal muscles are relaxed, the examiner may place the palpating fingers deep enough to feel the contraction of the psoas major when the subject lifts the foot off the floor, flexing the hip beyond 90 degrees.

Pectineus

The **pectineus** is a rather flat muscle bordering laterally to the iliopsoas and medially to the adductor longus. **Proximal attachments**: Superior ramus of the pubic bone and neighboring structures. **Distal attachment**: Along a line (pectineal line) on the upper posteromedial aspect of the femur, below the lesser trochanter. The area of the distal attachment of this muscle is approximately as wide as its proximal attachment, giving the muscle a quadrangular shape. **Innervation**: Femoral nerve (L_2-L_4). **Anatomic actions**: Adduction and flexion of the hip.

The pectineus belongs essentially to the adductor group of muscles, its fibers running approximately parallel to those of the adductor longus. Palpation of the pectineus as a separate muscle is difficult, but it may be felt contracting together with other muscles. It is suggested that the student palpate this muscle on himself or herself, as follows: In the sitting position, the palpating fingers are placed in the crotch, where some of the adductor tendons can be grasped from front to back. The hip is now flexed further with adduction and external rotation, and the motion is continued until the legs are crossed. The tendon of the adductor longus is prominent and easily recognized; the pectineus lies just lateral to the adductor longus.

Lateral Muscles

The muscles of this group—the **gluteus medius**, the **gluteus minimus**, the **tensor fasciae latae**, and the **piriformis**—are located laterally, on the abductor side of the hip. The tensor, described with the flexors, lies anterolaterally and the piriformis, posterolaterally.

Gluteus Medius

The **gluteus medius** is the largest of the lateral hip muscles. It is covered, in part, by the gluteus maximus and by the tensor, but its upper middle portion is superficial, covered only by thick fascia. **Proximal attachment**: In a fan-shaped fashion from the crest of the ilium and from a large area on the outer surface of the ilium, as far down as the anterior gluteal line, a line that separates its origin from that of the gluteus minimus. From this wide proximal attachment, the fibers converge to have their **distal attachment** on the greater trochanter, near its tip. This muscle, like the deltoid in the upper limb, has anterior, middle, and posterior portions, but these portions are not clearly separated from each other. The posterior portion is comparatively small and supplemented by the piriformis muscle. **Innervation**: Superior gluteal nerve (L_4-L_5, S_1). **Anatomic actions**: Abduction of the hip. The anterior portion flexes and medially rotates the hip, while the posterior portion extends and laterally rotates the hip.

INSPECTION AND PALPATION   The middle portion of the gluteus medius is palpated laterally below the crest of the ilium and just above the greater trochanter. Active abduction either in the side-lying or standing position (Fig. 8–15) produces a muscle contraction.

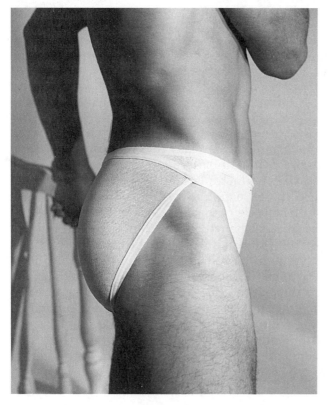

Figure 8–15 The gluteus medius and the tensor fasciae latae are seen contracting as the subject abducts the right hip, raising the right foot off the floor.

The anterior portion is palpated when the hip is internally rotated either in the supine position or in standing. This portion lies close to the tensor fasciae latae and acts together with the tensor in internal rotation. If the posterior margin of the tensor is first identified by the tests previously described, the gluteus medius may be palpated posterior to the tensor. The two muscles also may be identified by making them alternately contract and relax and by following the palpated muscle distally. If the muscle takes a direction toward the greater trochanter, it is the anterior portion of the gluteus medius; if the muscle takes a more anterior course, it is the tensor fasciae latae.

In palpating the anterior portion of the gluteus medius, it should be remembered that the gluteus minimus, which is covered by the medius, also participates in internal rotation and that the muscle tissue that is palpated represents the combined contraction of the two muscles.

The posterior portion of the gluteus medius is palpated in back of the middle portion when the hip is abducted. A part of the posterior portion is seen in Figure 8–15. This portion contracts strongly if the hip is abducted and externally rotated at the same time. However, with external rotation, other muscles in this region become active, so that the gluteus medius cannot be palpated in an isolated fashion.

The entire gluteus medius also may be felt as it contracts in supporting body weight on one leg, palpation being carried out on the side of the stance leg. In this case, the gluteus medius furnishes lateral stabilization of the pelvis to prevent dropping of the pelvis on the opposite side. This is the most important function of the gluteus medius.

Piriformis

The **piriformis**, the pear-shaped muscle (L. *pirum*, pear) belongs to the second layer of muscles in this region, as does the gluteus medius, both of which are covered here by the gluteus maximus. **Proximal attachments**: Ventral surface of the sacrum, sciatic notch, and sacrotuberous ligament. **Distal attachment**: The fibers take a downward lateral course, following the posterior border of the gluteus medius to have their distal attachment on the inner portion of the greater trochanter. **Innervation**: A branch derived directly from the first and second sacral nerves (L_5, S_1-S_2). **Anatomic action**: External rotation of the hip.

PALPATION The muscle is palpated in external rotation, especially if the gluteus maximus is relaxed, as when the limb is raised slightly forward. The palpating fingers are placed posterior to the greater trochanter and moved about somewhat until the best spot for palpation is located.

In palpating the piriformis, its close association with the posterior portion of the gluteus medius in regard to location and action should be kept in mind. The two muscles are likely to be felt contracting simultaneously.

Gluteus Minimus

The **gluteus minimus** belongs to the third and deepest layer of the muscles in the gluteal region. It lies close to the capsule of the hip joint and is covered by the gluteus medius. **Proximal attachment**: Fan-shaped, from the outer surface of the ilium, between the anterior and inferior gluteal lines, and from the septum between it and the medius. **Distal attachment**: Anterior border of the greater trochanter of the femur. **Innervation**: Superior gluteal nerve (L_4-L_5, S_1). **Anatomic actions**: Abduction, medial rotation, and flexion of the hip.

PALPATION   The gluteus minimus muscle cannot be very well differentiated from the medius since both muscles contract simultaneously in abduction and internal rotation. The anterior portion of the muscle is the thickest part and is felt, together with the medius, when the hip is internally rotated.

Medial Muscles

The adductor group is identified as the large muscular mass of the medial thigh, bordering anteriorly to the vastus medialis and the sartorius (see Fig. 8–12) and posteriorly to the hamstrings. This group comprises the following muscles: **adductor magnus, adductor longus, adductor gracilis, adductor brevis,** and **pectineus.** The obturator externus, the quadratus femoris, and the lower portion of the gluteus maximus also are capable of adducting the hip but do not belong to the adductor group proper.

In general, these muscles have **proximal attachments** on the ramus of the pubis and the ramus of the ischium and **distal attachments** posteriorly on the linea aspera of the femoral shaft. The line of action of these muscles in relation to the axis changes when the hip flexes, so that the action of each muscle can be determined only for a specific position of the joint.

The nerve supply to the adductor group is mainly from the obturator nerve. The adductor magnus also is innervated by a branch from the sciatic nerve and the pectineus also is supplied by the femoral nerve (L_2-L_5, S_1). **Anatomic actions**: Adduction of the hip. (In certain positions, different adductors may produce flexion, extension, or rotation of the hip.)

INSPECTION AND PALPATION   The adductor group can be palpated on the medial side of the thigh from the pubis to the distal thigh when resistance is given to adduction. This can be done on oneself by pressing the knees together. Palpating the individual muscles is difficult. The proximal attachment of the adductor longus is on the inferior ramus of the pubis, and the tendon becomes prominent with the motion of adduction. Lateral to this tendon is the muscular attachment of the adductor brevis. The pectineus has a muscular attachment that can be palpated on the superior ramus of the pubis. The adductor magnus can be palpated at its distal attachment on the adductor tubercle of the femur. The gracilis crosses the knee and attaches on the anteromedial side of the tibia beside the sartorius and the semitendinosus. Resistance to knee flexion activates the hamstrings and the gracilis. Proper identification requires palpating the muscles toward their proximal attachments. The hamstrings course laterally to the tuberosity of the ischium while the gracilis muscle belly remains medial to attach on the inferior ramus of the pubis.

FUNCTION OF MUSCLES ACTING AT THE HIP

Weight-Bearing and Non–Weight-Bearing Functions of Hip Muscles

In the lower extremities, muscles must be studied in both non–weight-bearing and weight-bearing situations. Non–weight-bearing, or open-chain, actions are important in the understanding of movements that can be produced by the muscles in the free extremity, limitations of motion produced by tightness or passive insufficiency of muscles, and positions used to elicit isolated contractions of muscles. Perhaps more important are the weight-bearing, or closed kinematic chain functions such as standing on one leg, climbing, rising up from a chair, or performing a sit-up. In these activities, the muscles of the lower extremity are required to perform forceful contractions upon the fixed distal extremity (sometimes called **reversed actions**). Slight to moderate weakness of the muscles is reflected by a decreased ability to perform closed-chain functions, while unresisted open-chain motions may still appear unimpaired.

Portions of a Muscle May Have Different Actions

Muscles such as the gluteus maximus and the gluteus medius cover large areas so that one portion of the muscle may be capable of an action different from another portion. Each of these muscles, however, has a main action that is shared by all portions of the muscle. The action of the gluteus maximus is extension, and the action of the gluteus medius is abduction. The upper portion of the maximus is located so that it acts in abduction; the location of the lower portion permits action as an adductor. The anterior portion of the medius is located well for internal rotation, while its posterior portion acts in external rotation.

Change of Action Because of Joint Angle

The leverage of the muscles of the hip about the three axes changes with the joint angle so that the effectiveness (torque) of a muscle, for a certain motion, may increase or decrease. These leverage changes are commonly found in the hip because of the large range of motion and the relatively long distances of the muscle force arms (movement arms or perpendicular distance from the line of pull of the muscle to the axis of joint motion). The gluteus medius and the tensor fasciae latae are considered internal rotators of the extended hip, but their leverage for internal rotation increases when the hip is flexed to 90 degrees. In some positions of the hip, the line of pull of a muscle may change so markedly (ie, from a position anterior to the axis of motion to one in which it is posterior to the axis) that the muscle can perform antagonistic muscle actions (Steindler, 1955). The piriformis is an external rotator when the hip is extended, but the same muscle becomes an internal rotator when the hip is flexed (Steindler, 1955; Kapandji, 1987). The best example of inversion of action occurs in the hip adductors. The line of pull of the muscles is anterior to the hip joint axis when the hip is in extension and posterior to the joint axis when the hip is in flexion. When the hip is in a position of flexion, as in climbing, the hip adductors are forceful hip extensors; and when the hip is extended, the adductors are flexors. The change from flexor to extensor action varies with the individual muscles between 50 and 70 degrees of hip flexion (Steindler, 1955).

Two-Joint Muscles Acting at the Hip

The hip muscles are either one-joint muscles acting at the hip only, or they pass two joints and have actions, or potential actions, over both joints.

Length-Tension Relationships

The efficiency of a two-joint muscle is substantially influenced by the positions of the two joints, in accordance with the principles governing length-tension relationships of muscle (see Chapter 4). Therefore, the rectus femoris can produce more force as a hip flexor if the knee flexes simultaneously with the hip, because this permits the muscle to contract within a favorable range. For the same reason, the rectus is more efficient as a knee extensor if the hip extends simultaneously with the knee. The hamstrings are more efficient as hip extensors when the knee extends simultaneously with the hip; the hamstrings are more efficient as knee flexors when the hip flexes simultaneously with the knee.

Muscles Acting in Flexion of the Hip

HIP FLEXION IN ERECT STANDING When a subject is standing with one hip flexed, that is, the knee pulled up toward the chest, it may be ascertained by palpation that the **iliopsoas**, the **rectus femoris**, the **sartorius**, and the tensor spring into action. The internal rotary action of the tensor appears to be compensated by the external rotary action of the sartorius, and the knee extensor action of the rectus appears to be checked by gravity and perhaps also by the action of some of the knee flexors. Both internal and external rotary actions have been ascribed to the iliopsoas, but for all practical purposes, this muscle should be considered as a pure flexor. The combined action of the iliopsoas, rectus femoris, sartorius, and tensor muscles (in proper proportion) results in pure flexion. The adductor muscles also act in hip flexion in the early part of the motion, and particularly when resistance is applied. Maximum isometric torque of the hip flexors is greatest when the muscles are stretched (hip is extended) and decreases with hip flexion (see Fig. 4–15).

HIP FLEXION IN THE SITTING POSITION Because, in the sitting position, the hip is already flexed to about 90 degrees, additional flexion necessitates actions by the hip flexors in the shortened range of their excursion. When flexion to an acute hip angle is carried out, the sartorius and the tensor can be felt contracting strongly, but in this range these muscles have lost much of their ability to develop tension and are incapable of carrying out the motion without the aid of the iliopsoas. In fact, as may be concluded from observation of individuals with isolated paralysis of the iliopsoas, this is the only hip flexor that can produce enough tension to flex the hip beyond 90 degrees in the sitting position. These persons can flex the hip sufficiently to walk, but when sitting, they must use their hands to lift and move the thigh.

In the sitting position, the hip flexors—in particular, the iliopsoas—control the vertebrae and pelvis on the femur as the person leans back and returns to the upright position. If the iliopsoas muscles are paralyzed bilaterally, the subject falls backward as soon as the center-of-gravity line of the head, arms, and trunk (HAT) falls behind the hip joint axis. Thus, persons with paraplegia must use hand support to prevent falling over backward when sitting without a backrest.

A general principle, which may be confirmed by observing the postural adjustments made by patients with paralysis of muscles ordinarily engaged in balancing the body or body segments, is that in the erect position—sitting or standing—**the trunk tends to incline toward the weak or paralyzed muscles and motion is controlled by the stronger antagonist with eccentric and concentric muscle contractions.**

SIT-UPS AND STRAIGHT LEG RAISING EXERCISES   A study of the actions of the hip flexors also
must include an analysis of muscle action in sit-ups and in raising one or both legs
in the supine position. In these activities, the abdominal muscles act synergisticly
with the hip flexors to furnish the necessary fixation to the pelvis and vertebrae.
In the sit-up, the neck flexors and abdominal muscles perform concentric contractions until the trunk is flexed (scapula clears the surface), and then they maintain
isometric contractions while the **iliopsoas** becomes the prime mover to raise the
trunk and pelvis on the fixed femur. The torque produced by the HAT is great and,
in turn, requires that the iliopsoas muscles produce large forces. If the abdominal
muscles are not strong enough to maintain lumbar flexion, the great force of the
psoas major pulls the lumbar spine into hyperextension (lordosis). Repetitive performance can lead to microtrauma and back problems. Patients with back injuries
should be taught to turn to the side and push up using the arms when rising from
the supine position (Kendall, Kendall, and Boynton, 1952).

Straight leg raising, and in particular bilateral straight leg raising, creates similar forces on the lumbar vertebrae. Figure 8–16 illustrates the great force that can
occur in the iliopsoas and be transmitted to its proximal attachments on the lumbar vertebrae and the ilium. Even though this value may be high, the force in the
hip flexors is high because they must match the torque of the lower extremity of
30 ft-lb (360 in-lb) for unilateral straight leg raising and 60 ft-lb for bilateral
straight leg raising. If the abdominal muscles cannot stabilize the proximal attachments of the hip flexors, the pelvis tilts anteriorly, and the lumbar vertebrae are
pulled into hyperextension.

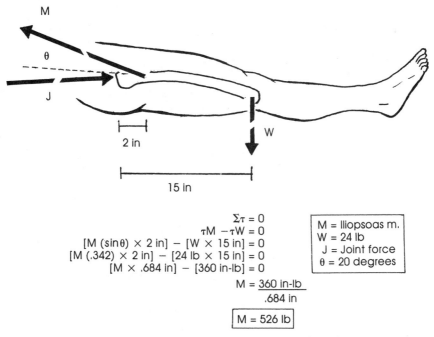

$$\Sigma_T = 0$$
$$\tau M - \tau W = 0$$
$$[M (\sin\theta) \times 2\ in] - [W \times 15\ in] = 0$$
$$[M (.342) \times 2\ in] - [24\ lb \times 15\ in] = 0$$
$$[M \times .684\ in] - [360\ in\text{-}lb] = 0$$
$$M = \frac{360\ in\text{-}lb}{.684\ in}$$

$$\boxed{M = 526\ lb}$$

M = Iliopsoas m.
W = 24 lb
J = Joint force
θ = 20 degrees

Figure 8–16   Illustration of the force occurring in the iliopsoas muscle at the initiation of straight leg
raising. The value of 526 lb is high because hip flexion is normally supplemented by the tensors fasciae
latae, the rectus femoris, the sartorius, and the hip adductors.

Muscles Acting in Extension of the Hip

Five important muscles pass behind the axis for flexion and extension of the hip and serve as extensors in all positions of the joint, namely, the **gluteus maximus**, the **biceps femoris** (long head), the **semimembranosus**, the **semitendinosus**, and the **adductors** (when the hip is in flexion). When the hip is flexed, as when the trunk is inclined forward in standing, the ischial tuberosities are carried backward in relation to the hip axis, and this improves the leverage of those extensor muscles that are attached to the tuberosities.

The hip extensors should be observed and palpated both when the lower extremities move in relation to the trunk and when the trunk moves in relation to the lower extremities. In many activities, both segments move simultaneously.

PRONE-LYING UNILATERAL HIP EXTENSION WITH KNEE EXTENDED   Palpation of the gluteus maximus and the medial hamstring group in the prone position has already been described. To obtain a larger range of motion than that seen in Figures 8–10 and 8–11, the subject should be prone on a table with the hips flexed over the edge of the table. A range of about 90 degrees in hip extension may then be observed. The changing muscular requirements when external or internal rotation is carried out simultaneously should again be observed: increased activity of the gluteus maximus in external rotation, decreased activity of the gluteus maximus in internal rotation, and increased activity of the medial hamstring group in internal rotation.

PRONE-LYING UNILATERAL HIP EXTENSION WITH KNEE FLEXED   When the hamstrings are palpated in hip extension while the knee is flexed, they can be felt "bunching up"; that is, they become short and thick. In this movement combination, length-tension relationships are most unfavorable, and the muscles may come close to, or arrive at, the point of active insufficiency. Subjectively, an uncomfortable cramp-like feeling is experienced in the posterior thigh region when full-range hip extension is attempted while the knee is maintained flexed to an acute angle. Children and young adults may not complain about discomfort, but in older subjects, this movement may be extremely uncomfortable and may produce a cramp. Therefore, it should be used with caution or be avoided.

Because very little tension can be produced by the hamstrings when they contract in their shortened range, hip extension with the knee flexed requires strong action of the gluteus maximus. This movement combination has been advocated as an isolated test for the gluteus maximus. Although it is true that, in hip extension with the knee flexed the gluteus maximus must be credited with doing most of the work, the hamstrings still contract to the best of their ability, so that an isolated action of the gluteus maximus is by no means achieved.

PRONE-LYING BILATERAL HIP EXTENSION, KNEES EXTENDED   In unilateral hip extension in the prone position, the pelvis remains comparatively stable; only mild synergistic contraction of the extensors of the vertebral column is required and may be observed and palpated. When both limbs are raised simultaneously, however, the leverage action on the pelvis (because of the contracting hip extensors and the weight of the limbs) becomes marked. Therefore, the demand on the extensors of the vertebral column, and in particular on the lumbar extensors, is much increased. The strong tension in these muscles should be observed and palpated.

HIP EXTENSORS IN THE SITTING POSITION   Forward inclination of the trunk and pelvis in the sitting or standing position is controlled at the hip joint by the hip extensors. An eccentric contraction permits forward movement to retrieve an object on the floor, and a concentric contraction of the hip extensors produces return to the erect position (see Fig. 11–10). Individuals with paralysis of the hip extensors fall forward unless the upper extremities are used to control the pelvis on the fixed femur (see Fig. 2–31B,C). Such hip extensor muscle activity can be seen in a more subtle form in ascending and descending stairs, in rising from a sitting position, and in walking. These activities are associated with simultaneous contraction of the quadriceps (acting as knee extensors) and the hamstrings (acting as hip extensors).

In these functional motions of leaning forward in the sitting position, bending over to touch the toes in the standing position, climbing the stairs, or rising from a chair, the hamstrings are primarily activated as hip extensors. When such motions are rapid or are accompanied by moderate or maximum resistance, the gluteus maximus also is activated (Basmajian, 1978).

Hip Abductors

The **gluteus medius, gluteus minimus, tensor fasciae latae,** and the upper fibers of the **gluteus maximus** abduct the hip. In certain positions other muscles also contribute to the force of abduction: **sartorius** (in abduction), **piriformis** and **obturators** (in flexion), and the **iliopsoas** in abduction. Using computed tomography, Clark and Haynor (1987) found the gluteus medius to have the majority of the cross-sectional area of the four abductor muscles measured: gluteus medius (60%), gluteus minimus (20%), and the tensor fasciae latae and piriformis (10% each). The mean total cross-sectional area of these abductors was 43 cm^2, which is small compared to the cross-sectional area of the quadriceps (175 cm^2) or the hamstrings (58 cm^2) as measured by Fick (1911). The hip abductors have, however, a large leverage advantage. The major abductors have their distal attachments on the greater trochanter or the shaft of the femur some 2 to 3 inches from the center of rotation of the hip, and they have large angles from the muscle lines of action to the joint axis: tensor fascia latae (83 degrees), gluteus medius (72 degrees), and gluteus minimus (61 degrees) (Clark and Haynor, 1987) as compared to the patellar tendon angle of 15 to 20 degrees.

Because of these leverage advantages, a large torque can be produced by the relatively small hip abductor muscles. Mean values of maximum isometric torques have been reported from 92 to 114 ft-lb for men and 58 to 76 ft-lb for women (Inman, 1947; Murray and Sepic, 1968; Halliday, 1979; Neuman, Soderberg, and Cook, 1988). Variations are due mainly to differences in positions, types of stabilization, and ages.

The hip abductors exert the greatest torque when contracting in the lengthened position, and the torque decreases linearly as the muscle shortens (see Fig. 4–16). In male subjects, Neumann and associates (1988) measured a maximum isometric mean torque of 100 ft-lb (SD = 19) when the muscles were on stretch in the position of 10 degrees of adduction. At 40 degrees of abduction, the torque decreased to 37 ft-lb (SD = 11).

Measurements to determine differences in strength between the right and left hip abductors have been equivocal. In right-handed individuals, the right hip abductors were found to have small but significantly higher maximum isometric torques than the left side (Neumann, Soderberg, and Cook, 1988). In a later study using EMG and submaximal torque testing, the authors did not find a significant difference between sides (Neumann, Soderberg, and Cook, 1989). No significant difference between the maximum isometric torques of the right and left or dominant and nondominant sides of 56 subjects from 20 to 29 years of age was found by Cope (1975). This question may well be indeterminant in normal subjects because of stabilization. The greatest maximum isometric forces of a muscle occur with the strongest stabilization of the fixed attachment of the muscle. Lateral motion of the pelvis is difficult to stabilize mechanically, and in the case of the hip abductors, the best stabilization of the pelvis is by the contralateral hip abductors. This requires a bilateral maximum isometric contraction, and the torques on the left and right sides are therefore the same.

Unilateral Stance

A major function of the hip abductors is in closed-chain motion to maintain a level pelvis in unilateral stance. In standing on one foot, which occurs with every step, 85 percent of the weight of the body (HAT and contralateral limb) must be balanced by the hip abductors around the femoral head (fulcrum), forming a first-class lever system (see Figs. 8–17 and 2–10). Because the lever arm (d) of the weight in Figure 8–17 is longer than the lever arm (l) of the muscles, the hip abductors are at a mechanical disadvantage and must produce a force greater than 85 percent of body weight to maintain equilibrium. The two downward forces (W and M) produce a high compression force (J) between the head of the femur and the acetabulum. The joint compression force in unilateral stance has been calculated to be approximately 2.5 times body weight (Inman, 1947; LeVeau, 1977; Frankel and Nordin, 1980).

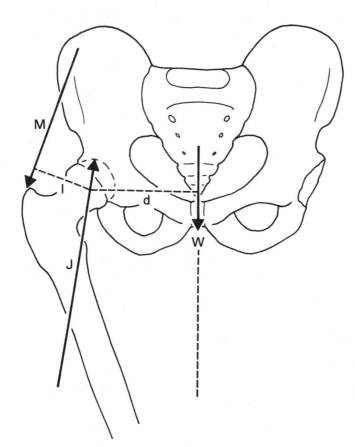

Figure 8–17 Forces on the pelvis when standing on one leg. W = 85% of body weight (head, arms, trunk, and opposite leg); M = force of the hip abductors required to maintain a level pelvis; J = joint reaction force between the head of the femur and the acetabulum; d = 4.25 in. (lever arm distance for W); l = 2.75 in. (lever arm for M). Lever arm distances were measured from x-rays and are provided so that the student can solve for the actual forces of M and W. This can be done in an approximate manner by making M and J into a parallel force system. For more precise values, the angle that M makes with the horizontal (71 degrees) must be used.

During the stance phase of walking, Maquet (1985) calculated a biphasic resultant or compression force on the head of the femur of over 4 times body weight with the foot flat. The resultant decreased to 1.3 times body weight at the midpoint of single leg support and rose to 3.4 times body weight near the end of single support.

The maximum isometric torque curves (see Fig. 4–16) demonstrate that the hip abductors produce the greatest torque at 15 degrees of hip adduction where length-tension relationships are most favorable. This point coincides with the high functional demands placed on the muscle in unilateral stance. As the center of gravity of the body is shifted laterally over the supporting foot, the hip assumes an adducted position, the hip abductors contract, and the opposite foot can be raised from the floor.

Muscles Acting in Adduction of the Hip

When adduction of the hip is carried out against resistance and with the thigh in a neutral position with respect to flexion, extension, and rotation, the five main adductors previously enumerated contract as a group. Their individual functional characteristics in various degrees of hip flexion have been described. Because some of these muscles, or parts of the same muscle, have opposite secondary actions, these actions counterbalance each other when pure adduction is carried out.

The total cross-section of the adductors far surpasses that of the abductors. At first glance, it might appear illogical that this is the case, because in the erect position the hip abductors have to work against gravity, whereas gravity does the work for the adductors. Activities such as squeezing an object between the knees and climbing a rope, which require force in adduction, are relatively rare and hardly warrant such a large cross-section. The explanation for the adductors' large bulk is found in their functions as flexors, extensors, and rotators and, in general, in their stabilizing action as co-contractors with the abductors. The electrical activities of these muscles in walking are illustrated in Figure 12–21.

Rotary Action of the Adductors

In years past, the adductors were thought to be external rotators of the hip. EMG studies, however, have shown them to act as internal rotators (Williams and Wesley, 1951; Basmajian, 1978). This action also can be identified by palpation with the subject in the sitting or standing position (careful attention should be paid to avoidance of active hip flexion). Even though the adductors attach on the posterior aspect of the femur (linea aspera), the axis of rotation does not go through the anatomic axis of the bone but rather through the mechanical axis from the head of the femur to the medial femoral condyle (see Fig. 8–9). When the femur is rotated medially, the linea aspera approaches the pubis. With lateral rotation, the distance between these attachments becomes longer. This phenomenon can be observed using a disarticulated pelvis and femur and measuring the distance between the ischial tuberosity and a midpoint on the linea aspera.

Muscles Acting in Rotation of the Hip

From previous discussions, it is obvious that most of the muscles about the hip joint have rotary actions. Which of these muscles are used for rotation depend on the position of the joint with respect to flexion, extension, abduction, and adduction. For example, the gluteus maximus, when extending the hip fully, also externally rotates the hip; but when the hip is flexed, the upper fibers have a line of pull for internal rotation (Steindler, 1955). The six small external rotators (piriformis, gemellus superior, gemellus inferior, obturator internus, obturator externus, and quadratus femoris) have a good angle of pull for external rotation; but the external rotary components of these muscles decrease in flexion of the hip, and at 90 degrees of hip flexion they possess a considerable abductor component. The piriformis changes from an external rotator in hip extension to an internal rotator in hip flexion (Steindler, 1955; Kapandji, 1987). The anterior portions of the gluteus medius and minimus and the tensor fasciae latae increase their leverage for internal rotation when the hip is flexed.

The maximum isometric torque for both the internal and external rotators occurs at their lengthened positions and decreases as the muscles contract in their shortened positions (May, 1966). Their forces were found to be equal when the leg was near the vertical (neutral) position. An interesting change in maximum torque of the internal rotators occurs when the hip is in flexion and extension. When the hip is flexed, the internal rotators can produce almost three times the torque that they can produce when the hip is extended (Jarvis, 1952; Woodruff, 1976). The external rotators show little difference with hip position. This large difference in the torque of the internal rotators is theorized to be the result of inversion of muscle actions, such as the increased internal rotation leverage of the gluteus medius, gluteus minimus, and piriformis when the hip is flexed. The conventional sitting position for testing the strength of the rotators of the hip may provide misleading information about the functional strength of this group when the subject is actually using the internal rotators in the erect position for walking or pivoting on one foot. A person with weak internal rotators may appear to have good strength in the sitting position but inadequate strength for the functions to be performed in the standing position.

CLINICAL APPLICATIONS

Hip Abductor Muscle Weakness

Persons with paralysis of muscles of the hips demonstrate a number of compensations in the attempt to maintain function. When the hip abductors are paralyzed, one-legged standing with the pelvis level becomes impossible (see Fig. 8–18B). However, the individuals may still manage to balance on one foot at least momentarily, and to do so well enough to permit walking with a limp. They shift the center of gravity of HAT laterally over the axis of motion of the hip (see Fig. 8–18C). The forces can be visualized in Fig. 8–17. If the weight of HAT and the swinging leg (W) is shifted closer to or over the hip axis of motion, the lever or movement arm of W becomes shorter and reduces the torque of W as well as the force that must be generated by the abductors (M). If W is brought directly over the axis, the lever arm distance is zero, W exerts no torque, and therefore the force of M is not needed. The system becomes a linear force system with the pressure on the femoral head reduced from 2½ times body weight to 85 percent of body weight. Walking in this manner is called the **gluteus medius limp**. This limp is seen also in people with pain in the hip, knee, or foot because the limp decreases joint com-

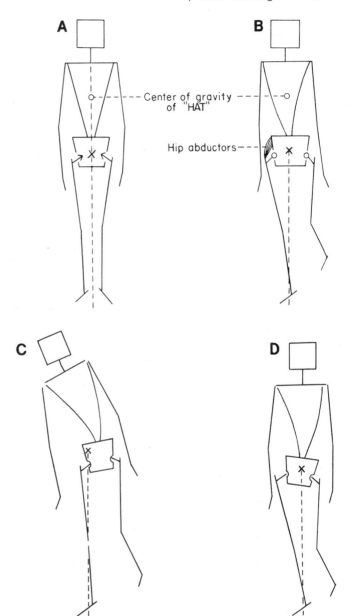

Figure 8–18 (*A*) Body alignment in standing on both feet. The pelvis is supported from both sides. The center-of-gravity line of the head, arms, and trunk (HAT) and of the body as a whole (X) falls in the center of the base of support. (*B*) Body alignment in standing on one foot. Body weight shifts over the stance limb. The hip abductors on the stance side become activated to balance the pelvis. (*C*) One-legged balance in the presence of hip joint pain or when the abductors of the hip are paralyzed. The upper part of the body inclines toward the side of paralysis. Weight of HAT counterbalances the weight of the raised leg, and the abductors at the stance hip are substantially relieved of their balancing function. (*D*) Trendelenburg's sign in paralysis or weakness of the hip abductors. The stance hip is adducted. Ligamentous tension is relied upon for hip balance.

pression forces throughout the entire stance limb. This type of gait, however, requires a marked increase in energy expenditure and creates abnormal forces in the trunk and lower extremities.

Compensation for weak, but not paralyzed, abductors is often made by allowing the pelvis to drop toward the unsupported side (see Fig. 8–18D). The hip on the supported side is in adduction, and motion is limited by the capsule and ligaments. This posture, which occurs in unilateral stance and in walking, is called **Trendelenburg's sign** or **gait**—a term originally used to describe the posture in congenital dislocations of the hip that render the hip abductors ineffective.

The most effective way to compensate for abductor muscle weakness and to prevent a limp is to supplement the muscle force by using a cane or forearm crutch in the opposite hand (weight bearing on the cane occurs simultaneously with the weak leg). Even a small upward force of 10 lb provides considerable assistance in reducing the force required by the gluteus medius because the force of the cane is applied at a long distance from the axis of motion.

The student is encouraged to calculate the muscle and joint forces in Fig. 8–17 and then to recalculate the forces with a short weight arm as in a gluteus medius limp. Forces that occur when using the cane can be calculated by adding the **positive** torque of the cane (τ_C) to the equation (eg, $-\tau_M + \tau_J - \tau_W + \tau_C = 0$). Values for the torque of the cane can be measured or approximated using 15 lb at 15 inches.

Paraplegia

People with paraplegia (paralysis of muscles in both lower extremities) can learn to use several compensations to help control their hips in functional activities. The iliofemoral or Y ligament, which limits hyperextension of the hip, is so strong that it permits persons with paraplegia to gain standing balance when the knees and ankles are stabilized with orthoses or braces (see Fig. 8–8). The person moves the center of gravity of HAT posterior to the axis of the hip joint and "hangs" on the Y ligaments to maintain the pelvis in extension on the femur. To use this balance skill for walking, parallel bars or crutches are required to move individual extremities or to lift the body as a whole. An effective compensatory muscle for these motions is the latissimus dorsi, which is innervated from C_6 to C_8. Closed-chain approximation of its distal attachments on the humerus and proximal attachments on the lower thoracic spinous processes, the thoracolumbar fascia, and the crest of the ilium produces hip elevation so that one extremity can be moved forward at a time. With bilateral contraction the entire body can be lifted and swung forward in a "swing-through" crutch gait. This is the fastest crutch gait but requires a high expenditure of energy and strong, well-conditioned upper extremities.

Laboratory Activities

HIP AND PELVIC REGION

1. On the bones, identify these landmarks. Which are palpable? Locate them on yourself and on a subject.

Femur	*Pelvis*	*Sacrum*
head	iliac crest	promontory
greater trochanter	anterior superior iliac spine	bodies of sacral
lesser trochanter	anterior inferior iliac spine	vertebrae
neck	posterior inferior iliac spine	sacral canal
intertrochanteric	posterior superior iliac spine	sacral foramina
crest (anterior)	posterior gluteal line	articulating surfaces with:
intertrochanteric	anterior gluteal line	body of fifth lumbar
line (posterior)	inferior gluteal line	vertebra

trochanteric fossa	acetabulum	inferior articulating
gluteal tuberosity	sciatic notch (greater	process of fifth lumbar
linea aspera	and lesser)	vertebra
	tuberosity of ischium	ilium (sacroiliac joint)
	ramus of ischium	coccyx
	ramus of pubis	
	obturator foramen	
	iliac fossa	

2. With your partner supine, perform passive range of the motions of hip flexion, rotation, abduction, and adduction. Describe the end-feels.

3. Differentiate hip extension and hyperextension from lumbar motion. Have subject on a treatment table in the prone position. Extend the subject's hip passively and have him or her do the motion actively while you observe where the motions are taking place. Then have the subject move to the side edge of the table so that the hip can be flexed to 90 degrees (let the foot be supported by the floor). This prevents pelvic and lumbar motion. Extend the opposite hip passively and note the range of motion and the end-feel. Then have the subject actively extend the hip.

4. Differentiate the range of motion of hip flexion with the knee flexed and then with it extended. Passively flex the hip through its full range permitting the knee to flex. Then passively flex the hip with the knee straight. Note the differences in range and end-feels. What are the structures that limit hip flexion when the knee is in extension?

5. On your partner, place the following muscles in their shortest position (contracture) and in their longest position (stretched):

iliopsoas	biceps femoris
pectineus	semimembranosus
rectus femoris	semitendinosus
tensor fasciae latae	sartorius

6. On your partner, palpate the hip musculature as described in Chapter 8:

iliopsoas	tensor fasciae latae
gluteus maximus	rectus femoris
gluteus medius	adductors
hamstrings	external rotators

7. Analyze hip muscle actions in weight bearing (closed chain):
   a. Sit sideways on a chair so that you can lean forward and backward. Palpate your hamstring muscles at their distal tendons behind the knee. As you lean back (hip extension) the tendons should be relaxed and when you lean forward they contract when you cross the vertical position. The hamstring muscles continue to contract with the forward lean (hip flexion) and on the return to the upright position (hip extension). What type of muscle contraction is occurring in the hamstrings as you lean forward and what type occurs to bring you back to the erect position? What muscle of the hip controls leaning back and then returning to the erect position? (It is difficult to palpate.)
   b. Stand upright and palpate the hamstrings at their proximal attachments on the ischial tuberosity. Lean the trunk back and feel the relaxation of the

muscles and then lean forward as in a. above. Note the relative inactivity of the gluteus maximus.

c. Stand upright and palpate your gluteus medius muscles just above the greater trochanters. When standing comfortably on both feet, the muscles should be relaxed. Gently shift your body weight to the right foot. Note the strong contraction of the gluteus medius. What is the purpose of this contraction?

d. Palpate the gluteus medius bilaterally when you walk. Do the muscles contract at the same time?

8. Analyze multiple actions of the hip adductors. Palpate the adductors on yourself during the following positions and motions:

a. Sit on a table with your feet unsupported and flex your hip. Then, **without any hip flexion**, externally rotate your hip followed by internal rotation.

b. Stand **erect** with the left foot on a block or a book and with the right foot hanging free and unsupported. Palpate the right adductors while you abduct the hip and then adduct it against the left leg. Note that the muscles do not contract until resistance is met. What muscle with what type of contraction is controlling the motion of adduction in this position? Then flex your hip, keeping the trunk erect. Then externally and internally rotate the hip (without flexing). What is the difference in the activity of the adductors when hip rotation is performed with the hip in flexion versus extension? Is there a contraction of the adductors when the motion of hip flexion is made?

c. Stand with one foot on a high step or a chair (to place the hip in flexion). Press down with your foot as if to lift your body up (eg, climbing) and note the strong contraction in the adductors.

d. Using the pelvis and a femur, attach a piece of string to the proximal attachment of the adductors and hold the free end near the middle or at different specific distal attachments. Keep the string taut but let it slide to represent the line of pull as you perform the motions in a., b., and c. above. Note the changing relationships between the axis of motion and the line of pull as you place the hip in flexion and extension. The axis for rotation of the hip is the mechanical axis rather than the anatomic axis.

CHAPTER 9

Knee Region

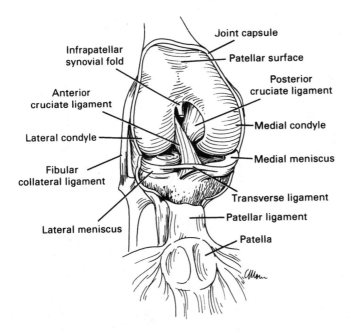

Figure 9–1 The right knee of a young adult flexed to about 90 degrees and viewed from the front. The anterior part of the capsule has been removed and the patella turned down. (Redrawn from *Acta Clinica: Osteoarthritis of the Knee*, Vol 1. Geigy Pharmaceuticals, Ardsley, NJ, 1963.)

The knee is a complex joint (Figs. 9–1 and 9–2) with three bones (**femur, tibia, and patella**), **two degrees of freedom of motion,** and **three articulating surfaces**: the **medial tibiofemoral, lateral tibiofemoral, and patellofemoral articulations**, which are enclosed by a common joint capsule. Functionally, the knee

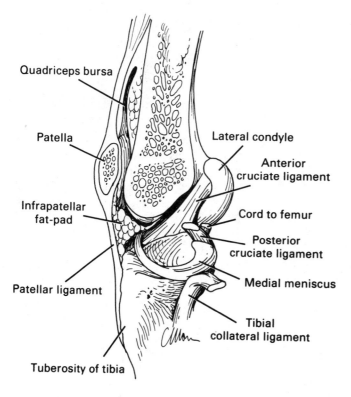

Figure 9–2 The right knee seen from the medial side. The femur and the patella have been split in half sagitally. (Redrawn from *Acta Clinica: Osteoarthritis of the Knee*, Vol 1. Geigy Pharmaceuticals, Ardsley, NJ, 1963.)

can support the body weight in the erect position without muscle contraction; it participates in lowering and elevating body weight (up to 0.5 M) in sitting, squatting, or climbing; and it permits rotation of the body when turning on the planted foot as a football player does when avoiding a pursuing tackler. In walking, the normal knee reduces energy expenditure by decreasing the vertical and lateral oscillations of the center of gravity of the body (Inman, Ralston, and Todd, 1981) while sustaining vertical forces equal to four to six times body weight (Morrison, 1970; Maquet, 1983). The multiple functions of the normal knees—to withstand large forces, to provide great stability, and to afford large ranges of motion—are achieved in a unique way. **Mobility** is primarily provided by bony structure, and **stability** is primarily provided by the soft tissues: ligaments, muscles, and cartilage. Athletic and industrial injuries to these stabilizing structures are common and are frequently caused by the larger torques developed by forces acting on the long lever arms of the femur and tibia.

PALPABLE JOINT STRUCTURES

The superficial structures of the knee can be palpated best with the subject sitting on a table and with the knee relaxed in 90 degrees of flexion. The distal enlargements of the femur, the **condyles** (Gr. *kondylos*, knuckle; a rounded projection on a bone), can be felt anteriorly on both sides of the patella and followed proximally to the **epicondyles** (Gr. *epi*, upon). When the palpating fingers then move inferiorly from the femoral condyles, the depression for the **tibiofemoral joint line** is encountered. This line can be confirmed by passively rotating or extending the knee while feeling the motion of the tibial condyles on the femur. Anteriorly on the tibia, and below the tibial condyles, is a large roughened area, the **tuberosity of the tibia**, which is the distal attachment of the patellar tendon of the quadriceps femoris muscle. The sharp **crest of the tibia** may be followed distally to the ankle.

The **medial (tibial) collateral ligament** spans the tibiofemoral joint on the medial side and may be felt by palpating along the joint line. This broad fibrous band obliterates the joint line as the ligament courses from the medial epicondyle of the femur to the medial condyle and shaft of the tibia. If the palpating finger is placed on the joint line at the anterior margin of the medial collateral ligament, the edge of the **medial meniscus** may be palpated. The medial edge of the meniscus can be made more prominent by passively internally rotating the tibia. With passive external rotation, the meniscus will retract.

If the index finger is placed on the lateral epicondyle of the femur and the middle finger on the head of the fibula, the attachments of the **lateral (fibular) collateral ligament** can be identified. This smaller ligament is difficult to palpate as it crosses the joint line. It becomes readily palpable, however, if the foot is placed on the opposite knee and the hip is permitted to fall into external rotation. The lateral meniscus cannot be palpated.

The patella is best palpated when the subject is supine with the knee extended and relaxed. The thick patellar ligament may be felt from the tuberosity of the tibia to the apex of the triangular patella. Normally, the patella can be easily mobilized laterally and distally and can be compressed on the femur without discomfort.

NONPALPABLE STRUCTURES

Note the following nonpalpable structures on the skeleton, models, and in Figures 9–1 and 9–2: **articular surfaces** and **patellar surfaces** on the condyles of the femur; **intercondyloid fossa; lateral and medial supracondylar lines**, extending proximally from the condyles and enclosing an area that forms the floor of the popliteal fossa (L. *poples*, back of the knee); **articular surfaces of the condyles of the tibia** ("tibial plateau"), separated by the intercondylar eminence; **lateral meniscus**, nearly circular in form (Gr. *meniskos*, crescent); **medial meniscus; anterior and posterior cruciate ligaments**; and **transverse ligament**, connecting the menisci anteriorly.

KNEE JOINT

Motions of the Knee

The knee joint (*articulatio genu*, L. *genua*, knee or any structure bent like the knee) possesses two degrees of freedom: flexion-extension and axial rotation. Flexion is from 120 to 150 degrees depending on the size of the muscle mass of the calf in contact with the posterior thigh. In normal males aged 18 months to 54 years, Boone and Azen (1979) found a mean value for flexion of 143 degrees (SD = 5.4). When the hip is in extension, the range of motion of knee flexion decreases because of limitation by the two-joint rectus femoris muscle, which has its proximal attachment on the anterior inferior spine of the ilium. Hyperextension is minimal and does not normally exceed 15 degrees.

Normal passive motion end-feel for knee flexion is soft from contact of the tissues of the posterior calf and the thigh or from a shortened rectus femoris muscle if calf-thigh contact is not made. The end-feel for extension or hyperextension is firm from tension on ligamentous and posterior capsular structures. If the hip is flexed to 90 degrees, knee extension may be free or limited by the length of the hamstring muscles.

Axes for Flexion and Extension

The axis of motion is located a few centimeters above the joint line passing transversely through the femoral condyles. Two methods to determine the axis of flexion and extension of the knee exist in the literature. The geometric center of the knee was found by Fisher in the 19th century by measuring successive points of contact between the femoral and tibial condyles in a series of x-rays taken at successive joint angles. By calculating the perpendiculars to the curvatures and connecting these centers, a curved line representing the path of the axis was obtained (Fig. 9–3).

The second method is the instant center of rotation of Reuleaux (1875). This axis represents the point of zero velocity on the femoral condyles during flexion and extension (Frankel and Burstein, 1907). The axis coincides with the center of the cruciate ligaments in the sagittal plane (Maquet, 1983; O'Connor et al, 1990). Using this method, Smidt (1973) measured the axis as moving through a pathway of 3.2 cm from extension to 90 degrees of flexion. Movement of the axis during joint motions occurs in most joints, but the magnitude is usually small. The size of the knee joint causes considerable translation of the axis.

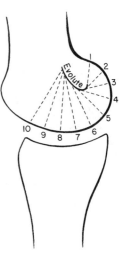

Figure 9–3   Changing radius of curves of the femoral condyles. The axis of motion for flexion and extension moves along an evolute. Number 1 represents the radius of curvature in flexion and number 10, the radius in extension. (Redrawn from Fick, 1911, p 538.)

Clinically, the axis of knee flexion and extension is approximated as directed through the center of the lateral and medial condyles of the femur.

Because of the shifting axis of motion of the human knee, problems occur when devices with mechanical hinge joints such as a goniometer, isokinetic dynamometer, knee-ankle-foot (long-leg) orthosis, or below-knee prosthesis are applied to the knee. When the knee joint is moved from extension to flexion, the anatomic axis of the knee moves about 2 cm, while the mechanical axis of the attached device remains fixed. Thus the arms of the mechanical device cannot remain parallel to the thigh and leg, and motions or pressures between the mechanical and anatomic parts will occur. Compromise and careful alignment are required to prevent discomfort and abrasions. Misalignment of an orthotic knee joint can cause pressure of cuffs on the extremity during knee flexion and gapping during knee extension (or vice versa).

Axial Rotation

Axial rotation occurs in the transverse plane when the knee is flexed. When the knee is fully extended, the medial and lateral collateral ligaments are relatively tense, contributing materially to the stability of the joint. These ligaments slacken when the joint flexes, and this is one of the reasons why a considerable amount of transverse rotation may take place in the flexed position. In Figure 9–4, the position of the medial epicondyle when the knee is extended (Me) is compared with its position when the knee is flexed (Mf). Note that the distance from the medial epicondyle to point A (representing the attachment of the medial collateral ligament) is less in flexion than in extension. During knee flexion, more slack is produced in the lateral than in the medial collateral ligament; hence, the movement between the femoral and tibial condyles is more extensive laterally than medially. Transverse rotation takes place about a longitudinal axis located medial to the intercondylar ridge of the tibia so that, roughly, it may be stated that the lateral condyle rotates around the medial one.

Although many conflicting values are reported for this motion, the results of

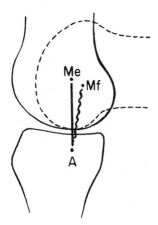

Figure 9–4 Slackening of the medial collateral ligament in flexion of the knee. Me = medial epicondyle in extension; Mf = medial epicondyle in flexion; A = point of attachment of medial collateral ligament. (Redrawn from Fick, 1911, p 542.)

published studies indicate the average total rotation to be approximately 40 degrees (Ross, 1932; Ouellet, Levesque, and Laurin, 1969). At 90 degrees of knee flexion, Mossberg and Smith (1983) found a mean total rotation of 40 degrees (SD = ± 8). External rotation was approximately twice as large as internal rotation. Axial rotation decreases as the angle of knee flexion becomes smaller and cannot be performed as the knee approaches extension. Rotation of the tibia on the femur can be performed voluntarily in the sitting position and is useful in placing and positioning the foot. The major functional importance of the motion, however, is in closed-chain motion, in which the femur rotates on the fixed tibia, as in turning from kneeling, sitting, or squatting positions and in sudden changes in direction while running.

Normal end-feels for passive internal and external rotation of the knee are firm. Motion is limited by capsular and ligamentous structures, including the collateral, cruciate, and oblique popliteal ligaments as well as the retinacula and the iliotibial tract.

Terminal Rotation of the Knee

Normally, when the knee moves into extension, the tibia externally rotates about 20 degrees on the fixed femur. This motion can be observed in the last 20 degrees of knee extension and is called **terminal rotation of the knee**, or the "screw home mechanism." It is purely a mechanical event that occurs with both passive and active knee extension and that cannot be produced (or prevented) voluntarily. In closed-chain motion such as rising from a chair, terminal rotation is seen as internal rotation of the femur on the fixed tibia. Although many species such as chimpanzees, orangutans, and birds walk on flexed knees, terminal rotation provides humans with an exquisite and energy-efficient mechanism for the extended knee. This screw mechanism provides a mechanical stability to withstand forces occurring in the sagittal plane. It permits humans to stand erect without quadriceps muscle contraction and to withstand anterior-posterior forces on the extended knee with reduced muscle force. Although the amount of terminal rotation of the knee is modest, it is, like axial rotation, a requisite for normal knee function. Both motions must be evaluated and regained for successful rehabilitation of the knee.

Accessory Motions

The closed-packed position of the knee is full extension, in which terminal rotation produces tightening of the ligamentous and capsular structures with strong stabilization of the joint. Accessory motions normally cannot be produced in this position. If, however, the knee is placed in 25 or more degrees of flexion and the femur is stabilized, the tibia can be distracted several millimeters on the femur, moved 1 to 3 mm in anterior or posterior glides and medial and lateral glides, as well as in abduction and adduction. An excessive glide is a possible indication of laxity in soft tissue structures, i.e., ligaments, menisci, or the capsule.

Anatomic Basis for Joint Motion

The tibiofemoral joints achieve their greatest stability and two degrees of freedom of motion in a remarkable way. The medial and lateral femoral condyles are convex both longitudinally and transversely. They are connected anteriorly by the patellar surface and separated distally and posteriorly by the intercondylar notch. These condyles articulate with the two smaller tibial condyles, which have only a slight concavity (the lateral tibial condyle is also convex anteriorly and posteriorly). The congruity of the articulations is increased slightly by the intercondylar eminence of the tibia and the wedge-shaped medial and lateral menisci (semilunar cartilages), which form an incomplete ring or crescent on each tibial condyle. The longitudinal articulating surface of the femoral condyles is approximately twice the length of the surface of the tibial condyles. Thus, the motions of knee flexion and extension cannot be pure rolling or hinge motions (see Fig. 1–8). Instead, the condyles execute both rolling and sliding movements, with the ratio of each varying in the range of motion. Rolling is predominant at the initiation of flexion, and sliding occurs more at the end of flexion (Kapandji, 1987). Because the length of the articular surface of the lateral femoral condyle is longer than that of the medial condyle, the movements of the two condylar surfaces differ also.

Menisci

MEDIAL AND LATERAL MENISCI   The **medial and lateral menisci** are fibrocartilages that serve to increase the congruency of the tibiofemoral articulations and to distribute pressure (see Figs. 9–1 and 9–2). Weight-bearing areas of the knee are almost equal on the medial and lateral tibiofemoral surfaces with the largest area occurring when the knee is in hyperextension (Maquet, 1983). With knee flexion, the weight-bearing area moves posteriorly on the tibial condyles and becomes smaller (Table 9–1). Surgical removal of the menisci decreases the surface area and causes pressure

Table 9-1   Weight-bearing Areas of the Tibiofemoral Articulations With Intact Menisci and With Meniscectomy

Knee Flexion in Degrees	Menisci Intact Mean in cm²	Meniscectomy Mean in cm²
−5	20	12
45	13	9
90	12	6

SOURCE: Data from Maquet, PGJ: Biomechanics of the Knee. Springer-Verlag, New York, 1984, p. 67.

to increase on the femoral and tibial condyles, which may lead to later osteoarthritis.

The only bony attachments of the menisci to the tibia are through their horns at the anterior and posterior intercondylar fossae and through the coronary ligaments, which are part of the capsule and which attach the peripheral edges of the menisci to the margin of the tibia. These cartilages are not attached to the articulating surfaces of the tibia and are therefore movable. They do have numerous other attachments:

1. The transverse ligament connects the anterior horns of the two menisci.
2. Fibrous bands connect the anterior horns of both menisci to the retinaculum of the patellar tendon (meniscopatellar fibers).
3. The medial collateral ligament is attached to the medial meniscus.
4. The tendon of the semimembranosus muscle sends fibers to the posterior edge of the medial meniscus.
5. The popliteus muscle sends fibers to the posterior edge of the lateral meniscus.
6. The meniscofemoral ligament extends from the lateral meniscus (posteriorly) to the inside of the medial condyle near the posterior cruciate ligament.

The menisci are moved and controlled on the tibia by both passive and active forces. Passively, they are pushed anteriorly by the femur as the knee extends and the contact of the femoral condyles is more anterior on the tibial condyles. Conversely, the menisci move posteriorly with knee flexion. According to Kapandji (1987), a total movement of 6 mm occurs in the medial meniscus and 12 mm in the lateral meniscus. In addition, the menisci move or deform according to the direction of movement of the femoral condyles during axial rotation. Edges of the menisci are moved by their ligamentous and muscular attachments. For example, anterior movement is caused by the meniscopatellar fibers to the extensor mechanism, and posterior movement is caused by their attachments to the knee flexors (the semimembranosus and the popliteus muscles). If a meniscus fails to move with the femoral condyles, as may occur with sudden twisting or forceful movement, the meniscus may be crushed or torn by the condyles.

Collateral Ligaments

TIBIAL AND FIBULAR COLLATERAL LIGAMENTS   Strong medial (tibial) and lateral (fibular) collateral ligaments prevent passive movement of the knee in the frontal plane. The medial collateral ligament prevents abduction of the tibia on the femur (genu valgum, or knock knee), and the lateral collateral ligament prevents adduction of the tibia (genu varum, or bowleg). Secondarily, the collateral ligaments restrain anterior and posterior displacement of the tibia as well as rotation when the knee is extended. The attachments of the collateral ligaments on the femoral condyles are offset posteriorly and superiorly to the axis for flexion. This offsetting causes the ligaments to become taut when the knee moves into extension and to become slack as the knee flexes (see Fig. 9–4). The collateral ligaments thus provide stability to terminal rotation of the extended knee and yet permit axial rotation in the flexed knee. Axial rotation also is facilitated by a decrease in the congruency of the joint surfaces when the knee is flexed. The posterior aspects of the femoral condyles have a greater convexity and the intercondylar notch is wider at this point. Thus, when the knee is flexed, the mating surfaces with the tibial intercondylar tubercles and the menisci are reduced, and the condyles have more freedom to rotate (see Table 9–1).

Cruciate Ligaments

ANTERIOR AND POSTERIOR CRUCIATE LIGAMENTS The **anterior and posterior cruciate ligament** (L. *crux*, cross) provide control and stability to the knee throughout the motions of flexion and extension. These ligaments lie in the center of the joint within the femoral intercondylar fossa (see Figs. 9–1 and 9–2). They receive their name because they form a cross when viewed from the side or from the front. If viewed from above, however, they are parallel (Fig. 9–5). Although intimately related to the joint capsule, they are not within the capsule and are extracapsular structures. The cruciate ligaments maintain a relatively constant length throughout the motions of flexion and extension even though not all of the parts are taut at the same time. In this way, these ligaments help to force the sliding motions of the condylar surfaces to occur.

The **anterior cruciate ligament (ACL)** attaches to the anterior intercondylar fossa of the tibia and courses laterally and superiorly to attach on the inside of the lateral condyle of the femur. Severance of this ligament allows anterior dislocation of the tibia on the femur (anterior drawer sign: Hoppenfeld, 1976; McCluskey and Blackburn, 1980). Severance of the ACL in cadavers demonstrated an anterior displacement of the tibia on the femur of 7 mm (McQuade et al, 1989; Shoemaker and Daniel, 1990). Such attempted movement in able-bodied subjects is far less. Mean values of the anterior drawer test in college students with, intact knees were measured from 1.2 to 2.7 mm at 90 degrees of flexion (Chandler, Wilson, and Stone, 1989).

Secondary functions of the ACL are generally considered to be that of limiting internal and external rotation (Shoemaker and Daniel, 1990). No significant differences, however, between the intact and ACL-deficient knees for internal and external rotation ranges of motion were found in an in vitro study by McQuade and associates (1989).

The **posterior cruciate ligament (PCL)** attaches on the posterior intercondylar fossa of the tibia and runs medially to attach on the inside of the medial femoral condyle (see Figs. 9–1 and 9–2). The PCL limits posterior displacement of the tibia on the femur (posterior drawer sign). Conversely, in closed-chain mo-

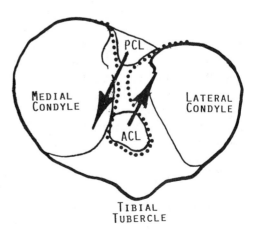

Figure 9–5 The tibia viewed from above. The *dotted line* is the attachment of the capsule as it folds in and around the attachments of the posterior cruciate ligament (PCL) and the anterior cruciate ligament (ACL). The *arrows* represent the direction of the ligaments as they course superiorly to attach to the inside of the femoral condyles.

tion, when the foot is planted in running, the PCL helps prevent anterior displacement (dislocation) of the femoral condyles on the tibial condyles. Normally the PCL permits only minimal passive movement. The average displacements in posterior draw tests for college students with intact knees were from 0.6 to 1.0 mm in men and from 1.2 to 1.9 mm in women when the knee was at 90 degrees of flexion (Chandler, Wilson, and Stone, 1989).

Joint Capsule

The **joint capsule** forms a sleeve around the joints, attaching just above the femoral condyles and below the tibial condyles. Anteriorly, there is a cutout for the patella and posteriorly, there is a central fold that almost divides the joint space (see Fig. 9–5). Retinacula and ligaments reinforce and become integral parts of the capsule. The proximal tendon of the popliteus muscle pierces the capsule to attach on the lateral femoral condyle. The semimembranosus muscle forms part of the oblique popliteal ligament and gives off fibers to the medial collateral ligament as well as to its large bony attachment. These are a few examples of the complex passive and active connections among the menisci, ligaments, retinacula, bones, muscles, and the capsule.

Patellofemoral Joint

The patella is a sesamoid bone set within the joint capsule to articulate with the anterior and distal saddle-shaped surfaces of the femoral condyles (trochlear surfaces). The articulating surface of the patella has a prominent vertical ridge dividing the medial and lateral articular facets. There is considerable variation, and the osseous shape does not always reflect the cartilaginous surface (Fulkerson and Hungerford, 1990). The purposes of the patella are to:

- Increase the leverage or torque of the quadriceps femoris muscle by increasing its distance from the axis of motion (force arm distance)
- Provide bony protection to the distal joint surfaces of the femoral condyles when the knee is flexed
- Decrease pressure and distribute forces on the femur
- Prevent damaging compression forces on the quadriceps tendon with resisted knee flexion such as deep knee bends. (Tendons are designed to withstand large tension forces but not compression or friction forces)

The extensor or quadriceps mechanism stabilizes the patella on all sides and guides the motion between the patella and the femur. Distally, the patella is anchored to the tuberosity of the tibia by the strong patellar tendon. Dense fibrous retinacula and muscles anchor the patella on each side. Laterally, the patella is stabilized by superficial and deep retinacula, the iliotibial band, and the vastus lateralis muscle. When the knee is flexed, these structures move posteriorly and create lateral and tilting forces on the patella. Normally, such motions are prevented by the balanced forces created by the medial stabilizing structures: the patellofemoral ligament, the medial meniscopatellar ligament, and the oblique fibers of the vastus medialis muscle (VMO). Superiorly, the rectus femoris and the vastus intermedius attach to the base of the patella. Thus, the patella is affected by both static (fascia) and dynamic (muscle) forces.

As the patella glides on the trochlear surfaces during knee flexion, the patellar articulating surfaces also change. At the beginning of the motion, the contact area is on the distal third of the patella. As flexion approaches 90 degrees, the articulating surface moves toward the base to cover the proximal one-half of the patella (Huberti and Hayes, 1984). Huberti and Hayes found contact pressures to be the same on the medial and lateral facets and to increase with knee flexion to 90 degrees. At 120 degrees of flexion, two areas of contact and pressure occur. One is at the patellofemoral articulation, and the other is between the quadriceps tendon and the femur.

Knee Alignment and Deformities

An anterior view of the extended knee reveals an angle, open laterally, between the shafts of the femur and the tibia. The size of the angle is variable; about 170 degrees (as measured from the longitudinal axis of each bone) is regarded as average (Fig. 9–6). This angle is due to the adducted position of the shaft of the femur and the compensatory direction of the tibia to transmit weight perpendicularly to the foot and ground. Thus, during weight bearing on one leg, forces are directed toward the medial side of the knee. If the angle becomes smaller than 170 degrees, the condition is referred to as **genu valgum**, or knock knee. Conversely, if the angle approaches 180 degrees or opens medially, the deformity is referred to as **genu varum**, or bowleg.

The tendons of the quadriceps femoris and the ligamentum patella also form an angle with the center of the patella. This is called the "Q angle" (Ficat and Hungerford, 1977; see Fig. 9–6). Normal values for college men were 11.2 degrees (SD = 3) and 15.8 degrees (SD = 4.5) for women (Horton and Hall, 1989). Q an-

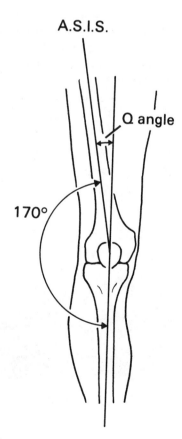

Figure 9–6 Alignment of the shaft of the femur with the tibia. The angle (on the lateral side) between the longitudinal axis of the femur and that of the tibia is usually about 170 degrees. The Q angle is formed by drawing a line from the tibial tuberosity through the center of the patella and drawing another line from the center of the patella to the anterior superior iliac spine (A.S.I.S.).

gles greater than 20 degrees are said to have a higher incidence of patellofemoral joint abnormalities such as chondromalacia patella and patellofemoral tracking problems. Excessive lateral displacement of the patella as it tracks on the trochlear surfaces is normally prevented by the congruence of the joint surfaces, the elevated lateral trochlear facet, and by the medial soft tissue stabilizers. Imbalances such as tightness of the iliotibial band or weakness of the VMO cause the patella to move laterally with muscle contraction of the quadriceps and may lead to changes in joint contact areas and pressures with resulting pain and dysfunction.

MUSCLES

Knee Extensors

The quadriceps femoris muscle group extends the knee and consists of four muscles: **rectus femoris, vastus lateralis, vastus medialis**, and **vastus intermedius**. These four muscles form a single, strong distal attachment to the patella, capsule of the knee, and anterior proximal surface of the tibia. In well-developed subjects in whom little adipose tissue is present, the rectus femoris, the vastus medialis, and the vastus lateralis may be observed as separate units (Figs. 9–7 and 9–8), while in other subjects, the boundaries of these muscles are less distinct. The vastus intermedius is deeply located and cannot be observed from the surface.

Rectus Femoris

The **rectus femoris** occupies the middle of the thigh, is superficial, and takes a straight course down the thigh. **Proximal attachments**: By two tendons: (1) the anterior or "straight" tendon, from the anterior inferior spine of the ilium; and (2) the posterior or "reflected" tendon from just above the brim of the acetabulum; as this tendon swings forward, it courses close to the hip joint and is blended with the capsule. The two tendons unite, covering part of the capsule anteriorly. **Distal attachment**: The muscle fibers attach to a deep aponeurosis narrowing to a broad

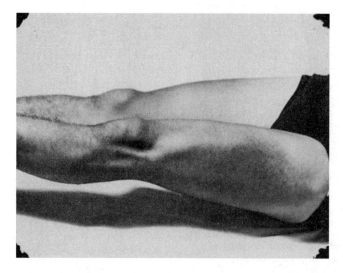

Figure 9–7 The vastus lateralis in contraction. The subject maintains extension of the knee while lifting the heel off the floor. The iliotibial tract is seen as it approaches its attachment on the tibia.

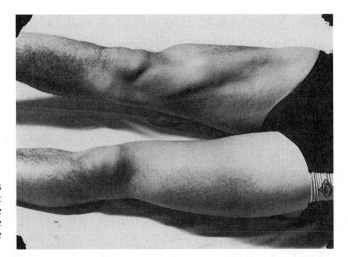

Figure 9–8 The vastus medialis in contraction. The subject's right knee is held extended while the heel is raised off the floor. Note the bulk of this muscle near the knee.

tendon that attaches to the superior border of the patella, and by means of the patellar tendon, into the tuberosity of the tibia. **Innervation**: Two branches of the femoral nerve (L_2-L_4). **Anatomic actions**: Hip flexion and knee extension. **Inspection and palpation**: When the hip is flexed, the tendon of origin may be observed and palpated in the V-shaped area between the sartorius and the tensor fasciae latae as seen in Figure 8–12. The muscular portion is superficial and may be followed down the thigh to its attachment on the patella (see Figs. 9–7 and 9–8).

Vastus Lateralis

The vastus lateralis is the largest of the four muscles and is located on the lateral side of the rectus femoris. **Proximal attachment**: By a broad aponeurosis on the lateral and posterior aspects of the femur, as high up as the greater trochanter and as far posterior as the linea aspera. **Distal attachments**: The lateral border of the patella, the lateral patellar retinaculum, and by means of the patellar tendon, the tuberosity of the tibia. The fibers converge toward the patella at a 12- to 15-degree angle, which is even greater in distal portions (Leib and Perry, 1968). **Innervation**: Branches of the femoral nerve (L_2-L_4). **Anatomic action**: Knee extension. **Inspection and palpation**: The muscle may be seen and palpated from just below the greater trochanter down to the patella (see Fig. 9–7).

Vastus Medialis

The vastus medialis lies in a position medial to the rectus. **Proximal attachments**: Medial and posterior aspects of the femur, as high up as the intertrochanteric line and as far posterior as the linea aspera. **Distal attachments**: Medial portion of superior border of patella, medial patellar retinaculum, and by means of the patellar tendon, the tuberosity of the tibia. **Innervation**: Branches of the femoral nerve (L_2-L_4). **Anatomic action**: Knee extension. **Inspection and palpation**: The distal portion of the muscle is quite bulky and is palpated medially in the lower third of the thigh (see Fig. 9–8).

Vastus Intermedius

Vastus intermedius, located underneath the rectus, is partially fused with the two other vasti muscles. **Proximal attachments**: Anterior and lateral surfaces of the femur, as high up as the lesser trochanter and as far posterior as the linea aspera. The muscle fibers are aligned parallel to the long axis of the femur. **Distal attachments**: Superior border of the patella, fused with the tendons of the two other vasti muscles, and directly into the capsule of the knee joint. **Innervation**: Branches of the femoral nerve (L_2-L_4). **Anatomic action**: Knee extension. **Palpation**: If the rectus is grasped and lifted somewhat, the vastus intermedius may be palpated underneath the rectus if approached from the medial or lateral side of the rectus.

The patella lies within the common tendon of the quadriceps, which extends above and on the sides of the patella as well as being attached to it. From the apex of the patella, the patellar ligament, the continuation of the quadriceps tendon extends to the tuberosity of the tibia. On the sides of the patella, tendinous fibers spread out to form the medial and lateral retinacula, which attach to the condyles of the tibia.

Articularis Genu

The **articularis genu** (subcrureus) is a small, flat muscle with attachments on the anterior lower portion of the shaft of the femur and the capsule of the knee joint or on the superior edge of the patella. The muscle lies beneath the vastus intermedius and is sometimes blended with it. This muscle is innervated by a branch of the nerve to the vastus intermedius. Neither the attachments of this muscle nor its purpose has been clearly described. The predominant theory is that the function of the articularis genu is to pull the joint capsule (and synovial membrane) superiorly as the knee extends, thereby preventing an impingement or crushing of these structures in the patellofemoral articulation. Perhaps more important than a controversy about the role of this muscle is the fact that the anterior-superior capsule must move and pleat with knee extension. When it does not do so, injuries to the capsule and plica (seams in the synovial membrane) may occur.

Knee Flexors

A number of muscles pass posterior to the axis for flexion and extension of the knee, contributing to a variable extent of knee flexion. The muscles are the **biceps femoris**, the **semitendinosus**, and the **semimembranosus** (collectively called the hamstrings); the **gastrocnemius**; the **plantaris**; the **popliteus**; the **adductor gracilis**; and the **sartorius**.

Biceps Femoris

The biceps femoris is a muscle of the posterior thigh, also known as the "lateral hamstring." **Proximal attachments**: By two heads: (1) The long head to the tuberosity of the ischium, having a common tendon of attachment with the semitendinosus; (2) the short head, to the lower portion of the shaft of the femur and to the lateral intermuscular septum. **Distal attachments**: The two heads unite to be attached to the head of the fibula, to the lateral condyle of the tibia, and to the fascia of the leg. **Innervation**: Branches of the sciatic nerve (L_4-L_5, S_1). **Anatomic**

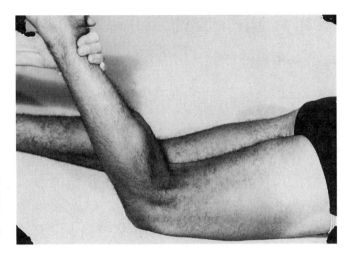

Figure 9–9 The tendon of the biceps femoris is seen on the lateral side of the posterior knee region when knee flexion is resisted. Note also the two heads of the gastrocnemius.

actions: Hip extension and external rotation as well as knee flexion and external rotation.

INSPECTION AND PALPATION When knee flexion is resisted (subject prone), the long head of the biceps femoris may be observed and palpated from its attachment on the head of the fibula to the ischial tuberosity (Fig. 9–9). The short head is covered largely by the long head and is, therefore, difficult to identify. The common tendon of the two heads also is seen in Figure 10–8 as it approaches its attachment to the head of the fibula. The biceps tendon is easily palpated with the subject in the sitting position if the leg is externally rotated with respect to the femur.

Semitendinosus

The **semitendinosus** is one of the medial hamstrings, the muscular portion of which lies medial to that of the long head of the biceps in the posterior thigh. **Proximal attachment**: Tuberosity of the ischium, having a common tendon with the long head of the biceps. **Distal attachment**: Medial aspect of the tibia near the knee joint, distal to the attachment of the gracilis. **Innervation**: Branches of the sciatic nerve (L_5, $S_{1,2}$). **Anatomic actions**: Hip extension and internal rotation as well as knee flexion and internal rotation.

INSPECTION AND PALPATION With the subject prone, the tendon may be observed and palpated posteriorly on the medial side of the knee when knee flexion is resisted (Fig. 9–10). Palpation of the tendon also may be done with the subject in the sitting position. The palpating fingers are placed in the "fold" of the knee, medially, where several relaxed tendons may be distinguished. If the muscles of this region are then tightened without joint movement, the tendon of the semitendinosus rises markedly from the underlying tissue, as it is the most prominent tendon in the back of the knee. The tendon may be followed proximally toward the muscle belly as it proceeds obliquely toward the ischial tuberosity. Once the tendon of the semitendinosus has been identified, another small, firm, and round tendon may be palpated medially to the semitendinosus. This is the tendon of the adductor gracilis. The adductor gracilis may be distinguished from the semitendinosus by palpating the muscle belly toward its proximal attachment. The gracilis remains

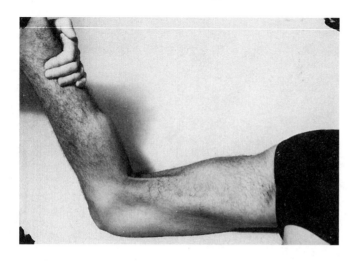

Figure 9–10 The prominent tendon of the semitendinosus is seen on the medial side of the posterior knee region when knee flexion is resisted.

medial in its course toward the pubis. In the sitting position, internal rotation of the leg with respect to the thigh also brings out the tendons of both the semitendinosus and gracilis.

Semimembranosus

The **semimembranosus** has a **proximal attachment** on the tuberosity of the ischium and a **distal attachment** on the medial condyle of the tibia. **Innervation:** Branches of the sciatic nerve (L_5, $S_{1,2}$). **Anatomic actions:** Knee flexion and internal rotation as well as hip extension and internal rotation.

PALPATION Although this muscle has the largest cross-section of the hamstrings, it is not easily palpated as an individual muscle because it is to a large extent covered by the semitendinosus and, proximally, by the adductor magnus. Together with these muscles, the semimembranosus makes up the large muscular mass of the medial and posterior thigh. The muscular portion of the semimembranosus extends farther distally than that of the semitendinosus; therefore, its lower portion may be palpated on both sides of the semitendinosus tendon. As the semimembranosus approaches its distal attachment, its tendon lies deep and can be palpated only with difficulty.

Gastrocnemius

The two heads of the gastrocnemius (Gr. *gaster*, belly, and *kneme*, leg) have their **proximal attachments** above the femoral condyles and span the knee joint on the flexor side. The muscular portion of the gastrocnemius may be seen contracting in resisted flexion of the knee (see Figs. 9–9 and 9–10). Because the gastrocnemius is more important as a plantar flexor of the ankle than as a knee flexor, it is discussed in more detail in Chapter 10.

Plantaris

The **plantaris**, a small muscle in the posterior knee region, has its **proximal attachment** above the lateral condyle of the femur, where it lies between the lateral head of the gastrocnemius and the popliteus, close to, and partially blended with, the capsule. Following the medial border of the soleus, it joins the Achilles tendon and attaches **distally** into the calcaneus. **Innervation:** Tibial nerve (L_5, S_1). The muscle belly is at times large and at times atrophied, and the specific function is unknown.

Popliteus

The **popliteus** is the most deeply located muscle in the back of the knee. It lies close to the capsule, covered by the plantaris and the lateral head of the gastrocnemius. **Proximal attachment:** By a strong tendon from the lateral condyle of the femur. The muscle fibers take a downward medial course and are attached into the proximal posterior portion of the body of the tibia. The **distal attachment** is widespread in a proximal-distal direction, giving the muscle a somewhat triangular shape. The location of the popliteus and the direction of its fibers are indicated in Figure 9–11. **Innervation:** Tibial nerve (L_4-S_1). **Anatomic actions:** Medial rotation and flexion of knee.

Rotators

The muscles that act in internal rotation of the tibia with respect to the femur are the **semitendinosus, semimembranosus, popliteus, gracilis**, and **sartorius**.

External rotation of the tibia with respect to the femur is accomplished by the **biceps femoris**, possibly aided by the tensor fasciae latae. That the biceps femoris is a strong external rotator may be ascertained by applying resistance to the motion with the subject in the sitting position. Contraction of the biceps femoris may be isolated from the medial hamstrings by placing the subject prone with the

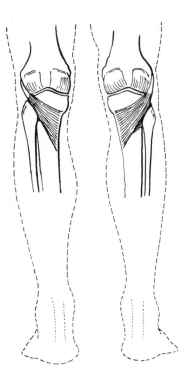

Figure 9–11   Location of the popliteus muscle.

knee flexed slightly beyond 90 degrees. The muscle will contract when performing external rotation of the knee.

The distal attachments of the tendons of the sartorius, gracilis, and semitendinosus are on the anterior medial surface of the tibia below the medial condyle, where they form the **pes anserinus** (L. *pes*, foot; *anserinus*, goose). Some of the fibers of these three tendons blend with each other and with the deep fasciae of the leg. The three muscles are thought to be important for medial stabilization of the knee.

FUNCTIONS OF MUSCLES OF THE KNEE

Knee Extensors

The quadriceps femoris is a large and powerful muscle capable of generating in excess of 1000 lb (4450 N or 2200 kg) of internal force. Such great force is needed in closed-chain motion to elevate and lower the body, as in rising from a chair, climbing, and jumping, and to prevent the knee from collapsing in walking, running, or landing from a jump. Here the quadriceps mechanism provides an active restraint to the femoral condyles on the tibial plateau to supplement passive restraints such as the posterior cruciate ligament and joint contours.

The rectus femoris crosses the hip and is a hip flexor as well as a knee extensor. As would be expected, the muscle becomes active as a knee extensor early in the range of motion when the hip is extended and the maximum torque output of the quadriceps is increased with hip extension. This effect can be observed when a seated subject is having difficulty extending the knee against resistance. If the subject leans back to place a stretch on the rectus femoris, increased force becomes available.

At one time it was thought that the vastus medialis was responsible for the last 20 to 30 degrees of knee extension. EMG studies have shown, however, that all four of the quadriceps muscles are active early and throughout the range of motion (Pocock, 1963; Leib and Perry, 1971). Basmajian (1978) found that while the onset of EMG activity in the four muscles was variable when knee extension was performed against little or no resistance, working against resistance caused all four muscles to be activated by 80 degrees of knee flexion. Anatomically and functionally, Leib and Perry (1968) further divide the vastus medialis into the vastus medialis longus (VML) and the vastus medialis oblique (VMO). The superior longitudinal fibers of the VML are directed 15 to 18 degrees medially from their attachment on the patella in the frontal plane. The prominent inferior fibers of the VMO are more obliquely directed to form an angle of 50 to 55 degrees. In a mechanical study on cadavers, the authors found that each of the quadriceps muscles **except** the VMO could extend the knee and that the vastus intermedius was the most efficient (required the least force). It was, however, impossible to extend the knee with the VMO regardless of the amount of force applied. The vastus medialis is believed to play an important role in keeping the patella on track in gliding on the femoral condyles (tracking mechanism). The medially directed forces of the VMO counteract the laterally directed forces of the vastus lateralis, thus preventing lateral displacement of the patella in the trochlear groove.

Knee Flexors

Open-chain motions of knee flexion and rotation are important for placement and movement of the foot but require little muscle force to execute (except for deceleration of the leg in walking or running). Great forces are required of these muscles, however, as they act on other joints or in closed-chain motion. The hamstring muscles are primary hip extensors and contract strongly to stabilize the pelvis during trunk extension (prone), and to control the pelvis on the femur as the seated or standing subject leans forward to touch the feet and then returns to the upright position (see Fig. 11–10). The hamstrings, sartorius, and the gracilis muscles have rotary actions at the hip and knee, and the popliteus is a rotator at the knee. After the foot is planted on the ground during the stance phase of walking, the knee and hip must rotate for forward motion of the body to occur over the supporting foot. The rotation is initiated and controlled by the rotator muscles. In activities such as running, turning, cutting, or maintaining balance on an unstable base of support (such as uneven ground or a rocking boat), the force required of the rotator muscles increases markedly. Activities carried out in the kneeling or squatting position (such as gardening, welding, mining, or playing football) require strong forces from the rotator muscles to initiate and control hip and knee motions on the fixed tibia in response to necessary twists of the trunk and upper extremities. Thus, injuries to the knee flexors (ie, hamstring "muscle pull") are more commonly due to their actions as rotators or as decelerators of limb motion than as flexors of the knee.

Popliteus

The popliteus muscle is deep set in the calf and difficult to palpate or study. Although considered a small muscle, it has a cross-sectional area larger than those of the gracilis or the sartorius muscles and an area approximately 70 percent as large as that of the semitendinosus. While the popliteus is classified as a knee flexor, its leverage is poor for this motion. Basmajian (1978) reported finding only 10 to 15 percent of maximum EMG activity of the popliteus associated with performance of knee flexion (prone) or knee extension (sitting). On the other hand, when these motions were performed with voluntary medial rotation of the knee, the activity of the popliteus increased to 40 to 70 percent of maximum activity. A greater amount of activity occurred during knee extension than during knee flexion!

An important function of the popliteus is considered to be its rotary action for unlocking the extended knee. Because terminal knee extension requires lateral rotation of the tibia on the femur, initiation of knee flexion requires the reverse action of medial rotation of the tibia on the femur. This action is thought to be performed by the popliteus muscle. An additional function of the muscle has been investigated electromyographically by Barnett and Richardson (1953). These investigators recorded large amounts of EMG activity from the popliteus when "knee bends" were performed from the standing position. When the knee approached a right angle, action potentials appeared in the popliteus, and the activity persisted as long as a crouching posture was maintained. The investigators point out that when the knee is bent, the weight of the body from above tends to cause the femoral condyle to slide forward on the tibial plateau, and "although the posterior cruciate ligament is generally credited with resisting this subluxation, it appears, in fact, that it has active support of the popliteus to stabilize the knee in this position."

The PCL attaches to the medial condyle of the femur, while the popliteus—by means of its strong tendon—attaches to the lateral condyle. The action of the popliteus, therefore, is an important complement to that of the posterior cruciate ligament in preventing a forward sliding of the condyles in weight bearing on flexed knees.

One-Joint and Two-Joint Muscles Acting at the Knee

Only five of the muscles that act on the knee are one-joint muscles: the three vasti, the popliteus, and the short head of the biceps femoris. The remaining muscles cross both the hip and knee (rectus femoris, sartorius, gracilis, semitendinosus, semimembranosus, long head of the biceps femoris, and the iliotibial tract of the tensor fasciae latae), or the knee and ankle (gastrocnemius). Thus, motions or positions of the hip and ankle influence the range of motion that can occur at the knee as well as the forces that the muscles can generate (passive and active insufficiency).

Under ordinary conditions of use, two-joint muscles are seldom used to move both joints simultaneously. More often, the action of two-joint muscles is prevented at one joint by resistance from gravity or the contraction of other muscles. If the muscles were to shorten over both joints simultaneously and to complete the range at both joints, they would have to shorten a long distance and would rapidly lose tension as the shortening progressed. In natural motions, however, the muscles are seldom, if ever, required to go through such extreme excursion. The two joints usually move in such directions that the muscle is gradually elongated over one joint while producing movement at the other joint. The result is that favorable length-tension relations are maintained.

Two-Joint Muscles of the Knee

The action of the two-joint muscles is considered in the following movement combinations:

KNEE FLEXION COMBINED WITH HIP EXTENSION If the subject is lying prone or standing erect and flexes the knee while extending the hip, the hamstring muscles must shorten over both joints simultaneously, and difficulty is experienced in completing knee flexion. Some subjects complain of a cramp in the muscles of the posterior thigh when performing this motion. All subjects lose strength rapidly as knee flexion proceeds while the hip is extended (see Fig. 4–8). The range of useful excursion becomes almost exhausted. Another factor that often limits full excursion of the hamstrings is the inability of the rectus femoris, which is being stretched over the hip and knee simultaneously, to elongate sufficiently. When spasticity of the rectus femoris is present, the interference of this muscle becomes marked, resulting in a forward tilting of the pelvis; in the prone position, the buttocks then become elevated in an awkward manner.

KNEE EXTENSION COMBINED WITH HIP FLEXION In a supine or standing position, straight leg raising—consisting of hip flexion with the knee maintained extended—may be performed. The movement proceeds without strain throughout a certain range; then difficulty arises mainly from the inability of the hamstrings to elongate sufficiently and, to a lesser extent, from the decrease in strength of the rectus muscle, which has to shorten over the hip and knee simultaneously. By performing a passive movement of hip flexion, first with the knee extended and then with the knee flexed, the effect of hamstring interference in hip flexion becomes obvious. If straight leg raising is limited by contracture or spasticity (eg, 30 degrees), normal step length is diminished in walking. The knee may be extended fully on one side when the hip is extended, but the opposite leg is not capable of reaching as far forward (hip flexion and knee extension) as usual. The subject is limited to short steps and usually walks with the knees flexed.

KNEE FLEXION COMBINED WITH HIP FLEXION   This combination provides for elongation of the hamstrings over the hip while knee flexion is carried out, resulting in favorable length-tension relations (see Fig. 4–17). During hip-knee flexion, the hip flexors and the hamstrings act synergistically to provide a functionally useful movement whereas in other movement combinations, these two muscle groups may act as antagonists.

KNEE EXTENSION COMBINED WITH HIP EXTENSION   This is a most useful combination that occurs in activities such as rising from the sitting position, climbing stairs, running, and jumping. The hamstrings then act as hip extensors, while the quadriceps extends the knee and, by doing so, elongates the hamstrings over the knee. In this movement, as in the previous one, an effective portion of the length-tension curve is used.

In closed-chain motion, co-contraction of the hamstrings and quadriceps occurs to elevate the body (knee extension and hip extension) or lower the body (knee flexion and hip flexion). When a person stands up from a chair, the quadriceps performs a concentric contraction to extend the knee, and the hamstrings perform a concentric contraction to extend the hip. When the person sits down, eccentric contractions of both muscle groups control the rate of knee flexion (quadriceps) and hip flexion (hamstrings).

KNEE FLEXION COMBINED WITH PLANTAR FLEXION OF THE ANKLE   The gastrocnemius is capable of performing these two motions simultaneously, but if full range at both joints is attempted, the muscle has to shorten a long distance, and tension falls rapidly. It is not a very useful movement.

KNEE EXTENSION COMBINED WITH PLANTAR FLEXION OF THE ANKLE   The quadriceps extends the knee while the gastrocnemius (and soleus) plantarflex the ankle. As the quadriceps extends the knee, the gastrocnemius becomes elongated over the knee, and optimal conditions result for plantar flexion of the ankle. This functional combination is commonly seen, for example, in rising on tiptoes, running, and jumping.

JOINT FORCES

Even in normal activity, the articulating surfaces of the knee sustain forces that far exceed body weight and are thus subject to microtrauma and its subsequent degenerative results (Davies, Wallace, and Malone, 1980). Maximum isometric knee extension was calculated by Smidt (1973) to produce a femorotibial compression force of 1.6 times the body weight when the knee was extended and three times the body weight when the knee was in a position of 60 degrees. In Figure 2–24, the joint force was calculated as 350 lb when holding a 30-lb weight on the foot. Symptomatic inflammatory responses may occur when these forces are accompanied by overuse of the knee (eg, gardening, jogging, or roofing) and by hypermobility or hypomobility of joint structures from the foot to the spine, which call for compensatory motion or stabilization at the knee during weight-bearing activities (Davies, Wallace, and Malone, 1980). For example, excessive pronation at the ankle produces increased medial rotation of the tibia and repetitive abnormal stresses on knee joint structures.

Tibiofemoral Joint Forces

When standing on both feet, the body weight vector passes between the knees, and each tibial plateau has a compressive force of 45 percent of body weight (68 lb in a 150-lb person). In unilateral stance, however, the compressive force increases to about twice the body weight (Fig. 9–12). This force is equally distributed over the weight-bearing surfaces of the tibia (Maquet, 1983). The knee supports the weight of the thigh, HAT, and the opposite lower extremity. This weight acts through a center of gravity that is slightly higher than S_2 and projects to the base of support, thus passing on the medial side of the knee causing a varus thrust (see Fig. 9–12A, B). The force of the weight is counterbalanced by dynamic and static forces of the iliotibial band. Dynamic forces occur at both the hip and knee in unilateral stance through the attachments of the gluteus maximus and the tensor fasciae latae muscles. Tension of the band can be palpated on the lateral thigh to the tibia when a person stands on one leg. Increase or decrease in the torque of the weight in a normal subject is counterbalanced by increase or decrease in the dynamic force of the iliotibial band so that weight bearing continues to be equally distributed on the tibial condyles.

Tibiofemoral joint forces during walking have been calculated to be up to six times body weight at the beginning of the single-leg stance phase. During the stance phase, the compression forces fall to equal body weight and then rise to four times body weight at the end of single-leg stance. In the swing phase, the compression on the joint surfaces is less than body weight (Maquet, 1983).

Abnormalities that alter the torque of the weight or the iliotibial band cause movement of the central joint force medially or laterally with unequal distribution of compression forces (Maquet, 1983). Areas receiving excessive physiologic pressure over many years may develop pain, destruction of cartilage, and osteoarthritis. Conditions that can change the forces or the lever arms to produce these problems include paralysis of the tensor fasciae latae muscle; iliotibial band tightness; obesity; genu varus or valgus; traumatic or surgical shortening of the neck of the femur; excessive pronation of the foot; or changes in alignment of the femur, tibia, or foot from fractures.

An example of biomechanical causes in the development of knee joint pathology can be seen in obesity. As the weight gain increases, the individual can be seen to shift the trunk more and more laterally with each step in walking. This maneuver decreases the force that the hip abductor muscles must generate to balance the increased weight (see Figs. 8–17C and 8–18). The tensor fasciae latae is one of these muscles and therefore the force and torque it contributes at the knee are decreased (see Fig. 9–12). In addition, the excessive lateral trunk shift causes the force of the weight to move from the medial side of the knee joint toward the lateral side, with the joint reaction force moving laterally as well. This produces asymmetric distribution of condylar pressures with excess pressure on the lateral condyles and a valgus thrust. In time, these abnormal forces can lead to a knee-knee deformity, cartilaginous and meniscal thinning and destruction, and osteoarthritis (Maquet, 1983).

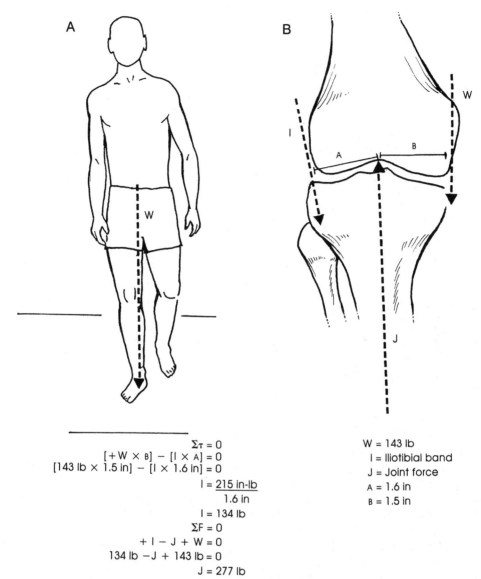

$$\Sigma\tau = 0$$
$$[+W \times B] - [I \times A] = 0$$
$$[143 \text{ lb} \times 1.5 \text{ in}] - [I \times 1.6 \text{ in}] = 0$$
$$I = \frac{215 \text{ in-lb}}{1.6 \text{ in}}$$
$$I = 134 \text{ lb}$$
$$\Sigma F = 0$$
$$+I - J + W = 0$$
$$134 \text{ lb} - J + 143 \text{ lb} = 0$$
$$J = 277 \text{ lb}$$

W = 143 lb
I = Iliotibial band
J = Joint force
A = 1.6 in
B = 1.5 in

Figure 9–12   Calculation of forces on the tibiofemoral joint in the frontal plane when a 150-lb person is standing on one leg shows compression forces of almost twice the body weight. (*A*) Projection of the center of gravity of the body to the base of support. (*B*) Vector diagram of the forces on the tibia during unilateral stance for a person weighing 150 lb. W = body weight minus the weight of the leg. A and B = perpendicular distance from the force vectors of W and I to the axis of motion (distances were measured on a femur).

Patellofemoral Joint Forces

For simplification, the patella can be considered to act like the rope on a pulley (trochlear surface of the femoral condyles), with the force generated in the quadriceps tendon equal to the force in the patellar tendon (Fig. 9–13). The result of these two forces is the patellofemoral joint compression force. Actually, the forces in patellar and quadriceps tendons differ because of the shape of the bones and the attachments of the tendons (Hehne, 1990). The large forces that can be created by the quadriceps muscle (eg, 380 lb with a 30-lb boot in Fig. 2–24) also pro-

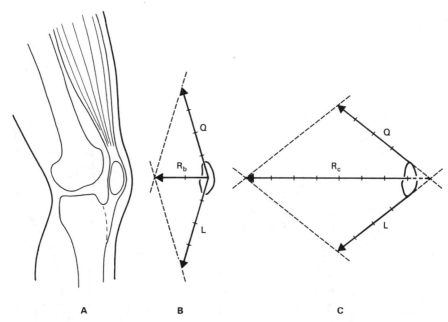

A   **B**   **C**

Figure 9–13 Patellofemoral joint compression forces. (*A*) Lateral view of the patellofemoral articulation. (*B*) Graphic composition of the forces on the patella during active contraction of the quadriceps muscle group when the knee is in slight flexion and (*C*) when in marked flexion. Q = quadriceps muscle force; L = force of the patellar ligament; R = resultant of Q and L, or the patellofemoral compression force. Even with a similar force in Q, R is seen to increase with the joint angle ($R_c > R_b$).

duce large compression forces between the patella and the femur. When the knee is in extension, the resultant force is small because the forces of the tendon and the ligament are almost on a straight line. When the knee is flexed, the resultant force becomes large and can easily exceed the force of the muscle. Smidt (1973) calculated patellofemoral joint reaction force in maximum isometric quadriceps contractions as 0.8 times body weight when the knee was in the 15-degree position. The force increased to 2.6 times body weight when the knee was at a 90-degree angle. During level walking, the joint reaction forces were calculated by Reilly and Martens (1972) to be one half or less of body weight. Patients with patellofemoral dysfunction find that pain is increased in ascending or descending stairs and in activities requiring kneeling or squatting. Quadriceps resistive exercises through a full arc of knee extension may be impossible to complete because of pain. When pain is present, quadriceps muscles may be strengthened by applying resistance with the knee in an extended position, or through a short arc of terminal extension (eg, 20 degrees).

Torque of Muscles Acting at the Knee

An example of maximum isokinetic torques for the quadriceps and hamstring muscles is shown in Figure 4–19. At slow speeds of motion (below 30 degrees per second), the peak torque values are similar to those obtained under isometric conditions. Peak torques decrease with the velocity of concentric muscle contractions at speeds from 30 to 360 degrees per second (see Fig. 4–19). Eccentric muscle contraction produces peak torques that are higher than maximum isometric torques and torques that do not change with velocity of motion (Westring and Seger, 1989).

Quadriceps Femoris Torque

Early investigators using isometric measurements found that maximum force of the knee extensors reached a peak at about 60 degrees of knee flexion and decreased with further extension of the knee as seen in Fig. 4–18 (Williams and Stutzman, 1959; Mendler, 1963; 1967b). In concentric isokinetic measurements, peak extensor torque also occurs near 60 degrees with slow velocities. Velocities above 60 degrees per second show that the peak torques occur progressively later in the range of motion (see Fig. 4–19). Westring and Seger (1989) have demonstrated, however, that when the quadriceps and hamstring torques are corrected for the effect of gravity on the weight of the leg and the dynamometer arm, the angle at which peak force occurs remains constant around 50 to 60 degrees of motion. Such gravity corrections for isokinetic knee flexion and extension in the sitting position require measuring and adding the torque of the weight of the leg and the dynamometer arm to the recorded torque of the quadriceps and subtracting this torque from that produced by the hamstring muscles (Fillyaw, Bevins, and Fernandez, 1986).

The increase in torque output while the quadriceps are losing favorable length-tension relationships is due to the changing patella lever arm distance within the range of motion. When the knee is fully flexed, the patella lies in the intercondylar groove and close to the axis of motion. (The quadriceps muscle is at this point stretched and has an advantageous length-tension position.) As the knee is extended, the patella moves out of the groove to reach a maximum lever arm distance at 45 degrees of flexion. Smidt (1973) measured mean patellar lever arm distances of 3.8 cm at 90 degrees of flexion and 4.9 cm at 45 degrees. The lever arm distance then decreased to 4.4 cm at full extension. In a cadaver study, however, Kaufer (1971) measured a consistent increase in patellar force arm distance from knee flexion to extension. With patellectomy (surgical removal of the patella), a 30 percent increase in quadriceps muscle force was required to extend the knee (Kaufer, 1971).

Functionally, the greater torque output of the quadriceps muscle at the 50- to 60-degree position coincides with a need for large torques in elevation of the body, as in rising from a chair and climbing. In these activities, a perpendicular line from the center of gravity of the body falls well posterior to the knee axis and therefore exerts a large resistance torque for the quadriceps to match. Very little torque is required of the quadriceps in erect standing.

Knee Flexor Muscle Torque

The maximum isometric torque measurement of the curves for the hamstring muscles shows the greatest torque to occur when the muscles are elongated at both the hip and knee (hip flexion and knee extension) and the lowest torque when the muscles contract in the shortened position of hip extension and knee flexion (see Fig. 4–17). The length-tension factor seems to predominate in torque production even though there are changes in the muscle force arm distances that are occurring. Smidt (1973) found mean force arm distances for the knee flexors of 2.5 cm at 90 degrees of flexion, 4.1 cm at 45 degrees, and 2.5 cm at full extension. Functionally, the need for great torque in the knee-extended–hip-flexing position occurs in closed-chain motion when the hamstring muscles are the primary muscle group used to lower and raise the weight of the trunk and arms when a person is reaching over to touch the floor or bending forward in the sitting position (see Fig. 11–10).

Hamstrings to Quadriceps Torque Ratio

The peak torques for the quadriceps muscles are greater than those of the knee flexors (see Fig. 4–19). This is not unexpected because the knee extensors have over twice the cross-sectional area of the knee flexors (Lehmkuhl and Smith, 1983), and the knee extensors have a longer force arm distance than the flexors (Smidt, 1973). Strength imbalance between these muscle groups has been suggested as a basis for injuries such as hamstring strains. Normative values for hamstring/quadriceps ratios (peak torque of hamstrings divided by peak torque of quadriceps) are 0.60 to 0.69 at 60 degrees per second increasing to 0.85 to 0.95 at 300 degrees per second not corrected for gravity (Davies, 1988). When corrected for gravity, the ratio is lower (ie, 0.45 to 0.55) and does not change with speed (Fillyaw, Bevins, and Fernandez, 1986; Westring and Seger, 1989).

INTERACTION OF MUSCLES AND LIGAMENTS IN FUNCTION

Although the static ligamentous and capsular structures of the knee can limit manual passive joint movements, these structures are unable to withstand the high forces that occur in even ordinary daily activities of standing, walking, ascending stairs, or rising from a chair. An example of such incompetency is illustrated in Figure 9–14, where ligaments and the posterior capsule have been used for years to attempt to limit hyperextension of the knee.

Normally, both the dynamic contraction of muscles and the static forces of the ligaments and capsule are used to stabilize the knee. The ligaments and other soft tissues additionally provide a sensory system for proprioception and kinesthesia (see Chapter 3), as well as input for producing reflex muscle contraction to unload and protect ligaments (Barrack and Skinner, 1990). Considerable basic information is available in the physiologic literature on neurology of animal joints. Clinicians, however, have previously focused on the passive and mechanical roles of the ligaments. The frequency of progressive instability and disability after ligament injuries and repairs, however, has directed attention to investigation of sensory functions of ligaments and joint tissues in human subjects.

Sensory Innervation and Reflexes

The ligaments, capsule, and other soft tissues of the knee are richly innervated with sensory nerve fibers and receptors (see Fig. 3–9). Mechanoreceptors have been found in human cruciate and collateral ligaments, the capsule, and synovial lining and on the outer edges of the menisci (Kennedy, Alexander, and Hayes, 1982; Schutte et al, 1987). Reflexes from joint mechanoreceptors to the muscles have been demonstrated in human subjects, including facilitation of the hamstrings and inhibition of the quadriceps with loading the ACL (Solomonow et al, 1987). Swelling in the joint capsule has long been known to produce inhibition of the quadriceps muscle and a sudden collapse of the knee. This inhibition has been considered to be caused by deformation of the mechanoreceptors in the ligaments and capsule. Infusion of only 60 mL of normal saline solution into the joint cap-

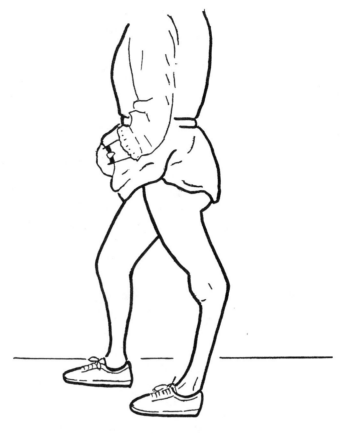

Figure 9–14 Genu recurvatum from long-term reliance on ligamentous and capsular structures for stability. This patient had poliomyelitis when she was a young woman, resulting in paralysis of her hamstring and gastrocnemius-soleus muscles (note atrophy). She has good but not normal strength in her quadriceps muscles. For 30 years she walked with hyperextension of the knee, which gradually stretched the ligaments and the posterior capsule. Recently she began to have pain in the knee.

sule produced a 30 to 50 percent decrease of the EMG amplitude of the quadriceps muscle (Kennedy, Alexander, and Hayes, 1982). Clinically, Barrack, Skinner, and Buckley (1989) demonstrated over a 25 percent increase in the threshold for proprioception (of slow passive motion) in knees with complete ACL tears compared to the normal knee. The last two groups suggest that people with complete tears of the ACL may lose the stabilizing reflexes of ligaments as well.

Static and Dynamic Connections

In addition to neural elements, there are important local connections between the dynamic and static structures that were described earlier in this chapter (anatomic basis for joint motion). These interconnections include the numerous attachments to the menisci, the reinforcement of the capsule by ligaments and retinacula, the extensive soft tissue attachments of the semimembranosus and the iliotibial band, and the penetration of the capsule by the popliteus muscle.

Balanced Torques

To simplify and find solutions, biomechanical problems are reduced to a minimum number of forces as in Figures 2–19 and 2–24, where only three forces were considered: the resistance, the muscle, and the joint reaction forces. In real movement, many muscle and ligament forces occur and vary so that balanced torques in each plane are maintained throughout the range of motion (see Balanced Forces, Chapter 6). Usually all the muscles that cross a joint participate in the motion to variable degrees, and co-contraction is common. O'Connor and coworkers (1990) propose that the body has many muscle and ligament combinations to provide balanced torques and that the individual can consciously or subconsciously select options. A simple example is the ability to stabilize a joint with only ligaments or with only isometric muscle contractions. More choices occur when the rotary component of the patellar tendon force vector causes an anterior translatory torque on the tibia (Fig. 9–15). This torque can be balanced by passive ACL force, active hamstring muscle contraction, or by a combination of ACL and hamstring forces. Experimentally, such anterior translation has been demonstrated in cadavers by applying quadriceps force with intact and severed anterior cruciate ligaments. Greater anterior displacement occurred in the ACL-deficient knee from 30 degrees of flexion to extension in the unloaded tibia. In the loaded tibia, the amount of anterior displacement increased and occurred at 70 degrees in the range of motion (Grood et al, 1984).

Muscle Protection of Ligaments

The use of muscles to unload ligaments is illustrated in walking at the termination of the swing phase. Here the hamstring muscles contract to decelerate the swinging leg and to unload the anterior cruciate ligament (see Fig. 12–21[4]). Such muscle contraction was not available to the lady in Figure 9–14 and thus was one of the factors leading to ligamentous laxity. In pathologic situations when muscles substitute for ligamentous action, there is an increase in muscle contraction and an increase in energy expenditure. EMG during level and grade walking in people with complete ACL ruptures showed significantly higher amplitudes in the medial head of the gastrocnemius as compared to normal subjects. This muscle, the hamstrings, and the vastus medialis and lateralis had earlier onsets of contraction in the gait cycle but were not significantly different at all grades. There was also a tendency for increased duration of contraction in the gait cycle (Lass et al, 1991). Although voluntary reaction time for muscular protection of the knee is too slow

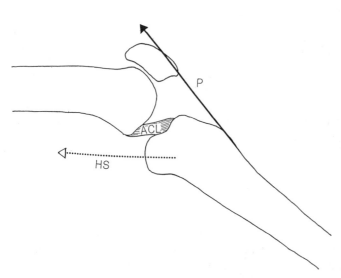

Figure 9–15 Longitudinal section through the knee at 40 degrees of flexion illustrates the line of action and direction of the patellar tendon force P when the quadriceps muscle contracts in open-chain motion. The direction of P produces a superior-anterior force on the tibia. This force causes anterior dislocation of the tibia during knee extension if the force is not counteracted by other forces. Forces that can prevent anterior dislocation of the tibia in this position are the anterior cruciate ligament (ACL), active contraction of the hamstring muscles (HS), or a combination of both the passive ligamentous force and the dynamic muscle force.

in many sports situations, the latter authors recommend that rehabilitation programs include coordination training. Decreased hamstring reaction time in individuals with knee injuries has been demonstrated with a 12-week dynamic closed-chain coordination program (Ihara and Nakayma, 1986).

CLINICAL APPLICATIONS

Quadriceps muscle paralysis occurs with severance of the femoral nerve from a gunshot or other trauma. The person is unable to extend the knee in the sitting position or perform straight leg raising when supine. When the person is prone, the knee can be flexed and extended by concentric and eccentric contractions of the hamstring muscles. Many compensations, however, can be used by adults so that they can walk and function in a safe manner without a noticeable limp.

In the upright position, momentum from the hip can be used to straighten the knee in walking. The big problem is to keep the knee from buckling when weight is placed on the extremity in stance phase. A very effective compensation is that of using the gluteus maximus to extend the knee in closed-chain motion. This occurs in the stance phase of walking at the time of and following heel strike. Some people develop such strength and control of the knee with the gluteus maximus that they can prevent the knee from buckling when they are standing, even if a strong push is applied to the back of the knee. When more force is needed, such as in stair climbing, the hand on the side of the weak quadriceps is used to push on the thigh. This can be done in a casual manner and is seldom noticed as an abnormality by others. Some individuals develop a form of hop-and-skip run by using the gluteus maximus together with the hand to keep the weak knee straight. Rising up from low chairs usually can be accomplished by the strong leg and by pushing up with the hands if needed. A very discrete compensation often seen in walking is a slight forward lean from the hips. This places the center of gravity of HAT in front of the knee axis of motion in the sagittal plane, and quadriceps muscle force is not needed to keep the knee extended. Instead, there is a hyperextension force that is limited by the posterior capsule, PCL, and hamstring muscles.

An orthosis (brace) may be needed for those who cannot learn these techniques, those who exert destructive forces on their knee joint when walking, or those who have pain. Even the very slight forward-leaning posture can cause low back pain over time. It is particularly important not to permit use of these quadriceps compensations in growing children. Instead, an orthosis is needed to prevent genu recurvatum and other ligamentous laxities and bony deformities. Compliance, however, is often a challenge because the child may be able to walk and run without the orthosis.

Laboratory Activities |

KNEE REGION

1. On the bones, identify the following bony landmarks and determine those that are palpable.

Femur	*Tibia*
medial and lateral condyles	medial and lateral condyles
epicondyles	tibial plateau
adductor tubercle	intercondylar eminence
linea aspera	tibial tuberosity
medial and lateral	anterior border
supracondylar lines	interosseous border
intercondylar notch	proximal articular surfaces
popliteal surface	
patellar surface	
distal articular surfaces	
Fibula	*Patella*
head, neck, shaft	anterior and posterior
	surfaces

2. While seated with the knee bent, palpate on yourself and then on a classmate the patella, anterior border of tibia, head of the fibula, tibial tuberosity, medial and lateral epicondyles of femur, and lateral condyle of tibia. Locate medially and laterally the joint space between the tibia and femur. With the knee extended, grasp your patella and move it passively from side to side and in an up-and-down movement from proximal to distal end. Keep the quadriceps muscle completely relaxed to accomplish this maneuver. Repeat this same procedure on a partner.

3. With a partner in the prone position, passively flex the knee. Note the range of motion and the end-feel. Have the partner turn on one side so that the hip can be flexed, and then repeat passive knee flexion. Why is there more motion when the hip is flexed? What is the limiting structure to knee flexion when the hip is flexed and when it is extended?

4. Have your partner sit in a chair. Observe terminal rotation of the tibia on the femur when the knee is slowly extended. Then observe the femur internally rotating on the fixed tibia as the partner slowly stands up.

5. Have your partner perform axial rotation of the knee sitting in a chair with the heel touching the floor. Observe and palpate the movement of the medial and lateal malleoli and then the tibial condyles. Note that as the knee is placed more toward extension, rotation is less, and when the knee is in full extension, axial rotation of the knee is impossible. Attempts cause rotation in the hip.

6. Select a partner. Following the descriptions in this chapter, palpate knee muscles and tendons:
   quadriceps femoris
   biceps femoris
   semimembranosus
   semitendinosus
   adductor gracilis
   proximal attachments of gastrocnemius
   distal attachments of sartorius and tensor fasciae latae

7. Have your partner stand in a normal (relaxed) manner with eyes straight ahead (if the subject looks down, the muscle activity changes). Palpate the quadriceps and hamstring muscles during the following activities. Note whether the muscles are relaxed or have a slight or strong contraction:

   a. Normal relaxed standing.

   b. Sway forward from the ankles, return, and then sway back slightly.

   c. Stand on one leg.

   d. Hyperextend the knees.

   e. Bend forward at the hips to touch floor. Return to erect position.

   f. Perform a deep knee bend (squat) and return.

8. Palpate the hamstrings and the quadriceps with the subject sitting in a chair, slowly rising to the standing position, standing, and then slowly returning to the sitting position. Why do both the quadriceps and the hamstrings contract when rising up and sitting down? What type of contraction is occurring in the vasti muscle on rising and on sitting down?

9. Analyze quadriceps and hamstring muscle activity in ascending and descending stairs for both the lead leg and the following leg.

CHAPTER 10

Ankle and Foot

The ankle, foot, and toes consist of a complex of 34 joints that, by bony structure, ligamentous attachments, and muscle contraction, can change in a single step from a flexible structure conforming to the irregularities of the ground to a rigid weight-bearing structure. The flexible-rigid characteristics of the ankle-foot complex provide multiple functions, including:

- Support of superincumbent weight
- Control and stabilization of the leg on the planted foot
- Adjustments to irregular surfaces
- Elevation of the body, as in standing on the toes, climbing, or jumping
- Shock absorption in walking, running, or landing from a jump
- Operation of machine tools
- Substitution for hand function in persons with upper extremity amputations or muscle paralysis

Ankle injuries and foot pain and dysfunction are common and stem from the large forces that occur in the foot and ankle even in standing (see Fig. 2–16). Ankle joint forces up to 4.5 times body weight while walking on a level surface were calculated by Stauffer and associates (1977). As the foot sustains these large forces, it is also making the final adjustment to the ground and must compensate for motions or deviations at the knee or hip to keep the center of gravity within the small base of support. When the foot is not protected by a shoe, the structures are subjected to trauma and temperature extremes. If the foot is enclosed in a shoe, the structures may be subjected to abnormal pressures and friction, as well as to a warm, humid environment conducive to bacterial and fungal growth and infection.

PALPABLE STRUCTURES

The malleoli of the ankle, like the epicondyles of the knee, serve as landmarks for their respective regions. The **medial malleolus** (L. diminutive of *malleus*, hammer) is a prominent process of the enlarged distal portion of the tibia on the inner side of the ankle. The **lateral malleolus** is found on the outer side of the ankle. It is the most distal portion of the fibula (see Fig. 10–5).

Palpation of the malleoli reveals that the lateral malleolus projects farther distally than the medial one. Thus, lateral motion of the ankle is more limited than medial motion. If the subject stands with the kneecap pointing straight forward (knee axis in frontal plane), palpation also reveals that the lateral malleolus has a more posterior location than the medial one. The axis of the ankle joint is identified by an imaginary line just distal to the tips of the malleoli (Inman, 1976).

Palpation on the medial side of the foot (Fig. 10–1C): Just distal to the tip of the medial malleolus, the edge of the **sustentaculum tali** (L. *sustenataculum*, a support) may be felt as a slight protuberance (about the distance of a finger width) (see Fig. 10–1C). The sustentaculum tali is like a shelf of the calcaneus, which supports the inferior medial aspect of the talus and where the two bones form one of their three articulations. If the finger is moved toward the toe, again about a finger width, the more prominent **tuberosity of the navicular** (L. *navicula*, diminutive of navis, ship) can be felt. The strong **calcaneonavicular or spring ligament** runs from the sustentaculum tali to the tuberosity of the

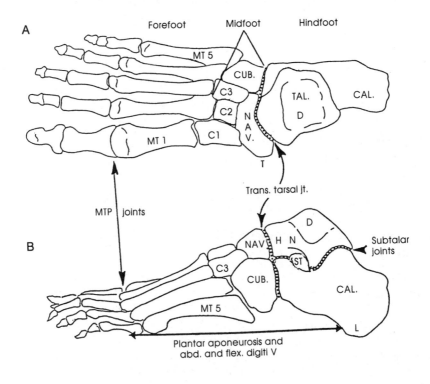

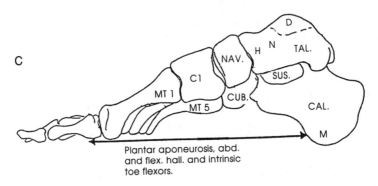

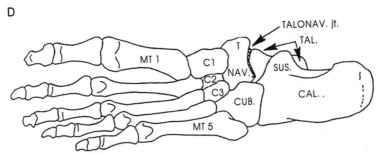

Figure 10–1 Schematic view of the bones of the foot, joints, and static and dynamic support of the arches. (*A*) Dorsal view. (*B*) Lateral view. (*C*) Medial view. (*D*) Plantar view. TAL. = talus; CAL. = calcaneus; NAV. = navicular; CUB. = cuboid; C1, C2, and C3 = medial, intermediate, and lateral cuneiforms; MT 1–5 = metatarsals 1–5. Areas of bones: D = dome of talus; N = neck of talus; H = head of talus; T = tuberosity of the navicular; ST = sinus tarsi; L = lateral tuberosity of the calcaneus; and M = medial tuberosity of the calcaneus. The line of action of the plantar aponeurosis is intended to represent the general direction of both static and dynamic support of the arches, which, in addition, include other ligamentous and extrinsic muscle contractions.

navicular. This ligament supports the head of the talus and, when overstretched, permits the talus to move medially and plantarward, thus reducing the amount of longitudinal arch and producing a flatfoot deformity. If the palpating finger is placed between the tuberosity of the navicular and the distal end of the medial malleolus, the **talus** can be felt. The bone becomes more prominent when the foot is passively everted and then disappears as the foot is inverted. Immediately posterior to the distal end of the medial malleolus, the small prominence of the **medial tubercule of the talus** can sometimes be palpated.

The four landmarks (the medial malleolus, the tuberosity of the navicular, the sustentaculum tali, and the medial tuberosity of the talus) are the attachments of the **medial collateral**, or **deltoid ligament** of the ankle. Within this triangle, the deltoid ligament may be palpated. Identification in the subjects is difficult; pain or tenderness in this area may be indicative of ligamentous tear or strain (Hoppenfeld, 1976). The deltoid ligaments of both ankles are composed of both deep and superficial layers, and they prevent lateral motion of the ankle or talocrural joint (talus-tibia-fibula). The deltoid ligaments are so strong that eversion sprains are unusual; with severe lateral motion, avulsion (L. *avulsio*, from *a*, away, plus *vellere*, to pull) of the ligamentous attachments or fracture may occur before ligamentous tears.

As the palpating finger proceeds from the tuberosity of the navicular toward the toe on the medial side of the foot, the **first cuneiform** is palpated followed by a prominence of the **first tarsometatarsal joint**, the concave shaft of the **first metatarsal**, and the prominence and joint line of the **first metatarsophalangeal (MTP) joint**.

Palpation on the lateral side of the foot: A large area of the lateral surface of the **calcaneus** may be palpated (see Fig. 10–1B). The posterior portion feels relatively smooth, but a small process may be felt below and slightly anterior to the tip of the lateral malleolus. This process is an attachment for a **lateral collateral ligament (calcaneofibular)** and separates the tendons of the peroneus longus and brevis. More anteriorly, the **tuberosity at the base of the fifth metatarsal bone** may be felt as a large, easily identified prominence on the lateral side of the foot near the sole. The **cuboid bone** may be palpated between the calcaneus and the tuberosity of the fifth metatarsal bone and may be followed dorsally toward its articulations with the lateral cuneiform and with the navicular bones. The cuboid extends dorsally to about the middle of the foot, but this area is covered by ligaments and tendons, and the various bones are difficult to distinctly recognize.

The **three cuneiform bones** (L. *cuneus*, wedge) that lie across the instep of the foot form the arched part of the dorsum of the foot. The height of this arched portion varies considerably in different individuals. The **medial cuneiform** bone is identified by its medial position between the tuberosity of the navicular bone and the base of the first metatarsal bone. The **intermediate** and **lateral cuneiform bones** lie in line with the second and third metatarsal bones, respectively, articulating proximally with the navicular bone (see Fig. 10–1A and D).

The **tarsometatarsal articulations** can be palpated on their dorsal surfaces if the metatarsal bones are passively moved up and down or rotated. The second tarsometatarsal joint is strongly mortised into the recess formed by the three cuneiforms and the third metatarsal and thus forms a very rigid part of the arch (see Fig. 10–1A).

The **heads of the metatarsal bones** are felt both on the dorsal and the plantar sides of the foot. By manipulating the toes in flexion and extension, the heads of the metatarsal bones are particularly well palpated from the plantar side. Their plantar surfaces constitute the ball of the foot on which weight is carried when standing on tiptoes. In the region of the head of the first metatarsal bone, the sesamoid bones, which are imbedded in the tendon of the flexor hallucis brevis, can sometimes be palpated and moved slightly from side to side. The **shafts of the metatarsal bones** are best palpated on the dorsum of the foot. The phalanges of the toes are easily recognized. The **interphalangeal** (IP) **joints** should be palpated and manipulated.

The **talus** (astragalus), articulating with the tibia and the fibula above, with the calcaneus below, and with the navicular bone in front, has only small palpable areas. If the finger is placed on the anterior side of the lateral malleolus, the **trochlea** (dome) of the talus becomes prominent with passive plantar flexion. Slightly distal to this point is a depression that lies over the **sinus tarsi**, which is a channel that runs between the articulations of the talus and the calcaneus. If the foot is inverted, the neck of the talus may become more prominent. Over the sinus tarsi lies the **anterior talofibular ligament**, one of the three lateral collateral ligaments of the ankle. The **calcaneofibular ligament** courses from the distal end of the lateral malleolus to the lateral aspect of the calcaneus, and the **posterior talofibular ligament** runs horizontally from the posterior portion of the lateral malleolus to the talus. The lateral collateral ligaments limit medial motion of the talus and calcaneus. The anterior talofibular ligament also limits anterior movement of the talus and is commonly sprained in inversion injuries of the ankle.

NONPALPABLE STRUCTURES

Because of the joint capsules and the many ligaments (short, long, transverse, longitudinal, and oblique) that cross the various joints of the foot, the shape of each individual bone cannot be palpated in detail. Shapes of the articulating surfaces should be studied on a disarticulated bone set. The attachments and course of the **long plantar ligament** should be noted from the plantar surface of the calcaneus (anterior to the tuberosity) to the bases of the third, fourth, and fifth metatarsals. The **tarsal canal** (between the talus and the calcaneus) should be explored and the strong interosseous (talocalcaneal) ligament visualized. This ligament becomes a major limiting factor in the motion between the two bones.

Several of the bones of the foot have grooves to accommodate tendons. A groove on the inferior surface of the cuboid bone contains the tendon of the peroneus longus; the tendon of the flexor hallucis longus is lodged in a groove on the talus, then courses below the sustentaculum tali of the calcaneus; the same tendon, nearing its digital attachment on the distal phalanx, passes through an osteofibrous groove on the plantar surface of the big toe.

JOINTS

Talocrural Joint

Type of Joint

The talocrural joint, between the talus and the **crus** (L. leg), is a hinge joint with one degree of freedom of motion. The talocrural joint is usually referred to as the "ankle joint." The trochlea of the talus possesses a superior weight-bearing surface that articulates with the distal end of the tibia and has medial and lateral surfaces that articulate with the medial malleolus of the tibia and the lateral malleolus of the fibula. The tibia and fibula are bound together by the anterior and inferior talofibular ligaments. Thus, the malleoli form a strong mortise for the trochlea of the wedge-shaped talus.

Axis of Motion

A line connecting points just distal to the tips of the malleoli identifies the approximate direction of the ankle joint axis (Fig. 10–2). When the horizontal axis (x axis) of the knee is perpendicular to the midline of the body (ie, sagittal plane) the tip of the medial malleolus is usually anterior and superior to the lateral malleolus. Thus, the axis of the ankle is oblique to both the sagittal and frontal planes, and, according to Inman (1976), the vertical axis (y) is also oblique to the horizontal plane.

   A single joint axis that is not perpendicular to the cardinal planes but intersects all three planes is called a **triplanar axis** (McPoil and Brocato, 1985). Motion around this axis occurs in all three planes. In the ankle joint, Lundberg and coworkers (1989a) produced 30 degrees of plantar flexion from the neutral position. They measured motions of up to 28 degrees in the sagittal plane (plantar flexion), one degree in the horizontal plane (in the direction of internal rotation), and 4 degrees in the frontal plane (pronation). With 30 degrees of dorsiflexion, these authors measured 23 degrees in the sagittal plane, 9 degrees in the horizontal plane (in the direction of external rotation), and 2 degrees in the frontal plane (supination).

   When a person is sitting, the horizontal axis (y) of the knee joint can be projected to the floor from the centers of the medial and lateral epicondyles of the femur. The axis of the ankle joint can be projected from the medial and lateral malleoli (Fig. 10–3 and Laboratory Activity 9 in this chapter). The angle formed between the horizontal axes of the knee and ankle is referred to as the **angle of tibial torsion**. Reports in the literature show average values in adults to be 20 to 23 degrees of tibial torsion with extensive variation of range from −4 to +56 degrees (Inman, 1976). Measurements by students in kinesiology classes, however, average between 10 and 15 degrees of tibial torsion.

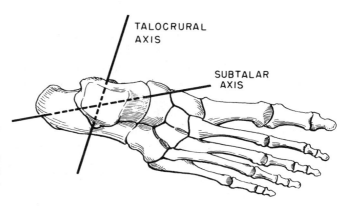

TALOCRURAL
AXIS

SUBTALAR
AXIS

Figure 10–2 Axes of the upper ankle joint (talocrural) and the lower ankle joint (subtalar). (Redrawn from Elftman, 1960.)

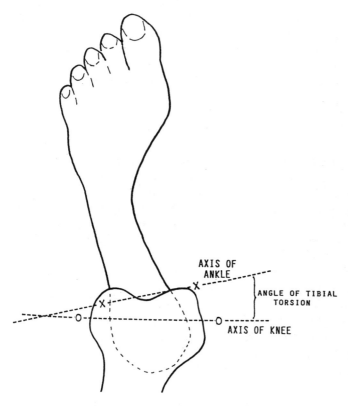

AXIS OF ANKLE

ANGLE OF TIBIAL TORSION

AXIS OF KNEE

Figure 10–3 Clinical measurement of tibial torsion. The subject is seated with the horizontal axis of the knee in the frontal plane and the foot on the floor. The position of the foot is traced and perpendiculars are projected to the outline from the medial and lateral centers of knee flexion (o) and from the centers of the medial and lat-eral malleoli (x). Lines drawn through these points represent the axes of the knee and ankle to form the angle of tibial torsion. In this example, the angle is 14 degrees.

Movements of the Ankle Joint

The triplanar motions are by convention described as dorsiflexion (movement of the dorsal surface of the foot toward the anterior surface of the leg) and plantarflexion (movement of the plantar surface of the foot toward the posterior surface of the leg). This agreement has occurred because the terms flexion and extension have led to misunderstandings. A few authors, however, prefer to use flexion and extension (Kapandji, 1987).

Normal range of dorsiflexion is stated to be from 0 to 30 degrees from the anatomic position (American Academy of Orthopaedic Surgeons, 1965; Hoppenfeld, 1976; Kapandji, 1987). Active range of dorsiflexion of 13 (SD = 4) degrees was measured in healthy male subjects age 18 months to 54 years by Boone and Azen (1979). This measurement was made in the supine position, which places the knee in extension and the gastrocnemius muscle, which crosses the knee and the ankle joints, in a lengthened position to limit dorsiflexion. While this is an important functional measurement related to walking, in which the knee extends and the ankle dorsiflexes in the stance phase, it is equally important to determine the range of motion permitted by joint structures alone. Ankle motion alone is best measured with the knee flexed as in a sitting position. With the gastrocnemius on a slack of the knee, the range of motion in dorsiflexion is larger.

Plantarflexion in the same group of male subjects was 56 (SD = 6) degrees with an average of 58 degrees for subjects under 19 years of age and 54 degrees for those over 19 (Boone and Azen, 1979). Plantarflexion range of motion is not altered by the position of the knee because there are no dorsiflexor muscles that cross the knee.

The normal end-feel for dorsiflexion of the joint is firm. When the knee is flexed, limitation is due to ligamentous structures; when the knee is extended, limitation is due to the length or resistance of the gastrocnemius muscle. The end-feel of plantarflexion is firm because of resistance of the capsule, ligaments, and dorsiflexor muscles.

Tibiofibular Articulations

The tibia and fibula are firmly connected at the superior and inferior tibiofibular articulations by the interosseous membrane, which is classified as a **syndesmosis** (Gr. *syndemos*, band or ligament). Motions at these synovial joints are limited to a few degrees but are essential for normal motions of dorsiflexion and plantarflexion. At the superior tibiofibular joint, motion is restrained by the distal attachments of the biceps femoris tendon, the lateral collateral ligament, and the tendon of the popliteus muscle as well as the tibiofibular ligaments and the fascia. Slight gliding movement in the joint can be felt with dorsiflexion of the ankle. Knee injuries or surgery treated with immobilization can lead to limitation of motion in the superior tibiofibular joint with resulting limitation of dorsiflexion of the ankle. The importance of the superior tibiofibular joint is described by Helfet (1974) and its clinical relevance is presented by Radakovich and Malone (1982) as the "forgotten joint."

The small motions of the superior tibiofibular joint are produced by dorsiflexion and plantarflexion at the lower tibiofibular joint. The malleoli are held together firmly by anterior and posterior ligaments of the distal tibiofibular joint. The dome of the talus, however, is wider anteriorly than posteriorly. Yet the malleoli maintain congruence with the talus throughout the range of plantarflexion and dorsiflexion (Inman, 1976). Such disparity requires motion to occur at the distal tibiofibular joint in the form of abduction or rotation and is reflected to the superior tibiofibular joint. Dorsiflexion causes the head of the fibula to move superiorly, and plantarflexion causes the head to move inferiorly. When this small motion is prevented by forceful compression of the malleoli, dorsiflexion can be seen to be limited.

THE FOOT

The bones of the foot are classified into three segments: the **hindfoot** (talus and calcaneus), the **midfoot** (navicular, cuboid, and the three cuneiforms), and the **forefoot** (metatarsals and phalanges) (see Fig. 10–1). These bones and the associated ligaments form three arches: the **medial longitudinal arch**, the smaller **lateral longitudinal arch**, and the **transverse arch**. Small but critical motions occur in all of the tarsal and metatarsal joints during open- and closed-chain motions of the ankle and foot to provide flexibility of the arches during weight acceptance in walking or running and rigidity of the foot during propulsion (Fig. 10–4). The importance of these small motions can be appreciated in pathologic situations with absence of tarsal motion, which occurs with surgical fusion of the tarsal joints and with artificial legs (prostheses), when the sole of the foot may tilt after heel strike. These abnormal forces lead to compensatory hypermobility at the knee and the metatarsal joints (Engsberg and Allinger, 1990).

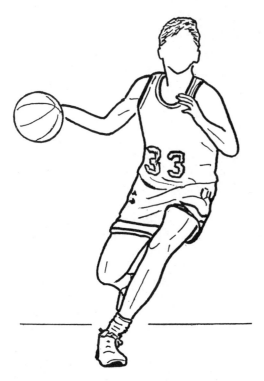

Figure 10–4 Closed-chain motion in the left foot, ankle, knee, and hip. The sole of the foot is planted on the floor and maintained there by adaptive motions in the ankle and foot as the knee and hip undergo rotations, flexion-extension, or abduction-adduction. The right lower extremity and the upper extremities are in open-chain motion.

Subtalar Joint

The superior surface of the calcaneus presents three facets (posterior, middle, and anterior) that articulate with corresponding facets on the inferior surface of the talus. The posterior calcaneal facet is convex (see Fig. 10–1B), while the middle and anterior facets of the calcaneus are concave, thus limiting anterior or posterior displacement of the talus on the calcaneus. This joint has two capsules. One encloses the posterior articular facets of the talus and the calcaneus. The second encloses the middle and anterior facets of the subtalar joint as well as the talonavicular joint. The later articulation, however, is considered a part of the transverse tarsal joint.

A sulcus (groove or trench) occurs between the posterior and middle articular surfaces of the talus to form the **sinus tarsi**, which communicates from the medial to lateral sides of the ankle (Fig. 10–1B). Short, thick, and strong **interosseous talocalcaneal ligaments** course the length of the sinus tarsi and bind the talus and the calcaneus firmly together. These ligaments and the adipose tissue in the sinus tarsi have been found to be richly endowed with neural receptors and nerve fibers traced to the cerebellum (Valenti, 1988). Valenti hypothesized from this and additional clinical and EMG evidence that the interosseous ligaments are the "proprioceptive subtalar center" responsible for rapid reflex response to closed-chain motion.

Joint Axis and Movements

The triplanar axis of the subtalar joint is represented by a line beginning on the lateroposterior aspect of the calcaneus and going in a forward-upward-medial direction through the sinus tarsi as seen in Figure 10–2 (Manter, 1941; Hicks, 1953; Elftman, 1960; Inman, 1976). Inman measured an angle of 42 degrees (SD = 9) in the sagittal plane and 23 degrees (SD = 11) in the transverse plane.

Motion is described by those who have studied the subtalar joint in cadavers and normal human subjects as a rotation or a screw-like motion around the triplanar axis. Kapandji (1987) describes inversion as movement of the calcaneus on the fixed talus as distal, medial, and a tilt (or plantar flexion, adduction, and supination). Inman (1976), using a specially designed spheric goniometer, measured an average of 40 degrees of subtalar motion from maximum inversion to maximum eversion.

Terminology for Motions of the Tarsal Joints

Descriptions of the motions of the foot are not well defined and are confusing. Some authors call motions in the frontal plane **inversion** (turning in) and **eversion** (turning out) (Kapandji, 1987; Norkin and Levangie, 1992); some authors use the terms **supination** (to turn up) and **pronation** (to turn down) (McPoil and Brocato, 1985; Oatis, 1988); others use the terms **pronation-supination** and **eversion-inversion** as synonyms (Inman, 1976). Throughout the literature, each term (ie, pronation) is frequently used to define the other term (ie, eversion), as, for example, pronation is dorsiflexion, abduction, and eversion (Table 10–1). In this text the terms will be used interchangeably with eversion-inversion used more frequently in open-chain motion and pronation-supination used more often in closed-chain motion.

The terms **abduction** and **adduction** when applied to the ankle and foot are particularly confusing because these motions are usually considered as occurring in the frontal plane. In the talocrual and tarsal joints, however, abduction and adduction are used for motions in the transverse plane around a vertical axis (see Table 10–1). Individual movements of the ankle joints in this plane are small (Lundberg et al, 1989a, b, c) and are rarely visible clinically. Some authors, however, are describing abduction and adduction of the foot and ankle from rotations that occur in the knee and the hip (Oatis, 1988; Bordelon, 1990). For example, when a person is sitting in a chair with his or her feet on the floor, the foot can be moved medially or laterally around a vertical axis through the tibia. Motion, however, is not occurring in the joints of the foot but rather between the tibia and femur by alternate activation of the medial and then lateral hamstrings (see Chap-

Table 10–1 Variations in the Terms Used to Describe Motions at the Subtalar Joint

Author	Transverse Plane (Vertical Axis)	Frontal Plane (Ant-Post Axis)	Sagittal Plane (Transverse Axis)
Cailliet (1963)	Abd – Add	Ever – Inver	DF – PF
Kapandji (1987)	Abd – Add	Pron – Sup	DF – PF
Lundberg et al 1989b	Ext – Int Rot (−1.8° +5.6°)	Pron – Sup (−2.7° +5.5°)	DF – PF (−2.7° +5.1°)*

Abd–Add = abduction and adduction; Ant – Post = anterior and posterior; DF – PF = dorsiflexion and plantarflexion; Ever–Inver = eversion and inversion; Ext – Int Rot = external and internal rotation; Pron – Sup = pronation and supination.
*Mean values (degrees) of the motion between the talus and the calcaneus with 20 degrees of medial tilt (pronation) and 20 degrees of lateral tilt (supination). Subjects were weight bearing in closed-chain motion.

ter 9 under Axial Rotation). Even greater motion is exhibited by the foot when the knee is extended and the hip is internally and externally rotated. This motion, which can be up to 90 degrees in each direction, occurs in the hip and knee joints (Kapandji, 1987).

Transverse Tarsal Joint

The transverse tarsal joint is also called the **midtarsal joint,** or the **Chopart joint,** relating to a surgical level of amputation (see Fig. 10–1). When viewed from above, the joint line is S-shaped and is formed by two articulating surfaces, the **talonavicular and calcaneocuboid joints.** The transverse tarsal joint participates in movement of the forefoot on the hindfoot to lower the longitudinal arch of the foot in pronation and to elevate the arch during supination. Independent motion, however, does not normally occur in these joints. Ligamentous attachments and bony structures mechanically link the transverse tarsal joint with the subtalar joint to form a triplanar axis of motion with one degree of freedom. In inversion, the navicular and the cuboid move medially and turn around and under the fixed talus. The calcaneus follows the cuboid by moving anteriorly and turning under the talus (Kapandji, 1987).

Average motion in the frontal plane with 20 degrees of medial tilt (supination) and 20 degrees of lateral tilt (pronation) was greater for the talonavicular joint (13 and 8 degrees) than for the subtalar joint (6 and 3 degrees) (Lundberg et al, 1989b). Total motion, a composite including flexion-extension, rotation, translation, and abduction-adduction, was measured in midfoot joints of fresh amputated specimens by Ouzounian and Shereff (1989). Average motion in the talonavicular joint with dorsiflexion–plantarflexion was 7 degrees and with supination-pronation, 17 degrees. The calcaneocuboid joint had an average of 2 and 7 degrees.

Tarsometatarsal Joints

The cuboid and the three cuneiform bones articulate with the bases of the five metatarsals to form the **tarsometatarsal joints** (see Fig. 10–1). The strong mortising of the second metatarsal by the cuneiforms and the adjacent metatarsals permits only slight motions of flexion and extension. The other metatarsal joints permit slight rotations in arcs around the more rigid second segment. The most mobile fourth and fifth metatarsal joints were found to average 9 and 11 degrees of total motion with dorsiflexion–plantarflexion and supination-pronation (Ouzounian and Shereff, 1989).

Metatarsophalangeal and Interphalangeal Joints

These joints correspond in structure to those in the fingers, but they possess some functional differences. The metacarpophalangeal (MCP) joints of the fingers permit 90 degrees of flexion and from 0 to 30 degrees of hyperextension. At the metatarsophalangeal (MTP) joints of the toes, however, these relationships are reversed. Hyperextension is 90 degrees, and flexion is only 30 to 45 degrees. The large range of hyperextension is used for standing on the toes and in walking (MTP joint hyperextension in late stance phase). Abduction and adduction movements of the toes have less range of motion and muscular control than in the hand.

The interphalangeal (IP) joints of the toes are similar to those of the fingers, with the great toe possessing one such joint and the four lesser toes having proximal and distal IP joints.

Accessory Motions of the Ankle and Foot

The closed-packed position of the talocrural joint is full dorsiflexion, and accessory motions are therefore performed in slight plantarflexion. With the medial and lateral malleoli stabilized in one hand, the talus can be moved passively in a posterior or anterior direction and distracted a few millimeters. Two to three millimeters of motion are considered normal (Harper, 1987). Excessive anterior or posterior movements are called **anterior drawer** or **posterior drawer signs** and are indicative of ligamentous laxity or disruption of ligaments.

With maximum supination (inversion) the tarsal bones form a rigid structure. This is the closed-packed position (Kaltenborn, 1980). In a neutral or pronated position, the tarsal bones are more flexible. Small gliding motions can be achieved by fixating one bone and moving the adjacent bone. With the talus stabilized, the calcaneus can be moved anteriorly, medially, or laterally, as well as distally (distraction). The talonavicular, calcaneocuboid, naviculocuneiform, and tarsometatarsal joints can be moved in dorsal and plantar gliding movements when one bone is stabilized and the adjacent bone moved on it. There is little intercuneiform motion.

The heads of the metatarsals normally can be moved in short arcs around each other or the rigid second segment. Motion is occurring at the tarsometatarsal joints and is limited by the joint structures as well as the transverse metatarsal ligaments. These ligaments attach between the heads of all the metatarsals to limit abduction or "splaying" of the metatarsal heads.

In the toes, the closed-packed position is hyperextension of the MTP joints, whereas in the MCP joints of the hand, the most mechanically stable position is in 90 degrees of flexion. The IP joints in both the fingers and toes are in a closed-packed position when they are in extension.

Deformities of the Foot

Foot deformities may develop from various causes, such as congenital malformations of bones, muscular paralysis or spasticity, stresses and strains in weight bearing, and poorly fitting shoes, or from a combination of several of these, as follows:

PES VALGUS   A more or less permanent pronation-eversion of the foot, in which body weight acts to depress the medial longitudinal and transverse arches. Several stages may be recognized, the last stage being known as pes planus or structural, rigid, flatfoot.

PES VARUS (CLUBFOOT)   A more or less permanent supination-inversion of the foot so that the weight is transferred to the outside of the foot and the medial border of the foot is off the ground.

PES CALCANEUS   Subject walks on heel. The front part of the foot does not touch the ground.

PES EQUINUS   In pes equinus (L. *equinus*, relating to a horse), subject walks on ball of foot with the heel off the ground.

PES CAVUS   Exaggerated high arch, or hollowness of the foot.

Combinations of two of the above deviations also occur, such as calcaneovalgus, equinovarus, and equinocavus.

HALLUX VALGUS   A lateral deviation of the great toe at the MTP joint. This condition is often accompanied by a bunion or inflammation of the bursa on the medial side of the toe joint.

MUSCLES OF THE ANKLE AND FOOT

The muscles that pass over the ankle joints have proximal attachments on the tibia and the fibula, with the exception of the gastrocnemius and the plantaris, which are attached to the femur. Because no muscles attach to the talus, the muscles passing from leg to foot act simultaneously on both the ankle and subtalar joints. The toes are activated both by extrinsic muscles, which originate above the ankle joints, and by intrinsic muscles originating below these joints.

The muscles that act on the ankle, or on the ankle and the toes, and that have proximal attachments mainly on the shank may be divided into three groups: posterior, lateral, and anterior.

Posterior Group of Muscles

Gastrocnemius

The **gastrocnemius** (G. *gaster*, belly, and *kneme*, knee) makes up the major portion of the muscles of the calf. **Proximal attachments:** By two tendinous heads, the medial and the lateral, from above the condyles of the femur, these attachments being partly adherent to the capsule of the knee joint. The medial head is the larger of the two and its muscular portion descends farther distally than that of the lateral head (Fig. 10–5). The muscle fibers of the two heads converge to have

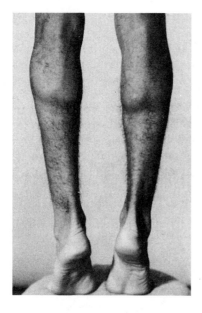

Figure 10–5 Both soleus and gastrocnemius muscles contract in rising on tiptoes. Note that the medial head of the gastrocnemius descends somewhat farther than the lateral head. Note the combined inversion of the heels.

distal attachments on a broad tendon aponeurosis, which begins as a septum between the two heads and which fuses with the aponeurosis over the soleus muscle. Distally, this tendon aponeurosis narrows to form the tendocalcaneus (Achilles tendon), which attaches to the calcaneus. **Innervation**: Branches of the tibial portion of the sciatic nerve (S_1-S_2). **Anatomic action**: Plantarflexion of the ankle and knee flexion.

INSPECTION AND PALPATION   The gastrocnemius is largely responsible for the characteristic contour of the human calf. It is seen contracting in rising on tiptoes, walking, running, and jumping. In athletic individuals, the muscle bellies of the gastrocnemius when contracting are short and bulky, and the tendinous portions are comparatively long.

Soleus

The **soleus** (L. *soles*, sole, sandal), like the gastrocnemius, belongs to the posterior group of the leg. These two muscles together are also called the **triceps surae**, or three-headed muscle of the calf. **Proximal attachment**: Popliteal line of the tibia and the upper one third of the posterior surface of the fibula. **Distal attachment**: By means of a tendinous aponeurosis covering the posterior surface of the muscle, which narrows distally and unites with the tendon of the gastrocnemius to form the tendocalcaneus. **Innervation**: Tibial portion of sciatic nerve (S_1-S_2). **Anatomic actions**: Plantarflexion of the ankle.

INSPECTION AND PALPATION   The soleus is covered largely by the gastrocnemius, but in the lower portion of the calf it protrudes on both sides of the gastrocnemius so that it may here be observed and palpated. When the subject rises on tiptoes, both gastrocnemius and soleus contract strongly (see Fig. 10–5). A comparatively isolated contraction of the soleus may be seen if the subject lies prone with knee flexed and plantarflexes the ankle against slight resistance (Fig. 10–6). The foot should be stabilized on the plantar side so that the subject may press lightly against the examiner's hand.

Function of the Triceps Surae

Plantarflexion of the ankle is performed mainly, and almost exclusively, by the **triceps surae**. These muscles have both a large cross-sectional area (43 cm^2 as compared with 33 cm^2 for all the other muscles of the ankle combined) and excellent leverage for plantarflexion. The perpendicular distance from the tendocalcaneus to the ankle joint axis is approximately 5 cm (2 inches). Measurement of the maximum forces and torques that can be produced by the plantarflexors is difficult because of the large forces that are imposed on the equipment, soft tissues, or intervening joints. Forces measured or calculated at the MTP area during maximum isometric plantarflexion range from 225 to 440 lb (1000 to 1780 N) in men (Reys, 1915; Cureton, 1941; Haxton, 1944; Beasley, 1958, 1961; Tornvall, 1963; Backlund and Nordgren, 1968). Beasley measured plantarflexion force in the sitting position in more than 3000 normal subjects ranging in ages from 5 to 70 years. He reported the mean value as 2.4 times body weight. After 30 years of age, the value decreases gradually, becoming about 1.7 times body weight at 70 years. Average values for young adult men were approximately 390 lb, and those for women were 280 lb. Even greater forces would be expected if the knee were extended so that the gas-

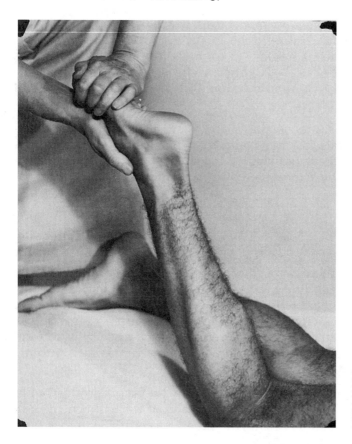

Figure 10–6 A comparatively isolated contraction of the soleus is obtained when plantar flexion is performed while the knee is flexed.

trocnemius has a more favorable length-tension relationship. This increase is demonstrated in two studies using young adult women: With subjects in the sitting position and knees flexed to 90 degrees, Bernard (1979) recorded a mean of 98 ft-lb of torque. When the subjects were in the long sitting position with the knee extended, Belnap (1978) recorded a mean of 122 ft-lb of torque. When the sitting values were converted to force (dividing the torque by the length of the forefoot lever arm), they were similar to the force values recorded by Beasley (1958).

Other muscles have tendons passing posterior to the axis of motion of the talocrural joint, but they have poor leverage and are quite ineffective as plantar-flexors. These muscles do not act on the calcaneus but attach to more distal parts of the foot and have specific actions at other joints. The tendons of the posterior tibialis and the peroneal muscles lie so close to the malleoli that they barely pass posterior to the axis. The tendon of the flexor digitorum longus lies only slightly farther back. The flexor hallucis longus has somewhat better leverage, but its action as a plantarflexor of the ankle still is insignificant compared with that of the triceps surae (Fig. 10–7).

The importance of the soleus as a postural muscle has been confirmed by EMG. Joseph (1960), in studying the activity of various muscles in the "standing-at-ease" position, found continuous electrical activity in the soleus in all of the 12 subjects investigated; activity in the gastrocnemius could be detected in only 7 of the 12 subjects. A force of one half the body weight was calculated for the soleus to maintain a unilateral stance (see Fig. 2–16).

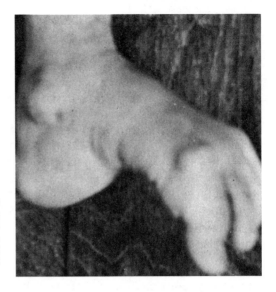

Figure 10–7 Postpoliomyelitic paralysis of the triceps surae. The long toe flexors, although passing posterior to the axis of the talocrural joint, are incapable of plantar-flexing the ankle. With the triceps surae out of action, the long toe flexors are instrumental in the development of a calcaneocaval deformity.

The soleus has been found to contain a higher proportion of slow-twitch muscle fibers than the gastrocnemius, which possesses predominantly fast-twitch muscle fibers (Denny-Brown, 1929; Edgerton, Smith, and Simpson, 1975; see also Chapter 3). This indicates that the soleus is concerned more with stabilization at the ankle and control of postural sway than is the gastrocnemius. Being composed of slow-twitch, fatigue-resistant motor units, the soleus operates economically, that is, with less fatigue for sustained contraction than the gastrocnemius, which contains predominantly fast-twitch and fast-fatiguing motor units.

The gastrocnemius and the soleus are both involved in activities requiring forceful plantar flexion of the ankle. In rising on tiptoes, both muscles are seen to contract simultaneously (see Fig. 10–5), and their state of contraction may be ascertained by palpation. In running and jumping, the action of the gastrocnemius is indispensable because its fibers possess the quality of producing a rapid rise in tension. (The function of the triceps surae in walking is discussed in Chapter 12.)

PARALYSIS OF THE TRICEPS SURAE   When the gastrocnemius-soleus group is paralyzed, the individual cannot rise on tiptoes, and gait is severely affected (see Chapter 12). The act of climbing stairs is awkward and slow, and activities such as running and jumping are all but impossible. The deep calf muscles and the peroneals, although passing posterior to the axis of the upper ankle joint, are incapable of substituting for the triceps surae.

The effect of paralysis of the triceps surae may be observed in persons with spina bifida (congenital defect in the vertebrae) who have lost innervation to the triceps surae but retain innervation to the posterior tibialis and the peroneals, and in persons with postpoliomyelitis in whom the deep calf muscles have been spared. If these individuals are children (whose feet are pliable), a calcaneocaval deformity tends to develop (see Fig. 10–7). It is obvious that the tibialis posterior, the flexor hallucis longus, and the flexor digitorum longus (although their tendons pass posterior to the joint axis) are incapable of plantarflexing the ankle. These muscles have poor leverage at the upper ankle joint and, furthermore, do not attach to the calcaneus. Their tendons pass to the sole of the foot, and when the muscles contract, they affect more distal joints rather than the talocrural joint.

The tendons of the flexor digitorum longus and flexor hallucis longus have a shortening effect on the foot in a front-to-back direction, and the calcaneus, having lost the counterbalancing effect of the triceps surae, assumes a dorsiflexed position. These elements all contribute to the development of a calcaneocaval deformity.

Bilateral paralysis of the triceps surae causes loss of standing balance because there is insufficient muscle force to prevent the tibia from dorsiflexing and collapsing on the foot. People with such weakness are often thought to be nervous because they do not stand still and are constantly moving their feet to get their base of support under their center of gravity. They can stand still only if they are holding onto a stable object or leaning against a wall. People with bilateral amputations have the same problem when standing in prostheses because they have no muscles to control closed-chain positions of the feet and ankles.

Tibialis Posterior

The **tibialis posterior** is the most deeply situated muscle of the calf. It lies close to the interosseous membrane between the tibia and the fibula, covered by the soleus and the gastrocnemius. **Proximal attachments**: Posterior surface of the interosseous membrane and adjacent portions of the tibia and the fibula. In the upper calf, it occupies a central position between the flexor digitorum longus medially and the flexor hallucis longus laterally. In the lower calf, it takes a more medial course. Its tendon lies in a groove on the medial malleolus and is held down by a broad ligament. It then continues to the sole of the foot. **Distal attachments**: The tuberosity of the navicular bone and, by means of fibrous expansions, adjacent tarsal bones and the bases of the metatarsals. The spreading out of its attachments provides a tendomuscular support on the plantar side of the foot. **Innervation**: Tibial nerve (L_5-S_1). **Anatomic actions**: Inversion and assists in plantarflexion of the ankle.

INSPECTION AND PALPATION   The tendon of the tibialis posterior is observable and well palpable both above and below the medial malleolus. It is particularly easy to identify just proximal to the tuberosity of the navicular bone, where it lies superficially. Above the malleolus, its tendon lies close to those of the flexor digitorum longus and the flexor hallucis longus. These tendons may be identified by inversion of the ankle (which brings out the toe flexors). For palpation of these tendons, have the subject seated on a chair, the limb to be tested crossed over the other so that the foot is relaxed and plantarflexed. Notice that the tendon of the tibialis posterior lies closer to the medial malleolus than do the other two tendons.

Flexor Digitorum Longus and Flexor Hallucis Longus

The **flexor digitorum longus** (FDL) is a deep muscle lying medially in the calf, covered by the soleus and the medial head of the gastrocnemius. **Proximal attachments**: Tibia, below the distal attachment of the popliteus, and the intermuscular septum between the popliteus and the tibialis posterior. In the lower leg, the FDL crosses over the tibialis posterior so that at the malleolus it comes to lie behind the tendon of the tibialis posterior. **Distal attachments**: The tendon enters the sole of the foot near the sustentaculum tali, crosses the tendon of the flexor hallucis longus, and divides into four parts that attach into the bases of the distal phalanges of the second to fifth toes. On the way to its attachment, each tendon perforates the corresponding tendon of the short toe flexor, an arrangement similar to that of the hand. **Innervation:** Tibial nerve (L_5–S_1). **Anatomic actions:** Flexion of the MTP joints and IP joints and plantarflexion of the ankle. **Palpation:** The tendon of the flexor digitorum longus can be palpated on the medial aspect of the medial malleolus when the toes are flexed.

The **flexor hallucis longus** (FHL) is located under the soleus on the lateral side of the calf. The FHL is a strong muscle, its cross-section almost two times that of the flexor digitorum longus. **Proximal attachments:** Posterior surface on the fibular and intermuscular septa. Its tendon passes behind the medial malleolus, through a groove in the talus, and then under the sustentaculum tali. After entering the sole of the foot, the FHL tendon crosses to the medial side of the tendon of the FDL. At the MTP joint, the tendon passes between the two sesamoid bones in the tendon of the flexor hallucis brevis. **Distal attachment:** Base of the distal phalanx of the great toe. **Innervation:** Tibial nerve (L_5-S_2). **Anatomic actions:** Flexion of the first MTP joint, IP joint, and ankle plantarflexion.

Isolated contractions of the FHL and FDL are best observed by stabilizing the proximal phalanges and then asking the subject to flex the distal IP joints of the toes.

Functions of the Deep Muscles of the Calf

The **tibialis posterior** is the invertor or supinator of the subtalar joint and produces this motion in either dorsiflexion or plantarflexion. Other muscles produce motion in a limited range or in open-chain motion only. Contraction of the triceps surae produces inversion of the calcaneus (see Fig. 10–5). The anterior tibialis, FDL, and FHL may invert weakly from an everted position to neutral.

The extensive distal attachments of the posterior tibialis on the sustentaculum tali, navicular tuberosity, cuneiforms, cuboid, and bases of the metatarsals indicate an important function in dynamic support of the arch of the foot (Kaye and Jahss, 1991). This occurs when increased loads are placed on the foot, and muscle contraction is needed to stabilize the arches during walking, standing on one foot, running, or jumping. In addition to providing stabilization of the joints of the hindfoot, midfoot, and forefoot, contraction of the posterior tibialis causes the navicular to move slightly inferior and medially to stabilize against the talus. This motion prevents the large torques of the triceps surae from producing motion in the talonavicular and tarsal joints. With paralysis of the posterior tibialis, the downward forces of the talus stretch the medial-plantar ligaments, and in time the arch may collapse into a flatfoot deformity with the navicular bearing weight on the floor.

The major functions of the FDL and the FHL muscles are in closed-chain motions of walking, running, and standing on the toes. In these activities, the long toe flexors contract to support the longitudinal arch and to apply force on the ground in the push-off phase of walking. The force exerted by these muscles can be felt by placing the fingertips under the toes of a person who is standing. When the person then sways forward slightly from the ankles, the powerful gripping force will be felt.

Lateral Group of Muscles

This group is located on the lateral side of the shank, anterior to the calf group, occupying a comparatively small area and being separated from the anterior and posterior groups by intermuscular septa. There are two muscles in this group: the peroneus longus and peroneus brevis.

Peroneus Longus and Brevis

In its location, the **peroneus longus** (Gr. *perone*, brooch, fibula) appears as a direct continuation of the biceps femoris. **Proximal attachments:** The principal attachment is to the head of the fibula near the distal attachment of the biceps femoris. The peroneus longus, however, has additional proximal attachments, including the neighboring area of the tibia, the shaft of the fibula, and intermuscular septa. The muscle fibers converge to form a tendon that passes in a groove behind the lateral malleolus and then to the cuboid bone, where it enters the sole of the foot. There, the tendon follows a groove of the cuboid bone; the groove has an oblique direction coursing forward and medially. **Distal attachments:** Plantar surface of first cuneiform bone and base of first metatarsal. **Anatomic actions:** Eversion and plantarflexion of the ankle and depression of the head of the first metatarsal.

The **peroneus brevis**, as its name indicates, is shorter than the peroneus longus. **Proximal attachments:** Fibula, lower than the longus, and intermuscular septa. Its tendon passes behind the lateral malleolus, then across the calcaneus and the cuboid. **Distal attachments:** The dorsal surface of the tuberosity of the fifth metatarsal bone. **Anatomic actions:** Eversion and plantarflexion of the ankle.

The two peronei muscles are innervated by the superficial branch of the common peroneal nerve (L_4-S_1). The common peroneal nerve becomes superficial as it winds around the neck of the fibula. At this point, the nerve is vulnerable to compression, which can cause loss of sensation and muscle paralysis. This frequently occurs if a person sits for a period of time with one leg crossed over the opposite knee. When the person stands up to walk, he or she is surprised that the leg has "gone to sleep," the foot cannot be controlled, and the ankle may collapse with weight bearing. Usually the person moves to relieve the pressure on the nerve, and sensation and muscle strength are rapidly recovered. Continued compression can occur, however, in a cast that is too tight under the head of the fibula. If the pressure is not relieved promptly, permanent loss of sensation and paralysis of the peroneal and dorsiflexor muscles may occur.

INSPECTION, PALPATION, AND FUNCTION OF THE PERONEAL MUSCLES The muscular portion of the peroneus longus is identified just below the head of the fibula and may be followed down the lateral side of the leg. From halfway down the leg to the ankle, the two peroneal muscles lie close together. Nearly all the brevis is covered by the longus, but in the lower part of the leg, it can be felt separately from the longus.

When eversion is resisted, as illustrated in Figure 10–8, both muscles contract. The tendon of the peroneus brevis stands out more than the tendon of the peroneus longus and can be followed to its attachment on the fifth metatarsal bone. At the malleolus, the tendons of the peroneal muscles appear as if they may slip over to the front side, but they are anchored firmly by retinacula. Above the malleolus, the tendon of the peroneus longus lies slightly posterior to that of the brevis, and, at least in some individuals, it is easily palpated. Below the malleolus, the tendon of the peroneus longus is held down close to the bone. It lies on the plantar side of the tendon of the peroneus brevis but is rather difficult to identify (see also Fig. 10–9B).

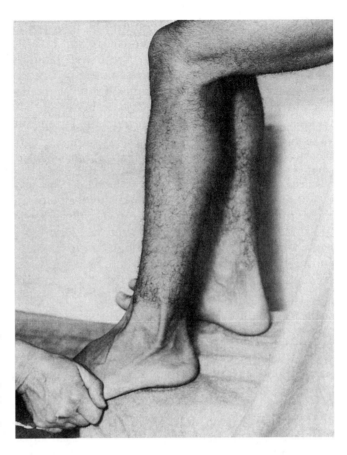

Figure 10–8 The tendons of the peroneus longus and peroneus brevis both pass posteriorly to the lateral malleolus. The tendon of the brevis may be followed to its attachment on the fifth metatarsal bone. Note also the tendon of the biceps femoris at the knee.

Note that when eversion of the foot is resisted in the sitting position, as in Figure 10–8, external rotation of the leg with respect to the thigh occurs simultaneously; the prominent tendon of the biceps femoris is seen at the knee.

In open-chain motion, the peroneus longus, brevis, and tertius (if present) are the main evertors of the subtalar joint and do so whether the ankle is in dorsiflexion or plantarflexion. Their major functions, however, occur in closed-chain motions of standing on one foot, walking, jumping, and running. In these activities, the peroneal muscles provide major support of the arches of the foot, adjustment

Figure 10–9 Severance of the tibial portion of the sciatic nerve with the common peroneal nerve preserved. (A) The patient is prone, knee flexed. Passive plantar flexion is performed. (B) When the patient attempts to plantar-flex the foot actively, the foot swings out in marked eversion. The tendons of the peroneus longus and peroneus brevis (plainly visible) course so close to the axis of the talocrural joint that their action in plantar flexion is practically nil. (Frames from a motion picture.)

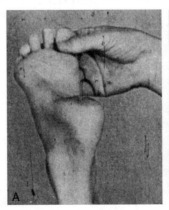

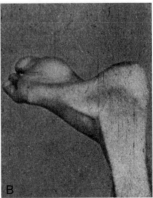

of the foot to the ground, and control of the leg on the planted foot. With paralysis of the peroneals, the ankle is unstable and inversion ankle sprains may occur.

Although the peroneals are classified as plantarflexors, their leverage is poor for the motion. The ineffectiveness of the peroneals as plantarflexors can be seen in Fig. 10–9. Nevertheless, normal torque of plantarflexion requires strong contraction of the peroneals (and the deep calf muscles) to stabilize the tarsal and metatarsal bones to make the force of the triceps surae effective through the foot to the floor.

Anterior Group of Muscles

The anterior group is located on the lateral side of the anterior margin of the tibia, the sharp, bony ridge palpable from the tuberosity of the tibia all the way down to the ankle. It is separated from the lateral group by an intermuscular septa but appears, on palpation, to be continuous with it. The muscles of the anterior group are the tibialis anterior, extensor hallucis longus, extensor digitorum longus, and peroneus tertius. This group is also called the **pretibial group.**

Anterior Tibialis

The **anterior tibialis** is responsible for the roundness of the shank anteriorly. When this muscle is paralyzed, a flatness or even slight concavity of this region results, so that the anterior margin of the tibia becomes even more prominent than normal. **Proximal attachments:** Lateral condyle and proximal half of the shaft of tibia, interosseous membrane, and fascia of the leg. The muscle becomes tendinous well above the ankle, and its tendon passes over the dorsum of the ankle, held down by the transverse and cruciate ligaments. **Distal attachments:** Medial cuneiform bone and base of the first metatarsal bone. **Innervation:** A branch from the common peroneal nerve and a branch from the deep peroneal nerve (L_4-S_1). **Anatomic action:** Dorsiflexion of the ankle.

INSPECTION AND PALPATION   Because the muscle is superficial throughout its course, it may be observed and palpated all the way from proximal attachment to distal attachment. The muscular portion is palpated proximally, on the lateral side of the anterior margin of the tibia when the foot is dorsiflexed. Its tendon is observed and palpated as it passes over the ankle, where it rises considerably when the foot is dorsiflexed (Fig. 10–10). In the illustration, the subject flexes the toes so that the tendon of the extensor hallucis longus muscle, which lies just lateral to that of the anterior tibialis, does not contract. If the student wishes to observe both tendons simultaneously, the ankle should be held dorsiflexed and the great toe should be flexed and extended.

Extensor Hallucis Longus

In its upper portion, the **extensor hallucis longus** (EHL) is covered by the anterior tibialis and by the extensor digitorum longus. **Proximal attachment:** Middle portion of shaft of the fibula and interosseous membrane. The tendon of the EHL passes on the dorsum of the ankle, lateral to the tendon of the tibialis anterior, and is held down by ligaments. **Distal attachment:** Base of distal phalanx of great toe. **Innervation:** A branch from the deep peroneal nerve (L_4-S_1). **Anatomic actions:** Extension of the first MTP and IP joints and ankle dorsiflexion.

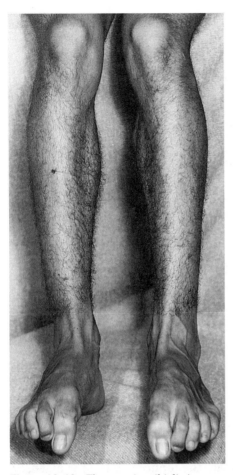

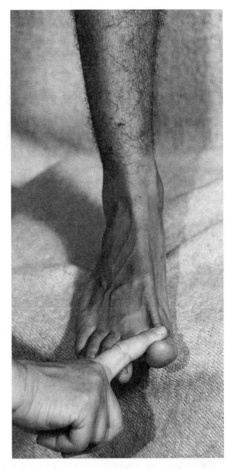

Figure 10–10 The anterior tibialis is superficial and can be observed all the way from proximal attachment to distal attachment. Its tendon is strong and prominent as it passes the ankle joint.

Figure 10–11 The tendon of the extensor hallucis longus is observed when the great toe is dorsiflexed against resistance. It lies just lateral to the tendon of anterior tibialis at the ankle.

INSPECTION AND PALPATION By resisting dorsiflexion of the great toe, as seen in Figure 10–11, the course of the tendon of EHL over the dorsum of the foot may be observed. The muscular portion is palpated in the lower half of the leg, but because it is almost entirely covered by the anterior tibialis and the extensor digitorum longus, it cannot be easily distinguished from these muscles.

Extensor Digitorum Longus

The **extensor digitorum longus** (EDL) and **peroneus tertius** muscles are described together because they usually are not well differentiated in their upper portions. The peroneus tertius is the most lateral part of the EDL but is sometimes described as a separate muscle. The EDL is superficial, bordering laterally to the peronei muscles and medially to the EHL and the anterior tibialis. **Proximal attachments**: The EDL attaches to the upper portion of the tibia and fibula, interosseous membrane, and intermuscular septa and fascia; the peroneus tertius attaches to the distal portion of the fibula and to the interosseous membrane. The

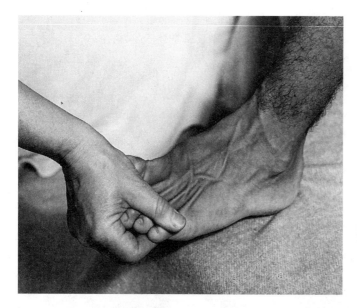

Figure 10–12 The tendons of the extensor digitorum longus are seen as they pass the ankle and proceed toward the four lesser toes. Examiner resists on the dorsum of the toes. In this subject, the tendon of the peroneus tertius, which passes laterally to the other tendons, could not be found.

common tendon passes on the dorsum of the ankle, and, like the other tendon in this region, it is held down by the transverse and cruciate ligaments. The tendon divides into five slips, the most lateral being the tendon of the peroneus tertius. **Distal attachments**: Four tendons go to the bases of the middle and distal phalanges of the four lesser toes; the tendon of the peroneus tertius goes to the dorsum of the fifth metatarsal bone. **Innervation**: A branch from the deep peroneal nerve (L_4-S_1). **Anatomic actions**: Extension of MTP and IP joints of the four lesser toes and dorsiflexion and eversion of the ankle.

INSPECTION AND PALPATION To better see and palpate the tendons of the toe extensors without simultaneous contraction of the anterior tibialis, have the subject sit on a chair and lift the toes off the floor while maintaining the sole on the floor. If resistance is given to the four lesser toes, the individual tendons stand out better (Fig. 10–12). The tendon of the peroneus tertius, when present and observable, is seen lateral to the tendon going to the fifth toe. The distal attachment of this tendon is variable, and the muscle may be missing altogether.

Function of the Pretibial Group

The anterior tibialis is the primary dorsiflexor of the ankle. It has good leverage, a straight line of pull, acts on the upper ankle joint only, and has twice the cross-sectional area of the toe extensors combined. The EHL and the EDL extend the toes first, and thus lose effectiveness in dorsiflexion of the ankle. When the anterior tibialis is paralyzed and the toe extensors are intact, a limited range of dorsiflexion of the ankle can be produced. If the EDL acts in isolation, a strong eversion of the ankle also occurs. Paralysis of the muscles results in a drop-foot during the swing phase of walking and requires excess hip and knee flexion to keep from tripping or dragging the toes on the floor.

The pretibial group moves the foot and toes in many important open-chain motions such as preventing the foot and toes from dragging in the swing phase of walking, placing the foot for driving, keeping time to the beat of music, or wiggling toes into shoes. Open-chain motions of the foot require little muscle force because the foot weighs only about 2 lb and the muscles have good leverage. Stronger contractions can be seen and palpated when a subject is standing on one foot in closed-chain motion. Here a constant interplay can be found between all of the muscles of the foot to keep the center of gravity within the small base of support.

Intrinsic Muscles of the Foot

While the intrinsic muscles of the foot have names similar to those of muscles in the hand, most differ in structure or function.

Four layers of intrinsic muscles occur on the plantar surface of the foot. Brief descriptions of the attachments of these muscles are given in Table 10–2. They should be studied using an anatomic atlas. In addition to bony attachments, these muscles have extensive connections with the plantar aponeurosis, ligaments, and tendons of the foot. These tissues form strong coupling of the static and dynamic structures. Although the muscles can perform motions such as abduction, adduction, and flexion of the toes, their major functions are supporting the arches in walking and running, supplementing the force of the long toe flexors, and main-

Table 10–2 Intrinsic Muscles on the Plantar Surface of the Foot

	Proximal Attachment	Distal Attachment	Innervation
Layer I			
Abductor hallucis	Calcaneal tuberosity Plantar aponeurosis	First toe—base of 1st phalanx	Medial plantar $(L_4$-$L_5)$
Flexor digitorum brevis	Calcaneal tuberosity Plantar aponeurosis	Second phalanges of lesser toes	Medial plantar $(L_4$-$L_5)$
Abductor digiti minimi	Calcaneal tuberosity Plantar aponeurosis	Fifth toe—base of 1st phalanx	Lateral plantar $(S_1$-$S_2)$
Layer II			
Quadratus plantae	Concave surface of calcaneus	Tendon of the flexor digitorum longus	Lateral plantar $(S_1$-$S_2)$
Lumbricals	Tendons of the flexor digitorum longus	Extensor hood of MCP joints 2–5	1 = Medial plantar 2–4 = Lateral plantar
Layer III			
Flexor hallucis brevis	Cuboid and lateral cuneiform	First toe—base of 1st phalanx	Medial plantar $(L_4$-$S_1)$
Adductor hallucis (two heads)	Bases of metatarsals 2–4, MTP ligaments	First toe—base of 1st phalanx	Lateral plantar $(S_1$-$S_2)$
Flexor digiti minimi brevis	Base of 5th metatarsal	Fifth toe—base of 1st phalanx	Lateral plantar $(S_1$-$S_2)$
Layer IV			
Dorsal interossei	Adjacent surfaces of metatarsals 1–5	Extensor hood of MCP joints 2–4	Lateral plantar $(S_1$-$S_2)$
Plantar interossei	Medial sides of metatarsals 3–5	Extensor hood of MCP joints 3–5	Lateral plantar $(S_1$-$S_2)$

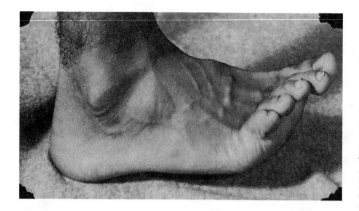

Figure 10–13 The muscular portion of the extensor digitorum brevis is seen on the lateral side of the dorsum of the foot. The tendons of distal attachment of this short muscle are hidden under those of the long toe extensors.

taining the toes in extension for the forceful pull of the flexors at push-off. If the toes are not maintained in extension, they curl and the force for push-off is not effective.

The **extensor digitorum brevis** is the only intrinsic muscle on the dorsum of the foot. Its proximal attachments and muscle belly are on the dorsolateral side of the foot just below the sinus tarsi (Fig. 10–13). Four tendons extend to attach to the base of the proximal phalanx of the great toe and to the lateral sides of the extensor digitorum tendons of the second to the fourth toes. **Innervation:** Branch of the deep peroneal nerve (L_5-S_1). **Anatomic action:** Extension of the MTP joints of the medial four toes. Contraction balances the medial pull of the extrinsic toe extensors.

Use of Toes for Skilled Activities

With one exception, movements performed by the human hand can potentially be performed by the foot. Opposition of the thumb is not represented in the foot. The possibilities of developing the feet for grasping objects and performing skilled sensorimotor tasks have been amply demonstrated by children with congenital amputations of the upper extremities, particularly if the entire limbs are missing. These children learn to use their feet in an extraordinarily skilled manner and are capable of doing practically everything with their feet that able-bodied children do with their hands.

FUNCTION OF LOWER EXTREMITY MUSCLES

The lower extremities have major functional requirements in high-energy closed-chain motion. For example, when a person is standing, it is impossible to move one leg in open-chain motion to take a step or to kick a ball unless the person can stand and support body weight on the opposite leg in closed-chain motion. Analysis of muscle forces needed in activities such as deep knee bends or stair climbing is dependent upon the external forces occurring, particularly gravity, rather than the direction of joint motion. Table 10–3 presents an analysis of the direction of sagittal plane motion, primary or essential muscle activation, and the type of muscle contraction used in common closed-chain activities.

Palpation of muscles along with observation of these activities demonstrates that raising and lowering the body weight uses the **same muscle groups with**

Table 10–3 Analysis of Lower Extremity Muscle Activity in Closed-Chain Motion (Sagittal Plane)*

Activity	Direction of Joint Motion	Muscle Prime Movers	Type of Contraction
Chairs			
(Arising)	Hip ext	Hamstrings	Concentric
	Knee ext	Quadriceps	Concentric
	Ankle PF	Gastro-Sol	Concentric
(Sitting)	Hip flex	Hamstrings	Eccentric
	Knee flex	Quadriceps	Eccentric
	Ankle DF	Gastro-Sol	Eccentric
Standing on toes			
(Up)	Hip stabilized	Co-cont	Isometric
	Knee stabilized	Co-cont	Isometric
	Ankle PF	Gastro-Sol	Concentric
(Down)	Hip stabilized	Co-cont	Isometric
	Knee stabilized	Co-cont	Isometric
	Ankle DF	Gastro-Sol	Eccentric
Deep knee bends			
(Down)	Hip flex	Hamstrings	Eccentric
	Knee flex	Quadriceps	Eccentric
	Ankle DF	Gastro-Sol	Eccentric
(Up)	Hip ext	Hamstrings	Concentric
	Knee ext	Quadriceps	Concentric
	Ankle PF	Gastro-Sol	Concentric
Standing			
(Bend forward to touch toes)	Hip flex	Hamstrings	Eccentric
	Knee stabilized	Co-cont	Isometric
	Ankle stabilized	Co-cont	Isometric
(Return to standing)	Hip. ext	Hamstrings	Concentric
	Knee stabilized	Co-cont	Isometric
	Ankle stabilized	Co-cont	Isometric

Co-cont = co-contraction; DF = dorsiflexion; ext = extension; flex = flexion; Gastro-Sol = gastrocnemius-soleus; PF = plantar flexion.
*In these activities almost all muscles in the lower extremities may be activated depending on the imposed load. Eccentric and concentric contractions are essential for the motion, and co-contraction and isometric contractions are necessary synergists.

concentric and eccentric muscle contractions. These contractions are not related to anatomic actions of muscles that are defined for open-chain motion. In addition to analysis of these activities, it is helpful to analyze in slow motion stair climbing for muscle activation in the moving extremity in open-chain motion, and in the fixed extremity in closed-chain motion. Solution of the muscle activity that is required explains why therapists teach patients with asymmetric lower extremity weakness to go upstairs leading with the "good leg" and downstairs leading with the "weak leg" or "up with the good, down with the bad."

Arches of the Foot

The ability of the foot to change from a flexible to a rigid structure within a single step is dependent upon the bony structure of the three arches of the foot, static ligament-fascial support, and dynamic muscle contraction. In closed-chain motion, such as standing, superincumbent body weight is distributed through the talus posteriorly to the tuberosity of the calcaneus and anteriorly to the heads of the metatarsal bones and the toes. Body weight is distributed to these points through the three arches. The medial longitudinal arch is the longest and the highest. It is composed of the calcaneus, the talus, the navicular, the medial cuneiform, and the first metatarsal bones. The lateral longitudinal arch is lower and composed of the calcaneus, the cuboid, and the fifth metatarsal. The transverse arch is concave from medial to lateral in the midtarsal and tarsometatarsal areas. Distally, the heads of the metatarsal bones are flexible and conform to the contour of the ground.

Structurally, the arches of the foot have some of the properties of the mechanical arch, such as wedge-shaped bones, but lack the peripheral buttresses (fixed supports) needed to prevent collapse of the arch. Ligaments, however, connect the tarsal and metatarsal bones on the dorsal and plantar surfaces to bind the bones of the arches into a structure with properties of the solid curved beam. When loaded, the curved beam bends, and compression forces occur on the top (convex side) and tension forces occur on the plantar surface (concave side). As the amount of load increases, the beam eventually collapses. Larger forces can be supported by the beam if a tie-rod is placed across the base of the beam to prevent the two ends from moving apart. Mechanically, this is the truss, which is a variant of the arch. In the foot, the tie-rod is represented by the plantar aponeurosis as well as by contraction of intrinsic and extrinsic muscles of the foot (see Fig. 10–1B,C; Sarrafian, 1987).

The **plantar aponeurosis** is a strong series of fascial bands that invest the sole and sides of the foot from a 2- to 3-cm proximal attachment on the tuberosity of the calcaneus to the toes. The aponeurosis is an attachment for intrinsic muscles of the foot (eg, flexor digitorum brevis) and is the fascial covering for others (eg, abductor hallucis). Tendon and neurovascular bundles perforate the aponeurosis on their way to the toes. Complex vertical septa (walls) and lateral mooring structures connect the longitudinal bands to deep structures, the skin, and each other. Distal attachments of the plantar aponeurosis are associated with the sheaths of the flexor tendons, plantar plates, and deep structures of the toes. These attachments are distal to the MTP joints, and when the joint is hyperextended, tension is placed on the plantar aponeurosis. This tension prevents the displacement of the calcaneus from the metatarsal heads and collapse of the arches in addition to compressing the tarsal and metatarsal bones into a rigid structure. Such rigidity is needed when standing on the toes and in the terminal stance phase of walking.

Mechanically, the MTP aponeurotic mechanism is similar to the **windlass**, which is a drum with rope wound around it and with a crank to turn it. The quarter turn produced by the MTP joints in hypertension converts the tarsal joints into a rigid structure and a flexible structure when the MTP joint is in a neutral or flexed position. This can be experienced when a person stands on a step or a large telephone book with the edge of the book at the MTP joint. Weight bearing on the foot is seen to be flexible in pronation to conform to the surface and the MTP joint goes into flexion. When the MTP joint is manually placed in about 45 degrees of hyperextension, however, the arches of the foot become rigid, and the plantar aponeurosis can be felt to be firm.

Dynamic Muscle Forces

All the extrinsic and most of the intrinsic muscles on the plantar surface of the foot cross under the arches. When the muscles contract in closed-chain motion, the forces that are produced tighten the arches. The posterior tibialis and the peroneus longus with their extensive plantar attachments have major effects on the transverse arch but also tighten the longitudinal arches. The flexor hallucis longus and the abductor hallucis span the medial arch, and the abductor digiti minimi runs the length of the lateral arch. The flexor digitorum brevis, quadratus plantae, and flexor digitorum longus run the midplantar length and tighten the longitudinal arches. The adductor hallucis affects the transverse arch. Thus, the muscles of the toes, which, compared to the fingers, have limited function and use in open-chain motion, have great importance in closed-chain motions of walking and running.

Loading of the Foot

Conventionally, weight distribution in standing is stated to be in a 50-50 percent manner on the calcaneus and the metatarsal heads with the first metatarsal head absorbing twice the weight that each of the four lateral metatarsal heads supports in a proportion of 2:1:1:1:1. There is, however, considerable variation in the distribution of pressure on the structures of the foot. Cavanagh, Rodgers, and Iiboshi (1987), for example, found an average of 60 percent of the weight distributed to the heel, 8 percent to the midfoot, 28 percent to the ball of the foot, and 4 percent to the toes. There was a high degree of variability among subjects. Variations in the distribution of weight on the forefoot and the heel during standing can be felt (and measured) with postural sway as well as with different heel heights on shoes.

Vertical loading of the medial longitudinal arch of the foot in bilateral standing can be measured clinically by the distance of the tuberosity of the navicular from the floor when the person is sitting (non-weight bearing) and standing (weight bearing). The difference in young adults varies from 1 to 10 mm. Normally, during relaxed standing no EMG activity occurs in the muscles of the arches or the toes (Basmajian and Latif, 1957). The foot is supported by osseous and ligamentous structures using the curved beam and truss mechanics. As the load increases and the arches are stressed, the muscles become the second line of stability. In the normal foot that was statically loaded with up to 400 lb, Basmajian (1978) recorded EMG activity in the muscles that support the arches. In persons with flat feet, Gray (1969) demonstrated abnormal EMG activity in the anterior and posterior tibialis and in the peroneal muscles during standing.

With walking, running, and standing on the toes, muscle contraction and the windlass mechanism are added to support the arches. EMG activity of the extrinsic and intrinsic muscles that support the arches begins shortly after the foot contacts the ground in the stance phase and continues as the heel rises and the MTP joint hyperextends to tighten the plantar aponeurosis (Sarrafian, 1983). The muscle activity and the tension on the aponeurosis continue until the toe leaves the ground. These mechanisms can be observed and palpated on another person during standing and rising up on the toes. Note the marked supination of the longitudinal arch and inversion of the calcaneus when standing on the toes (see Fig. 10–5).

CLINICAL APPLICATIONS

An example of a common sports-related injury of the arches of the foot is plantar fasciitis (*-itis*, inflammation) or heel spur. This problem has a high incidence in runners and aerobic dancers. Those with the problem complain of pain in the arch of the foot near the heel when they walk and that the pain becomes worse with jumping or running. The pain can be reproduced by deep palpation at the proximal attachment of the plantar aponeurosis or by passively hyperextending the MTP joints to stretch the aponeurosis.

The cause of the pain is considered to be repetitive stress of the supporting mechanisms of the arches with cumulative microtrauma to the plantar aponeurosis (it also can be caused by a sudden tear). This condition is usually due to a combination of factors, including insufficient strength in the muscles that support the arches, marked increase in the load placed on the arches, and faulty alignment of the foot. Malalignment of the foot is not uncommon. For example, an inverted calcaneus requires a pronation compensation at the calcaneotalonavicular joint to place the metatarsal heads parallel to the ground for weight bearing (Tiberio, 1988). Such malalignment, however, may never become a problem until the arches are overloaded and compensatory motions and muscle contractions fail to provide support. A careful history usually reveals a marked increase in intensity of the activity or a change of running surfaces or shoes before the onset of pain.

Another cumulative trauma problem in running activities is posterior tibial shin splint, which causes pain with contraction or stretch of the muscle. The pain can be reproduced by palpation of the proximal attachment of the muscle along the inner edge of the shin. This problem is usually associated with overpronation of the ankle, which requires more work from the posterior tibialis to support the arch in activity. DeLacerda (1980) measured the amount of depression of the navicular tuberosity before subjects started a running program. He found that those who later developed shin splints had an average depression of the navicular tuberosity of 9 mm between sitting and standing, whereas those who did not develop problems had a depression averaging 6 mm.

Laboratory Activities

ANKLE AND FOOT

1. On the skeleton, identify the following bones and bony landmarks. Locate on yourself and on a subject those that are palpable:

tibia	cuboid
fibula	three cuneiform bones
medial and lateral malleoli	metatarsal bones
tuberosity of navicular	(heads, bases, shafts)
talus	phalanges
calcaneus	tuberosity of fifth metatarsal
sustentaculum tali	

2. With disarticulated bones of the tibia, fibula, and foot, observe the articulating surfaces and simulate the motions of the:
   a. Talocrural joint
   b. Talocalcaneal joint (subtalar)
   c. Talonavicular and calcaneocuboid joints, which form the transverse tarsal joint
   d. Tarsometatarsal joints

  e. MTP joints

  f. Interphalangeal (IP) joints

3. Perform passive motion of the joints above on your partner's foot and describe the range of motion, the end-feels, and the limiting structures. Subject's leg and foot must be relaxed.

4. Measure the amount of active dorsiflexion that occurs when the knee is flexed to 90 degrees, and compare it to the amount possible when the knee is extended. What structure limits dorsiflexion when the knee is extended?

5. Palpate the sole of the relaxed foot between the calcaneous and the metatarsal heads. Then hyperextend the MTP joints and palpate to feel the tightening of the plantar aponeurosis (windlass mechanism).

6. Palpate around the head of the fibula to feel motion as the subject actively dorsiflexes the ankle. Place your fingers on each malleolus and feel the slight spreading that occurs with dorsiflexion. If you can hold the malleoli together, dorsiflexion will be limited.

7. Grasp around the calcaneus and hold it in eversion (subtalar motion) and move the transverse tarsal joint. Then hold the calcaneus in inversion and move the transverse tarsal joint. Notice the relative difference in the rigidity and flexibility of the midfoot in the two positions of the calcaneus. What is the importance of these two states of the transverse tarsal joint?

8. Measure the amount of depression of the navicular from sitting to standing. This is easier to do if a chair is placed on a treatment table. Have the subject sit in the chair with feet flat on the table. Mark the tuberosity of the navicular and measure the distance to the surface. Have the subject stand and measure the distance again. Compare results with others.

9. Measure the amount of tibial torsion present and compare angles with other subjects (see Fig. 10–3 for illustration):

  a. Have the subject sit in a chair with feet on the floor and with the knee caps pointing straight ahead. Place a piece of paper under the foot. Passively lift the relaxed leg and foot up and set it down on the paper. Identify the knee axis (x axis) running through the medial and lateral epicondyles of the femur and project it to the paper (draw the line of the knee axis on the paper).

  b. Trace around the outline of the foot and mark projections of the medial and lateral malleoli on the paper. Remove the paper and draw a line through the projections for the malleoli to represent the axis of the talocrural joint.

  c. With a protractor or a goniometer, measure the angle formed by the two axes (angle of tibial torsion). Compare with measurements on other subjects.

10. On yourself and on a subject, palpate ankle muscles and tendons following descriptions in Chapter 10:

gastrocnemius	peroneus longus
soleus	peroneus brevis
tibialis posterior	anterior tibialis
flexor digitorum longus	extensor hallucis longus
flexor hallucis longus	extensor digitorum longus
extensor digitorum brevis	

11. Analyze by observation and palpation the synergistic muscle actions in weight bearing (make sure that the subject is standing upright and looking straight ahead):
    a. Normal comfortable standing.
    b. Sway forward slightly from the ankles [observe first, then palpate, including the longitudinal arch and placing your finger(s) under the toes].
    c. Sway backward slightly from the ankles. Why is it possible to sway farther forward than backward?
    d. Rise up on the toes. Observe from behind and note the supination of the calcaneus occurring with plantarflexion.
    e. Stand on heels. Why is balance so poor compared to standing on toes?
    f. Stand on one foot. How long can you stand on one leg? What implications does this have for persons who have had an amputation of one leg?
    g. Deep knee bend, keeping heels on floor and then letting heels rise.

12. Analyze jumping up. What muscles in the lower extremity are stretched in preparation for the jump? What muscles are the prime movers for the jump? What type of contraction is made? Analyze landing.

13. Have a standing subject perform open-chain rotation of the lower limb with the knee extended. Determine by palpation at which joints (in the lower extremity) motion is occurring. Then have the subject perform closed-chain rotation with the knee extended and analyze where motion is occurring.

CHAPTER 11

Head, Neck, and Trunk

The vertebrae, ribs, and jaw have multiple purposes that frequently must be carried out simultaneously: protecting organs (spinal cord and viscera); providing the vital functions of breathing, chewing, and swallowing; supporting head, arms, and trunk (HAT) against the force of gravity; transmitting forces between upper and lower extremities; and providing stability and mobility for hand function, locomotion, and other activities. The anterior portion of the vertebral column (bodies and disks) provides for weight bearing, shock absorption, and mobility in all directions. The posterior portion of the column provides for protection of the spinal cord, guidance and limitation of motion, and elongated processes to increase the leverage of muscles of the trunk and extremities.

BONES

Normal Curves of the Vertebral Column

In posterior view, the normal spine is vertical. The linear alignment remains when the subject flexes the trunk. Laterally, the normal spine exhibits anterior and posterior physiologic curves that increase the resistance of the vertebral column to axial compression (Kapandji, 1974). At birth, the vertebral column is a single curve that is convex posteriorly. As the infant raises the head from the prone position and develops the ability to sit, the cervical vertebrae become convex anteriorly. As the child achieves standing and walking, the lumbar vertebrae develop an anterior convexity largely because of the tension of the psoas muscles (Cailliet, 1981). At about 10 years of age, the physiologic curves are similar to those found in the adult (Kapandji, 1974), with three curvatures: cervical (concave posteriorly), thoracic (convex posteriorly), and lumbar (concave posteriorly). The center of gravity of the head and subsequent superimposed segments falls on the concave side of all three curves (see Figure 12–3). In the standing position, the lumbar spine is normally in a position of lordosis. In the erect sitting position, the pelvis and sacrum are rotated posteriorly and the lumbar curve is decreased.

When the normal subject stands and slowly flexes HAT, a lateral view of the spinous processes reveals an unfolding of a posterior convexity without flattened areas or angulations. Lateral flexion to each side (viewed posteriorly) also produces symmetric curves of the spinous processes. Lack of symmetry, straight areas, or angulations indicate skeletal deviations. Although these deviations are considered abnormal, they may or may not be accompanied by back pain and dysfunction.

Nonpalpable Structures

The vertebral column is imbedded in muscles posteriorly and laterally and not available for palpation anteriorly; therefore, its general structure and the characteristics of its individual parts should be studied using a disarticulated bone set and an anatomic atlas. **An anatomic orientation must precede clinical palpation.** It is recommended that the preliminary study include the following: (1) The **physiologic curves** of the vertebral column: cervical, thoracic, lumbar, and sacrococcygeal. (2) The **general structure of a vertebra**: body and arch, enclosing the vertebral foramen; laminae; transverse, articular, and spinous processes; **specific characteristics** of the 7 cervical, 12 thoracic, and 5 lumbar vertebrae; the intervertebral disks. (3) **Ligaments** that bind the vertebrae together: anterior and posterior longitudinal ligaments, extending the entire length of the column; ligamenta flava (L. *flavus*, yellow) between the laminae of adjacent vertebrae; ligamenta intertransversaria, interspinalia, and supraspinalia; and ligamentum nuchae.

On the skull, the following structures should be identified: the **inferior nuchal line of the occipital bone**, which is almost parallel with the superior nuchal line but is hidden from palpation by muscles; the **occipital condyles**, one on each side, which go into the formation of the atlanto-occipital joints; the **jugular processes** of the occipital bone, which are located lateral to the occipital condyles and serve as attachments to one of the short posterior neck muscles (rectus capitis lateralis); and the **foramen magnum** of the occipital bone, which transmits the medulla oblongata.

On the anterior side of the foramen magnum is the **basilar part of the occipital bone**. This portion of the bone lies on the anterior side of the axis of motion of the atlanto-occipital joints and serves as an attachment for the deep flexor muscles of the head (longus capitis, rectus capitis anterior).

On the mandible (lower jaw), the following parts should be identified: the **body, ramus, convex condyles**, and **coronoid process** for attachment of the temporalis muscle. At rest, the condyles of the mandible lie in the glenoid fossa of the temporal bone. When the mouth is opened, the condyles move down and forward to lie beneath the **articular tubercle** on the **zygomatic process** of the temporal bone (see Fig. 11–11).

Palpable Structures

If the fingers are placed behind the earlobes, the mastoid portion of the temporal bone can be palpated, its lowest part being the **mastoid process** (Gr. *mastor*, breast; *eidos*, resemblance). In the erect position, this process is best felt if the head is bent forward slightly so that the sternocleidomastoid (SCM) muscle, which attaches to it, is relaxed. When the head is tipped backward, the muscle tightens, and only part of the process may be palpated.

If the fingers are moved in a posterior direction from the mastoid process, the **occipital bone** with its **superior nuchal line** is reached. The lateral portion of this ridge serves, in part, as a site for attachments of the SCM muscle and its medial portion, in part, as a site for attachment of the trapezius.

At the point where the two superior nuchal lines of the right and the left sides meet in the median line is a small eminence, the **external occipital protuberance**; the external occipital crest extends from the protuberance to the foramen magnum, also in the median line. These bony eminences, which are not too easily palpable, serve as sites for attachment of the **ligamentum nuchae**, a strong ligamentous band extending from the seventh cervical vertebra to the skull. This ligament is attached to the trapezius muscle and to a number of posterior neck muscles. It is best palpated when it is slack—when the head is tilted backward.

Just anterior to the external auditory canals, the **condyles of the mandible** can be palpated. When the subject opens the mouth or deviates the jaw, the condyles can be felt to move on the glenoid fossa and tubercle of the temporal bones. The mandibular condyles also can be felt by placing the finger in the ear canal and pressing anteriorly.

For clinical orientation, the following landmarks may be used to determine the height of specific vertebrae: C-3—level with the hyoid bone, which can be palpated anteriorly just below the mandible; C-4 and C-5—level with the thyroid cartilage; C-6—level with the arch of the cricoid cartilage; body of T-4—height of the junction of the manubrium and the body of the sternum; body of T-10—level with the tip of the xiphoid process; spinous process of L-4—level with the highest portion of the crest of the ilium; S-2—height of the posterior superior iliac spines.

First and Second Cervical Vertebrae

The first cervical vertebra, the **atlas**, has a transverse process that protrudes more laterally than do those of the other vertebrae in this region. This process may be palpated and is found just below the tip of the mastoid process. This region is rather sensitive to pressure, and it is recommended that the process be identified on one's self before palpating it on another person. The **posterior tubercle of the atlas** (its rudimentary spinous process) lies deep but may be found in its relation to the second cervical vertebra. The **spinous process of the axis**, the second cervical vertebra, is strong and prominent and is therefore easy to identify.

Third to Sixth Cervical Vertebrae

The lateral portions of these vertebrae present a number of processes and tubercles that are best palpated with the subject supine to relax the muscles of the neck. These vertebrae have short and perforated transverse processes for the vertebral arteries, and their articular processes protrude laterally; therefore, the palpable areas of these vertebrae feel very uneven. Their short, bifid spinous processes may be felt in the median line, although they are covered by ligamentum nuchae.

Vertebra Prominens (C-7)

Because of the prominence of its spinous process, which is longer and sturdier than those of the other cervical vertebrae and not bifid, the vertebra prominens can be identified easily in most individuals. Often, however, the spinous process of the first thoracic vertebra is equally prominent. When the subject bends the head forward, identification of these processes is facilitated. When two processes in this region seem to be equal in size, they are identified as those of C-7 and T-1.

Thoracic and Lumbar Vertebrae

When the subject bends forward, flexing the entire spine, the spinous processes of the vertebral column become somewhat separated from each other and may be palpated throughout the thoracic and lumbar regions. The vertebra prominens is used as a starting point for counting the vertebrae, which can be done accurately in most subjects, particularly if the subject is told to "make the back round." Vertebral columns, however, present a great deal of individual variations. One or the other spinous process may be less developed and more difficult to locate, and minor lateral deviations of the processes are common also.

In the thoracic region, the spinous processes are directed downward and overlap each other, so that the spinous process of one vertebra is located approximately at the height of the body of the next lower one. In the lumbar region, the spinous processes are large and directed horizontally, so that the height of the spinous process more nearly represents the height of its body. The change from one type to another is gradual. The two lowest thoracic vertebrae resemble the lumbar vertebrae, having rather horizontally directed spinous processes that are approximately at the height of the intervertebral disk between its own body and the body of the next lower vertebra.

Sacrum and Coccyx

The exterior surface of the sacrum is palpated as a direct continuation of the lumbar spine. The medial sacral crest represents the rudimentary spinous processes of the sacral vertebrae, the processes being fused with the rest of the bone. On both sides of the crest are rough areas serving as sites for attachment of ligaments, fascia, and muscles. The approximate boundaries of the sacrum may be determined by following the crests of the ilia in a posterior direction, where the sacrum is interposed between the two ilia. The "dimples" medial to the posterior superior spines of the ilia indicate the posterior approach to the sacroiliac joints.

Caudally, the sacrum is continuous with the coccyx, and the two bones form a marked posterior convexity so that the tip of the coccyx has a deep location between the two gluteal eminences. If a subject sits on the front portion of a hard chair and then leans against the back of the chair, the coccyx may be felt contacting the chair.

Thorax (Rib Cage)

The thorax consists of the 12 thoracic vertebrae in back, the sternum in front, and the 12 ribs. Most of the external surfaces of the thorax may be palpated. Some difficulty arises in palpating the upper ribs, which are hidden by structures of the neck and by the clavicle. In obese individuals, palpation of the last two, or "floating," ribs may be difficult also. Those portions of the ribs that lie close to the vertebral column are covered by muscles, but, beginning at their angles, the ribs may be palpated in their lateral, forward, and downward courses. It should be recalled that the 1st to 7th ribs attach to the sternum, the 8th to 10th ribs join with each other by means of cartilage, and the 11th and 12th ribs have free ends.

When the ribs on the left side are being palpated, it is recommended that the subject place the left hand on top of the head and stretch the left side so that the ribs become somewhat separated from each other. In stretching the side of the thorax, the distance increases between the lowest part of the rib cage laterally and the crest of the ilium, permitting the floating ribs to be more or less easily located. In the ordinary erect position, this distance is very short. In pathologic conditions, as in advanced states of lateral curvature of the spine, the ribs may actually come to rest on the ilium and nerves may become pinched, causing pain.

Sternum

The sternum may be palpated from the xiphoid process below to the manubrium and the sternoclavicular joints above.

JOINTS

The motion segment of the spine consists of two adjacent vertebrae, three intervertebral joints, the soft tissues of the intervertebral disk, longitudinal and intersegmental ligaments, and the capsules of the facet joints (White and Panjabi,

1978). The disk and the bilateral facet joints form a triangle whereby motion at one joint always produces motion at the other two joints. In most of the vertebral joints, six degrees of freedom of motion are permitted. These are forward and backward bending (flexion-extension), side bending (lateral flexion), rotation, anterior-posterior shear, lateral shear, and distraction-compression. Biomechanically, the bony and ligamentous structures of the vertebrae are divided into anterior and posterior vertebral structures. The anterior structures function primarily to bear weight, and the posterior structures are responsible primarily for controlling motion.

Anterior Vertebral Joint Structures

The weight-bearing bodies of the vertebrae, intervertebral disks, and the longitudinal ligaments form the anterior vertebral structures (Fig. 11–1). Biomechanical functions of the vertebral bodies include resistance to the compressive forces of superincumbent weight; muscle contractions; and external loads that occur in lifting, pulling, or pushing. The intervening disks protect the facet joints from compression injury and permit as well as limit motions of the vertebrae. Each disk is composed of three parts: the **annulus fibrosus**, a series of fibroelastic cartilaginous rings that enclose the **nucleus pulposus**, a gel with an 80 percent or more water content; and two hyaline **cartilaginous plates**, which separate the nucleus and the annulus from the vertebral bodies. The fibers in the annulus run obliquely from the inferior edge of the upper vertebrae to the superior margin of the lower

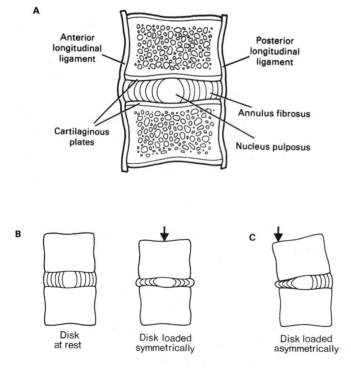

Figure 11–1 Anterior vertebral structures. (*A*) Sagittal view of two vertebral bodies and associated soft tissues. (*B*) Response of disk to loading.

vertebrae. Fiber direction is opposite in alternate layers, forming crossing patterns so that motions in opposite directions can be restrained. The circumference of the disk is basically the same as the bodies, but the height becomes greater in the lumbar area. In total, the intervertebral disks account for approximately 25 percent of the length of the vertebral column.

With weight bearing or muscle contraction, forces are transmitted from the bodies of the vertebrae to the disk. The fluid nucleus is normally confined, and the pressure increases to exert forces on the elastic annulus, which bulges (stretches) to absorb the force and limit motion (see Fig. 11–1B). In most loading situations, the force is not applied in the center but rather on the anterior, posterior, or lateral parts of the body. This produces compression of the annulus near the force and tension on the opposite side, with each serving to limit vertebral compression.

The nucleus pulposus is composed largely of water and is hydrophilic (loves water). Compression forces produced by standing and walking during the day cause the nucleus to lose small quantities of water, which are restored during sleep and recumbency, when pressures inside the nucleus are reduced. Thus, changes in standing height of an individual may amount to as much as 2 cm between morning and evening. The supply of blood vessels to the disk disappears in the second decade of life (Cailliet, 1981), and the ability of the nucleus to restore lost water begins to decrease. Repeated microtrauma from lifting heavy objects, as well as the aging process, causes an increase in fibrous elements of the annulus and a decrease in the relative number of resilient elastic elements. The aging process causes mature adults (30 to 50 years) to become prone to injuries of the annulus and to herniation of the nucleus onto the nerve roots. Older adults (50 to 90 years) may lose trunk height and be prone to develop thoracic kyphosis (Gr. *kyphos*, a hump), a prominent convex curvature of the spine.

Longitudinal Ligaments

Anterior and **posterior longitudinal ligaments** (ALL and PLL) cover the front and back of the vertebral bodies from the axis to the sacrum (see Figs. 11–1 and 11–2). The broad and strong ALL attaches to the annulus and the edge of the vertebral body. Between the body and the ligament are veins and arteries that pass into foramina to the body. The ALL limits backward bending, and in the lumbosacral area supports the anterior convexity. The narrower PLL attaches to the annulus and the superior margin of the vertebral body. The ligament does not attach to the body but covers a plexus of arteries, veins, and lymphatics and the nutrient foramina through which these vessels pass to the cancellous bone of the body. Forward bending is somewhat restrained by the PLL but its leverage is poor, and the tensile strength is relatively low (Myklebust et al, 1988). With forward bending, however, the PLL becomes taut to close the nutrient foramina and trap fluid in the cancellous vertebral body. This mechanism is thought to increase the vertebral body's ability to withstand compression forces.

When these ligaments (as well as the ligamentum flavum) were removed from the spine, Tkaczuk (1968) found them to retract. He suggested that normal disks are prestressed by the ligaments. Thus, the disk and the ligaments present a system of balanced forces and resistance to motion.

Table 11-1   Some Examples of Forces on the Lumbar (L-3) Intervertebral Disk

	Newtons	Ratio to Standing
Supine in traction (300 N)	100	−0.2
Supine	250	−0.5
Supine arm exercises (20 N)	600	+1.2
Standing at ease	**500**	**1.0**
Sitting unsupported	700	+1.4
Sitting in office chair	500	1.0
Cough in standing	700	+1.4
Standing forward bent 40 degrees	1000	+2.0
Lifting 100 N (knees ext, back flex)	1700	+3.4
Lifting 100 N (knees flex, back ext)	1900	+3.8

Source: Data from Nachemson, A: Disc pressure measurements. Spine 6:93, 1981; Nachemson, A: Lumbar intradiscal pressure. In Jayson, M (ed): *The Lumbar Spine and Back Pain.* Churchill Livingstone, Edinburgh, 1987.

Disk Pressures

Recording of pressures within the lumbar disk has been studied in both cadavers and live human subjects by Nachemson (1960, 1981, 1987). His work demonstrated that in normal disks (1) the center of the nucleus pulposis acts hydrostatically; (2) disk pressure is linearly related to the compressive force up to 450 lb; (3) the nucleus supports about $1\frac{1}{2}$ times the compressive load and the annulus supports $\frac{1}{2}$ of the imposed load; (4) pressures exerted on the sides of the annulus reach 4 to 5 times the compressive load; and (5) the bilateral facet joints can support $\frac{1}{5}$ of the imposed load. More recent studies by McNally and Adams (1992) confirm that compressive forces are generally distributed across the nucleus in normal disks and that the annulus may behave either as a fluid or as a tensile structure. Detailed exploration of pressures in different areas of the disk suggest that it functions with multiple fluid compartments possessing mechanical properties that vary with the load and the loading history.

Examples of approximate disk loads recorded by Nachemson at L-3 in different postures and activities are found in Table 11–1. The prestress of the disk by the ligaments can be seen in the supine position. Traction in the area of 500 N was needed to reduce the force to zero. Many seemingly mild activities, such as arm exercises in the supine position and unsupported sitting, create greater forces on the disk than occur while standing.

Posterior Vertebral Joint Structures

Posterior vertebral structures comprise the arches, the transverse and spinous processes, the bilateral facet joints, joint capsules, and ligaments. The facet joints (apophyseal or zygoapophyseal joints) are formed by the inferior articulating process of one vertebra with the superior articulating process of the vertebra below (see Fig. 11–4C). The major functions of facet joints are to control vertebral motions and to protect the disk from excessive shear, flexion, side bending, and rotation. The direction and amount of motion permitted are determined by the planes of the joint surfaces, which change in their orientation from the cervical through the lumbar areas.

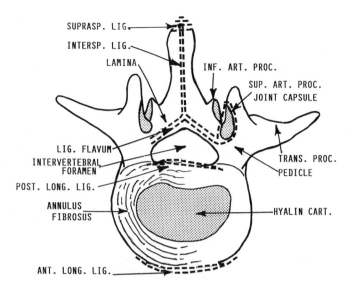

Figure 11–2 Superior view of a lumbar vertebra, illustrating the schema of the longitudinal ligaments of the vertebral bodies and the intersegmental ligaments of the vertebral arches from C2 to the sacrum. Note the continuity of the supraspinous ligament, the interspinous ligament, the ligamentum flavum, and the capsular ligaments, as well as the continuity of the posterior longitudinal ligament and the annulus fibrosus. Articulating surfaces of the lumbar vertebral body and facet joints on the inferior and superior articular processes are illustrated. Note the sagittal-frontal orientation of the lumbar facet joint articulations.

Ligaments

The **ligamenta flava** (L., *flavus*, yellow) are a series of 23 intersegmental ligaments that connect the lamina of two adjacent vertebrae from C-2 to the sacrum (Fig. 11–2). The yellow color reflects the high elastic content, which contributes to the pre-stress of the disk and resistance to forward bending. Ligamentum flavum fibers cover the anterior surface of the capsule of the facet joint and provide tension on the capsule to prevent nipping and injury by the facet joints in movement. In addition, the fibers of the ligamentum flavum are continuous with the **interspinous ligaments**, which attach between adjacent spinous processes. The interspinous ligaments are continuous with the **supraspinous ligament**, a strong, fibrous cord attaching to the tips of the spinous processes and continuous with the thoracodorsal fascia. In the cervical area, the supraspinous ligament becomes the **ligamentum nuchae** (L., *nucha*, nape or scruff of the neck). **Intertransverse ligaments** are segmental with attachments between adjacent transverse processes.

The interspinous and the supraspinous ligaments resist motions of forward bending very efficiently. This ligamentous system is attached farther from the vertebral bodies than the spinal muscles and thus has a leverage advantage. In addition, the supraspinous ligament has great tensile strength, especially in the lumbar area (Myklebust et al, 1988).

Coupling Motions

Motions in the vertebral joints seldom occur in pure planar motion but rather in combined motions called **coupling**. A simple example of coupling occurs when an anterior force in the horizontal plane is applied to a vertebra. This vertebra translates forward on the z axis (anterior shear) and rotates forward around the x axis (flexion). Coupling occurs because of the orientation of the planes of the bilateral facet joints and limitation of motion by the annulus, vertebral ligaments, fascia, and muscles. Grieve (1988) states that tripling is more appropriate. He gives the example of turning the head to look over the shoulder while sitting. For individual cervical vertebrae, this view requires motions of backward bending, rotation, and side bending.

The greatest complexity of coupling in the spine is with side bending and rotation. After one or two degrees of motion, side bending is always accompanied by rotation, and rotation is always accompanied by side bending (Grieve, 1988). MacConaill and Basmajian (1969) present the basis of this in a mechanical principle that says, "If a flexible rod is bent first in one plane and then, while it is in this bent position, is bent again in a plane at right angles to the first, it always rotates on its longitudinal axis at the same time." If this principle is applied to movements in the vertebral column, the "rod" (the spine) is normally "bent"—with an anterior concavity in the thoracic region and a posterior concavity in the lumbar region, causing compression on the concave side and soft tissue tension on the convex side. Thus, the "spinal column is already bent by its normal curves and lateral bending approaches a right angle to these curves" (Kent, 1974). The direction of vertebral rotation as lateral bending occurs is regulated by tension put on the ligaments and by the direction of the normal physiologic curves in combination with the direction of the lateral bend. The concave side of the normal curve turns to the convex side of the lateral curve (MacConaill and Basmajian, 1969). A lateral bend to the left would cause rotation of the thoracic vertebral bodies to the right. Lumbar bodies would tend to rotate left, but because the articular surfaces in this region are directed in a nearly sagittal plane, rotation here is limited.

The effects of coupling of vertebral motions can be seen in the extreme in pathologic lateral curvature of the spine (scoliosis). In severe right thoracic–left lumbar lateral curvature, a hump (or gibbus) may be seen on the right side of the posterior rib cage with a depression of the rib cage on the left side. This hump is due to rotation of the vertebrae to the convexity of the lateral curvature. The ribs, in turn, follow the vertebrae and form the hump. In mild or early cases of scoliosis, the hump is not obvious in the standing position. If lateral curvature is present, asymmetries of the sides in the thoracic area are sighted by the examiner when the subject flexes the trunk to reach toward the floor.

Cervical Region

The occiput, atlas (C-1), and axis (C-2) form the **craniovertebral area**. Here the facet joints are specialized, only two or three degrees of freedom exist, and the planes are nearly horizontal. The **atlanto-occipital joints** have two degrees of freedom of motion. The two joints work in unison to provide movements between the head and the vertebral column. The shallow, concave joint surfaces on the atlas, one on each side of the vertebral canal, support the two convex condyles of the occipital bone. This structure permits support of the head from below without interfering with the passage of the medulla oblongata into the vertebral canal, while still providing needed mobility of the head.

Movement of the head at the atlanto-occipital joints is mainly a nodding movement in the sagittal plane about a transverse axis through the two condyles. The approximate location of this axis is demonstrated by placing the tips of the two index fingers pointing toward each other on the mastoid processes. Small lateral bending movements also are permitted, but these are quite limited.

The **atlanto-axial joints** (C-1 to C-2) are formed by one centrally located articulation and two facet joints (inferior articular processes of the atlas and the superior articular processes of the axis). Centrally, the dens of the axis (odontoid process) fits into a ring formed by the anterior arch of the atlas and its transverse ligament posteriorly, so that the atlas pivots around the dens. The axis of motion is vertical through the dens. Approximately 50 percent of rotation in the cervical area occurs at the atlanto-axial joints.

In the typical **cervical vertebral articulations** (C-2 to C-3 through C-6 to C-7), the articulating surfaces of the facet joints change from horizontal to a 45-degree angle between the horizontal and frontal planes. This facet orientation, along with loose and elastic capsules, permits motion in each plane. The superior articular facets slide up and forward in forward bending and down the back in backward bending. In side bending right, the left superior facet goes up and forward while the right superior facet goes down and backward, producing a rotation of the body of the vertebrae to the right and the spinous process to the left (White and Panjabi, 1978).

Normally, the erect posture of the cervical spine is lordotic (concave posteriorly). Flexion occurs to a straight line, and extension occurs until the spinous processes contact to limit motion.

Specific joint ranges of vertebral motion cited in the literature vary considerably. White and Panjabi (1978) present representative angles based on literature review and their experimental work (Fig. 11–3). In each intervertebral articulation from C-2 to C-7, flexion-extension varied from 8 to 17 degrees, side bending varied from 7 to 10 degrees, and rotation varied from 9 to 12 degrees.

In addition to permitting and controlling motion, the facet joints in the cervical area also share some of the weight-bearing forces of the head because of their 45-degree orientation to the frontal plane. This function is significant because the head (10 lb) may be supported by the long lever arm of the cervical vertebrae dur-

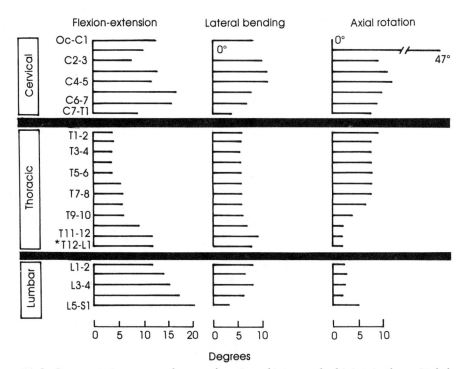

Figure 11–3 Representative average degrees of motion of intervertebral joints in the sagittal, frontal, and horizontal planes. These values are based on the author's review of the literature as well as on analysis of motion. (Adapted from White and Panjabi: The basic kinematics of the lumbar spine. *Spine* 3:12, 1978.)

ing sitting and standing postures for periods up to 16 or more hours per day without rest.

Thoracic Region

The thoracic vertebrae support and permit motion of the head and trunk; provide protection of the heart, lungs, and great vessels; supply articulations for respiration; and provide attachments for muscles of respiration, the trunk, and the extremities.

The plane of the facet joints moves toward the vertical or frontal plane (see Fig. 11–4C). This orientation limits flexion and anterior shear motions and permits side bending. The ribs and the sternum, however, limit the potential motions of the thoracic vertebrae. Extension of the thoracic spine also is limited by contact of the spinous processes. Total extension is to a straight line. Representative angles at typical thoracic vertebrae for forward and backward bending combined were 4 to 6 degrees; for side bending, 6 degrees; and for rotation, 8 degrees (see Fig. 11–3). The lower thoracic vertebrae have fewer restrictions from the ribs, and their facet joint planes are more sagittally oriented. Intervertebral motions more resemble lumbar motions, with increased flexion-extension and side bending and less rotation.

Costal Joints

Two synovial joints are formed by the ribs on each side of the thoracic vertebrae posteriorly (see Fig. 11–4). The typical ribs 2 through 9 articulate with the adjacent body, the body above, and the disk between to form the costovertebral joint, while the atypical ribs 1, 10, 11, and 12 articulate with the corresponding body

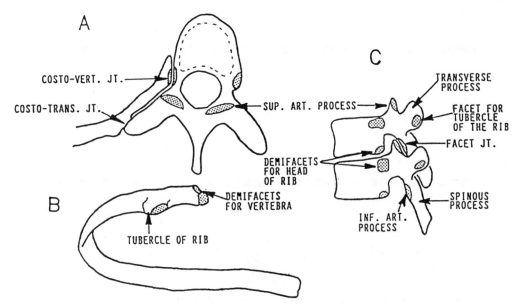

Figure 11–4 Articulating surfaces of a typical thoracic vertebra and rib. (*A*) Superior view with horizontal section through the superior articular processes and the neck of the rib. (*B*) Posterior inferior view of a typical left rib. (*C*) Left side view of the costal and facet joint articulating surfaces.

only. Ribs 1 through 10 articulate with the same transverse process to form the costotransverse joint. Both of these joints are reinforced by strong ligaments. Anteriorly, the cartilages of ribs 2 through 7 form synovial joints with the sternum (the first rib is cartilaginous only). The costal cartilages of ribs 8 through 10 articulate with the cartilage above, and the lateral ends of ribs 11 and 12 are free or floating.

Elevation and depression of the ribs occur by a pivoting motion through an axis crossing the costovertebral and costotransverse joints. The orientation of the upper ribs is more horizontal, and the motion of elevation produces an increased anterior diameter of the rib cage. The lower ribs have a more oblique downward orientation, and elevation of the ribs increases the transverse diameter of the rib cage. Increase in the anterior diameter can be felt by placing one hand on the upper part of the sternum and the other hand on the back in the upper thoracic area and asking the subject to perform a vital capacity maneuver (maximum inspiration followed by a maximum expiration). The larger changes that occur in the transverse diameter can be felt by placing both hands over the lateral surfaces of the lower ribs and asking the subject to perform the same vital capacity maneuver.

In addition to participating in the function of respiration, the articulations and structures of the rib cage protect vital organs and make significant contributions to the stability of the thoracic spine.

Lumbar Region

The large bodies and the intervertebral disks of the lumbar vertebrae, along with the strong anterior longitudinal and iliolumbar ligaments, normally bear most of the weight of HAT in erect posture. Lumbar facet joints are half-moon–shaped with articulating surfaces in both sagittal and frontal planes. The proportion of sagittal surface is greater at T-12 to L-1. This progressively changes to more frontal plane orientation at L-5 to S-1. This facet joint orientation prohibits motions of rotation and anterior shear. Although rotation is described as being 1 to 3 degrees, Porterfield and DeRosa (1991) consider this to be cartilage deformation rather than true joint motion. Facet joint damage was demonstrated in a cadaver study when the lumbar spine was loaded and subjected to 1 to 3 degrees of rotation (Adams and Hutton, 1983).

Forward bending of the lumbar spine occurs to a straight line in adults. Representative motions for backward bending from this position increase from 12 degrees at T-12 to L-1 to 20 degrees at L-5 to S-1. Side bending decreases from 6 to 3 degrees (see Fig. 11–3).

With narrowing of the intervertebral disk, the tips of the facet joints rest on the lamina of the vertebrae above or below. This occurs with degenerative disk disease and results in up to 70 percent of the compression force being transmitted through the articular processes, which are not designed for weight bearing (Adams and Hutton, 1983). Contact of the facet tips also may occur with prolonged standing in normal subjects because of the decrease in disk height combined with the lordotic position in standing. Adams and Hutton postulate that the dull ache that can occur in the low back may be due to pressure and microtrauma on the facet joint capsules.

Forward bending of the trunk in the standing position creates major forces on the articular surfaces of the facet joints and capsular structures. In cadavers, the capsular ligaments of the facet joints were found to provide 39 percent of the passive resistance to forward bending, the disk 29 percent, the supraspinous and interspinous ligaments 19 percent, and the ligamenta flava 13 percent (Adams, Hutton, and Stott, 1980).

Lumbosacral Junction

Angulation of the vertebral column at the lumbosacral junction is marked in standing (see Fig. 8–3), and the joint is subjected to a great deal of anterior shear by the superimposed body weight. This joint is reinforced by strong iliolumbar ligaments from L-4 to L-5 and by sacrolumbar ligaments, which primarily restrict motions of lateral bending but also limit flexion, extension, and rotation (Yamamoto et al, 1990). The near frontal plane orientation of the L-5 to S-1 facet joints prevents excessive anterior shear of the fifth lumbar vertebra. Anatomic variations that weaken the joint may permit the lumbar vertebra to slide forward on the sacrum, a pathology known as **spondylolisthesis** (Gr. *spondylos*, vertebra; *olisthesis*, a slipping or falling).

Thoracolumbar Fascia

The **thoracolumbar fascia** (also called thoracodorsal fascia) is a strong, complex structure that acts like a huge ligament to connect the ribs, vertebrae, and sacrum; the posterior intervertebral ligamentous system; and three trunk muscles. This fascial system provides humans with the unique ability to lift heavy weights overhead and to stabilize the trunk for throwing objects with high velocities (Farfan, 1988). Detailed anatomic description of the fascia and biomechanical considerations are presented by Bogduk and Macintosh (1984).

The thoracolumbar fascia is composed of anterior, middle, and posterior layers. The **anterior layer** is deep and attaches to the transverse processes of the lumbar vertebrae to cover the quadratus lumborum muscle. The **middle layer** is composed of strong, transverse fibers attaching to the lumbar transverse processes medially and the 12th rib and the transverse abdominis muscle at the lateral raphe (Gr. seam). The **posterior layer** covers the back and is attached to the spinous processes and the supraspinous ligament medially. Superiorly, the fascia blends with that of the splenius muscles and distally attaches to the sacrum and fuses with the fascia of the gluteal muscles. Laterally, the posterior layer attaches to the ribs and the ilia and at the lateral raphe forms attachments with the internal abdominal oblique muscle.

The posterior layer of the thoracodorsal fascia is further divided into superficial and deep lamina. The superficial lamina is the broad aponeurosis of the latissimus dorsi muscle with fibers directed inferiorly and medially from the lateral raphe to attach the latissimus muscle to the spinous processes. The deep lamina is fused to the superficial lamina and crosses it in the opposite direction. Together they form a series of strong triangular structures with apices on the lateral raphe and bases covering two vertebral levels (Bogduk and Macintosh, 1984). In addition, the thoracodorsal fascia provides a retinaculum (L. a net) to envelop the erector spinae and multifidus muscles.

These connections permit a number of forces to be applied to the lumbodorsal fascia, the spinous processes, and the posterior ligamentous system to cause lumbar extension and resistance to lumbar flexion. These forces include contraction of the latissimus dorsi muscles when the hands are fixed; contraction of the transverse abdominis and internal abdominal oblique muscles; contraction of the erector spinae to make the fascial envelope rigid; and the motion of forward bending as in leaning over to pick something up from the floor. The ways in which the thoracodorsal fascial system is thought to function are discussed later in this chapter in the section on forward bending and lifting.

MUSCLES

Head, neck, and trunk muscles are paired with a muscle on each side of the midline. When both muscles contract and movement occurs, the motion is forward or backward bending in the sagittal plane. If only one of the muscles contracts, side bending or rotation occurs in the frontal or transverse planes. Most frequently, the neck and trunk muscles participate in co-contractions to stabilize the vertebrae to withstand applied weight, extremity muscle contractions, and ground reaction forces.

Kinesiologic knowledge of functions of the superficial muscles of the neck and trunk is almost equal to our knowledge of extremity musculature. Knowledge of the actions and functions of the deep neck and trunk musculature, however, is limited because the three to five layers of muscles are difficult to differentiate by manual palpation or surface electrode (EMG) recording. Insertion of fine wire electrodes into the deep muscles of the neck and the trunk may endanger vital structures, and the risk may be unacceptable for normal studies. Even when fine wire electrodes can be inserted safely, it is difficult to determine from which muscle the electrode is recording. Unfortunately, lack of knowledge of muscle actions has been equated to lack of importance of those muscles.

Anterior Cervical Muscles

The two short **rectus capitis anterior** and **rectus capitis lateralis muscles** have their **proximal attachments** along the length of the transverse processes of the atlas. The fibers of the rectus capitis anterior are directed medially to **attach** on the occipital bone anterior to the foramen magnum. The fibers of the lateralis are directed laterally to **attach** on the jugular process of the occipital bone. **Innervation:** C_1 to C_2. **Anatomic action:** Bilateral contraction of these muscles produces flexion of the head on the atlas. The rectus capitis lateralis has excellent leverage for me-diolateral control of the head or lateral flexion with unilateral contraction.

Longus Capitis and Longus Colli Muscles

The **longus capitis** has its **proximal attachments** on the transverse processes of cervical vertebrae 3 to 6, and the fibers run superiorly to cover the rectus capitis anterior and **attach** just in front of it on the basilar part of the occipital bone. **Innervation:** C_1-C_3. **Anatomic actions:** Acting bilaterally, the muscles can produce flexion of the head and the upper cervical spine. With unilateral action, the muscles are in positions to produce lateral bending and rotation of this area.

The **longus colli** is a complex three-part muscle covering the anterolateral surface of the vertebrae from the arch of the atlas to the third thoracic vertebra. The fibers of the vertical portion of the muscle extend from the bodies of the upper cervical vertebrae (C-2 to C-4) to the bodies of the distal vertebrae (C-5 to T-3). The superior and inferior oblique portions of the muscle have attachments on the third to the sixth cervical transverse processes. The fibers of the superior portion **ascend** to attach to the anterior arch of the atlas, and the fibers of the inferior portions **descend** to attach to the bodies of the thoracic vertebrae (T-1 to T-3). **Innervation:** C_2-C_7. **Anatomic action:** Flexion of the cervical spine. Basmajian (1978) states that EMG studies show the longus colli to be a strong flexor of the cervical spine. He hypothesized that the increase in longus colli activity found during talking, coughing, and swallowing represents stabilization of the neck for these functions.

PALPATION The longus capitis and longus colli can be palpated by placing the fingers medial and deep to the SCM muscle near the anterolateral surface of the cervical vertebrae. Have the subject rotate the head to the same side to relax the SCM muscle and then resist neck flexion with the other hand so that the muscle contraction can be felt by the palpating fingers.

Scalenus Anterior, Medius, and Posterior Muscles

The **scalene muscles** (Gr. *skalenos*, uneven triangle) have **superior attachments** on the transverse processes of the lower six cervical vertebrae and their **inferior attachments** on the anterior inner border of the first or second rib (scalene posterior). The superior attachments of the scalenes are adjacent to the inferior attachments of the longus capitis and the oblique portions of the longus colli so that there are direct lines of pull from the anterior aspects of the occiput through the cervical vertebrae to the first and second ribs. **Innervation:** C_3-C_8. **Anatomic action:** With bilateral contraction, the scalene muscles flex the cervical spine, and with unilateral contraction, they produce lateral flexion and rotation to the same side. When the cervical spine is stabilized, the scalene muscles elevate the first and second ribs. In the absence of longus colli contraction to initiate cervical forward bending, bilateral contraction of the scalene muscles increases the cervical lordotic curve (Kapandji, 1974).

PALPATION The scalenus anterior and scalenus medius attach to the first rib and may be palpated during forced inspiration by placing the fingertips just above the clavicle and behind the SCM muscle. They are also felt in the erect position when rotation of the head is resisted to the same side to relax the SCM.

The ventral roots of C_5-T_1 spinal nerves and the subclavian artery and vein pass between the scalenus anterior and the scalenus medius and above the first rib. Anatomic variation, hypertrophy, or spasm of these muscles can cause compression of the vessels or nerve roots, resulting in pain and dysfunction. This has been termed **thoracic outlet syndrome** and, more recently, **thoracic inlet syndrome**.

Sternocleidomastoid Muscles

The **sternocleidomastoid muscles (SCM)** are the most superficial of the anterior neck muscles (Fig. 11–5). **Proximal attachments:** By two heads, with one head from the upper border of the manubrium sterni, partly covering the sternoclavicular joint, and the other head from the upper border of the clavicle. **Distal attachments:** Mastoid process of the temporal bone and the superior nuchal line of the occipital bone. **Innervation:** Spinal accessory nerve (XI) C_1-C_3. **Anatomic actions:** Unilateral contraction combines rotation of the head (face) to the opposite side, lateral flexion to the same side, and extension of the head and cervical vertebrae.

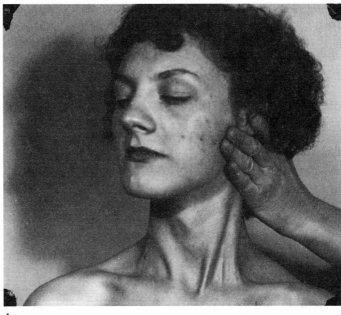

A

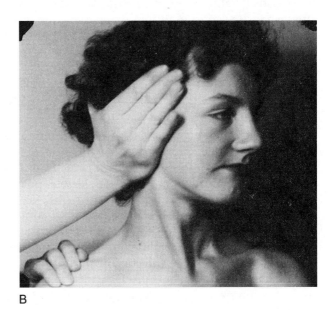

Figure 11–5 Testing the sternocleidomastoid muscle unilaterally. (*A*) For strong activation of the left sternocleidomastoid muscle, the head is rotated to the right and resistance is given to lateral flexion of the head to the left. Both sternal and clavicular portions are seen. (*B*) In this patient, the clavicular portion of the right sternocleidomastoid muscle is missing. The sternal portion is seen contracting.

B

Most anatomic texts state that the bilateral action of the SCM is neck flexion. Kapandji (1974), however, points out that the SCM, which completely bridges the cervical vertebrae, requires synergistic contractions of the vertebral muscles to stabilize the cervical spine so that the SCM can produce a flexion motion. In the absence of these synergistic contractions, isolated contraction of the SCM causes extension of the head and an increase in the lordotic cervical curve.

Because of the attachments on the sternoclavicular joint, the SCM are considered accessory muscles of inspiration. Persons with attacks of asthma or other respiratory distress exhibit contractions of the SCM and other accessory muscles on inspiration.

Accessory Neck Flexors

A large number of small muscles essential for chewing, swallowing, and speaking also are classed as accessory neck flexors. These include the **platysma, suprahyoid muscles** (digastric, stylohyoid, mylohyoid, and geniohyoid), and **infrahyoid muscles** (sternohyoid, thyrohyoid, sternothyroid, and omohyoid). The primary action of these muscles is positioning of the hyoid bone, the thyroid cartilage, and the mandible. When the jaw is stabilized by the masseter muscles, the suprahyoid and infrahyoid muscles can be felt to contract with resisted neck flexion. With paralysis of the long neck flexors, however, the accessory muscles produce some stabilization of the neck but cannot lift the head in the supine position. These muscles also are seen to contract ineffectively during inspiration when a person is in respiratory distress.

Posterior Cervical Muscles

Numerous muscles are on the posterior aspect of the cervical spine and as a group have considerably more bulk than the anterior group, indicating that greater strength is needed to maintain extension. Cervical nerves exit between these muscles and are sometimes compressed, causing tension headaches or neck and shoulder pain.

Suboccipital Muscles

Four short, deep muscles connect the upper two cervical vertebrae and the occipital bone. The **rectus capitis posterior major** attaches to the spinous process of the axis, and the **rectus capitis posterior minor** attaches just above on the atlas. The muscles ascend and fan out to attach on the inferior nuchal line of the occiput. The **inferior oblique** goes from the spinous process of the axis to the transverse process of the atlas where the **superior oblique** attaches and goes up to the occiput. **Innervation:** Suboccipital nerve (C_1). **Anatomic actions:** Bilateral contractions produce head extension at the atlanto-occipital joint, whereas unilateral contractions produce lateral flexion and, at the atlantoaxial joint, rotation.

These and the short anterior muscles are thought to provide precise fine control of head posture. The muscles can be palpated with the fingertips when the subject is supine and the muscles of the neck are relaxed.

Transversospinal Muscles

The transversospinal muscles are so named because they attach between the transverse and spinous processes. The **rotatores** are the deepest and attach to the transverse process of one vertebra and to the base of the spinous process above. These small muscles are difficult to distinguish from the **multifidus** (L. multifid, many parts), which cover the rotatores. The multifidus attach to the transverse processes and traverse two to five vertebrae above to attach to a spinous process. The next layer consists of the **semispinalis capitis** and **cervicis** with attachments on the transverse processes of the upper six thoracic vertebrae. The superior attachment of the capitis is on the head above the inferior nuchal line of the occiput. The semispinalis cervicis attaches superiorly to the spinous processes of C-2 to C-5.

Erector Spinae Muscles

A large number of posterior spinal muscles are called **erector spinae**, or **sacrospinalis muscles**. These muscles are continuous from the sacrum to the occiput, and their combined action is vertebral extension or prevention of flexion. They are named from medial to lateral as **spinales, longissimus,** and **iliocostalis** and from their attachments from head to sacrum as **capitis, cervicis, thoracis** (dorsi), or **lumborum**, but not all are represented in each area.

The **iliocostalis cervicis** has attachments on the angles of the third to sixth ribs and on the transverse processes of C-4 to C-6. The **longissimus capitis** and **cervicis** have attachments on the transverse processes of the upper five thoracic vertebrae, with superior attachments on the mastoid process and the transverse processes of C-2 to C-6. In the cervical area, the superficial layer of the erector spinae is the **splenius capitis** and **cervicis**, which attach to the lower part of the ligamentum nuchae and the spinous processes of the upper three thoracic vertebrae. The capitis courses laterally to attach to the mastoid process and the superior nuchal line of the occiput, and the cervicis goes to the transverse processes of the upper cervical vertebrae. All of these muscles are then covered by the upper trapezius and the levator scapulae, which can exert forces on the head and cervical spine as well as on the scapula. These muscles are described with the shoulder (see Fig. 7–4). **Innervation:** C_1 to T_4. **Anatomic actions:** With bilateral contraction of the cervical erector spinae group, backward bending at the atlanto-occipital joint and the cervical spine occurs. Unilateral contraction can produce lateral flexion, and lines of pull in some of the muscles have a vector in the direction of rotation.

Deep Muscles of the Back

The intrinsic muscles of the back are continuous with the posterior cervical muscles and include the deep transversospinal group and the more superficial erector spinae group. Their function is control of extension and prevention of collapse of the vertebral column. These functions are supplemented by the quadratus lumborum, psoas major, latissimus dorsi, internal abdominal oblique, and transverse abdominis muscles as well as the thoracodorsal fascia.

Transversospinal Muscles

The transversospinal muscles are multiple, small muscles between transverse or spinous processes, or both, with fasciculi (L. small bundles) crossing from one to five vertebral segments.

The **intertransversalii** attach between adjacent transverse processes, and the **interspinalis** muscles attach between the spinous processes on each side of the interspinous ligaments. Actions of these muscles are theorized from their mechanical lines of pull as lateral flexion and extension of the trunk. The muscles, however, are of small cross-sectional area and often have poor leverage because attachments are near the axis of motion. It seems unlikely that these muscles can produce the forces or torques required for movement or stabilization of the trunk. Some investigators have proposed that these small muscles function in proprioception to provide precise monitoring of intervertebral positions and length-tension relationships of muscles (Abrahams, 1977; Macintosh and Bogduk, 1987; Porterfield and DeRosa, 1991).

The **multifidus muscles** are composed of fasciculi from a common tendon on the spinous processes, which cross two to four segments to attach distally on the transverse processes in the thoracic region, the mammary processes in the lumbar area, the posterior iliac crest, and the sacrum. The deep **rotatores** are often included with the multifidus. In the lumbar area, the multifidus is a large muscle mass occupying the space between the spinous and transverse processes and the sacral groove. The fascicles have a nearly vertical line of pull at right angles to the spinous processes. Thus, both by size and leverage, the multifidus can exert high torques in lumbar extension. Macintosh and Bogduk (1987) consider the muscles to have only the "rocking" component of lumbar extension, whereas Porterfield and DeRosa (1991) propose that, in standing, the multifidus creates torques to prevent both flexion and anterior shear forces. Deep fasciculi of the multifidus also attach to the capsule of the facet joints, thus protecting the capsule from being nipped in movement (Lewin, Mofett, and Viedik, 1962).

Thoracic and Lumbar Erector Spinae Muscles

Strong tendons and fascia anchor the erector spinae or sacrospinalis distally to the spinous processes from T-11 through S-5, the sacrum, the sacrotuberous and sacroiliac ligaments, the posterior iliac crest, and muscle fibers of the gluteus maximus. From these attachments, deep and superficial muscles ascend through the lumbar, thoracic, and cervical areas. The deep part of the **lumbar longissimus** and the **lumbar iliocostalis** consist of muscle fascicles attaching near the posterior superior iliac spine and crest of the ilium. The fascicles run lateral to the multifidus, with the longissimus attaching to the medial part of the lumbar transverse processes and the iliocostalis attaching to the tips from L-1 to L-4. Porterfield and DeRosa (1991) suggest that these muscles function to provide strong stabilization and compression of the lumbar vertebrae on the ilium as well as posterior shear forces, particularly in the lower lumbar area.

Superficial to these muscles are the **thoracic longissimus** and the **thoracic iliocostalis**, which have long tendons from the sacrum, iliac crest, and lumbar spinous processes. Muscle fascicles arise on the tendons and are attached to all the ribs and transverse processes of the thoracic vertebrae (longissimus) and the lower six to eight ribs (iliocostalis). The long tendons in the lumbar area form the aponeurosis that covers the deep layer of the erector spinae (Macintosh and Bogduk, 1987). These muscles have good leverage for lateral flexion of the trunk when acting unilaterally and for backward bending of the spine when acting bilaterally.

INSPECTION AND PALPATION   The action of the erector spinae as a group may be observed best in the lumbar and lower thoracic regions when the subject, in the prone position, raises the upper part of the body off the floor (Fig. 11–6). These muscles should also be palpated in erect standing, and the effect of swaying the upper part of the body forward and backward should be observed (during forward sway, the muscles become tense; during backward sway, the muscles are relaxed). These muscles are also active in lateral bending and in rotation of the trunk; the

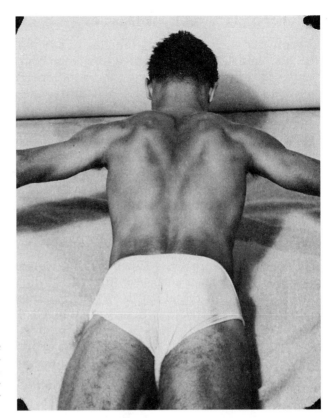

Figure 11–6 The erector spinae group is best observed in the lumbar region. In the thoracic region, this group is covered by the rhomboids and the trapezius. The trapezius is seen contracting strongly.

muscles should be palpated in these movements and their actions analyzed. In walking, the erector spinae group in the lumbar region may be felt contracting on each step (see Chapter 12).

Quadratus Lumborum

The **quadratus lumborum** is a large muscle on the posterior abdominal wall between the psoas major and the erector spinae. The muscle attaches to the crest of the ilium lateral to the attachments of the erector spinae and sends attachments to the 12th rib and the transverse processes of L-1 to L-3. **Innervation**: T_{12} to L_3. **Anatomic action**: Depression of the 12th rib and lateral flexion of the trunk. In the erect position, lateral flexion of the trunk to the opposite side occurs with an eccentric contraction of the ipsilateral quadratus lumborum and the return by a concentric contraction. These muscles have excellent leverage along with size to prevent collapse of the vertebral column in the frontal plane (ie, scoliosis).

PALPATION   The muscle is best palpated with the subject in a supine position to relax the erector spinae muscles. The palpating fingers should be placed above the iliac crest just lateral to the attachments of the erector spinae. The subject is asked to elevate or "hike" the hip. This motion is not unique to the quadratus lumborum, but also can be performed by the erector spinae and lateral abdominal muscles and the latissimus dorsi if the humerus is stabilized.

Anterior and Lateral Trunk Muscles

The anterior and lateral trunk muscles, in addition to functioning as supporters of the abdominal viscera and breathing, are concerned with movements of the trunk—flexion, lateral bending, and rotation. They consist of large sheaths of muscles in several layers. The fibers of the various layers run in different directions, a factor that contributes to the strength of the combined layers. A similar arrangement of fibers is seen in the thoracic region where the external and internal intercostals represent two layers corresponding to the external and internal oblique abdominal muscles.

The linea alba is a fibrous band in the median line of the abdominal region, extending from the xiphoid process above to the pubis below. This line unites the aponeuroses of the muscles of the right and left sides.

Rectus Abdominis

The **rectus abdominis** is a superficial muscle and consists of two parts, one on each side of the linea alba. **Proximal attachments**: Xiphoid process of the sternum and adjacent costal cartilages. **Distal attachments**: Pubic bones, near the symphysis pubis. The longitudinally arranged muscle fibers are interrupted by three tendinous inscriptions (L. a mark or line), the lowest one at, or slightly below, the level of the umbilicus. **Innervation**: Ventral portions of the 5th through the 12th intercostal nerves. **Anatomic actions**: Trunk flexion.

INSPECTION AND PALPATION   In well-developed subjects, the rectus abdominis may be observed and palpated throughout its length in flexion of the trunk (Fig. 11–7).

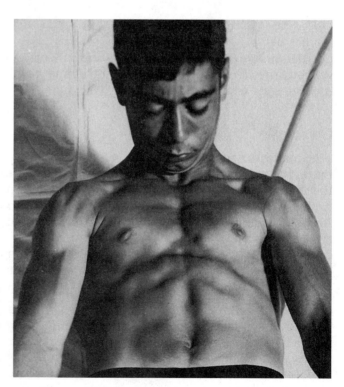

Figure 11–7 Activation of the rectus abdominis. In the supine position, the head and the shoulders are raised so that the spine flexes. The three tendinous inscriptions across the muscle are seen, the lowest slightly below the umbilicus.

The tendinous inscriptions and the muscular portions between them are well recognized. In the subject shown, the lowest inscription is well below the level of the umbilicus, and three "muscle hills" above this inscription can be seen (see Fig. 11–8). The widest portion of the linea alba (it is unusually wide in this subject) is found above the umbilicus. The lowest portion of the rectus is usually uninterrupted by inscriptions; in the illustration, however, the lowest portion of the rectus is hidden by the subject's shorts.

In obese individuals, the tendinous inscriptions and the boundaries of the muscle cannot be recognized very well but, when the subject raises the head while in the supine position, the tension in the muscle can always be palpated.

External Abdominal Oblique

The **external abdominal oblique muscle** constitutes the superficial layer of the abdominal wall. It is located lateral to the rectus abdominis and covers the anterior and lateral regions of the abdomen. **Proximal attachments**: Anterolateral portions of the ribs, where it interdigitates with the serratus anterior and, at its lowest point of attachment, with slips from the latissimus dorsi. **Distal attachments**: The upper fibers have a downward-forward direction and attach into an aponeurosis by which they are connected to the linea alba; the lower fibers are attached to the crest of the ilium. **Innervation**: Lower intercostal nerves (T_7 to T_{12}). **Anatomic actions**: Unilateral contraction produces trunk rotation to the opposite side and side bending to the same side.

INSPECTION AND PALPATION   Because of the oblique direction of the fibers of the externus, flexion of the trunk combined with rotation brings out a strong contraction of this muscle, particularly if the movement is opposed by the weight of the upper part of the body (Fig. 11–8). To activate the muscle on the right side, the trunk is rotated to the left; the muscle on the left side contracts in trunk rotation to the right. Bilateral action helps to produce flexion of the trunk without rotation. The muscles are also active bilaterally when one is "straining" or coughing.

Internal Abdominal Oblique

The **internal abdominal oblique muscle**, being covered by the external oblique, belongs to the second layer of the abdominal wall. The muscle extends essentially over the same area as the externus, but its fibers cross those of the externus. **Proximal attachments**: Inguinal ligament, crest of ilium, and thoracolumbar fascia. From this region, the fibers fan out to distal attachments on the pubic bone, on an aponeurosis connecting with the linea alba, and on the last three or four ribs where the direction of the fibers is continuous with those of the internal intercostals. **Innervation**: Lower intercostal nerves and branches from the iliohypogastric nerve (T_9-L_1). **Anatomic actions**: Unilateral contraction causes side bending and trunk rotation leading with the opposite shoulder.

INSPECTION AND PALPATION   In palpation, the internal oblique cannot be well differentiated from the other layers of the abdominal wall. However, the tension of the abdominal wall (seen and felt on the left side of the abdomen when the trunk is rotated to the left, as in Fig. 11–8) is due, at least in part, to the internal oblique. In this movement, the line of action of the external oblique on the right side and

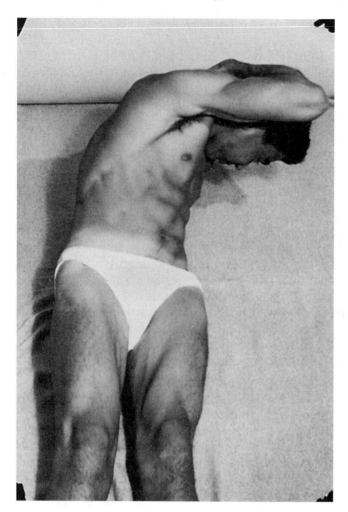

Figure 11–8 Activation of the right external oblique abdominal muscle. In the supine position, the head and the shoulders are raised and the trunk rotated to the left. The interdigitations of the right external oblique with the latissimus dorsi and serratus anterior are seen. The rectus abdominis is also contracting. (From Smith, LK and Mabry, M: *Poliomyelitis and the postpolio syndrome.* In Umphred, DA (ed): *Neurological Rehabilitation*, ed 3. Mosby-Yearbook, St. Louis, 1995, with permission.

the internal oblique on the left side is a continuous one, both muscles contributing to the rotation.

Transverse Abdominis

The transverse abdominis composes the innermost layer of the abdominal wall. This muscle has been named the "corset muscle" because it enclosed the abdominal cavity like a corset. The direction of its fibers is transverse. **Proximal attachments**: Lower ribs, thoracolumbar fascia, crest of ilium, inguinal ligament. **Distal attachment**: By means of an aponeurosis, partly fused with those of the other abdominal muscles, into the linea alba. **Innervation**: Lower intercostal nerves, iliohypogastric, and ilioinguinal nerves (T_7-T_{12}). **Anatomic action**: Abdominal compression.

PALPATION   In forced expiration, a tightening of the abdominal wall is felt anterolaterally between the lower ribs and the crest of the ilium. The transverse abdominis is partly responsible for this tension, which involves all the layers of the abdominal wall.

External and Internal Intercostals

The **external and internal intercostal muscles**, as their names indicate, are located between the ribs. They may be looked upon as the thoracic continuation of the external and internal oblique abdominal muscles. Each intercostal muscle extends between two adjacent ribs, but all of them together compose a two-layered muscle sheath enclosing the thoracic cavity. **Innervation**: Intercostal nerves. **Anatomic actions**: Elevation and depression of the ribs.

PALPATION If an attempt is made to insert the fingertip between two ribs, the intercostals offer resistance. The muscles also may be felt in movements of the trunk involving a widening or narrowing of the intercostal spaces. For example, in sitting or standing, the subject reaches overhead with the left arm, then flexes the trunk to the right while spreading the ribs apart on the left side. The subject then returns the trunk to the upright position. The intercostals on the left side may be felt in both parts of this movement as they oppose the action of gravity, and in particular during the return movement.

Diaphragm

The **diaphragm** is a musculotendinous dome that separates the thoracic from the abdominal cavity. The muscle is perforated by openings (hiatus, foramina, and arches), which permit passage of the aorta, vena cava, esophagus, nerves, psoas major, and the quadratus lumborum muscles. **Peripheral attachments**: Inner surface of the xiphoid process of the sternum, the inner surface of the costal cartilages and adjacent parts of the lower six ribs, the tendinous lumbocostal arches covering the psoas and quadratus muscles, and two tendinous crura (L. legs) attaching to the anterior longitudinal ligament and the bodies of the first three lumbar vertebrae. **Central attachments**: The muscular fibers of the right and left parts of the diaphragm ascend to form the dome with central tendinous attachments to each other. **Innervation**: Phrenic nerve (C_3-C_5). **Anatomic action**: Inspiration.

PALPATION The diaphragm can be palpated directly by placing the fingertips just under the anterior surface of the rib cage on one side and placing the thumb under the opposite side. When the person breathes in using the diaphragm, the central portion descends and puts pressure on the abdominal contents, causing the abdomen to rise. This is often mistakenly called "abdominal breathing." The subject should be supine and may need to be taught how to breathe with the diaphragm. When attention is called to breathing, it is common for subjects to voluntarily change their pattern to upper chest breathing.

FUNCTIONS OF THE HEAD, NECK, AND TRUNK MUSCLES

Balancing of the Head and the Vertebral Column

The function of the muscles of HAT in maintaining the upright position may be compared to guy wires supporting an upright pole. As long as the pole remains vertical, the forces in the wires are balanced and minimal. If the pole starts to tilt, increased force occurs in the guy rope on the opposite side to maintain stability. Another way to maintain stability is to increase forces on several wires and compress the pole into the ground. In the body both of these mechanical examples are used, often simultaneously. Among the muscles involved in this equilibration are:

- **Anterior**: suboccipital, longus capitis and colli, scalenes, SCM, rectus abdominis, internal and external abdominal obliques, and psoas major
- **Posterior**: suboccipital, transversospinal, and erector spinae
- **Lateral**: scalenes, SCM, quadratus lumborum, psoas major, internal abdominal oblique, and intercostals

In normal, relaxed upright sitting or standing, these muscles show only minimal periodic activity related to postural sway (see Fig. 11–10A). Movement of the center of gravity of the head or of HAT or a push or pull on the trunk immediately activates greater muscle contraction to resist the force and return the trunk to balance.

If one of these groups of muscles is paralyzed, the body assumes a posture in relation to gravity that eliminates the necessity for contraction of this group. For example, if the abdominal muscles are paralyzed, the person sits or stands with slight trunk flexion so that the erector spinae control anterior motion of the trunk with eccentric and concentric contractions. The rule is that the head or trunk deviates toward the weakness for postural control. If, in this example, the person leans back to the point at which the center of gravity of HAT falls posterior to the vertebral axis, control of the motion is lost, and the person may fall. The interplay between the trunk flexors and extensors can be palpated by placing the fingers of one hand into the lumbar erector spinae and those of the other hand into the upper rectus abdominis when sitting on the edge of a chair. The muscles are felt to alternately contract and relax with slight forward and backward sway from the hips.

Trunk Motions and Stabilization of the Vertebrae

The transversospinal and erector spinae muscles have lines of pull with force vector components in the directions of extension, rotation, and side bending of the vertebrae. It has been demonstrated by EMG that maximum activity of these muscles occurs during extension of the spine against gravity or in eccentric contraction to control flexion. With paralysis of these muscles, the person is unable to extend the spine in the prone position or straighten it in the upright position (Fig. 11–9).

Although the transversospinal and erector spinae muscles may have high activity during motions of side bending, rotation, maximum inspiration, and forced expiration, this does not mean that the muscles are prime movers for these activities. Most frequently, the back muscles are acting as synergists to stabilize the vertebrae in extension to prevent unwanted motion of the prime movers. For example, the external oblique muscles have excellent leverage for trunk rotation but also cause trunk flexion. Increased EMG activity of the lumbar multifidus on the contralateral side is found with trunk rotation. The activity, however, is the same for both the rotation and the return to the midline position, indicating that this activity may be more for stabilization than for rotation (Valencia and Munro, 1985). During side bending, EMG activity of the erector spinae and multifidus can

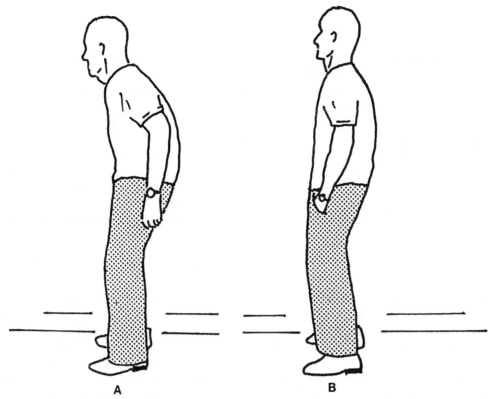

A   **B**

Figure 11–9 This man has paralysis of his abdominal and back extensor muscles that was caused by poliomyelitis when he was a young man. Illustration (*A*) demonstrates his inability to extend the spine. He is supporting his trunk with the posterior ligamentous system. Note that he has a posterior pelvic tilt to increase tension on the thoracolumbar fascia and the ligaments. (*B*) He maintains a more erect posture when he can push down on his hands. Here he appears in a casual posture with his hands in his pockets. In reality, he is pushing down on his hips to extend his spine. He has precarious trunk balance unless he is grasping stable objects or supporting his trunk with his elbows or hands. He is unable to produce an effective push or pull on another object, such as a drawer or a door. He cannot lift or carry objects such as a plate of food because even this slight amount of weight changes the center of gravity of the head, arms, and trunk (HAT) beyond his control.

be found throughout the motion. If, however, care is taken to maintain the motion exactly in the frontal plane, electrical silence is found in these muscles (Pauly, 1966). Again, this evidence indicates that the back extensors are not prime movers for side bending. Instead, the motion is accomplished by a contralateral eccentric contraction of the lateral abdominals, quadratus lumborum, and the psoas major going down and a contralateral concentric contraction of the same muscles to return to the erect position.

The psoas major is a large muscle with attachments on the vertebral bodies, disks, and transverse processes from T-12 to L-5. In closed-chain motion, the psoas is a major prime mover and stabilizer of the trunk. For example, the iliopsoas muscles elevate HAT in a sit-up and prevent HAT from falling backward in unsupported sitting. Analysis of the lines of pull of the psoas major in lumbar flexion were found to be anterior or through the vertebral axes of flexion, and in extension, the lines run posterior to the axes (Sullivan, 1989). Sullivan states that, regardless of the position of the lumbar spine, the psoas is active in stabilization.

An important function of the trunk musculature is to fixate the thorax, pelvis, and vertebrae to stabilize the proximal attachments of the muscles of the neck, shoulders, and hips as the extremities are moved. In the supine position, head and neck flexors are synergistically accompanied by a strong isometric contraction of the rectus abdominis to stabilize the rib cage. During leg raising, all the abdominal muscles are activated to stabilize the pelvis and lumbar vertebrae. By varying the lever arm length of the lower extremity (flexing or extending the knees) and by using one or both extremities, a finely graduated exercise program for weak abdominal muscles can be developed. Manual resistance to shoulder motions such as extension-adduction (an action of the pectoralis major) causes abdominal muscle activity, particularly of the external oblique on the same side and the internal oblique on the opposite side.

In the prone position, similar activation of the erector spinae occurs. Hip extension produces a synergistic contraction of the back extensors to stabilize the pelvis. If the arms are placed over the head and then lifted, the back extensors automatically contract.

Forward Bending and Lifting (Knees Straight)

When a standing person bends forward at the hips to touch the toes, eccentric contractions of the hip extensor muscles (primarily the hamstrings) and the erector spinae muscles occur to control hip flexion and forward bending of the vertebrae. Concentric contractions of these same muscles return the trunk to the upright position (Fig. 11–10B). An unusual phenomenon of sudden muscle inhibition of the erector spinae can be seen on the EMG record when the trunk has completed about two-thirds of the range of trunk flexion on the way down. EMG silence continues until the trunk has been extended about one-third of the range on the return to standing. This point of inhibition has been named the "critical point" and has been found to have a mean value of 81 degrees of trunk flexion (Kippers and Parker, 1984). The authors found this value to occur at 60 percent of maximum hip flexion and 90 percent of maximum vertebral flexion. When a weight was lowered or lifted from the floor, the angle of the critical point increased slightly. Fine wire EMG studies of the deeper lumbar multifidus muscles have shown a decrease in activity at the critical point but not always electrical silence (Valencia and Munro, 1985). Inhibition of the erector spinae muscles during the highest torque requirements of forward flexion and extension of the vertebral column suggests that load bearing is produced by structures in addition to the extensor muscles of the spine, such as the facet joints and posterior ligaments.

The "inflated balloon theory" was first proposed as a spring load bearing mechanism. With lifting, contraction of abdominal muscles occurs along with closure of the muscles of the glottis and the floor of the perineum with increase in intra-abdominal and intrathoracic pressure. Increased abdominal pressure in turn converts these closed chambers into rigid-walled cylinders that provide substantial support to columns like an elongated balloon or the abdominal and thoracic cavities (Morris, Lucas, and Bresler, 1961). The validity of this theory is questioned in subsequent studies of the role of abdominal muscles in lifting. Strengthening the abdominal muscles does not increase intra-abdominal pressure. Futhermore, deliberately increasing the intra-abdominal pressure with a Valsalva maneuver does not decrease the load on the lumbar spine.

Current theory attributes the ability of the trunk to withstand large flexion moments to a complex of passive and dynamic forces produced by the posterior

A. NORMAL RELAXED STANDING

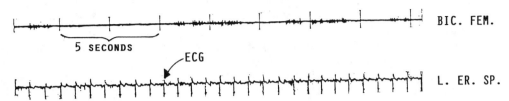

BIC. FEM.

5 SECONDS

ECG

L. ER. SP.

B. STANDING -- FORWARD BEND TO TOUCH TOES -- RETURN TO STANDING

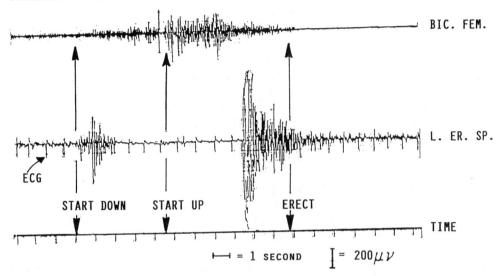

BIC. FEM.

L. ER. SP.

ECG

START DOWN   START UP   ERECT

TIME

⊢—⊣ = 1 SECOND   ⌶ = 200 μν

C. MAXIMUM ISOMETRIC CONTRACTION -- PRONE

KNEE FLEXION   TRUNK EXTENSION

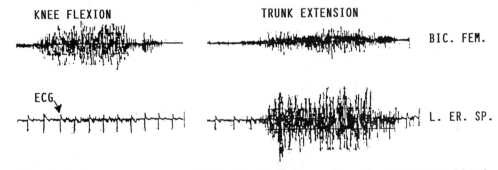

BIC. FEM.

ECG

L. ER. SP.

Figure 11–10 Surface electromyograms (EMG) of the left lumbar erector spinae (L. ER. SP.) at L3 and of the left biceps femoris (BIC. FEM.) muscles. (*A*) Normal, relaxed standing shows minimal intermittent activity in the biceps femoris. The erector spinae shows barely perceptible activity. The regular spikes in the baseline of this muscle are due to the electrocardiogram. (*B*) Forward bending to touch the toes demonstrates the eccentric contraction in the biceps to lower the body and the concentric contraction to raise the trunk. The erector spinae also shows eccentric and concentric contractions at the beginning and ending of the maneuver. The muscle becomes electrically silent about two-thirds of the way down and remains silent until about one-third of the ascent has been completed. (*C*) Maximum isometric contractions produced by manual resistance demonstrate a standard for comparison of amplitude and frequency of the EMG activity. Note the contraction of the biceps femoris during trunk extension to stabilize the pelvis on the thighs.

spinal ligaments, the thoracolumbar fascia, and the transverse abdominis and internal oblique muscles (Bogduk and Macintosh, 1984; Gracovetsky, Farfan, and Helleur, 1985; Macintosh and Bogduk, 1987; Gracovetsky et al, 1990). This theory is based on the hip extensor muscles (hamstrings, gluteus maximus, hip adductors, etc) providing the major forces to lower or elevate the trunk. Large forces can be generated by these muscles because of their size and leverage advantages. These forces must be transmitted to the upper body through the lumbar spine, which has relatively smaller muscles with shorter lever arms. When the lumbar spine is in flexion, the line of pull of the erector spinae muscles is almost parallel to the vertebrae with a minimal extension component. Erector spinae muscle contraction in this position would not be effective in producing lumbar extension but would increase disk compression to injurious levels.

Passively, the posterior ligaments (facet joint capsules, interspinous ligaments, supraspinous ligament, and thoracolumbar fascia) can support large forces when the lumbar spine is in the forward bent position. The trunk can then be elevated by the hip extensor muscles, and, as the center of gravity of HAT and any added weight moves closer to the axis of hip motion, the erector spinae are activated to complete vertebral extension. A dynamic lateral force on the thoracolumbar fascia is added by contraction of the transverse abdominis and internal oblique muscles through their attachments on the lateral raphe. This bilateral force and the increased intra-abdominal pressure prevents the passive elongation of the thoracolumbar fascia by the imposed load of HAT.

Additional forces are provided by the geometry of the attachments of the thoracolumbar fascia to the lumbar spinous processes. The superficial and deep lamina of the fascia cross to form a series of strong triangles with apices on the lateral raphe and bases covering two vertebral levels. Forces from contraction of the transverse abdominis and the internal abdominal oblique are transmitted to cause approximation of the spinous processes (an extension torque on the lumbar vertebrae and a possible "bracing" force in the thoracic spine). Contraction of the latissimus dorsi when the arm is fixed as in a pull-up creates similar forces on the thoracolumbar fascia (Nachemson, 1981, 1987; Gracovetsky et al, 1985). This theory also includes the "hydraulic amplifier mechanism." When the erector spinae muscles contract, they expand and put tension on the aponeurosis and fascial coverings of the muscles. This additional tension provides an antiflexion force during forward bending and an extension force during trunk elevation similar to pressure forces in an elongated balloon.

Squat Lifting and Lowering

Another way to lift objects from the floor is to flex at the knees and hips and dorsiflex at the ankles. Squat lifting can be used with two positions of the pelvis and vertebrae: (1) anterior tilt of the pelvis with lordotic position of the lumbar spine or (2) posterior tilt of the pelvis with kyphotic position of the vertebrae. EMG activity of the erector spinae muscles in lifting differs according to the position of the trunk. When the trunk is in the lordotic position, EMG activity is greater than in the flexed position, and the maximum activity occurs at the initiation of the lift (DeLitto and Rose, 1992). Lowering requires eccentric contractions of the gastrocnemius-soleus, quadriceps, and hip extensor muscles with isometric contraction of the erector spinae when the trunk is in the lordotic position. When the spine is in kyphosis, erector spinae EMG activity is decreased and inhibited as in bending with the knees straight. When the lift is performed in the kyphotic position of the back, there is no contraction of the erector spinae at the initiation of the lift, and the peak activity occurs in the middle of the lift (Holmes, Damser, and Lehman, 1992).

Thus, although lifting with the back in flexion decreases disk pressure, and lifting with the back in extension provides muscle control to protect the facet joints, there is a lack of agreement on which posture is better. This may mean that each posture is of value in different situations. Many authorities advocate squat lifting with the pelvis in anterior tilt and the lumbar spine in extension (Delitto and Rose, 1992). Some bending and lifting activities, however, cannot be performed with the back in extension. This includes lifting from the floor or bending when squatting is impossible, such as when lifting an object out of a crate. It should be noted that weight lifters and furniture movers can be seen to use both the ligamentous and muscular systems. Important factors in both types of lifting are to bring the object close to the body's center of gravity to minimize the torque on the back and to avoid twisting, which can injure the lumbar facet joints as well as further increase disk pressure (Adams and Hutton, 1983; Nachemson, 1981).

Functional Activities (Muscles of the Extremities and Trunk)

Lifting the body using the arms includes chin-ups, pull-ups, prone push-ups, sitting push-ups, and crutch-walking. The prime movers for these motions are concentric contractions of the elbow flexors (for pull-ups), the elbow extensors (for push-ups), the glenohumeral adductors and extensors, and the scapular depressors. Equally important are synergistic isometric contractions of the abdominal and trunk extensor muscles to prevent distraction of the intervertebral joints with lengthening of the trunk. When the abdominal muscles and erector spinae are paralyzed as in spinal cord injuries, the person may not be able to lift the body for transfers regardless of the strength in the arms. The latissimus dorsi (C_5 to C_7) and the quadratus lumborum (T_{12} to L_3), if innervated, provide strong forces to approximate the pelvis to the arms or rib cage when the arms are fixed in closed-chain motion. Both are important crutch-walking muscles to "hike" the hip. Lowering the body from the elevated positions requires eccentric contractions of the same muscles.

Rising up and sitting down, deep knee bends, and ascending and descending stairs have similar patterns of muscle activity. If the fingertips of each hand are placed on the patellar tendon and the hamstring tendons when the extremity is relaxed, strong contractions are felt in both muscle groups when the person is asked to stand up. Elevating the body from a sitting or squatting position or ascending a step (lead leg) requires knee extension with a concentric contraction of the quadriceps and hip extension with a concentration contraction of the hip extensors, particularly the hamstring muscles. A relatively isometric contraction of the erector spinae maintains the head and spine in the erect position. Lowering the body to sit, squat, or descend a step (following leg) requires knee flexion and hip flexion with eccentric contractions of the quadriceps and the hamstring muscles and isometric contractions of the erector spinae.

While the quadriceps and the hamstring muscles may have agonist-antagonistic relationships in open-chain motion, these relationships change to co-contraction in closed-chain motion of supporting, lifting, or lowering of the body.

Pushing or pulling on external objects such as a drawer or a door require strong stabilization of the trunk to develop an effective force. Pushing activates the abdominal muscles and the hip flexors so that the trunk is not driven into extension. Pulling activates the back and hip extensors so that the trunk does not flex. This principle is the same in the prone push-up. The prime movers for the push-up phase are the elbow extensors, glenohumeral adductors and extensors, and scapular abductors with concentric contractions. To maintain a rigid trunk, strong isometric contractions occur anteriorly in the abdominal, hip flexor, and knee extensor muscles. The posterior muscles are relatively inactive except for cervical erector spinae to maintain neck extension. Returning the body to the floor is accomplished by eccentric contractions of the upper extremity musculature and continued isometric contractions of the anterior trunk and leg muscles.

Breathing and Coughing

The primary muscles that are used in inspiration are the diaphragm (which produces about two-thirds of maximum inspiratory capacity), the external intercostals, and the scaleni. Muscles of forced expiration are the abdominals and the internal intercostals. In normal, quiet breathing, the only muscles that contract are those of inspiration. Expiration is accomplished by the relaxation of these muscles (or eccentric contraction of inspiratory muscles) and the passive recoil of the lung (elastic tissues and the surface tension produced by the fluid interface on the 3 million alveoli).

During exercise or forceful breathing activities such as a vital capacity maneuver or in coughing, all the primary muscles of respiration are activated, along with accessory muscles and stabilizing muscles. Accessory muscles of inspiration are the SCMs, the pectoralis minor, and the suprahyoid and infrahyoid muscles. The pectoralis major and the serratus anterior have also been found to be active in forced inspiration. During exercise or forced ventilation, expiration occurs by contraction of the abdominal muscles. The latissimus dorsi can assist with expiration when the arms are stabilized by placing the hands on the thighs or a table. During coughing, the latissimus dorsi can be seen to contract sharply.

The upper trapezius, erector spinae, and the quadratus lumborum are activated in forced breathing, probably more as stabilizers than as primary muscles of respiration. The erector spinae contract strongly in coughing to prevent trunk flexion that would occur with abdominal muscle contraction. Persons with back injuries often feel severe pain when they cough, sneeze, or strain because of the reflex stabilizing contraction of the back extensors.

TEMPOROMANDIBULAR JOINTS

The temporomandibular joints (TMJ) or the craniomandibular articulations are among the most frequently used in the body. In their functions of chewing, talking, yawning, swallowing, and sneezing, the TMJs are estimated to move 1500 to 2000 times per day. These joints provide motions of opening, closing, protrusion, retraction, and lateral deviation of the mandible on the temporal bone. Normally, opening and closing should be in a straight line without lateral deviations of the mandible on the temporal bone. The person should be able to place the width of three fingers between the teeth with opening. There should be no clicking or popping with joint motion or pain from palpation of the muscles of mastication.

The bilateral TMJs or the craniomandibular articulations are synovial joints formed by the convex condyles of the mandible, the concave glenoid fossa (mandibular fossa), and the convex articular eminence of the temporal bone (Fig. 11–11). In the adult, the mandibular condyles are about two times as wide in the frontal plane as in the sagittal plane, providing a large articular area. The bony articulating surfaces are covered with fibrous cartilage and separated by a movable articular disk forming an upper and a lower joint space (see Fig. 11–11B,C). Posteriorly, the disk is attached to thick connective tissue called the bilaminar zones, which are separated by spongy tissue with an extensive neural and vascular supply that normally is not subjected to large joint forces. The disk is attached medially and laterally to the sides of the condyles and anteriorly to the joint capsule and the lateral pterygoid muscle. These attachments cause the disk to move forward with the condyle when the mouth is opened. The joint is surrounded by a capsule that is reinforced laterally by the temporomandibular ligament running from the articular eminence and the zygomatic arch posteriorly to the neck of the mandible. The capsule and its ligaments limit motions of the mandible, particularly depression and retrusion. Protrusion of the mandible is limited by the stylomandibular ligament (the styloid process is seen below the TMJ in Fig. 11–11A).

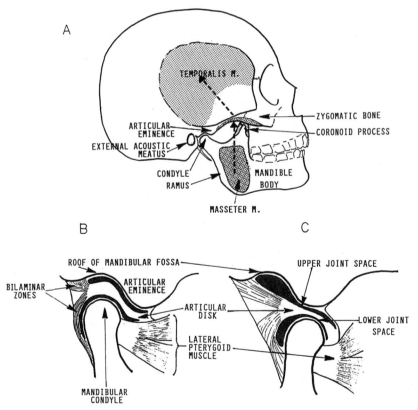

Figure 11–11   The temporomandibular joint (TMJ). (*A*) Bony landmarks and attachments of the temporalis (*light shading*) and the masseter muscles (*darker shading*). Approximate lines of pull of these muscles (*dotted vectors*) that close the TMJ illustrate the leverage advantage of these powerful muscles. Note the close proximity of the TMJ to the ear. (*B*) Schematic midsagittal section of the TMJ when the jaw is closed and the mandibular condyle is in the mandibular fossa of the temporal bone. (*C*) The jaw is open and the mandibular condyle is beneath the articular eminence.

Motions of the Temporomandibular Joint

Opening of the mouth occurs with rotation of the mandibular condyles around the lower joint space, followed by translation of the articular disk on the upper joint space down to the articular eminence. Thus the TMJ has been described as a hinge joint on a movable base. Closing of the mouth requires reversal of the translatory and rotational motions. These motions of the condyles can be felt by placing the index fingers flat against the side of the jaw with the fingertips touching the tragus of the ear and asking the subject to open the mouth slowly. The posterior part of the condyles can be felt by placing the fingertips inside the ears and pressing forward. When the mouth is opened, the condyles move away from the fingertips and then return with closure of the jaw. Other motions that can be made by the mandible are protrusion, retrusion, and lateral shift, which includes mediolateral translatory motion. Functional movements of the jaw are combinations of these motions. In chewing, they are called incision for cutting food and mastication for crushing and grinding.

Muscles

Jaw Closure

Three powerful muscles that are all innervated by the trigeminal nerve (cranial nerve V) close the jaw. The **temporalis** muscle attaches to the temporal fossa and its fibers converge into a tendon running under the zygomatic arch to attach on the coronoid process of the mandible (see Fig. 11–11A). The muscle can be palpated by placing the fingers over the temporal fossa and asking the subject to bite down. The muscle is felt to contract with retrusion and lateral shift of the mandible as well. The **masseter** attaches to the zygomatic arch and divides into superficial and deep parts that attach to the angle and ramus of the mandible (see Fig. 11–11A). To palpate the superficial part of the muscle, place the index finger just under the zygomatic arch and over the ramus of the mandible and then ask the subject to bite down. The deep part can be palpated by placing the gloved index finger inside the mouth. The finger is placed between the teeth and the cheek as close to the ear as it will go. Have the subject bite down gently and the masseter can be felt to contract strongly. The masseter also has a small lateral force component.

The **medial pterygoid** muscle (on the inside of the mandible) is almost a mirror image of the masseter. The medial pterygoid attaches to the pterygoid (G. *pteron*, wing) fossa of the sphenoid bone and to the medial side of the ramus and angle of the mandible often interdigitating with fibers of the masseter. Together, these muscles form a "sling" around the ramus of the mandible. In addition to the large vertical force component, the medial pterygoid has a medial force component to match the lateral component of the masseter. The medial pterygoid can be palpated by placing the gloved index finger upward against the medial side of the angle of the mandible and having the subject gently close the jaw.

Jaw Opening

The normal rest position of the mandible in the erect position is with the lips closed and the teeth several millimeters apart. This is maintained by low levels of activity of the temporalis muscles (Basmajian, 1978). Reduction of this activity and the force of gravity are sufficient to cause the mouth to open. Rapid or resisted opening of the jaw is performed by a part of the lateral pterygoid, the digastric, and the suprahyoid and infrahyoid muscles.

The **lateral pterygoid** muscle has a horizontal direction of pull relative to the vertical direction of the masseter and the medial pterygoid (see Fig. 11–11B,C). The muscle attaches to the neck of the mandibular condyle and frequently the articular disk. Two heads are formed with the superior head located medially and upward at about a 45-degree angle to attach on the greater wing of the sphenoid bone. The inferior head fans out in a more horizontal direction to attach on the distal lateral pterygoid plate of the sphenoid bone. **Innervation:** Trigeminal nerve (cranial nerve V).

Because the lateral pterygoid muscles are deep and difficult to palpate or record EMG activity, their actions have been described from anatomic lines of pull to include protrusion, depression, and lateral shift of the mandible (Gray, 1966). Some EMG findings, however, have shown activity in the superior head with closing of the jaw and activity in the inferior head with opening of the jaw. This has led to the proposal that the two heads have different actions (McNamara, 1973; and Sarnat and Laskin, 1992). These authors propose that the probable function of the superior head of the lateral pterygoid is protrusion to stabilize the mandibular condyle against the posterior aspect of the articular eminence during mastication. The primary action of the inferior head is depression and protrusion of the mandible.

The **digastric** muscle is composed of two muscle bellies lying on the underside of the chin. The anterior belly attaches to the inner border of the mandible near the midline, and the posterior belly attaches to the mastoid notch of the temporal bone. The two muscle bellies are joined in a tendinous loop attached to the hyoid bone. Marked EMG activity was recorded for jaw opening in both bellies of the muscle, and moderate activity was found with protrusion, retrusion, and lateral shift (Widmalm, Lillie, and Ash, 1988). In swallowing, the authors found a complex pattern with high-amplitude, short-duration bursts of activity. In parts of the swallowing act, the two bellies of the digastric muscle contracted antagonistically. **Innervation:** Posterior belly by the facial nerve (VII) and anterior belly by the trigeminal nerve (V).

The **mylohyoid** and the **geniohyoid** muscles may also participate in depression of the mandible when the hyoid bone is stabilized and may elevate the hyoid when the mandible is stabilized.

CLINICAL APPLICATIONS

Temporomandibular Dysfunction

Abnormal signs or symptoms of TMJ involvement have been reported from 20 to 80 percent in a review of 25 studies of healthy subjects (Burakoff, 1991). The incidence of problems is greater in females than in males and increases with age. The TMJs along with the muscles of mastication are a complex area to evaluate because of their close relation and attachments to head, neck, shoulder, and thoracic structures (upper quarter). Dysfunction in the TMJs is frequently unrecognized because pain may be referred to the ear, head, face, or other upper quarter areas (Travell and Simons, 1983). Abnormalities in the other areas may in turn contribute to TMJ dysfunction. Although the causes of TMJ abnormalities are in most cases multiple, there is a high association of previous trauma (Pullinger and Monteiro, 1988) and postural abnormalities in the head and neck (Mannheimer and Dunn, 1991).

Injuries can be produced by blows to the head such as whiplash in an auto accident, hitting the chin on bicycle handlebars, or falling and landing on the back of the head. Often problems with the TMJ go unrecognized and untreated at the time because of more serious vascular and cerebral concerns. Long-term repetitive microtrauma can occur from clenching and grinding the teeth (bruxism), constant gum chewing, cracking hard candy or nuts with the teeth, cervical traction, prolonged thumb-sucking or mouth breathing, malocclusion, or dental procedures with wide and prolonged opening of the mouth. Repetitive, abnormal forces in occupational and athletic activities can lead to TMJ pain and dysfunction. These include the extended head position of the professional scuba diver, the clenched jaw forward-tilted head position of the symphony violinist, the clenched jaw of the weight lifter, and the asymmetric mouth breathing of the freestyle swimmer (Goldman, 1991).

Postural deviations such as pronation in one foot, a short leg, or scoliosis (lateral curvature of the spine) cause asymmetry in shoulder height and head tilt with altered craniovertebral forces. In the sagittal plane, the forward head posture produces major alterations in craniovertebral relationships. The forward-head position is a common postural abnormality that can be a result of low back pain and loss of lumbar lordosis, thoracic kyphosis or dowager's hump, habitual or occupational slumped sitting postures, or craniocervical injury. Usually the forward-head posture shows a straight cervical spine on x-ray with loss of the normal lordosis. The longus capitis and colli are shortened and often in contraction. To see anything other than the ground, the head is hyperextended on the neck. This position then causes the suboccipital extensor muscles to shorten, the suprahyoids to shorten, and the infrahyoids to lengthen, with mandibular repositioning and hyperactivity of the muscles of mastication. Compression may occur posteriorly in the C-1 to C-2 area with craniofacial pain (Mannheimer and Dunn, 1991). Such complexities illustrate that the TMJ cannot be considered in isolation and that in many instances a multidisciplinary treatment approach of dentists and physical therapists can be effective in restoring function.

Laboratory Activities

HEAD, NECK, AND TRUNK

1. On a skeleton and on a partner, observe and palpate the cervical, thoracic, and lumbar curves in the sagittal plane in standing. Have your partner bend forward and note that the thoracic curve increases in flexion, but that the cervical and lumbar areas move to a straight line. Have the subject bend backward (extend the trunk) and note that the lumbar curves increase and the thoracic curve moves to a straight line. Have your partner sit in a chair. Note the difference in the curves from the standing position.

2. Have your partner take off one shoe and stand while you view and palpate relative heights for symmetry:

a. Shoulders
b. Anterior superior iliac spines
c. Crests of the ilia
d. Posterior superior iliac spines
e. Inferior angles of the scapula

Trace by palpation the spines of the vertebrae from C-7 to the sacrum to see if there is any lateral deviation of the vertebrae. Have the subject put on the shoe and repeat the measurements.

3. With the subject standing in front of you, ask him or her to raise the right arm over the head and side bend the trunk to the left. Palpate the spines of the vertebrae from C-7 to the sacrum to determine if there is a smooth curve to the left without any straight segments. Repeat with side bending to the right.

4. Have a subject sit on a stool or table so that the pelvis is stabilized, and have the subject rotate the trunk to the right and then to the left. Where does the majority of the rotation occur?

5. On a disarticulated bone set, identify the following parts of the atlas; axis; and one each of a cervical, thoracic, and lumbar vertebrae: body, vertebral foramen, transverse processes, spinous process, lamina, pedicle, and all articulating surfaces.

6. Articulate pairs of the vertebrae (and the ribs) and simulate all the possible motions. Visualize the bony and ligamentous limiting structures.

7. On a partner, palpate the neck and trunk muscles as described in this chapter.

8. Palpate the abdominal and the lumbar erector spinae muscles in a subject who is lying down (supine). Have subject perform the following activities:
   a. Lift the head. Why do the abdominal muscles contract?
   b. Raise one lower extremity a few inches. Why do the abdominal muscles contract?
   c. Cough. Why do the abdominal muscles contract? The erector spinae muscles?

9. Palpate the erector spinae muscles in a subject who is prone with forehead resting on the table and arms flexed beside the head.
   a. Raise the arm a few inches. Why do the erector spinae contract?
   b. Lift one lower extremity a few inches and determine why the erector spinae contract.

10. Palpate the abdominal and erector spinae muscles on a subject sitting on a table or a stool and perform the following activities of the trunk (keep the hip position at 90 degrees of flexion):
    a. Trunk flexion. Which muscle group is contracting and with what type of contraction while flexing and what type while returning to the upright posture?
    b. Perform side bending to the right and return to the upright position. Which side is contracting and with what type of contraction? Note that the contraction can be in either the abdominal or the erector spinae muscles with a small change in the position of the hips or trunk in the sagittal plane.

11. Analyze the following activities for the total body. State the prime mover(s) for each joint motion, the type of muscle contraction, and the essential stabilizing muscles:

a. Supine: Perform a sit-up and return.

b. Prone: Raise head and shoulders and extend the trunk.

c. Prone: Perform a push-up.

d. Standing: Perform a chin-up.

e. Standing: Bend forward and touch the floor and return.

f. Standing: Sit down in a chair and return.

g. Ascending stairs for lead leg and for following leg. Descending stairs.

12. On the skull, identify bony structures around the TMJs—temporal bone, acoustic meatus, glenoid fossa, articular eminence, and zygomatic arch. On the mandible, identify the coronoid process, ramus, body, and condyles. Note the shape and the angle of the condyles, and simulate articulation with the glenoid fossa and the articular eminence in opening and closing the jaw.

13. On a partner, palpate the condyles of the mandible as the jaw is slowly opened and then closed. Feel for rotation followed by descent on the eminence, presence of symmetry of motion and absence of jerks or pops. Observe whether the path of the lower teeth on opening is straight or deviates. Palpate the condyles and the tip of the chin while the subject slowly protracts and retracts the mandible and then deviates the mandible to each side.

14. Palpate the masseters and the temporalis muscles and ask the subject to clench the teeth to feel the muscles when they contract. Palpate the digastric muscle under the chin and give some resistance to jaw opening to feel the muscle contract.

CHAPTER 12

Standing and Walking

Posture is a general term that is defined as a position or attitude of the body, the relative arrangement of body parts for a specific activity, or a characteristic manner of bearing one's body. Postures are used to perform activities with the least amount of energy. Thus, posture and movement are intimately associated; movement begins from a posture and may end in a posture—as when a person is in a sitting position and then moves to a standing position. In normal function, postural "sets" and adjustments are rapid and automatic.

Postural relationships of body parts can be altered and controlled cognitively and voluntarily, but such control is short-lived because it requires concentration. Changing abnormal postures is difficult and requires extensive evaluation and treatment, which may include increasing range of motion, stability, muscle strength, and endurance as well as training and cueing.

STATIC OR STEADY POSTURES

The body can assume a multitude of postures that are comfortable for long periods, and many accomplish the same purposes. In many cultures, for example, people do not sit in a chair to rest the body but rather use a variety of floor-sitting postures such as crossed legs, side sitting, or the deep squat. Normally, when discomfort occurs from joint compression, ligamentous tension, continuous muscle contraction, or circulatory occlusion, a new posture is sought. If a joint has been in one position for a long time, the able-bodied person moves and stretches the joint and muscles. Habitual postures without positional changes can lead to tissue damage, limitation of motion, or deformity. Individuals with sensory losses (eg, peripheral nerve injuries, spinal cord transection) fail to perceive the discomfort of vascular occlusion. If this is not alleviated by relieving the pressure periodically, tissue destruction may occur, leading to pressure sores. Persons with lower-extremity amputations are especially prone to adaptive shortening (contractures) of the hip and knee flexors caused by resting the residual limb on a pillow and by prolonged sitting. Furthermore, if the joints of persons with muscle paralysis are not passively moved through their ranges of motion, the joint structures and muscles adaptively shorten to the habitual position.

STANDING POSTURE

Perpendicular Standing Posture

A perpendicular or rigid standing posture is assumed when one is standing at attention or told to "stand up straight." The weight is shifted posteriorly so that a lateral plumb line falls through the ear, tip of the shoulder, center of the hip and knee, and very close to the axis of the ankle joint. This is an unnatural posture requiring conscious effort, increased contraction of muscles, and increased energy expenditure.

Unfortunately, perpendicular posture has been equated with good or desirable posture. This has come about because of translation errors and misinterpretation of the work of Braune and Fischer (1889). This position was used by the authors to locate points of the body on the coordinate system. The position was called *normalstellung*, meaning upright reference, not normal posture. Comfortable relaxed standing was called *bequeme haltung*, meaning comfortable hold.

Asymmetric Standing

If standing must be maintained for any length of time, the normal person has a variety of options. A common choice is to stand first with the weight on one leg and then shift to the opposite leg (Fig. 12–1). The contralateral foot is on the ground but bears little weight. The hip posture is of the Trendelenburg type, in which the abductor muscles are inactive and the support comes from the ligaments of the hip joint. The knee on the weight-bearing leg is fully extended, with the center of gravity falling anterior to the knee axis of motion to reduce quadriceps muscle contraction. The arm postures are more variable, with hands at sides, held behind the back, on hips, in pockets, or folded on the chest. Another common standing posture is with weight distributed over both feet in a wide base, the knees and hips in extension, and the hands held behind the back or folded on the

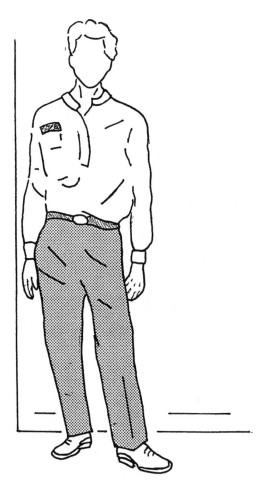

Figure 12–1 One example of a normal asymmetric standing posture. Support in the lower extremity is mainly through the right leg, using ligamentous and bony support at the hip and knee.

chest. Many people stand very comfortably on one leg with the opposite foot used to brace the knee. This type of one-leg posture is called the **nilotic stance** (belonging to the Nile) and is commonly practiced in Africa and among sheep herders, who often use a staff for balance (Fig. 12–2).

Symmetric Stance

Evaluation of body alignment in standing is performed using a symmetric, relaxed stance with the feet at approximately the width of the hip joints, the arms relaxed at the side of the body, and the eyes directed forward. A more natural position is achieved if the subject takes a few steps in place before assuming the posture. Alignment of the head, shoulders, trunk, hips, knees, and ankles are assessed from the side (Fig. 12–3) and from the front and back.

Although this position is called comfortable, relaxed standing, it is not comfortable for any length of time, and the individual will soon choose an alternative posture that is less tiresome. Nevertheless, the standing position of humans is extremely efficient as compared to that of animals who stand on flexed extremities. In the human, the line of gravity falls very close to (or through) the joint axes (see Fig. 12–3). Only minimal contraction of a few muscles such as the soleus, erector

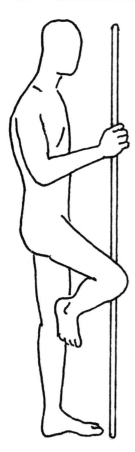

Figure 12–2 The nilotic stance (from the Nile) is an energy-efficient posture used by many people. The left knee is stabilized by the right foot and balance is maintained by light hand support.

spinae, trapezius, and the temporalis (jaw closure) are needed to maintain the erect posture. Discomfort with need to change position is caused more from vascular insufficiency in compressed joint cartilage and tense ligaments than from muscle fatigue. Another factor leading to change in standing posture is that of maintaining adequate return of venous blood to the heart. Contraction of muscles in the legs compresses the veins and assists in propelling blood and lymph toward the right atrium of the heart to maintain cardiac output. This muscle activity in the legs is referred to as the "muscle pump." A person standing still or at attention for a period of time who does not perform isometric contractions of the calf and thigh muscles may have pooling of venous blood in the extremities, inadequate venous return, insufficient cardiac output to the brain, and an episode of fainting.

Postural Sway

The high center of gravity of the human (S2) and the small base of support in standing place the body in unstable equilibrium. The constant displacement and correction of the position of the center of gravity within the base of support is called **postural sway** (Fig. 12–4). Electromyograms (EMGs), particularly in the leg muscles, show low-level alternating contractions in antagonistic muscles (eg, anterior tibialis and soleus). Contraction and relaxation of the biceps femoris muscle during standing can be seen in Fig. 11–10A.

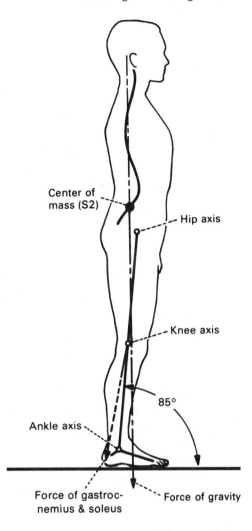

Figure 12–3 In the relaxed, standing posture, the gravitational force line through the center of mass falls behind the hip joint, in front of the knee joint, and in front of the ankle joint. In the lower limbs, active muscle contraction for balance is required, but only in the gastrocnemius-soleus muscles. (Redrawn from Rosse, C and Clawson, K: *The Musculoskeletal System in Health and Disease.* Harper & Row, Hagerstown, MD, 1980.)

There is a multisensory control of postural sway with afferent input from the visual, vestibular, proprioceptive, and exteroceptive organs. In children up to 2 years of age, vision plays a minor role in postural stability. The visual role gradually increases in importance in adults ages 20 to 60, when stability decreases by 30 percent when the eyes are closed. In those over 60 years of age, 50 percent of stability is lost with eye closure, thus making vision a major factor in balance of the elderly (Pyykko, Pirkko, and Aalto 1990). Poor visual acuity in people averaging 82 years of age was found to have a significant correlation with both increased postural sway on soft surfaces and incidence of falls (Lord, Clark, and Webster, 1991).

Standing posture is most stable in adults from about 20 to 60 years of age, whereas those younger and older have increased mean values and variability for all measurements of the center of pressure in the base of support: area, length of path, velocity, and maximum amplitude of sway (Pyykko et al, 1988). Both the younger and older age groups also have slowed reaction time (of muscle activity) to disturbances of posture as compared with the adult age group (Woollacott, 1988). Children approach adult values of postural stability by ages 12 to 15 but display a high variability until adulthood (Taguchi and Tada, 1988).

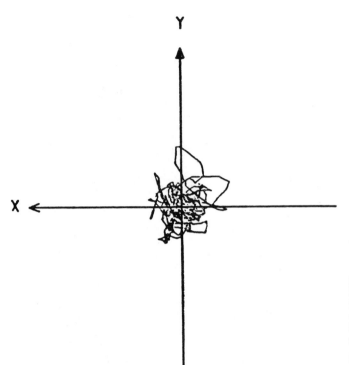

Figure 12-4 Postural sway. Recording of the movement of the center of pressure for 60 seconds in a subject standing on a balance platform. Values: mean amplitude of sway in inches = .13 × .15 Y; length of path = 32.2; velocity = .54 in./sec.

Increase in postural sway in the elderly has a high relationship to incidence of falls. An example is the significant increase found in postural sway in a group of 50- to 76-year-old people who had sustained Colles' fractures of the distal radius and ulna from falls (Crilly et al, 1987). Environmental alterations to provide compensation for diminished visual acuity and avoidance of soft or uneven surfaces are important interventions to prevent falls in the elderly.

Forces Occurring in Symmetric Stance

Balance at Ankle Joint

The vertical projection of the center of gravity of the body mass above the ankle joints falls anterior to the axis of the upper ankle joint (see Figures 2–11A and 2–16). A rotary force is thus set up at the ankle that would cause the tibia to dorsiflex (closed chain) unless opposed by a muscular force. The calf muscles furnish this equilibrating force, thereby preventing dorsiflexion of the ankle (excessive forward inclination of the shank with respect to the foot). The soleus muscle, in particular, is thought to be responsible for this equilibration (Denny-Brown, 1929; Joseph, 1960). During postural sway, the body weight seldom, if ever, passes behind the axes of the ankle joints, and consequently the calf muscles remain continuously, although variably, active (Smith, 1957). The normal ankle and foot are supported by bony and ligamentous structures, and no EMG activity is found in the other intrinsic or extrinsic muscles of the foot during bilateral stance.

EFFECT OF BILATERAL CALF MUSCLE PARALYSIS   If the calf muscles are paralyzed bilaterally, the subject is forced to keep the weight in vertical alignment with the axes of the upper ankle joints, or nearly so. If the body weight passes farther to the rear, the dorsiflexors of the ankle spring into action, but the safe range of backward sway is extremely limited. A subject with calf muscle paralysis tends to keep the feet a certain distance apart, to hold on to a nearby object to provide stability, or to move constantly from one foot to the other.

Balance at Knee Joints

The body mass above the knee joints consists of the head, arms, trunk, and thighs. A vertical line through the center of gravity of this body mass falls slightly in front of the axis for flexion and extension of the knees (see Fig. 12–3). During postural sway, this vertical line may occasionally, though rarely, move behind the axis of the knee joints. Most of the time, therefore, a rotary force in the sense of extension is present at the knees. What, then, prevents the knees from being extended and hyperextended?

This question was investigated by Smith (1957), who found that the counterbalancing force had three components of variable size, depending on the knee angle. As an example, in a subject who stood with the knees 6 degrees short of full extension (knee angle 174 degrees), the proportion of the three components were 50 percent, passive resistance in extra-articular tissues; 30 percent, postural activity of the knee flexor muscles (EMG studies usually show slight activity of either the hamstrings or the gastrocnemius muscles); and 20 percent, resistance by an articular mechanism.

FUNCTION OF THE QUADRICEPS IN STANDING   In most subjects, no EMG activity is detected in the quadriceps during bilateral standing (Basmajian, 1978). However, a short burst of quadriceps activity does appear if, during postural sway, the center-of-gravity line momentarily passes behind the knee axis. This has been confirmed by statography and by EMG (Åkerblom, 1948; Joseph and Nightingale, 1954). Continuous quadriceps action is required only in subjects who stand in such a manner that the center-of-gravity line of the supratibial mass falls posterior to the axis of the knee joint; such subjects are exceptions.

Hyperextension increases knee stability, but it has a delaying effect in activity situations when quick flexion of the knee is required. The "readiness position" in athletics, therefore, avoids complete knee extension. The failure of some individuals to make a quick start is due, to a great extent, to the knees being somewhat hyperextended; "being caught flat-footed" depends as much on knee alignment as on ankle position.

STABILITY VERSUS MOBILITY   Clinically, in the rehabilitation of the disabled, the individual's requirements with respect to stability and mobility must be carefully evaluated. If stability is the prime requirement, as may be the case in elderly persons with amputations, the prosthetic knee must have a large margin of safety. However, a young, active person who has an amputation and whose skill in controlling the prosthetic knee may develop to a remarkable extent, prefers mobility, which requires a readiness position of the prosthetic knee for quick starting and for ease and grace in walking.

BILATERAL QUADRICEPS PARALYSIS   Because of the stabilizing effect of gravity on the knee joints, an individual with bilateral paralysis of the quadriceps muscle is capable of standing erect without braces, provided that there are no other complicating factors. To minimize the danger of collapse at the knee during postural sway, the individual tends to keep the knees maximally extended, which may lead to hyperextension and **genu recurvatum**. The person may also choose to incline the trunk somewhat forward, increasing the stabilizing effect of gravity.

EFFECT OF CALF MUSCLE PARALYSIS ON KNEE STABILITY A prerequisite for stabilization of the knee by gravity is that the body weight be kept forward as in normal, erect posture, which is possible only if the calf muscles are functioning. Indirectly, therefore, these muscles are responsible for knee stability. A subject with a combination of calf muscle and quadriceps paralysis benefits from wearing a foot-ankle orthosis with dorsiflexion limited at 90 degrees because this materially improves knee stability. Similarly, a blocking of dorsiflexion of the prosthetic foot in the above-knee artificial limb improves knee stability, whereas allowing dorsiflexion beyond 90 degrees causes the knee to become unstable.

Balance at Hip Joints

As previously stated, the center of gravity of head, arms, and trunk (HAT) is located inside the thorax, approximately at the height of the xiphoid process. A vertical line through this center may fall directly through, in front of, or in back of the common hip axis, depending on the individual's stance. Muscle action varies accordingly.

There has been much controversy with respect to the location of the center-of-gravity line of HAT in relation to the common hip axis in standing. In the latter half of the 19th century, anatomists (Meyer, 1853; Braune and Fischer, 1889; Fick, 1911) differed considerably in their opinions. Schede (1941), in his analysis of common ways of standing, showed that the center-of-gravity line may fall on either side of the common hip axis or directly through it. He stressed that incomplete extension of the hip is essential if the knees are to be stabilized by gravity because, when the hip is completely extended, a backward sway of the center of gravity of HAT can no longer be absorbed at the hip and, therefore, results in flexion of the knees.

Åkerblom (1948) reported that 22 subjects (out of 25 studied) stood with incomplete extension at the hip, varying from 2 to 15 degrees. His subjects stood "comfortably," with the feet slightly apart and the arms hanging relaxed. Variations of the center-of-gravity line with respect to the hip axis from one measurement to the other were found, indicating postural sway at the hip as well as at the ankle. He concluded that, in comfortable symmetric standing, the upper body is usually balanced over the hip joint in unstable equilibrium. Basmajian (1978) registered slight electrical activity in the iliacus in standing at ease, thus substantiating Åkerblom's findings of incomplete hip extension.

HIP POSTURE WHEN KNEE CONTROL IS LACKING It is of particular importance for individuals who have lost their ability to control the knee activity (such as patients with above-knee amputations and patients with paralysis of certain muscles, eg, the quadriceps) to stand with the hips short of full extension so that some postural sway can be absorbed at the hip. As pointed out by Schede (1941), when an above-knee prosthesis is worn, equilibration at the hip is mandatory for knee stability. These patients tend to have some increase in the lumbar curve, but a backward tilt of the pelvis for the purpose of decreasing the lumbar curve is contraindicated, because it would cause the artificial knee to buckle.

HIP POSTURE OF PATIENTS WITH PARAPLEGIA The patient with paraplegia, having lost control of the muscles of the ankles, knees, and hips, needs bracing to stand erect.

Bracing at ankles and knees is essential to maintain the knees in extension and to provide stability at the ankle, but the hips may be left free. Such a patient assumes a characteristic posture with the upper part of the body inclined backward so that the center-of-gravity line of HAT comes to fall well behind the hip axis (Fig. 12–5). The upright posture of the patient standing in bilateral knee-ankle-foot orthoses (KAFO) is supported at the hips by the iliofemoral (Y) ligaments. If the ligaments have been permitted to shorten, or if hip flexor spasticity exists, the hips will be in flexion. The patient demonstrates lordosis as he or she attempts to maintain the erect position. The patient is unable to bring the center of gravity of HAT posterior to the hip axis and requires constant support for HAT from the upper extremities. Crutch-walking will be laborious and impractical.

If a patient with paraplegia wishes to lean forward, as when picking up an object from the floor, the patient must brace himself or herself on a firm object with one hand while picking up the object with the other hand. Otherwise, the patient collapses at the hip as soon as the center of gravity of HAT moves in front of the hip axis.

Balance of the Trunk and Head

In the erect position, slight EMG activity is recorded from the erector spinae muscles. The rectus abdominis is inactive, and in some subjects slight activity may be recorded from the internal abdominal oblique muscles (Basmajian, 1978).

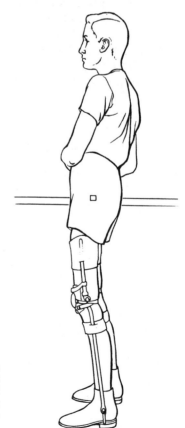

Figure 12–5 Characteristic posture of a paraplegic standing in knee-ankle-foot orthoses that stabilize the knees and ankles but leave the hips free. The center-of-gravity line of the upper part of the body falls well behind the common hip axis. The square on the shorts is positioned over the greater trochanter, which represents the approximate location of the center of the hip joint.

The center of gravity of the head is located about 1 inch (2 to 3 cm) above the transverse axis of the atlanto-occipital joints so that the head is in unstable equilibrium, much like that of a seesaw. When the head is erect, a perpendicular line through the center of gravity of the head falls somewhat anterior to the transverse axis for flexion and extension (Fig. 12–6A). Therefore, in ordinary standing and sitting, the posterior neck muscles are moderately active to prevent the head from dropping forward. When the head is inclined forward, as in reading, writing, and sewing, the demands on these muscles increase (see Fig. 12–6B). When the head is allowed to drop all the way forward, however, the ligamentum nuchae becomes taut, and muscular activity is no longer needed. If the head is tipped backward, the center-of-gravity line falls posterior to the transverse axis (see Fig. 12–6C), and the head tips all the way back unless the flexors of the head spring into action. By palpating the anterior neck muscles (sternocleidomastoid, scalenus anterior), the point at which the center of gravity passes behind the transverse axis can be ascertained.

AMBULATION

Ambulation can be defined in a broad sense as a type of locomotion (L. *locus*, place, plus *movere*, to move; in this case, moving from one place to another). Other types of locomotion include crawling or using a wheelchair. In humans, a bipedal (L. *bi*, two, plus *pes*, foot) pattern of ambulation is acquired during infancy. With practice (training), the sensorimotor system becomes very adept at automatically generating a repeating set of motor control commands to permit an individual to walk without conscious effort. Disease or injury of the nervous system or of the musculoskeletal system can disrupt the normal pattern of ambulation. A variety of compensatory mechanisms may be called into action in an effort to maintain functional ambulation. These compensations manifest themselves as abnormal patterns of walking and are invariably less efficient and more costly in terms of energy expenditure than the normal mechanisms.

Methods of Studying Locomotion

Humans have long appreciated the more apparent distinction between activities such as walking and running, but analysis of their fundamental mechanics was not possible before the development of the science of physics. With so many other important problems awaiting physical analysis, locomotion received only sporadic attention from pioneers such as Borelli (1679) and the Weber brothers

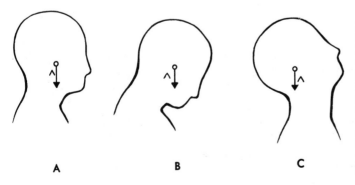

A   B   C

Figure 12–6 Relation of the center-of-gravity line of the head to the axis of the atlanto-occipital joints in different head positions. (*A*) Head erect, center of gravity slightly anterior to axis, posterior neck muscles moderately active. (*B*) Head forward, increased activity of posterior neck muscles. (*C*) Head backward, center of gravity posterior to axis, anterior neck muscles active.

(1836). Extraordinary advancements of the kinematics and kinetics of locomotion occurred in the latter part of the 19th century because of socioeconomic interest in the ability and limits of men and animals for work, racing, and military activities and, of course, flying. Innovative methods for studying locomotion were developed; some of these have not been exceeded to this time. Marey (1890), the eminent French physiologist, recorded locomotion photographically with methods that led to the development of motion pictures. This method consisted of making a series of exposures on a photographic plate of a walking subject. By means of a rotating shutter, exposures were made at intervals of 0.1 second. Because superimposition of several pictures on one another gave a confused record, "geometric chronophotography" was subsequently employed. The subject was dressed in black, and brilliant metal buttons and shining bands were attached to the clothing to represent joints and bony segments. The subject, strongly illuminated by the sun, was photographed as he or she walked in front of a black screen. Dots and lines thus appeared on the photographic plate because the rest of the body did not show against the black background. The principles of this method of recording have been used extensively by subsequent investigators.

In 1887, Muybridge published the most remarkable photographs of humans walking, running, jumping, climbing, and lifting; the gaits of over 30 animals, and the flight of birds (Fig. 12–7). He used 48 electrophotographic cameras arranged in three batteries that could make simultaneous lateral, anterior-

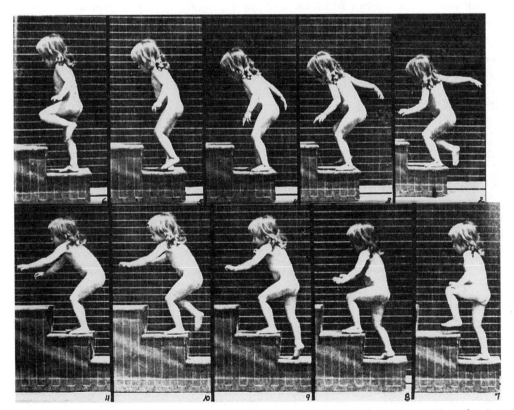

Figure 12–7   Serial photographs of a child ascending steps, showing the changes in position of various joints (circa 1880). The action proceeds from right to left in each row of photographs. (From *The Human Figure in Motion* by E. Muybridge, 1955. Dover Publications, Inc., with permission.)

posterior, and oblique exposures of the moving subject using camera speeds ranging up to $\frac{1}{6000}$ of a second. Over 4000 photographs of his work on humans and 4000 photos of birds and animals have since been reprinted (Muybridge, 1955, 1957).

In the early 1900s, a German mathematician, Otto Fischer, together with Wilhelm Braune, an anatomist, calculated the trajectories, velocities, accelerations, forces, and torques of joints and segments of the body in 31 phases of the gait cycle to establish the scientific basis of the kinematics and kinetics of human gait (Fig. 12–8). Among their many findings were calculations proving that the swinging leg was not a pendular action but required muscle forces for movement. This monumental work, published over the years from 1890 to 1907 is extensively cited in the literature. The work was not readily available until the recent English translations were published (Braune and Fischer, 1984, 1987).

Photographic Techniques

An interrupted light technique has been used to measure the amount of displacement of a particular part (or parts) of the body. Because the time between each adjacent pair of white dots is equal, a greater distance between dots indicates that the part is moving at a faster velocity.

Sutherland and Hagy (1972) developed a photographic method using motion picture cameras in front and on both sides of the subject. Black tape is placed on the subject over anatomic landmarks of the hip, knee, and foot, and a motion analyzer camera superimposes an x-y coordinate system on the walking subject.

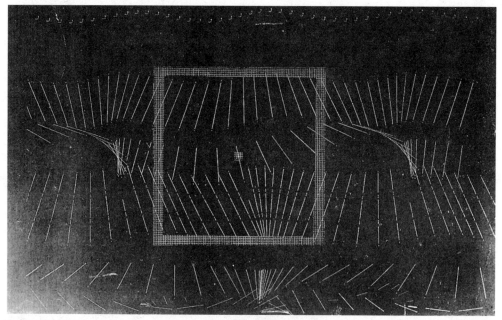

Figure 12–8 Chronophotographic plate (circa 1900) from the right side of the subject walking with Geisler tubes aligned to body segments and with the rectangular coordinate system superimposed. Four cameras took instantaneous exposures to calculate trajectories, velocities, and accelerations in the three planes of motion. Coordinates of the anatomical points were measured by an optical-mechanical instrument with an accuracy of some thousandths of a millimeter. (Adapted from Braune and Fischer: *The Human Gait.* Springer-Verlag, Berlin 1987.)

Lines are drawn between the landmarks to form right triangles, and the angle of joint motion is calculated trigonometrically from the measurements of two sides of the triangle (Fig. 12–9). EMGs can be filmed simultaneously with the walking subject by one of the side cameras. The advantage of this method is that walking patterns are not altered by invasive procedures, the attachment of apparatus to measure joint motion (electrogoniometers), or walking in a darkened room. Disadvantages are the time-consuming measurements and calculations.

The SELSPOT apparatus (Lindholm, 1974; Florence et al, 1978; Larsson, Sandlund, and Oberg, 1978) provides a means for automatically recording movement with the aid of small sources of light attached to the body parts. In many respects, this is similar to photographic techniques, but a photosensitive transducer (photocell) is used instead of film. A special television camera containing the photocell is focused on the light-emitting spot. Movement of the lightspot image over the

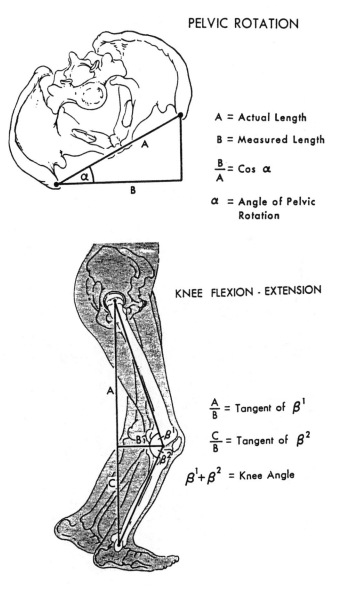

PELVIC ROTATION

A = Actual Length

B = Measured Length

$\dfrac{B}{A}$ = Cos α

α = Angle of Pelvic Rotation

KNEE FLEXION - EXTENSION

$\dfrac{A}{B}$ = Tangent of β^1

$\dfrac{C}{B}$ = Tangent of β^2

$\beta^1 + \beta^2$ = Knee Angle

Figure 12–9 Examples of the trigonometric method used by Sutherland to measure joint motions from motion picture film of the walking subject. (Adapted from Sutherland and Hagy: Measurement of gait movements from motion picture film. *J Bone Joint Surg* 54-A:787–797, 1972.)

photocell generates an electric signal that is easy to record on magnetic tape and to analyze with a computer. The movement of several lightspot sources can be tracked by the same photocell, and the output displayed on a television monitor as a moving stick figure (Fig. 12–10). The stick figure is generated by electronically connecting each of the dots representing the original light sources affixed to the body. Computer programs can be used to automatically detect and display the angle at each joint and to compute angular velocities of motion.

Videography

A single video camera can be used for a visual presentation of gait. An alternative is to use a variable speed treadmill with a backdrop. Treadmill walking is different from floor walking but more in muscle activity than in visible motions. The video can be viewed on the screen, and with stop action the joint angles and segment displacements can be manually measured with a goniometer and a ruler.

Automated video-computerized digital systems record reflective markers placed on segments and joint centers of the body (Kadaba, Ramakrishan, and Wootten 1990). Two or more cameras are needed to record the three planes, and marker placement requires a great deal of precision for accurate results. Problems occur with difficulty in identifying landmarks, obesity, skin motion, short distances between markers, and covering of markers by the arm swing (Perry, 1992).

Electrogoniometry

Electrogoniometry is a technique for continuous recording of joint motion. Figure 12–11 shows a simple electrogoniometer (elgon), in which motion of one arm of the goniometer with respect to the other arm changes the voltage output of a potentiometer mounted over the axis of rotation of the goniometer. The output signal is amplified and recorded on a strip chart to provide a permanent record of the rate and amount of angular motion. The goniometer is a hinge with a fixed axis of

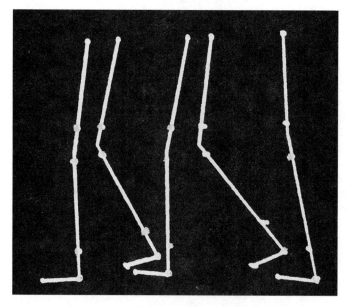

Figure 12–10 Computer-generated stick figures of a subject walking. Data for producing the stick figures came from tracking the movement of six light-emitting diodes (LED) taped to the subject's leg.

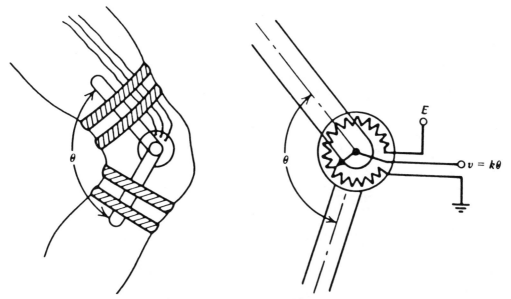

Figure 12–11   Mechanical and electric arrangement of a goniometer located at the knee joint. Voltage output is proportional to the joint angle and can be recorded on a moving strip chart. (From Winter, DA: *Biomechanics of Human Movement*. John Wiley & Sons, New York, 1979, p 12, with permission.)

motion superimposed over the anatomic joint, which has a moving axis. Maintaining accurate alignment is difficult for large ranges of motion. Single axis parallelogram elgons were developed to better approximate the instant center of joint motion (Perry, 1992). At the knee, thin parallelogram frames project forward from cuffs above and below the knee and are joined together well in front of the extended knee. The parallelograms are free to move and the junction between the two follows the path of the instantaneous joint axis. Triaxial parallelogram goniometers for recording joint motion in three planes also have been developed.

Patterns of Walking

Gait Cycle

Gait is defined as the manner or style of walking. One of the attributes of normal walking, as compared with most pathologic gait patterns, is the wide latitude of safe and comfortable walking speeds that are available. Thus, a description of an individual's gait pattern ordinarily includes the speed of locomotion (meters per second) and the number of steps completed per unit of time (steps per minute; this is also called **cadence**), as well as other characteristics of the gait pattern (Larsson et al, 1980).

During a walking cycle, a given foot is either in contact with the ground (**stance phase** of the gait cycle) or in the air (**swing phase**). The duration of the gait cycle for any one limb extends from the time the heel contacts the ground (called **heel-strike** or **heel-on**) until the same heel contacts the ground again as illustrated in Figure 12–12. The stance phase begins with initial contact of the foot (usually heel-strike, but in some pathologic conditions, other parts of the foot may contact the ground first) and ends with the foot (usually the ball of the foot and the toes) leaving the ground (called **toe-off**, or **ball-off**). The swing phase begins

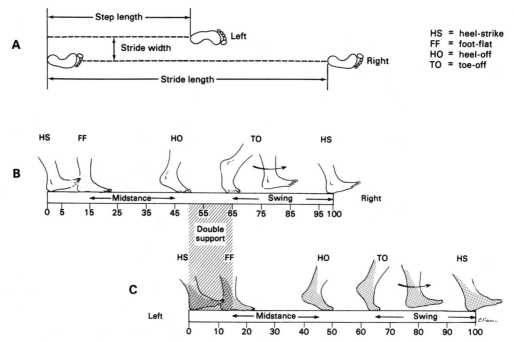

Figure 12–12   Phases of the gait cycle are shown on the same time axis for the left and right leg. (*A*) Representation of the stride dimensions as viewed from above or beneath the subject. (*B*) Side view of one complete cycle of the right leg. (*C*) Side view of one complete cycle of the left leg. The time axes indicate the percentage of the gait cycle completed, starting and ending with heel-strike (HS). Note that two steps occur during each stride. (Adapted from Rosse, C and Clawson, K: *The Musculoskeletal System in Health and Disease.* Harper & Row, Hagerstown, MD, 1980.)

with toe-off and ends with heel-strike. At ordinary walking speeds, the stance phase occupies approximately 60 percent and the swing phase 40 percent of a single gait cycle. Figure 12–12 depicts a full gait cycle for the left and right legs along the same time axis. A typical cycle can be expected to last 1 to 2 seconds, depending on walking speed. Figure 12–12 shows that a period of double support exists when both limbs are in a stance phase. The duration of double support varies inversely with the speed of walking. In slow walking, this period is comparatively long in relation to the swing phase; but as the speed increases, the period becomes shorter and shorter. In running, double support is no longer present. In fact, for a brief time, both feet may be off the ground simultaneously. Each of the two primary phases of the gait cycle can be subdivided into various stages called the **subphases** of gait. For example, the stance phase is comprised of heel-strike, foot-flat, heel-off, and toe-off subphases.

In pathologic gait, however, some of these subphases, such as heel-strike, may not occur. Perry (1974, 1992) has developed a functional classification that describes the phases of gait in both normal and pathologic gaits: stance phase includes initial contact, loading response, midstance, terminal stance, and preswing; the swing phase includes initial swing, midswing, and terminal swing.

Recording of the Walking Cycle

A record of the duration of foot contact with the ground in walking was first accomplished by a pneumatic method (Marey, 1873). Electric contacts attached to the sole of the shoe or foot or incorporated into a shoe insert are now commonly used. A contact on the heel and toe records heel-strike and toe-off to delineate stance and swing phases of the extremity. Contacts on the heel, metatarsal heads, and the great toe additionally record the points of foot-flat and heel-off so that walking speed, step, and stride length and the stance duration can be measured. In addition to determining time and distance factors in gait, these indicators are essential in identifying the phases of gait for simultaneous EMG and force recording of walking.

WALKING SPEED   Walking speed is an important factor in gait analysis because changes in speed are accompanied by changes in every aspect of walking, including time and distance measurements, energy expenditure, and muscle activity. A simple way to measure average speed, stride length, and cadence is to time the subject walking across a measured distance of at least 15 M and to count the number of steps taken. Normal subjects have the ability to alter their speed of walking from a stroll to a fast walk and into a run, thus making comparisons difficult. Each person, however, has a free or comfortable walking speed on a smooth, level surface that is most energy efficient for that individual. Perry (1992) measured the mean velocity of adults walking a free pace as 82 M per minute, or approximately 3 miles per hour. Their stride length averaged 1.4 M and the mean cadence was 113 steps per minute. Men walked faster and had a longer stride length and a slower cadence than women (Table 12–1). Only a part of the variability of stride is due to leg length. The free walking speed is often used in gait studies because it represents optimal efficiency for each individual, and the able-bodied subject reproduces the same values if the walking surface and the footwear remain the same (Inman, Ralston, and Todd, 1981). The authors classify medium walking speed for men as 100 to 120 steps per minute and for women, 105 to 125 steps per minute. Rates above or below these values are classified as fast or slow walking speeds.

Changes in walking speed are made by altering stride length or cadence, and usually the normal subject changes both parameters. Increased speed results in diminished duration of all of the component phases of the walking cycle (stance, swing, double support), with the double support phase decreasing toward zero and the swing phase decreasing the least. In the running subject, there is no double support period and the swing phase is longer than the stance phase.

Kinematics of Walking

The kinematics, or "geometry," of locomotion may be studied objectively by recording movements of points on the body, such as the summit of the head or the crest of the ilium, surface landmarks representing joint centers, and the long axes of bones. If movement paths of these landmarks are projected on the sagittal, frontal, and horizontal planes, a three-dimensional record is obtained.

Table 12-1   Mean Stride Values in Normal Adults 20 to 80 Years of Age Walking at Free or Customary Walking Speed on a Smooth Level Surface

	Males	Females	Total
Number of subjects	135	158	293
Velocity (meters per minute)	86	77	82
Stride length (meters)	1.46	1.28	1.41
Cadence (steps per minute)	111	117	113

Source: Data from Perry, J: *Gait Analysis: Normal and Pathological Function.* Slack, Thorofare, NJ, 1992.

Displacements in the Sagittal Plane

Vertical oscillations of the body occur twice in the gait cycle when viewed in the sagittal plane. These points follow a smooth sinusoidal curve with the highest level at midstance for each foot and the lowest level at double support (Fig. 12–13A). Oscillations of the body's center of gravity (S2) vary from 2 to 5 cm, depending on stride length and speed. These oscillations can be observed by viewing the walking subject from the side and focusing on a point such as the top of the head in relation to a horizontal line in the background. Studying subjects walking on a treadmill is helpful in learning to focus on joints or segments and to develop observational skills in gait analysis.

Large **angular motions** occur at the hip, knee, and ankle in the sagittal plane. (The reader will find it helpful to observe one joint of the dark leg throughout the gait cycle in Fig. 12–14 and then make comparisons with the graphic presentation in Fig. 12–15.)

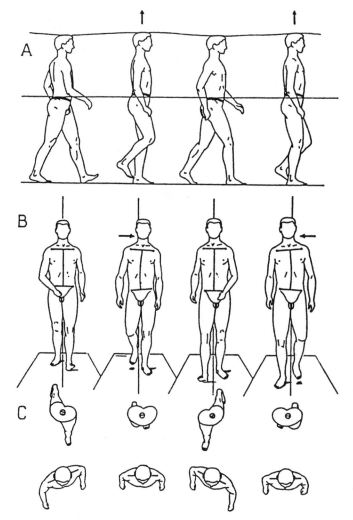

Figure 12–13 Line drawings from film sequences of human gait. (*A*) Sagittal plane. Vertical oscillations of the head and pelvis in the gait cycle. (*B*) Frontal plane. Lateral oscillations of the head and trunk and lateral pelvic tilt during unilateral stance. (*C*) Horizontal plane. Rotations of the pelvis and shoulders. (Adapted from Ducrochet et al., *Walking and Limping*. Masson et Cie, Paris, 1965. JB Lippincott, trans, Philadelphia, 1968.)

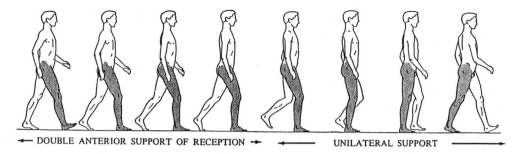

← DOUBLE ANTERIOR SUPPORT OF RECEPTION →   ←—— UNILATERAL SUPPORT ——→

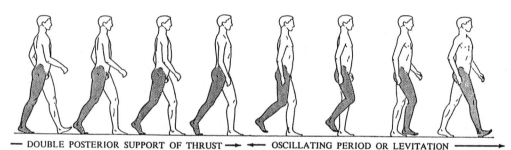

— DOUBLE POSTERIOR SUPPORT OF THRUST → ← OSCILLATING PERIOD OR LEVITATION ——→

Figure 12–14 Sagittal view of the human gait cycle (line drawings from film sequences). Functional descriptors from the French to English translation have been retained. (Adapted from Ducrochet et al., *Walking and Limping*. Masson et Cie, Paris, 1965. JB Lippincott, trans, Philadelphia, 1968.)

The **pelvis** remains relatively level in the sagittal plane and shows a mean excursion of only 3 degrees. The hip joint exhibits one cycle of flexion and extension, with approximately 30 degrees of hip flexion needed at heel-strike, and as the trunk moves forward over the foot, the hip (combined with the lumbar vertebrae) extends to an average of 10 degrees more than in the standing posture. The total angle was found to increase from 40 degrees in slow walking to 54 degrees in fast walking (Smidt, 1971).

The **knee joint** shows two cycles of flexion and extension in the gait cycle. Heel-strike occurs on an extended knee and is immediately followed by about 15 degrees of knee flexion, which is important for shock absorption. The knee extends again during the stance phase and begins to flex at heel-off. The second flexion cycle occurs in the swing phase, with an average of 70 degrees required to clear the swinging foot from the floor.

At the moment of heel-strike, the ankle joint is in a neutral position between dorsiflexion and plantarflexion, and the joint rapidly plantarflexes to provide contact of the entire foot with the floor (foot-flat). In this closed-chain motion, the tibia moves forward over the fixed foot to place the ankle in about 10 degrees of dorsiflexion. The heel rises (heel-off) and a second wave of plantarflexion occurs, peaking at about 20 degrees. At toe-off, the foot dorsiflexes in open-chain motion but only to the neutral position. Note that, in the gait cycle, most of the sagittal plane motion occurs in the range of plantar/flexion (0 to −20 degrees) and that motion in the range of dorsiflexion (0 to +10 degrees) occurs only in the stance phase (see Figs. 12–14 and 12–15).

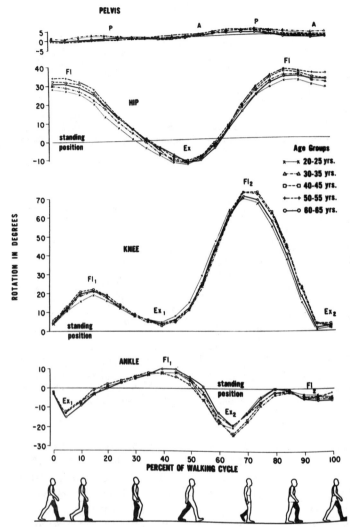

Figure 12–15 Mean patterns of sagittal rotation for the five age groups, 12 men in each group, two trials for each man. The zero reference positions for the hip, knee, and ankle excursions are the angular positions of the joints in the standing posture. Flexion (Fl) in these three curves is always represented by an upward deflection; extension (Ex), by a downward deflection. The reference position for pelvic tipping is the angle formed by the pelvic target and the horizontal at the time of the preceding heel-strike. P is the upward and backward movement of the anterior aspect of the pelvis; A is the downward and forward movement of the anterior aspect of the pelvis. Note that the hip has one wave of flexion-extension, while the knee and ankle have two each. (From Murray, MP, Drought, AB, and Kory, RC: Walking patterns of normal men. J Bone Joint Surg [Am] 46:335, 1964, with permission.)

An essential but often overlooked sagittal plane motion of the metatarsophalangeal joints (MTP) occurs during the stance phase from heel-off to toe-off. During foot-flat the MTP joints are in the neutral position. When the ankle starts to plantarflex at heel-off, the MTP joints hyperextend and move to approximately 55 degrees at the point of toe-off (see Fig. 12–14). During the swing phase, hyperextension of the MTP joints is maintained for toe clearance but gradually decreases to 25 degrees by the time of heel-strike. Pain or restriction of motion of the MTP joints can have devastating effects on the ability to walk.

Displacements in the Transverse Plane

Rotations around vertical axes occur at the vertebrae and hips. These rotations are seen as reciprocal motions of the shoulders and pelvis as the right arm and opposite left leg swing forward (see Fig. 12–13C and Fig. 12–16). The upper vertebrae and shoulders are rotating counterclockwise with reversal of direction on the next step. Inman, Ralston, and Todd (1981) found the magnitudes of these rotations to

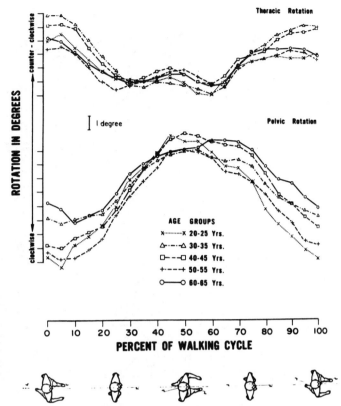

ROTATION IN DEGREES

counter - clockwise

clockwise

Thoracic Rotation

I degree

Pelvic Rotation

AGE GROUPS
x·······x 20-25 Yrs.
△-·-·△ 30-35 Yrs.
□--□ 40-45 Yrs.
+--+ 50-55 Yrs.
○—○ 60-65 Yrs.

0   10   20   30   40   50   60   70   80   90   100
PERCENT OF WALKING CYCLE

Figure 12–16 Mean patterns of transverse rotation of the thorax and pelvis for five age groups, 12 men in each age group and two trials for each man. (From Murray, MP, Drought, AB, and Kory, RC: Walking patterns of normal men. J Bone Joint Surg [Am] 46:335, 1964, with permission.)

increase with walking speed and the point of minimal rotation to be near the seventh thoracic vertebra.

At the **hip**, the pelvis rotates forward around the stance extremity, with the motion clinically called the **pelvic step**. The magnitude of this pelvic obliquity is about 5 to 7 degrees in slow walking and increases to 10 to 20 degrees with increased speed (Inman, Ralston, and Todd, 1981). Extreme shoulder and pelvic rotations are seen in world-class race walkers, who are required to maintain one foot in contact with the ground throughout the gait cycle.

Accompanying the pelvic rotation are internal and external rotations of the femur and the tibia-fibula. The entire lower extremity rotates inward during the swing phase and into the stance phase until foot-flat occurs. Then, in closed-chain motion, the extremity rotates externally to reach a maximum at toe-off (Fig. 12–17). Values for these rotations have large individual variation as well as variation of the means with different recording methods. Inman, Ralston, and Todd (1981) show a mean value of 14 degrees for thigh rotation and 20 degrees for tibial rotation.

Displacements in the Frontal Plane

The **head and trunk** shift laterally over the base of support during the stance phase of walking (Fig. 12–13B). Maximum lateral displacement occurs at unilateral stance and is about 2 cm in each direction. When visualized in both the sagittal

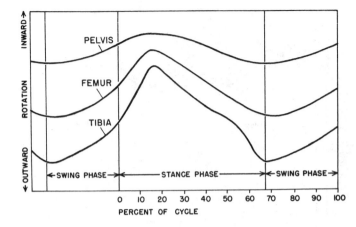

Figure 12–17 Transverse rotations of bony segments of the lower extremity during the walking cycle. (Composite curves for all subjects; redrawn from Eberhart, H et al: *Fundamental Studies of Human Locomotion and Other Information Relating to Design of Artificial Limbs*. University of California, Berkeley, 1947.)

and frontal planes during walking, the center of gravity at S2 is high and lateral on right unilateral stance, becomes low and crosses the midline at double support, and goes high and lateral again on left unilateral stance.

In unilateral stance, the **pelvis** on the contralateral swing leg tilts down about 8 degrees (Eberhart et al, 1947). This small motion serves two purposes: (1) It places a stretch on the hip abductor muscles of the stance leg to increase their force (length-tension) and (2) it decreases the rise of the center of gravity of the swing leg and therefore decreases energy expenditure.

Complex triplanar motion in the **subtalar and transverse tarsal joints** occurs in normal gait, with the majority of the motion occurring in the frontal plane as pronation and supination (or eversion and inversion of the calcaneus).

At heel-strike, closed-chain motion begins. The leg rotates internally, carrying the talus with it and causing the planted calcaneus to evert at the subtalar joint and the foot to pronate. Eversion of the calcaneus also causes the axes of the talonavicular and the calcaneocuboid joints to become parallel, permitting flexibility of the transverse tarsal joint and lowering of the longitudinal arch. Maximum pronation is about 5 degrees and occurs right after foot-flat. Flexibility of the foot in the early part of the stance phase is essential for shock absorption and for adaptation of the foot to uneven surfaces.

At midstance, the tarsal joints change to become a rigid structure necessary for propulsion. The leg begins to rotate externally at foot-flat, and the talus follows, causing the fixed calcaneus to invert and the foot to supinate. Inversion of the calcaneus causes the axes of the talonavicular and calcaneocuboid joints to diverge and to produce locking or rigidity of the transverse tarsal joint. As the heel rises, the MTP joints go into hyperextension and the plantar aponeurosis becomes taut to further increase supination and promote foot rigidity (see windlass mechanism, Chapter 10). Maximum inversion occurs at toe-off and is about 5 degrees.

Although the tarsal joint motions are small, they are a critical part of the gait cycle. If the motions are excessive, diminished, or occur at the wrong phase in the gait cycle, pain and dysfunction may occur not only in the foot but up the kinetic chain. For example, with excessive pronation, the leg and thigh have excess internal rotation after heel-strike, and the knee points toward the midline as it performs the first flexion cycle. In time, motion in such an abnormal plane can cause knee pain and patellofemoral tracking problems.

Kinetics of Ambulation

For an analysis of the contribution of muscles to movement, a more extensive knowledge of physics than that usually included in the background requirements for students of physical therapy and occupational therapy is required. The present chapter, therefore, does not attempt such an analysis, but some of the general features are described so that the reader may become somewhat familiar with methods used in the study of locomotion and may become aware of the difficulties that arise if the student is to go beyond an evaluation of muscles in static conditions to an understanding of how they control the body in motion.

When the body is stationary, the torque produced by the muscles about each joint must balance the torque produced by gravity, and the contribution of each muscle fiber is determined by the length-tension relationship, by the angle of pull, and by the lever arm relationships. When the body is in motion, these factors are still present, but more difficult ones are added. The tension produced by each muscle fiber decreases with its speed of shortening, and the faster the muscle fiber is stretched, the more the tension increases (see Chapter 4). The torque exerted by the muscle does not move the body directly but changes its acceleration. The change in acceleration changes its velocity, which finally results in displacement. To gauge the participation of muscles in movement, one must be able to visualize the movement in terms of its acceleration, a characteristic not readily appreciated.

Ground Reaction Forces

When the foot strikes the ground, the ground produces equal and opposite forces on the foot and body (Newton's third law). The resultant of these ground reaction forces (GRFs) is useful in visualizing the muscle contractions and orthotic forces needed to prevent the joints of the extremity and trunk from collapsing.

The force platforms (or plates) described by both Hellebrandt and Elftman in 1938 are still widely used (with technological improvements, of course) to record postural sway of a stationary subject and the GRF transmitted through the foot of a walking subject. These force platforms were comprised of a metal plate approximately 1 M^2 resting on four short pillars on each side. Strain gauges bonded to each pillar detected changes in the load supported by that pillar. When a load (mass) was placed anywhere on the force platform, the strain gauges generated voltage signals in proportion to the load supported by each pillar. By amplifying and recording the output signals of the strain gauges, the magnitude and direction of the forces being transmitted to the supporting surface were determined. Newer force platforms may use quartz (piezoelectric) force transducers.

The three rectangular components of the GRF in the stance phase of a single step are illustrated in Fig. 12–18. The largest component (Z) is the vertical force directed at a right angle to the floor. This component rises rapidly after heel contact and has two peaks that exceed body weight (horizontal dotted line). The first peak occurs as the supporting limb decelerates the body mass, and the second occurs as the body is accelerated. The decrease between the peaks to below body weight at midstance is due to elevation of the center of gravity by the opposite swinging leg. The X component represents anterior-posterior forces or fore-and-aft shear, with negative values indicating a forward direction and positive values indicating a posterior direction. The Y component represents medial-lateral shear, with the negative sign representing the lateral direction.

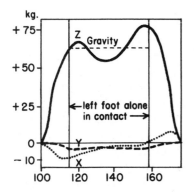

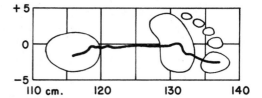

Figure 12–18 Vertical and horizontal components of ground reaction on the foot, as obtained from force plate studies. The second vertical line represents left heel-strike and the third vertical line represents left toe-off. Z = vertical component of GRF; X = fore and aft shear; Y = medial and lateral shear. Gravity represents the subject's body weight of 63 kg. (Redrawn from Elftman, H: The force exerted by the ground in walking. Arbeitsphysiol 10:485, 1939.)

Figure 12–19 Path of the point of application of the ground reaction on the foot, as obtained from force plate studies. (Redrawn from Elftman, H: The force exerted by the ground in walking. Arbeitsphysiol 10:485, 1939.)

Movement of the GRF from the heel to great toe during the stance phase is shown in Fig. 12–19. This has been named the **center of pressure**, which is an average point in time and space and does not always describe the location of force on the foot. For example, during midstance, weight bearing is on the calcaneus and the metatarsal heads, but the center of pressure is recorded at the midfoot, which may not be bearing any weight at all.

Composition of the vertical (Z) and the fore and aft (X) shear components form the resultant GRF in the sagittal plane (see Chapter 2 under Composition of Forces). Figure 12–20 provides some examples of the location of this resultant in relation to the ankle, knee, and hip axes. Study of the location of the GRF is helpful in understanding the complex muscle activity of gait. At heel-strike, GRF is posterior to the ankle axis creating a plantarflexor torque that is decelerated by the dorsiflexor muscles. The GRF runs through the axis of the knee in this instance and does not create a torque. At the hip, the GRF is anterior, creating a flexion torque that is counterbalanced by contraction of the hip extensors. In foot-flat, the GRF is posterior to the knee, requiring activity of the quadriceps to prevent the knee from buckling. At midstance, the GRF is well ahead of the ankle axis, creating a dorsiflexion torque that is controlled by the gastrocnemius and soleus muscles.

The GRF in the frontal plane is the resultant of the vertical (Z) and the horizontal (Y) components. For details on the location and magnitudes of the GRF, see Perry (1992).

Muscle Activity in the Gait Cycle

Electromyography

Electromyography (EMG) has been used to determine when muscles are contracting and relaxing during the gait cycle. Surface electrodes placed on the skin have the advantage of being noninvasive but the disadvantage of recording action potentials from deeper or adjacent muscles including antagonists (cross-talk). These electrodes are useful for recording activity from muscle groups such as the plantar flexors and from large superficial muscles. The other types of electrodes

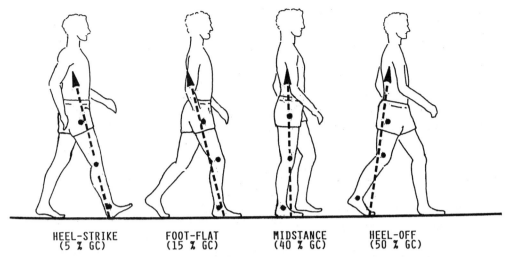

HEEL-STRIKE (5 % GC) FOOT-FLAT (15 % GC) MIDSTANCE (40 % GC) HEEL-OFF (50 % GC)

Figure 12–20 Schematic of the direction of the ground reaction force in the sagittal plane at four points in the stance phase. The percentages are the approximate time in the gait cycle (GC). Circles have been placed over the axes of motion for the ankle, knee, and hip.

used in EMG are fine wires 50 microns in diameter. Small needles are used to insert the fine wires into muscle bellies. The needle is then removed and electrodes are not felt with muscular contraction. The advantage of fine wire electrodes is that they record from a limited area and are the electrodes of choice to differentiate individual muscles or record deep muscle activity (Perry, 1992).

The onset, duration, and peaks of muscular activity are seen on the EMG, but such records do not provide quantitative values in terms of muscle tension except under very limited conditions. Muscle tension (force) includes muscle fiber contraction but is affected by noncontractile fascial forces, type and speed of muscle contraction, and length-tension relationships, as well as changes in lever arm distances and torques that occur with motion. The EMG records only the electrical activity of muscle fiber contraction and is rarely related to muscle tension (Winters, 1990). For example, with the same resistance, concentric contractions show higher EMG amplitudes than eccentric contractions (see Fig. 11–10B, EMG records of eccentric followed by concentric contractions of the biceps femoris and lumbar erector spinae muscles). For the same force, the amplitude of the EMG is greater at shorter muscle lengths (Heckathorne and Childress, 1981). With fatigue, the EMG shows increased motor unit recruitment and higher amplitudes when muscle tension decreases. Only under very limited conditions is the EMG amplitude linearly related to muscle force. This is most easily demonstrated with isometric contractions at the same point in the range of motion (Ralston, 1961). In addition, only the same electrode application can be used, because no two applications pick up the same sample of muscle fibers or motor units (Perry, 1992).

Nevertheless, several methods have been used to try to make quantitative comparisons of the EMG recording for a single muscle and between different muscles. Eberhart and associates (1947) described the EMG activity of the main muscle groups in the lower limb (see Fig. 12–21). The raw EMG record was filtered and rectified to produce the "integrated EMG," which shows the total amount of both positive and negative electrical activity "seen" by the recording electrodes at each instant. The point of maximum activity in the gait cycle for each muscle was set at 100 percent, the absence of activity was set as 0, and intermediate amplitudes were given proportional percentages. Quantitative comparisons between muscles cannot be made because each peak tension is different. The scale of percent electrical activity does not relate to muscle force because the extremity is undergoing accelerations and decelerations with concentric and eccentric contractions.

Normalization is a technique used to compare EMG activity in gait or other activity to the EMG activity of a maximum voluntary contraction (MVC) using the same electrode application. The MVC may be made against a dynamometer, which records a quantitative torque for that muscle group. A simpler method is to use the manual muscle test, which requires the muscle to move the extremity against gravity and hold it against maximum manual resistance (Daniels and Worthingham, 1986). This is also called the "break" test because the examiner usually exceeds isometric tension, causing the muscle to give with an eccentric contraction (see Fig. 11–10C for reference maximum isometric contractions of the biceps femoris and lumbar erector spinae). The reference EMG amplitude during an MVC is set at 100 percent, and the amplitudes in the gait cycle are rated proportionally and sometimes exceed the MVC. Limitations of normalization for quantification in a single muscle is that the MVC is usually an isometric contraction at one point in the range of motion, whereas the gait EMG contains both concentric and eccentric contractions at high velocity. Comparisons of EMG amplitudes of concentric or eccentric contractions with isometric contractions as an indicator of muscle force is inappropriate.

Regardless of the limitations of EMG in quantification of muscle force, it is a valuable tool in providing information on the timing of muscle activity and points of peak forces. The integrated EMGs in Figure 12–21 are summary curves from

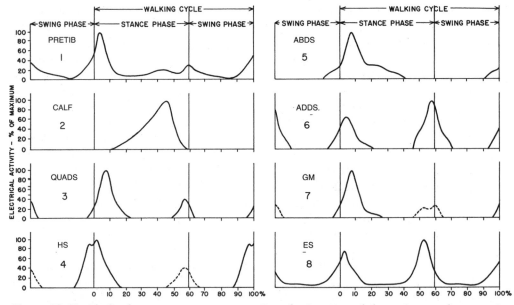

Figure 12–21 Idealized summary curves representing phasic action of the major muscle groups in level walking at 90 steps/min. (*1*) Pretibial group; (*2*) calf muscles; (*3*) quadriceps; (*4*) hamstrings; (*5*) abductors; (*6*) adductors; (*7*) gluteus maximus; (*8*) erector spinae. The amount of electric activity recorded from the muscle group is expressed as a percentage of the maximum electric activity recorded from that group while walking. It is not the maximum amount of activity that the particular muscle group is capable of producing with a maximum contraction. (Redrawn from Eberhart, H et al: *Fundamental Studies of Human Locomotion and Other Information Relating to Design of Artificial Limbs.* University of California, Berkeley, 1947.)

10 normal adult male subjects. General inspection of all the curves shows peak activity to occur during the stance phase, particularly around heel-strike, with minimal activity in the swing phase. The sharp rise and fall of the curves indicate a burst of activity followed by a period of inactivity. Such alternation between short periods of activity and relatively long periods of recovery accounts in part for the ability to walk comparatively long distances without experiencing fatigue. In some clinical conditions, muscles may contract throughout the gait cycle as the quadriceps do in a person who walks with flexed knees. Without any rest period in the gait cycle, these muscles fatigue rapidly.

Dorsiflexors of the Ankle

The **tibialis anterior, extensor hallucis longus,** and **extensor digitorum longus** are slightly active during the swing phase to prevent the foot and toes from dropping (see Fig. 12–21 [1–pretibial group]). Peak activity occurs in the stance phase just after heel-strike with an eccentric contraction to lower the foot to the ground. This contraction provides shock absorption and, in the case of the anterior tibialis, which has distal attachments on the medial cuneiform and the first metatarsal, deceleration of pronation. The tibialis anterior is the largest and strongest of the dorsiflexors. With paralysis of this muscle, strong contractions of the two long toe extensors can clear the foot from the floor in the swing phase. The ankle, however, tends to evert and the toes hyperextend at the MCP joints, often causing corns on the top of the toes from striking the shoe. With fine wire electrodes, the pretibial group showed a biphasic pattern with electrical silence at midstance rather than the low level activity seen in Figure 12–21 (1) (Inman, Ralston, and Todd 1981).

Calf Group

Activity of the **gastrocnemius** and **soleus** begins at foot-flat with an eccentric contraction to slow and control the advance of the tibia over the foot in closed-chain dorsiflexion (see Fig. 12–21 [2–calf muscles]). Peak activity occurs just after heel-off as the muscle contraction becomes concentric and then isometric to produce plantarflexion and stabilize the foot in supination. Because activity in the soleus begins before heel-off and ends before toe-off, Basmajian (1978) states that the muscle function is to support the body rather than to propel it forward (ie, push-off). The importance of the eccentric contraction of the calf muscles to control the advance of the tibia from foot-flat through midstance can be seen in persons with severe weakness or paralysis of the calf groups. At foot-flat, the tibia advances rapidly into dorsiflexion and the knee bends with each step, even though the quadriceps muscles are strong.

The **posterior tibialis, flexor digitorum longus,** and **flexor hallucis longus** are classified as calf muscles and as plantarflexors but are ineffectual forces for plantarflexion because of their small size and poor leverage. Perry (1992) estimates that altogether they can generate 10 percent of the plantarflexion torque of the soleus. They have, however, important activity at the tarsal joints and the toes. The **posterior tibialis** contracts at heel-strike, has peak activity just after heel-off, and is inactive through the swing phase (Perry, 1992). This activity decelerates pronation, adjusts the foot to the ground, and helps stabilize the tarsal joints in supination in late stance. The **flexor digitorum longus** and the **flexor hallucis**

longus are activated after foot-flat, peak just before toe-off, and are inactive in the swing phase. These muscles affect the longitudinal arch as it flattens and elevates, and they stabilize the toes to the ground.

Peroneals

The **peroneus brevis and longus** have phasic activity similar to the gastrocnemius-soleus muscles with contraction beginning in the stance phase after foot-flat and peaking after heel-off when support is on the toes (Inman, Ralston, and Todd 1981). These muscles, along with the posterior tibialis, are important in providing adjustment of the foot to the surface and mediolateral stability of the ankle through control of the tarsal joints and the arches of the foot. The peroneus longus, with its distal attachments on the plantar surface of the foot, is the main muscular support of the three arches and stabilizes the first metatarsal head to the ground (Kapandji, 1987).

Intrinsic Muscles of the Foot

An EMG study of six of the intrinsic muscles of the foot by Mann and Inman (1964) showed activity in all six during the last half of the stance phase and no activity in swing or early stance (abductor digiti minimi, abductor hallucis, extensor digiti brevis, flexor digitorum brevis, flexor hallucis brevis, interossei). Intrinsic activity occurs when the flexible foot must be transformed into a rigid structure. The plantar intrinsic muscles and the extrinsic toe flexors supplement the plantar fascia in this function. Gray and Basmajian (1968) recorded EMGs from six muscles supporting the arches in persons with flatfeet and those with normal arches (tibialis anterior and posterior, flexor hallucis longus and brevis, peroneus longus, and abductor hallucis). In persons with flat feet, the activity of the muscles started earlier in the stance phase. Gray and Basmajian attributed this to recruitment of muscles to compensate for lax ligaments and stresses in the walking cycle.

Quadriceps

The **quadriceps** group demonstrates biphasic activity in the gait cycle as seen in Figure 12–21 (3–quadriceps). With fine wire electrodes, however, the **vastus medialis, intermedius, and lateralis** have been found to have activity from only just before heel-strike through the first 15 percent of the stance phase (Perry, 1992). The activity recorded at toe-off is from the **rectus femoris**, which crosses both the hip and the knee and initiates the motion of hip flexion and knee extension. The vasti initiate a concentric contraction just before heel-strike to extend the knee. At heel-strike, the contraction becomes eccentric to decelerate knee flexion and stop it at 15 degrees. This prevents the knee from buckling and provides shock absorption. Then the knee extends and the vasti muscles are electrically silent throughout midstance and early swing.

Hamstrings

The **semitendinosus, semimembranosus,** and **long head of the biceps femoris** act at both the hip and the knee, and any activity of these muscles influence both joints (see Fig. 12–21 [4–hamstrings]). As a group, activity begins in late swing (before the quadriceps) and peaks at heel-strike. This is an eccentric contraction in open-chain motion (the knee extends 70 degrees while the hip flexes 30 degrees in the same time period). This force decelerates hip flexion and the rapidly swinging leg. At heel-strike the motion becomes closed-chain, and the muscle contraction is nearly isometric and stops by foot-flat. Perry (1992) suggests that the function at this point is to stabilize and protect the knee from hyperextension (see Fig. 9–14 of genu recurvatum thought to be caused by paralysis of the knee flexors). In closed-chain motion, the hamstring muscle activity also may help the gluteus maximus to maintain hip extension after heel-strike (Inman, Ralston, and Todd, 1981).

Knee flexion and hip flexion during the swing phase are the essential motions to lift the foot for toe clearance. Muscles that contribute to knee flexion in early swing are the **short head of the biceps femoris, the gracilis**, and the **sartorius**. The muscles relax during midswing (Perry, 1992).

Hip Abductors

The **gluteus medius and minimus, tensor fasciae latae**, and the **upper part of the gluteus maximus** stabilize the pelvis in the frontal plane during unilateral stance (see Fig. 12–21 [5–abductors]). Activity of the gluteus medius begins during terminal swing and rises sharply to peak at midstance when the extremity is in unilateral stance. The muscle becomes electrically silent at heel-off and as the weight is shifted to the other foot. In this closed-chain motion, the hip adducts about 5 degrees, while the gluteus medius contracts eccentrically to decelerate and limit the drop of the pelvis on the non–weight-bearing side.

The **tensor fasciae latae** are composed of anteromedial and posterolateral fibers that are independently active and have different functions (Pare, Stern, and Swartz, 1981). This study found the posterolateral fibers to become active at heel-strike, whereas the anteromedial fibers were inactive throughout the gait cycle. Inman, Ralston, and Todd (1981) suggest that the activity at heel-strike is to stabilize the iliotibial band against the contraction of the gluteus maximus. With increased speed, the anteromedial fibers became active after toe-off for hip flexion and internal rotation.

Hip Adductors

Although the **pectineus, gracilis**, and **adductors magnus, brevis, and longus** are classified as hip adductors, they have marked individual differences, and limited information is available about their activity. In Figure 12–21 (6–adductors), the adductors are shown to have two peaks of activity that occur in early and late stance. The early peak is almost synchronous with the peaks of the quadriceps, hamstrings, abductors, and gluteus maximus at a time when deceleration and transfer of body weight is occurring. Individually, the adductor magnus was found to be active in early stance, the adductor longus, in late stance, and the gracilis, in initial swing (Green and Morris, 1970; Perry, 1992).

Interpretation of the function of the adductors in gait is difficult because of leverage changes in the range of motion and the multiple actions that the muscles can produce, including hip flexion and extension, internal and external rotation, and in the case of the gracilis, knee flexion. This group represents a large mass of muscle that can exert great forces. Their importance may be more in the activities of running, jumping, climbing, and supporting the body on both legs, as in skiing.

Gluteus Maximus and Hip Extensors

Muscles that can extend the hip are the **gluteus maximus** (particularly the lower half), **hamstrings**, and **adductors** when the hip is flexed. Activity of the gluteus maximus (see Fig. 12–21 [7–gluteus maximus]) begins in terminal swing and rises sharply to peak as body weight is being transferred to the forward foot. The muscle acts synchronously with the quadriceps and adductors and partly with the hamstrings. The function is to decelerate the forward momentum of the trunk by preventing closed-chain hip flexion and stabilization of the hip after heel-strike. Persons with paralysis of the hip extensor muscles lean back 15 to 20 degrees in hip extension at initial stance to place the center of gravity behind the hip joint and prevent the pelvis and trunk from falling forward.

The gluteus maximus, through its attachment on the iliotibial tract, contributes force to decelerate hip adduction and knee flexion in early stance (Perry, 1992).

Hip Flexors

A number of muscles have actions as hip flexors: the **iliopsoas, tensor fasciae latae, sartorius, rectus femoris,** and **adductors**, especially the **adductor longus**. All of these muscles have shown brief activity at the beginning of the swing phase with electrical silence by midswing (Close, 1964; Green and Morris, 1970; Inman, Ralston, and Todd, 1981; Pare, Stern, and Swartz, 1981; Perry, 1992). Close (1964), however, found the iliopsoas silent in many subjects, indicating that initiation of hip flexion was performed by other muscles.

Trunk Muscles

The **transversospinal, erector spinae,** and **quadratus lumborum** muscles show biphasic activity in the gait cycle (see Fig. 12–21 [8–erector spinae]). Most investigators have found the activity to occur at ipsilateral and contralateral heel-strike (Eberhart et al, 1947; Waters and Morris, 1972; Winter and Yack, 1987; Perry, 1992). It is proposed that the muscle contractions counterbalance the trunk flexion torque that occurs when parts of the body are decelerating at heel-strike (Anderson and Winters, 1990). These two peaks of muscle contraction can be self-palpated by placing the thumb in the lumbar sacrospinalis on one side and walking in a normal manner (forward lean will cause the muscles to contract continuously and obscure the biphasic contraction).

Electromyographic activity reported for the **rectus abdominis, external oblique,** and **internal oblique** muscles in walking is variable. Sheffield (1962), using fine wire electrodes, demonstrated inactivity of these muscles during slow walking. In walking at comfortable speed, inactivity of the rectus abdominis was found in half of the subjects, and biphasic activity before heel-strike in the others (Waters and Morris, 1972). In fast-speed walking, all subjects demonstrated biphasic activity. The authors found the internal and external obliques to have continuous and often phasic activity before heel-strike during both comfortable and fast speeds of walking. The variability found at comfortable walking speeds is probably due to the low intensity of the muscle contractions of 5 to 10 percent of the MVC (Perry, 1992), and to the fact that just a few degrees of forward lean of the trunk can alter the abdominal muscle activity.

One of the functions of the trunk muscles during walking is to minimize the oscillations of the head and eyes. This is normally accomplished on a pelvic base that is moving up and down, shifting from side to side, tilting foward and backward, and rotating to each side as it moves forward. Despite the complex and continuous movement of the pelvic base and the fact that HAT makes up 60 percent of the body weight, the average trunk angle in the sagittal plane varies only 2 to 5 degrees over the stride (Winter, Ruder, and MacKinnon 1990; Krebs et al, 1992). Amplitude of the vertical oscillations of the head are similar to those of the center of gravity of the body, indicating that no shock absorption occurs in this direction. Medial-lateral and horizontal accelerations of the head, however, are markedly decreased from those occurring in the pelvis. Winter, Ruder, and MacKinnon (1990) hypothesized that the function of the trunk muscles in gait is to minimize horizontal accelerations of the head and provide a stable platform for the eyes.

Arm Muscles

Reciprocal motion of the arms in walking was once thought to be a passive ballistic movement produced by lower extremity and trunk motion. Kinetic studies of angular momentum, torque, and power as well as clinical observations of persons who have muscle paralysis in their arms have demonstrated that motions of the upper extremities in walking are under muscular control (Hinrichs, 1990). EMG studies of the arms of normal subjects show moderate activity in the posterior and middle deltoid to begin slightly before the arm starts its backward swing and to continue through the backward swing; no activity of the shoulder flexors occurs when the shoulder and elbow are flexing (Hogue, 1969; Hinrichs, 1990). Other muscles showing activity in shoulder extension are the latissimus dorsi and teres major. With increased speed of walking, slight and moderate activity of the triceps brachii occur. The posterior muscles are thought to decelerate the forward swing and accelerate the backward swing. The forces producing forward swing at low speeds of walking occur from passive joint structures and gravity.

Effect of Age on Walking

Investigations of the average age of independent walking in infants show a variation from 11 to 15 months (Wyatt, 1990). At this time, the infants contact the floor with the foot flat, have a wide base of support with a prolonged stance phase, show marked external rotation at the hips with toe out at the feet, exhibit a high guarding position of the arms, and crash frequently. By 2 years of age, heel-strike and the first wave of knee flexion in stance appear, the arms are lower, and most infants show reciprocal arm swing. External rotation of the hips decreases and the base of support narrows (Sutherland et al, 1988). The authors found the joint angles and timing of muscle activity in children to be similar to adult patterns by age 4. GRFs in children demonstrate adult patterns after age 5 (Beck et al, 1981).

There have been many studies of the influence of age (up to 87 years) on gait, including those by Murray and associates (1964, 1966, 1969, 1970), Gabell and Nayak (1984), Hageman and Blanke (1986), Blanke and Hageman (1988), Smidt

(1990), Winter, Patala, Frank, et al (1990), and Leiper and Craik (1991). A clear-cut picture of the time of age changes has not emerged because of the many other variables affecting gait (ie, speed, leg length), the difficulty of excluding individuals with pathologies affecting gait, and differing methodologies. Slight changes start to appear in some subjects after 60 to 65 years of age. There is a tendency to walk at a slower, comfortable pace, with fast speeds performed more by increasing cadence than stride length. Joint excursions and stride length may decrease, and the period of double support may increase, making for a more stable gait. When elderly subjects were carefully screened to eliminate anyone with a pathology that affects gait, few significant differences in gait parameters occurred between the older and younger groups (Gabell and Nayak, 1984; Blanke and Hageman, 1988). The clinical implications of these studies are that gait abnormalities in the elderly should not be considered as caused by normal aging but rather as some type of pathology that may need to be addressed.

Energy Cost of Walking

Muscles affect the rate of energy expenditure during movement partially by doing work on the body to increase and decrease the speed of motion or to lift the body against gravity. An equally important role of muscles is to decelerate different parts, to stabilize joints so that they do not move, and to lower the weight of the body. The overall metabolic cost of walking can be assessed by measuring oxygen consumption and carbon dioxide production and converting the results to energy units such as calories or METs (metabolic equivalents; see Chapter 3). In walking, oxygen rate and oxygen cost are frequently used to compare subjects.

Oxygen rate is the volume of oxygen consumed each minute (O_2 ml/min) divided by body weight in kilograms (O_2 ml/kg $\times$ min). Oxygen rate is related to time and intensity of walking and increases linearly with normal walking speeds from 40 to 100 M per minute (Ralston, 1958; Waters, 1992). Average comfortable walking speed for adults is 80 M per minute (3 miles per hour), with an average oxygen rate of 12 ml per kilogram per minute (Perry, 1992). In terms of METs this would be between 3 and 4 times the resting rate. **Oxygen cost** is the oxygen rate (O_2 ml/kg $\times$ min) divided by the speed of walking (M/min). This value represents the oxygen used for the task of walking a standard distance of 1 M (O_2 ml/kg $\times$ M). A person with a less efficient gait has a higher energy cost.

At **comfortable walking** speed, the average oxygen rate in healthy adults 20 to 80 years of age was the same at 12 ml/kg $\times$ min (Waters, 1992). Subjects from 20 to 60 years walked at an average speed of 80 M per minute, whereas subjects over 60 years walked at the slower speed of 74 M per minute. The oxygen cost for the seniors was therefore slightly higher. Children and teenagers were not as efficient and had higher oxygen rates and costs than the adults and seniors at comfortable walking speeds.

Saunders, Inman, and Eberhart (1953) described **six major determinants of gait** that minimize energy expenditure in walking by limiting displacement of the center of gravity and abrupt changes in its direction. The first determinant is **transverse pelvic rotation**. The pelvis on the swing side moves forward, making the leg segment effectively longer and preventing the center of gravity from having to drop to place the heel on the ground (compared to hip flexion without pelvic rotation). If the body's center of gravity can be prevented from dropping, energy is not needed to elevate it again. Race walkers demonstrate this determinant in the extreme.

The second and third determinants serve to depress the rise of the center of gravity by **downward tilt of the pelvis** on the swing side (5+ degrees) and by **knee flexion** on the stance side (15 to 20 degrees). These motions keep the center of gravity low and prevent the need to expend energy to lift the center of gravity. These three determinants conserve energy expenditure by decreasing the rise and the fall of the body's center of gravity in walking.

The fourth and fifth determinants are the effect of **motions and muscle activity of the knee, ankle, and foot** on the sagittal pathway of the knee. These mostly transverse plane motions change the abrupt arcing of the knee to a smooth sinusoidal curve, which is then reflected upward to the hip and the body's center of gravity.

The sixth determinant of gait is the **adducted position of the shaft of the femur** and the tibiofemoral angle (neck-shaft angle of 125 degrees; see Fig. 8–2a). This structure decreases the magnitude of the lateral excursions of the center of gravity over the supporting feet in the frontal plane. If the neck-shaft angle is less, for example, 90 degrees, wide lateral trunk shifts occur to place the body over the supporting feet. These excessive shifts require a marked increase in energy expenditure.

CLINICAL APPLICATIONS

The human body has extraordinary compensatory ability to walk in the presence of abnormalities such as joint sprains, casts for fractures, muscle paralysis, pain, or amputation. This compensation includes limping to avoid foot pain, use of ligaments to substitute for muscles in stabilizing joints, use of orthoses and prostheses, and use of the arms to provide locomotion (eg, canes, crutches, or wheelchairs). Regardless of the ability of the body to compensate for abnormalities, a price is paid through increased energy expenditure and often joint trauma. Normal human walking is so energy efficient that any gait abnormality increases energy expenditure for the same speed or distance. Energy expenditure is increased because (1) abnormal gait produces excessive displacements of the body's center of gravity, (2) muscles may have to act at higher intensities and for prolonged periods in the gait cycle, and (3) additional muscles may be recruited to help carry out the stance and swing phases of walking. Joint problems and pain are often due to repetitive microtrauma from long-term abnormal alignment, with overstretching of ligaments and wearing of cartilage.

In the presence of a gait impairment, the body usually compensates by decreasing the speed of walking to maintain the lowest possible oxygen rate. This increases the oxygen cost per meter walked, and therefore the efficiency of walking is decreased. People with stroke (hemiplegia), walking at their comfortable but very slow speed, were found to have close to the same oxygen rate as normal subjects (Bard, 1963). From an energy standpoint, walking was not unsafe, and they could walk short distances around the home. Distance walking could be exhausting, however, because of their low energy efficiency.

Even healthy young men walking with casts to immobilize the ankle, knee, or both joints show marked changes in energy expenditure (Waters et al, 1982). When walking at comfortable speeds with casts, the oxygen rates and the heart rates of these subjects were similar to their values during normal comfortable walking without casts (12 ml/kg × minute and 90 beats per minute). Their speed of walking, however, decreased from 10 to 30 percent, and the oxygen cost increased from 25 to 60 percent depending on the number of joints immobilized. Bard and Ralston (1959) found that a person with an above-knee amputation wearing a well-fitted suction socket prosthesis and walking at a comfortable speed used only slightly more energy than normal subjects walking at the same slower speed. Waters and associates (1976) compared the energy cost of walking using a prosthesis with the level of amputation and found performance significantly better the lower the level of amputation. Most of the subjects kept energy expenditure within normal limits by adjusting their gait velocity, and it was this slower speed that reflected loss of efficiency.

The use of crutches for locomotion can pose a major challenge to the energy, muscular, and cardiovascular systems, especially in people who are sedentary, have been confined to bed, or are recovering from trauma or illness. When able-bodied, healthy young men walked on crutches using one leg for weight bearing, their oxygen rate increased from 12 to 21 ml/kg × minute and their heart rates increased from 90 to 135 beats per minute (Waters et al, 1982). Their speed decreased and their oxygen cost more than doubled over normal walking (0.15 to 0.35 ml/kg × minute). Patients who recently suffered a fracture in one leg and who used crutches and their other leg for locomotion were found to have heart rates averaging 150 beats per minute (Waters et al, 1987). These rates of energy expenditure and cardiac response for crutch-walking may be classified as heavy work or strenuous activity.

For those who have lost control of more of the determinants of gait, the physiologic stress of walking can be even greater. Examples are children with cerebral palsy who are fighting spasticity and people with paraplegia (paralysis of both lower extremities) who use KAFO (long leg braces) and crutches to walk (see Fig. 8–8). Depending on the level of innervation, energy expenditure of walking (usually with a swing-through crutch gait) can be from three to nine times higher than in normal gait (Gordon and Vanderwalde, 1956; Clinkingbeard, Gersten, and Hoehn, 1964; Waters and Lunsford, 1985). Sometimes people spend so much of their energy on walking that they have little energy left for school, family, or work.

Thus, many activities in clinical kinesiology are directed to decreasing excessive energy expenditure of abnormal locomotion. Such activities include hands-on alterations of forces to high-technology applications of materials and instrumentation such as methods for measuring muscle force and joint motion, training to minimize gait deviations, improving the efficiency of prostheses and orthoses, developing lightweight wheelchairs, and using motorized and electronic devices for locomotion.

Laboratory Activities

STANDING AND WALKING

1. Palpate the muscles of the legs, thighs, and trunk on a subject assuming a variety of standing postures such as:
   a. Perpendicular military stance.
   b. Comfortable relaxed symmetric stance.

   c. Symmetric and asymmetric stances that people assume when standing in lines or for long periods. Include the many different arm positions seen.
   d. Nilotic stance on one leg with opposite foot on the knee. May need slight hand support.
2. Analysis of the motions of normal walking and identification of abnormal gait deviations require the development of skill in selectively focusing on one joint or segment at a time in a rapid manner to cover all extremities and trunk. This skill can be learned quickly by watching a subject walking on a treadmill. The observer should view from the side (sagittal plane) and from behind (frontal plane). If a suitable elevated platform is available, the subject may be observed from above (transverse plane). The observer should roll up a piece of paper to form a viewer to focus on the following parts of the body:
   a. Top of the head to see the vertical and lateral oscillations.
   b. A point on the lateral side of the hip to observe the vertical oscillations near the center of gravity of the body. A point over the sacrum to observe the lateral oscillations.
   c. In the sagittal plane, observe the near side hip motions, then the knee, then the ankle, and then the toes. Go to the opposite side of the treadmill to view the motions of the other leg.
   d. In the frontal plane (view from the back), observe the normal hip drop during the period of single limb support and then observe pronation and supination of the foot.
   e. Rotations of the hip and knee are best viewed from the front but are often obscured by the treadmill.
   f. Discard the viewer and observe each area in a systematic manner.
   g. Have the subject remove one shoe and walk on the treadmill. Observe and list all the gait deviations you see even if they are subtle.
3. Palpate muscles during walking.
   a. You can palpate your own gluteus medius, erector spinae, and abdominal muscles bilaterally when you walk.
   b. With care you can palpate the quadriceps and the hamstrings on a subject walking on a treadmill. Place your hands on the subject's leg and get into the rhythm so that you maintain constant contact but do not hinder motion. Then move your fingers to palpate the tendons.
   c. You can see the tendons of the dorsiflexors contract, and with care, you can palpate the calf muscles.

References

Abbott, BC, Bigland, B, and Ritchie, JM: The physiological cost of negative work. J Physiol [Lond] 117:380, 1952.

Abrahams, VC: The physiology of neck muscles: Their role in head movement and maintenance of posture. Can J Physiol Pharm 55:332, 1977.

Adal, MN and Barker, D: Intramuscular diameters of afferent nerve fibres in the rectus femoris muscle of the cat. In Barker, D (ed): *Symposium on Muscle Receptors*. Hong Kong University Press, 1962, p 249.

Adams, MA and Hutton, WC: The mechanical function of the lumbar apophyseal joints. Spine 8:327, 1983.

Adams, MA and Hutton, WC: The relevance of torsion to the mechanical derangement of the lumbar spine. Spine 6:241, 1981.

Adams, MA, Hutton, WC, and Stott, JRR: The resistance to flexion of the lumbar intervertebral joint. Spine 5:245, 1980.

Adrian, ED and Bronk, DW: The discharge of impulses in motor nerve fibers, Part II. J Physiol [Lond] 67:119, 1929.

Åkerblom, B: *Standing and Sitting Posture*. Nordiska Bokhandeln, Stockholm, 1948.

Alderink, GJ and Kuck, D: Isokinetic shoulder strength of high school and college-aged pitchers. J Sports Phys Ther 7:163, 1986.

Amadio, PC, Lin, GT, and An, K: Anatomy and pathomechanics of the flexor pulley system. J Hand Ther 2:138, 1989.

American Academy of Orthopaedic Surgeons: Joint motion: Method of measuring and recording. American Academy of Orthopaedic Surgeons, Chicago, 1965.

Anderson, GBJ and Winters, JM: Role of muscle in postural tasks: Spinal loading and postural stability. In Winters, JM and Woo, SL (eds): *Multiple Muscle Systems*. Springer-Verlag, New York, 1990.

Arvidsson, I: The hip joint: Forces needed for distraction and appearance of the vacuum phenomenon. Scand J Rehabil Med 22:157, 1990.

Atkinson, WB and Elftman, H: The carrying angle of the human arm as a secondary sex character. Anat Rec 91:49, 1945.

Aura, O and Komi, PV: Effects of prestretch intensity on mechanical efficiency of positive work and on elastic behavior of skeletal muscle in stretch-shortening cycle exercise. Int J Sports Med 7:137, 1986.

Backhouse, KM and Catton, WT: An experimental study of the function of the lumbrical muscles in the human hand. J Anat 88:133, 1954.

Backlund, L. and Nordgren, L: A new method of testing isometric muscle strength under standardized conditions. Scand J Clin Lab Invest 21:33, 1968.

Bagg, SD and Forrest, WJ: A biomechanical analysis of scapular rotation during arm abduction in the scapular plane. Am J Phys Med 67:238, 1988.

Bard, G: Energy expenditure of hemiplegic subjects during walking. Arch Phys Med Rehabil 44:368, 1963.

Bard, G and Ralston, HJ: Energy expenditure during ambulation with special reference to assistive devices. Arch Phys Med Rehabil 40:415, 1959.

Barnett, CH and Richardson, AT: The postural function of the popliteus muscle. Ann Phys Med 1:177, 1953.

436

Barrack, RL and Skinner, HB: The sensory functions of knee ligaments. In Daniel, DM, Akeson, WH, and O'Connor, JJ (eds): *Knee Ligaments: Structure, Function, Injury and Repair.* Raven Press, New York, 1990.

Barrack, RL, Skinner, HB, and Buckley, SL: Proprioception in the anterior cruciate deficient knee. Am J Sports Med 17:1, 1989.

Basmajian, JV: Electromyography. University of Toronto Medical Journal 30:10, 1952.

Basmajian, JV: *Muscles Alive: Their Function Revealed by Electromyography*, ed 4. Williams & Wilkins, Baltimore, 1978.

Basmajian, JV and Latif, A: Integrated actions and functions of the chief flexors of the elbow: A detailed electromyographic analysis. J Bone Joint Surg [Am] 39:1106, 1957.

Bayley, JC, Cochran, TP, and Sledge, CG: The weight-bearing shoulder. J Bone Joint Surg [Am] 69:676, 1987.

Beals, RD: The normal carrying angle of the elbow: A radiographic study of 422 patients. Clin Orthop 119:194, 1976.

Bearn, JG: An electromyographic study of the trapezius, deltoid, pectoralis major, biceps and triceps muscles, during static loading of the upper limb. Anat Rec 140:103, 1961.

Beasley, WC: *Ontogenetics and Biomechanics of Ankle Plantar Flexion Force.* American Congress of Physical Medicine and Rehabilitation, Philadelphia, 1958.

Beasley, WC: Quantitative muscle testing: Principles and applications to research and clinical services. Arch Phys Med Rehabil 42:398, 1961.

Bechtol, C: Biomechanics of the shoulder. Clin Orthop 146:37, 1980.

Beck, O: Die gesamte kraftkurve des tetanisierten froschgatrocnemius und ihr physiologisch ausgenutzter anteil. Pfluegers Arch Ges Physiol 193:495, 1921–1922.

Beck, RJ, Andriacchi, TP, Kuo, KN, et al.: Changes in the gait patterns of growing children. J Bone Joint Surg [Am] 63:1452, 1981.

Beevor, C: *Croonian Lectures on Muscular Movement.* Delivered in 1903. Edited and reprinted for the Guarantors of Brain. MacMillan, New York, 1951.

Belnap, B: Maximum Isometric Torque of the Plantar Flexors. Unpublished Thesis, Texas Woman's University, Denton, TX, 1978.

Belson, P, Smith, LK, and Puentes, J: Motor innervation of the flexor pollicis brevis. Am J Phys Med 55:122, 1976.

Bennett, RL and Knowlton, GC: Overwork weakness in partially denervated skeletal muscle. Clin Orthop 12:22, 1958.

Bernard, BA: Maximum Isometric Torque of the Plantar Flexors in the Sitting Position. Unpublished Thesis, Texas Woman's University, Denton, TX, 1979.

Bethe, A: Beiträge zum Problem der willkurlich beweglichen Armprothesen: Part I. Die Kraftkurve menschlicher Muskeln und die reziproke Innervation der Antagonisten. Münch Med Wochenschr 65:1577, 1916.

Binder, MD and Stuart, DC: Motor unit-muscle receptors interactions: Design features of the neuromuscular control system. In Desmedt, JE (ed): *Progress in Clinical Neurophysiology, vol 8*. S Karger, Basel, 1980, p 72.

Blakely, RL and Palmer, ML: Analysis of rotation accompanying shoulder flexion. Phys Ther 64:1214, 1984.

Blanke, DJ and Hageman, PA: Comparison of gait of young men and elderly men. Phys Ther 69:144, 1988.

Blix, M: Die Länge und die Spannung des Muskels. Skand Arch f Physiol 3:295, 1891; 4:399, 1892–1893; 5:150, 175, 1895.

Bloom, W and Fawcett, DW: *A Textbook of Histology*, ed 8. WB Saunders, Philadelphia, 1969.

Bloom, W and Fawcett, DW: *A Textbook of Histology*, ed 10. WB Saunders, Philadelphia, 1975.

Bobath, B: *Abnormal Postural Reflex Activity Caused by Brain Lesions*, ed 3. Aspen Systems Corporation, Rockville, MD, 1985.

Bobath, B: *Adult Hemiplegia: Evaluation and Treatment*, ed 2. William Heinemann, London, 1978.

Bobath, B: The treatment of neuromuscular disorders by improving patterns of coordination. Physiotherapy 55:1, 1969.

Bogduk, N and Macintosh, JE: The applied anatomy of thoracolumbar fascia. Spine 9:164, 1984.

Bohannon, RW, Gajdosik, RL, and LeVeau, BF: Isokinetic knee flexion and extension torque in the upright sitting and semi-reclined sitting positions. Phys Ther 66:1083, 1986.

Boone, D and Azen, S: Normal range of motion of joints in male subjects. J Bone Joint Surg [Am], 61:756, 1979.

Bordelon, RL: Clinical assessment of the foot. In Donatelli, R and Wolf, SL: *The Biomechanics of the Ankle*. FA Davis, Philadelphia, 1990.

Borelli, GA: *De Motu Animalium*. Lugduni Batavorum, 1679.

Boyes, JR: *Bunnell's Surgery of the Hand*, ed 5. JB Lippincott, Philadelphia, 1970.

Brand, P and Hollister, A: *Clinical Mechanics of the Hand*, ed 2. Mosby Year Book, St. Louis, 1992, p. 83.

Braune, W and Fischer, O: Ueber den Schwerpunkt des menschlichen Korpers mit Rücksicht auf die Ausrustung des deutsche Infanteristen. Abh d Kgl Sachs, Ges. d. Wissensch., Math Phys Klasse 26:562, 1889.

Braune, W and Fischer, O: *On the Centre of Gravity of the Human Body*. Translated by PGJ Maquet and R Furong. Springer-Verlag, Berlin, 1984.

Braune, W and Fischer, O: *The Human Gait*. Springer-Verlag, Berlin, 1987.

Brewer, B: Aging of the rotator cuff. Am J Sports Med 7:102, 1979.

Brodal, A: *Neurological Anatomy*, ed 3. Oxford University Press, New York, 1981, p 56.

Brown, LP, Neihues, SL, Harrah, A, et al.: Upper extremity range of motion and isokinetic strength of the internal and external shoulder rotators in major league baseball players. Am J Sports Med 16:577, 1988.

Browse, NL: *The Physiology and Pathology of Bed Rest*. Charles C Thomas, Springfield, IL, 1965.

Brunnstrom, S: Muscle testing around the shoulder girdle. J Bone Joint Surg [Am] 23:263, 1941.

Brunnstrom, S: *Movement Therapy in Hemiplegia*. Harper & Row, New York, 1970.

Buchthal, F and Schmalbruch, H: Motor unit of mammalian muscle. Physiol Rev 60:90, 1980.

Burakoff, R: Epidemiology. In Kaplan, AS and Assael, LA: *Temporomandibular Disorders: Diagnosis and Treatment*. WB Saunders, Philadelphia, 1991.

Burke, RE: Motor units: Anatomy, physiology and functional organization. In Brooks, VS (ed): *Motor Systems (Handbook of Physiology, Section I, The Nervous System)*. Williams & Wilkins, Baltimore, 1981.

Burkhead, WZ: The biceps tendon. In Rockwood, CA and Matsen, FA (ed): *The Shoulder, Vol 2*. WB Saunders, Philadelphia, 1990.

Burt, AM: *Textbook of Neuroanatomy*. WB Saunders, Philadelphia, 1993.

Cailliet, R: *Low Back Pain Syndrome*, ed 3. FA Davis, Philadelphia, 1981.

Cailliet, R: *Foot and Ankle Pain*, ed 2. FA Davis, Philadelphia, 1983.

Carr, J and Shepherd, R: *A Motor Relearning Programme for Stroke*, ed 2. Aspen, Rockville, MD, 1987.

Cavagna, GA: Storage and utilization of elastic surgery in skeletal muscles. Exerc Sports Sci Rev 5:89, 1977.

Cavanagh, PR, Rodgers, MM, and Iiboshi, A: Pressure distribution under symptom-free feet during barefoot standing. Foot Ankle 7:262, 1987.

Chandler, TJ, Wilson, GD, and Stone, MH: The effect of squat exercises on knee stability. Med Sci Sports Exerc 21:299, 1989.

Chang, DE, Buschbacher, LP, and Edlich, RF: Limited joint mobility in power lifters. Am J Sports Med 16:280, 1988.

Chen, W, Su, F, and Chou, U: Significance of acceleration period in dynamic strength testing study. J Orthop Sports Phys Ther 19:324, 1994.

Citron, N and Foster, A: Some aspects of lumbrical function. J Hand Surg [Br] 13:54, 1988.

Clark, JM and Haynor, DR: Anatomy of the abductor muscles of the hip as studied by computed tomography. J Bone Joint Surg [Am] 69:1021, 1987.

Clarkson, PM and Tremblay, I: Exercise-induced muscle damage, repair and adaptation in Humans. J Appl Physiol 65:1, 1988.

Clauser, CE, McConville, JT, and Young, JW: *Weight, volume and center of mass of segments of the human body*. AMRL-TR 69-70, Wright-Patterson Air Force Base, OH, 1969.

Clemmesen, S: Some studies of muscle tone. Proc R Soc Med 44:637, 1951.

Clinkingbeard, JR, Gersten, JW, and Hoehn, D: Energy cost of ambulation in traumatic paraplegia. Am J Phys Med 43:157, 1964.

Close, JR: *Motor Function in the Lower Extremity: Analyses of Electronic Instrumentation*. Charles C Thomas, Springfield, IL, 1964.

Colachis, SC, Worden, RE, Bechtol, CO, et al.: Movement of the sacroiliac joint in the adult male: A preliminary report. Arch Phys Med Rehabil 44:490, 1963.

Coon, V, Donato, G, Houser, C, et al.: Normal ranges of hip motion in infants six weeks, three months and six months of age. Clin Orthop 110:256, 1975.

Cope, D: Development of a Clinical Method for the Quantitative Measurement of Maximum Isometric Muscle Torque. Unpublished thesis, Texas Woman's University, Denton, TX, 1975.

Craik, RL: Abnormalities of motor behavior. In *Contemporary Management of Motor Control Problems: Proceedings of the II STEP Conference*, 1991.

Crilly, RG, Richardson, LD, Roth, JH, et al.: Postural stability and Colles' fracture. Age Aging 16:133, 1987.

Cureton, TK: Fitness of the feet and legs. Res Q Am Assoc Health Phys Educ 12:368, 1941.

Daniels, L and Worthingham, C: *Muscle Testing: Techniques of Manual Examination*, ed 5. WB Saunders, Philadelphia, 1986.

Davies, GJ: Isokinetic approach to the knee. In Mangine, RE (ed): *Physical Therapy of the Knee*. Churchill Livingstone, New York, 1988.

Davies, GJ, Wallace, LA, and Malone, T: Mechanisms of selected knee injuries. Phys Ther 60:1590, 1980.

Davis, WJ: Organizational concepts in the central motor networks of invertebrates. In Herman, RM, Grillner, S, Stein, PSG, et al. (eds): *Neural Control of Locomotion: Advances in Behavioral Biology, Vol 18*. New York, Plenum Press, 1976, p 265.

DeLacerda, FG: A study of anatomical factors involved in shin splints. J Orthop Sports Phys Ther 2:55, 1980.

DeLitto, SR and Rose, SJ: An electromyographic analysis of two techniques for squat lifting and lowering. Phys Ther 72:438, 448, 1992.

DeMauro, GJ: Personal Communication, June 1994.

Dempster, WT: *Space Requirements of the Seated Operator*. WACD Technical Report 55-159, July 1955. Office of Technical Services, US Dept of Commerce, Washington, DC, 1955.

Denny-Brown, DE: Histological features of striped muscle in relation to its functional activity. Proc R Soc Med 104B:371, 1929.

Departments of the Army and the Air Force: Joint Motion Measurement. TM 8-640/AFP 160-14, Washington, DC, 1968.

Dick, RW and Cavanagh, PR: An explanation of the upward drift in oxygen uptake during prolonged sub-maximal downhill running. Med Sci Sports Exerc 19:310, 1987.

DonTigny, RL: Function and pathomechanics of the sacroiliac joint. Phys Ther 65:35, 1985.

DonTigny, RL: Anterior dysfunction of the sacroiliac joint as a major factor in the etiology of idiopathic low back pain syndrome. Phys Ther 70:250, 1990.

Doody, SG, Freedman, L, and Waterland, JC: Shoulder movements during abduction in the scapular plane. Arch Phys Med Rehabil 51:595, 1970.

Drillis, R: Objective recording and biomechanics of pathological gait. Ann NY Acad Sci 74:86, 1958.

Drillis, R, Contini, R, and Bluestein, M: Body segment parameters. A survey of measurement techniques. Art Limb 8:44, 1964.

Dubs, L and Gschwend, N: General joint laxity: Quantification and clinical relevance. Arch Orthop Trauma Surg 107:65, 1988.

Duca, CJ and Forrest, WJ: Force analysis of individual muscles acting simultaneously on the shoulder joint during isometric abduction. J Biomech 6:385, 1973.

Ducroquet, R, Ducroquet, J, and Ducroquet, P: *Walking and Limping: A Study of Normal and Pathological Walking*. JB Lippincott, Philadelphia, 1965.

Eberhart, HD, et al.: *Fundamental Studies of Human Locomotion and Other Information Relating to Design of Artificial Limbs: Report to National Research Council, Committee on Artificial Limbs*. University of California, Berkeley, 1947.

Edgerton, VR, Smith, JL, and Simpson, DR: Muscle fibre type populations of human leg muscles. Histochem J 7:259, 1975.

Edman, KAP: Mechanism underlying double-hyperbolic force-velocity relation in vertebrate skeletal muscle. Adv Exper Med Biol 332:667, 1993.

Edwards, RHT: Human muscle function and fatigue. In *CIBA Foundation Symposium #82 Human Muscle Fatigue: Physiological Mechanisms*. Pittman Medical, London, 1981, p 1.

Einthoven, W: Un nouveau galvanometre. Archives Neerlandaises des Sciences Exactes et Naturelles, Ser II. 6:625, 1901.

Elftman, H: Measurement of external force in walking. Science 88:152, 1938.

Elftman, H: The force exerted by the ground in walking. Arbeitsphysiol 10:485, 1939.

Elftman, H: Knee action and locomotion. Bull Hosp Joint Dis 16:103, 1955.

Elftman, H: The transverse tarsal joint and its control. Clin Orthop 16:41, 1960.

Ellison, JB, Rose, SJ, and Sahrmann, SA: Patterns of hip rotation range of motion: A comparison between healthy subjects and patients with low back pain. Phys Ther 70:537, 1990.

Engsberg, J and Allinger, T: A function of the talocalcaneal joint during running support. Foot Ankle 11:93, 1990.

Farfan, HF: Biomechanics of the lumbar spine. In Kirkaldy-Willis, WH and Burton, CV (eds): *Managing Low Back Pain.* Churchill Livingstone, Edinburgh, 1988.

Faulkner, JA, Brooks, SV, and Opiteck, JA: Injury to skeletal muscle fibers during contractions: Conditions of occurrence and prevention. Phys Ther 73:911, 1993.

Feltz, D and Landers, D: The effects of mental practice on motor skill learning and performance: A meta-analysis. J Sports Psychol 5:25, 1983.

Ferrari, DA: Capsular ligaments of the shoulder. Am J Sports Med 18:20, 1990.

Fess, EE: Convergence points of normal fingers in individual flexion and simultaneous flexion. J Hand Ther 2:12, 1989.

Fiatarone, MA, Marks, EC, Ryan, ND, et al.: High-intensity strength training in nonagenarians. JAMA 263:3029, 1990.

Ficat, RP and Hungerford, DS: *Disorders of the Patello-Femoral Joint.* Williams & Wilkins, Baltimore, 1977.

Fick, R: *Anatomie und Mechanik der Gelenke: Teil III, Spezielle Gelenk und Muskel Mechanik.* Fisher, Jena, 1911.

Fillyaw, M, Bevins, T, and Fernandez, L: Importance of correcting isokinetic peak torque for the effect of gravity when calculating knee flexor to extensor muscle ratios. Phys Ther 66:23, 1986.

Fiorentino, MF: *Reflex Testing Methods for Evaluating CNS Development,* ed 2. Charles C Thomas, Springfield, Ill, 1973.

Fischer, O: *Kinematik Organischer Gelenke.* R Vierweg, Braunschweig, 1907.

Florence, JM, Brooke, MH, and Carroll, JE: *Evaluation of the child with muscular weakness.* Orthop Clin North Am 9:409, 1978.

Frankel, VH and Burstein, AH: *Orthopaedic Biomechanics.* Lea & Febiger, Philadelphia, 1970.

Frankel, VH and Nordin, M: *Basic Biomechanics of the Skeletal System,* ed 2. Philadelphia, Lea & Febiger, 1989.

Freedman, L and Munro, R: Abduction of the arm in the scapular plane: A roentgenographic study. Scapular and glenohumeral movements. J Bone Joint Surg [Am] 48:1503, 1966.

Friden, J and Lieber, RL: Structural and mechanical basis of exercise-induced muscle injury. Med Sci Sports Exerc 24:521, 1992.

Frisiello, S, Gazaille, A, O'Halloran, J, et al.: Test-retest reliability of eccentric peak torque values for shoulder medial and lateral rotation using the biodex isokinetic dynamometer. J Ortho Sports Phys Ther 19:341, 1994.

Frontera, WR, Hughes, VA, Dallal, GE, et al.: Reliability of isokinetic muscle strength testing in 45- to 78-year-old men and women. Arch Phys Med Rehabil 74:1181, 1993.

Frontera, WR, Meredith, CN, O'Reilly, KP, et al.: Strength conditioning in older men: Skeletal muscle hypertrophy and improved function. J Appl Physiol 64:1038, 1988.

Fulkerson, JP and Hungerford, DS: *Disorders of the Patellofemoral Joint.* Williams & Wilkins, Baltimore, 1990.

Gabell, A and Nayak, USL: The effect of age on variability in gait. J Gerontol 39:662, 1984.

Gerhardt, JJ and Russe, OA: *International SFTR Method of Measuring and Recording Joint Motion.* Distributed by Year Book Medical Publishers, Hans Huber, Bern, Switzerland, 1975.

Golden, C and Dudley, GA: Strength after bouts of eccentric or concentric actions. Med Sci Sports Exerc 24:926, 1992.

Goldman, JR: Soft Tissue Trauma. In Kaplan, AS, and Assael, LA: *Temporomandibular Disorders: Diagnosis and Treatment.* WB Saunders, Philadelphia, 1991.

Gollnick, PD, Armstrong, RB, Saubert, CW, et al.: Enzyme activity and fiber composition in skeletal muscle of untrained and trained men. J Appl Physiol 33:312, 1972.

Gordon, EE and Vanderwalde, H: Energy requirements in paraplegic ambulation. Arch Phys Med Rehabil 37:276, 1956.

Goss, C (ed): *Gray's Anatomy of the Human Body*, 29th Am ed. Lea & Febiger, Philadelphia, 1973.

Gracovetsky, S, Farfan, H, and Helleur, C: The abdominal mechanism. Spine 10:317, 1985.

Gracovetsky, S, Kary, M, Levy, S, et al.: Analysis of spinal and muscular activity during flexion/extension and free lifts. Spine 15:1333, 1990.

Grafstein, B and Forman, DS: Intracellular transport in neurons. Physiol Rev 60:1167, 1980.

Grant, JC: *An Atlas of Anatomy*, ed 7. Williams & Wilkins, Baltimore, 1978.

Gray, ER: The role of leg muscles in variations of the arches in normal and flat feet. Phys Ther 44:1084, 1969.

Gray, ER and Basmajian, JV: Electromyography and cinematography of leg and foot ("normal" and flat) during walking. Anat Rec 161:1, 1968.

Gray, H: *Anatomy of the Human Body*, ed 28. Lea & Febiger, Philadelphia, 1966.

Green, DL and Morris, JM: Role of adductor longus and adductor magnus in postural movements and ambulation. Am J Phys Med 49:223–240, 1970.

Green, LB: Developing self talk to facilitate the use of imagery among athletes. In Sheikh, AA and Korn, ER (eds): *Imagery in Sports and Physical Performance*. Baywood Publishing, Amityville, NY, 1994a.

Green, LB: The use of imagery in the rehabilitation of injured athletes. In Sheikh, AA and Korn, ER (eds): *Imagery in Sports and Physical Performance*. Baywood Publishing, Amityville, NY, 1994b.

Greenfield, BH, Donatelli, R, Wooden, M, et al.: Isokinetic evaluation of shoulder rotational strength between the plane of the scapula and the frontal plane. Am J Sports Med 18:124, 1990.

Grieve, GF: *Common Vertebral Joint Problems*. Churchill Livingstone, Edinburgh, 1988.

Grieve, GF (ed): *Modern Manual Therapy of the Vertebral Column*. Churchill Livingstone, Edinburgh, 1986.

Griffin, JW, Tooms, RE, Zwaag, RV, et al.: Eccentric muscle performance of elbow and knee muscle groups in untrained men and women. Med Sci Sports Exerc 255:936, 1993.

Grillner, S: Control of locomotion in bipeds, tetrapods, and fish. In Brooks, VB (ed): *Handbook of Physiology: The Nervous System*. American Physiological Society, Bethesda, MD, 1981.

Grood, ES, Suntay, WJ, Noyes, FR, et al.: Biomechanics of the Knee-Extension Exercise: Effect of Cutting the Anterior Cruciate Ligament. J Bone Joint Surg [Am] 66A:725, 1984.

Guth, L: "Trophic" influences of nerve on muscles. Physiol Rev 48:645, 1968.

Gutmann, E: Neurotrophic relations. Annu Rev Physiol 36:177, 1976.

Gutmann, E and Hnik, P (eds): *The Effect of Use and Disuse on Neuromuscular Functions*. Elsevier, New York, 1963.

Guyot, J: *Atlas of Human Limb Joints*. Springer-Verlag, New York, 1981.

Hageman, PA and Blanke, DJ: Comparison of gait of young women and elderly women. Phy Ther 66:1382, 1986.

Hakkinen, K, Komi, PV, and Kauhanen, H: Electromyographic and force characteristics of leg extensor muscles of elite weight lifters during isometric, concentric and various stretch-shortening cycle exercises. Int J Sports Med 7:144, 1986.

Haley, SM and Inacio, CA: Evaluation of spasticity and its effect on motor function. In Glenn, MB and Whyte, J: *The Practical Management of Spasticity in Children and Adults*. Lea & Febiger, Philadelphia, 1990.

Halliday, M: Maximum Isometric Muscle Torque of the Hip Abductors Measured Bilaterally and Unilaterally. Unpublished Thesis, Texas Woman's University, Denton, TX, 1979.

Hanson, J and Huxley, HE: Structural basis of the cross-striations in muscle. Nature 172:530, 1953.

Harper, M: Deltoid ligament: An anatomical evaluation of function. Foot Ankle 8:19, 1987.

Hass, S, Epps, C, and Adams, J: Normal ranges of hip motion in the newborn. Clin Orthop 19:114, 1973.

Haxton, HA: Absolute muscle force in the ankle flexors of man. J Physiol 103:267, 1944.

Heckathorne, CW and Childress, DS. Relationships of the surface electromyogram to the force, length, velocity and contraction rate of the cineplastic human biceps. Am J Phys Med 60:1, 1981.

Hehne, HJ: Biomechanics of the patellofemoral joint and its clinical relevance. Clin Orthop 258:73, 1990.

Helfet, AJ: *Disorders of the Knee*. JB Lippincott, Philadelphia, 1974.

Helgeson, K and Gajdosik, RL: The stretch-shortening cycle of the quadriceps femoris muscle group measured by isokinetic dynamometry. J Ortho Sports Phys Ther 17:17, 1993.

Hellebrandt, FA: Standing as a geotropic reflex: Mechanism of asynchronous rotation of motor units. Am J Physiol 121:471, 1938.

Hellebrandt, FA, Tepper, RH, and Braun, GL: Location of the cardinal anatomical orientation planes passing through the center of weight in young adult women. Am J Physiol 121:465, 1938.

Henneman, E: Recruitment of motoneurones: The size principle. In Desmedt, JE (ed): *Progress in Clinical Neurophysiology, Vol 9*. S Karger, Basel, 1981, p 26.

Herring, D, King, AI, and Connelly, M: New rehabilitation concepts in management of radical neck dissection syndrome. A clinical report. Phys Ther 67:1095, 1987.

Hickok, RJ: Physical therapy as related to peripheral nerve lesions. Phys Ther Rev 41:113, 1961.

Hicks, JH: The mechanics of the foot: I. The joints. J Anat 87:345, 1953.

Hinrichs, RN. Whole body movement: Coordination of arms and legs in walking and running. In Winters, JM and Woo, SL (eds): *Multiple Muscle Systems*. Springer-Verlag, New York, 1990.

Hinton, RY: Isokinetic evaluation of shoulder rotational strength in high school baseball pitchers. Am J Sports Med 16:274, 1988.

Hislop, HJ: Response of immobilized muscle to isometric exercise. J Am Phys Ther Assoc 44:339, 1964.

Hislop, HJ and Perrine, JJ: The isokinetic concept of exercise. Phys Ther 47:114, 1967.

Hogue, RE: Upper extremity muscular activity at different cadences and inclines during normal gait. Phys Ther 49:963, 1969.

Holmes, JA, Damser, MS, and Lehman, SL: Erector spinae activation and movement dynamics about the lumbar spine in lordotic and kyphotic squat-lifting. Spine 17:327, 1992.

Holt, GA and Kelsen, SG: Dyspnea. In Tierney, DF (ed): *Current Pulmonology: 14*. Mosby–Year Book, 1993.

Hoppenfeld, S: *Physical Examination of the Spine and Extremities*. Appleton-Century-Crofts, New York, 1976.

Horak, FB: Assumptions underlying motor control for neurologic rehabilitation. In *Contemporary Management of Motor Control Problems: Proceedings of the II STEP Conference*, 1991.

Horton, MG and Hall, TL: Quadriceps femoris muscle angle: normal values and relationships with gender and selected skeletal measures. Phys Ther 69:897, 1989.

Houk, JC, Crago, PE, and Andrymer, WZ: Functional properties of the Golgi tendon organs. In Desmedt, JE (ed): *Progress in Clinical Neurophysiology, Vol 8*. Karger, Basel, 1980, p 33.

Housh, DJ and Housh, TJ: The effects of unilateral velocity-specific concentric strength training. J Orthop Sports Phys Ther 17:252, 1993.

Howell, S, Imobersteg, A, Seger, D et al.: Clarification of the role of the supraspinatus in shoulder function. Bone Joint Surg [Am] 68:398, 1986.

Huberti, HH and Hayes, WC: Patellofemoral contact pressures. J Bone Joint Surg [Am] 66:715, 1984.

Huxley, HE: The mechanism of muscular contraction. Science 164:1356, 1969.

Huxley, HE: Sliding filaments and molecular motile systems. J Biol Chem 265:8347, 1990.

Ihara, H and Nakayma, A: Dynamic joint control training for knee ligament injuries. Am J Sports Med 14:309, 1986.

Inman, VT: Functional aspects of the abductor muscles of the hip. J Bone Joint Surg [Am] 29:2, 1947.

Inman, VT: *The Joints of the Ankle*. Williams & Wilkins, Baltimore, 1976.

Inman, VT and Ralston, HJ: The mechanics of voluntary muscle. In Klopsteg, PE and Wilson, PD: *Human Limbs and Their Substitutes*. Hafner Publishing, New York, reprinted 1968, chap 11.

Inman, VT, Ralston, HJ, and Todd, F: *Human Walking*. Williams & Wilkins, Baltimore, 1981.

Inman, VT, Saunders, JB de CM, et al.: Observations on function of the shoulder joint. J Bone Joint Surg [Am] 26:1, 1944.

Ivey, F, Calhoun, JH, Rusche, K, et al.: Isokinetic testing of shoulder strength: Normal values. Arch Phys Med 66:384, 1985.

Jackson, H: The Croonian lectures on evolution and dissolution of the nervous system. Br Med J 1:591, 1884.

James, B and Parker, AW: Active and passive mobility of lower limb joints in elderly men and women. Am J Phys Med 68:162, 1989.

Jansen, JKS and Rudjord, T: On the silent period and Golgi tendon organs of the soleus muscle of the cat. Acta Physiol Scand 62:364, 1964.

Jarit, P: Dominant-hand to nondominant-hand grip-strength ratios of college baseball players. J Hand Ther 4:123, 1991.

Jarvis, DK: Relative strength of the hip rotator muscle groups. Physiol Ther Rev 32:500, 1952.

Jiang, CC, Otis, JC, Warren, RF, et al.: Muscle excursion measurements and movement arm determinations of rotator cuff muscles. Orthop Trans 12:496, 1988.

Jobe, CM: Gross anatomy of the shoulder. In Rockwood, CA and Matsen, FA (ed): *The Shoulder, Vol 1*, WB Saunders, Philadelphia, 1990a.

Jobe, FW, Tibone, JE, Jobe, CM, et al.: The shoulder in sports. In Rockwood, CA and Matsen, FA (eds): *The Shoulder, Vol 2*, WB Saunders, Philadelphia, 1990b.

Jobe, FW, Tibone, JE, Perry, J, et al.: An EMG analysis of the shoulder in throwing and pitching. Am J Sports Med 11:3, 1983.

Johnson, EW and Braddom, R: Over-work weakness in facio-scapulo-humeral muscular dystrophy. Arch Phys Med Rehabil 52:333, 1971.

Johnson, MA, Polgar, J, and Weightman, P: Data on the distribution of fibre types in thirty-six human muscles: An autopsy study. J Neurol Sci 18:111, 1973.

Joseph, J: *Man's Posture: Electromyographic Studies*. Charles C Thomas, Springfield, IL, 1960.

Joseph, J and Nightingale, A: Man's posture, electromyography of muscles of posture: Thigh muscles in males. J Physiol 126:81, 1954.

Kadaba, MP, Ramakrishnan, HK, and Wootten, ME: Measurement of lower extremity kinematics during level walking. J Orthop Res 8:383, 1990.

Kaltenborn, FM: *Mobilization of the Extremity Joints*. Olaf Norlis Bokhandel, Oslo, 1980.

Kandel, ER, Schwartz, JH, and Jessell, TM: *Principles of Neural Science*, ed 3. Appleton & Lange, Norwalk, CT, 1991.

Kapandji, IA: *The Physiology of Joints, Vol 3, The Trunk and Vertebral Column*. Churchill Livingstone, Edinburgh, 1974.

Kapandji, IA: *The Physiology of the Joints, Vol 1, Upper Limb*, ed 5. Churchill Livingstone, Edinburgh, 1982.

Kapandji, IA: *The Physiology of the Joints, Vol 2, Lower Limb*, ed 5. Churchill Livingstone, Edinburgh, 1987.

Kaplan, E B: *Functional and Surgical Anatomy of the Hand*. JB Lippincott, Philadelphia, 1965.

Kaufer, H: Mechanical function of the patella. J Bone Joint Surg [Am] 53:1551, 1971.

Kaye, RA and Jahss, MH: Tibialis posterior: A review of anatomy and biomechanics in relation to support of the medial longitudinal arch. Foot Ankle 11:244, 1991.

Kelsey, DD and Tyson, E: A new method of training for the lower extremity using unloading. J Orthop Sports Phys Ther 19:218, 1994.

Kendall, HO, Kendall, FP, and Boynton, DA: *Posture and Pain*. Williams & Wilkins, Baltimore, 1952.

Kendall, HO, Kendall, FP, and Wadsworth, GE: Muscles: Testing and Function, ed 2. Williams & Wilkins, Baltimore, 1971.

Kennedy, JC, Alexander, IJ, and Hayes, KC: Nerve supply of the human knee and its functional importance. Am J Sports Med 10:329, 1982.

Kent, BE: Anatomy of the trunk: A review—Part I. Phys Ther 54:722, 1974.

King, BG and Showers, MJ: *Human Anatomy and Physiology*, ed 6. WB Saunders, Philadelphia, 1969.

Kippers, V and Parker, AW: Posture related to myoelectric silence of erectores spinae during trunk flexion. Spine 9:740, 1984.

Klopsteg, PE and Wilson, PD: *Human Limbs and Their Substitutes*. Hafner Publishing, New York, reprinted 1968.

Knapik, JJ, Wright, JE, Mawdsley, RH, et al.: Isometric, isotonic, isokinetic torque variations in four muscle groups through a range of joint motion. Phys Ther 63:938, 1983.

Komi, PV and Karlsson, J: Physical performance, skeletal muscle enzyme activities and fibre types in monozygous and dizygous twins of both sexes. Acta Physiol Scand (Suppl) 462:1, 1979.

Komi, PV: Physiological and biomechanical correlates of muscle function: Effects of muscle structure and stretch-shortening cycle on force and speed. Exerc Sports Sci Rev 12:81, 1984.

Krebs, DE, Wong, D, Jevsevar, D, et al.: Trunk kinematics during locomotor activities. Phys Ther 72:505, 1992.

Kues, JM, Rothstein, JM and Lamb, RL: The relationships among knee extensor torques produced during maximal voluntary contractions under various test conditions. Phys Ther 74:674, 1994.

Kuhlmann, JN and Tubiana, R: Mechanism of the normal wrist. In Razemon, JP and Fisk, GR (eds): *The Wrist*. Churchill Livingstone, Edinburgh, 1988.

Kumar, VP and Balasubramaniam, P: The role of atmospheric pressure in stabilizing the shoulder. J Bone Joint Surg 67b:719, 1985.

Landsmeer, JM and Long, C: The mechanism of finger control: Based on electromyograms and location analysis. Acta Anat (Basel) 60:330, 1965.

Larsson, BE, Sandlund, B, and Oberg, PA: Selspot recording of gait in normals and in patients with spasticity. Scand J Rehabil Med (Suppl) 6:21, 1978.

Larsson, LE, Odenrick, P, and Sandlund, B,: The phases of the stride and their interaction in human gait. Scand J Rehabil Med 12:107, 1980.

Lass, P, Kaalund, S, LeFevre, S, et al.: Muscle coordination following rupture of the anterior cruciate ligament. Acta Orthop Scand 62:9, 1991.

Lee, D: *The Pelvic Girdle*. Churchill Livingstone, Edinburgh, 1989.

Lehmkuhl, LD, and Smith, LK: *Brunnstrom's Clinical Kinesiology*, ed 4. FA Davis, Philadelphia, 1983.

Leib, FJ and Perry, J: Quadriceps function: An anatomical and mechanical study using amputated limbs. J Bone Joint Surg [Am] 50:1535, 1968.

Leib, FJ and Perry, J: Quadriceps function: Electromyographic study under isometric conditions. J Bone Joint Surg [Am] 53:749, 1971.

Leiber, RL and Bodine-Fowler, SC: Skeletal muscle mechanics: implications for rehabilitation. Phys Ther 73:844, 1993.

Leiper, CI and Craik, RL: Relationships between physical activity and temporal-distance characteristics of walking in elderly women. Phys Ther 71:791, 1991.

Leivseth, G and Reikeras, O: Changes in muscle fiber cross-sectional area and concentrations of Na, K-ATPase in deltoid muscle in patients with impingement syndrome of the shoulder. J Orthop Sports Phys Ther 19:146, 1994.

LeVeau, B: *Williams and Lissner: Biomechanics of Human Motion*, ed 3. WB Saunders, Philadelphia, 1992.

Lewin, T, Mofett, B, and Viedik, A: The morphology of the lumbar synovial intervertebral joints. Acta Morphol Neerl Scand 4:299, 1962.

Lewis, MM, Ballet, FL, Kroll, P, et al.: En block clavicular resection: Operative procedure and postoperative testing of function. Clin Orthop 193:214, 1985.

Lin, G, Amadio, PC, An, K, et al.: Functional anatomy of the human digital flexor pulley system. J Hand Surg [Am] 14:949, 1989.

Lindholm, LE: An optical instrument for remote on-line movement monitoring. *Conference Digest for European Conference on Electrotechnics*. Eurocon, Amsterdam, 1974, p E5.

Lombardi, V and Piazzesi, G: The contractile response during steady lengthening of stimulated frog muscle fibers. J Physiol 431:141, 1990.

Long, C: Intrinsic-extrinsic control of the fingers: Electromyographic studies. J Bone Joint Surg [Am] 50:973, 1968.

Long, C and Brown, ME: Electromyographic kinesiology of the hand: Muscles moving the long finger. J Bone Joint Surg [Am] 46:1683, 1964.

Long, C, Conrad, PW, Hall, EA, et al: Intrinsic-extrinsic muscle control of the hand in power grip and precision handling. An electromyographic study. J Bone Joint Surg [Br] 52:853, 1970.

Lord, SF, Clark, RD, and Webster, OW: Visual acuity and contrast sensitivity in relation to falls in an elderly population. Age Aging 20:175, 1991.

Lundberg, A, Goldie, I, Kalin, B, et al.: Kinematics of the ankle/foot complex: Part 1. Plantarflexion and dorsiflexion. Foot Ankle 9:194, 1989a.

Lundberg, A, Svensson, OK, Bylund, C et al.: Kinematics of the ankle/foot complex: Part 2. Pronation and supination. Foot Ankle 9:248, 1989b.

Lundberg, A, Svensson, OK, Bylund, C, et al.: Kinematics of the ankle/foot complex: Part 3. Influence of leg rotation. Foot Ankle 9:304, 1989c.

Lunnen, JD, Yack, J, and LeVeau, B: Relationship between muscle length, muscle activity and torque of the hamstring muscles. Phys Ther 61:190, 1981.

MacConaill, MA and Basmajian, JV: *Muscles and Movements: A Basis for Human Kinesiology*. Williams & Wilkins, Baltimore, 1969.

Macintosh, JE and Bogduk, N: The anatomy and function of the lumbar back muscles and their fascia. In Twomey, LT and Taylor, JR (eds): *Physical Therapy of the Low Back*. Churchill Livingstone, New York, 1987.

Mair, J, Koller, A, Artner-Dworzak, E, et al.: Effects of exercise on plasma myosin heavy chain fragments and MRI of skeletal muscle. J Appl Physiol 72:656, 1992.

Maitland, GD: *Peripheral Manipulation*, ed 2. Butterworths, Boston, 1977.

Mann, R and Inman, VT: Phasic activity of intrinsic muscles of the foot. J Bone Joint Surg [Am] 46:469, 1964.

Mannheimer, JS and Dunn, J: Cervical spine-evaluation and relation to temporomandibular disorders. In Kaplan, AS and Assael, LA: *Temporomandibular Disorders: Diagnosis and Treatment*. WB Saunders, Philadelphia, 1991.

Manter, JT: Movements of the subtalar and transverse tarsal joints. Anat Rec 80:397, 1941.

Maquet, PG: *Biomechanics of the Knee*. Springer-Verlag, Berlin, 1983.

Maquet, PGJ: *Biomechanics of the Hip as Applied to Osteoarthritis and Related Conditions*. Springer-Verlag, Berlin, 1985.

Marey, EJ: De la locomotion terrestre chez les bipedes et les quadrupedes. Journal d'Anatomie et de Physiologie 9:42, 1873.

Marey, EJ: *Animal Mechanism: A Treatise on Terrestrial and Aerial Locomotion*. D Appleton & Co, New York, 1890.

Marey, EJ and Demeny, G: Etude experimentale de la locomotion humaine. Comptes Rendus Hebdomadoires des Seances de l'Academie des Sciences 105:544, 1887.

Markhede, G, Monastyrski, J, and Stener, B: Shoulder function after deltoid muscle removal. Acta Orthop Scand 56:242, 1985.

Matthews, PBC: Proprioceptors and the regulation of movement. In Towe, AL and Luschel, ES (eds): *Handbook of Behavioral Neurobiology, Vol 5, Motor Coordination*. Plenum Press, New York, 1981, p 93.

May, WW: Maximum isometric force of the hip rotator muscles. Phys Ther 46:233, 1966.

May, WW: Relative isometric force of the hip abductor and adductor muscles. Phys Ther 48:845, 1968.

McCluskey, G and Blackburn, TA: Classification of knee ligament instabilities. Phys Ther 60:1575, 1980.

McNally, D and Adams, M: Internal intervertebral disc mechanics as revealed by stress profilometry. Spine 17:66, 1992.

McNamara, JA: The independent functions of the two heads of the lateral pterygoid muscle. Am J Anat 38:197, 1973.

McPoil, TJ and Brocato, RS: The foot and ankle: Biomechanical evaluation and treatment. In Gould, JA and Davies, GJ (eds): *Orthopedic and Sports Physical Therapy*. CV Mosby, St. Louis, 1985.

McQuade, KJ, Crutcher, JP, Sidles, JA, et al.: Tibial rotation in anterior cruciate deficient knees: An in vitro study. J Sports Phys Ther 11:146, 1989.

Menard, MR, Penn, AM, Jonathan, WK, et al.: Relative metabolic efficiency of concentric and eccentric exercise determined by P magnetic resonance spectroscopy. Arch Phys Med Rehabil 72:976, 1991.

Mendler, HM: Postoperative function of the knee joint. J Am Phys Ther Assn 43:435, 1963.

Mendler, HM: Knee extensor and flexor force following injury. Phys Ther 47:35, 1967a.

Mendler, HM: Effect of stabilization on maximum isometric knee extensor force. Phys Ther 47:375, 1967b.

Mennell, JB: *Physical Treatment by Movement, Manipulation and Massage*. The Blakiston Company, Philadelphia, 1947.

Mennell, JM: *Joint Pain: Diagnosis and Treatment Using Manipulative Techniques*. Little, Brown & Co, Boston, 1964.

Merton, PA: How we control the contraction of our muscles. Sci Am 226:30, 1972.

Meyer, H: Das aufrechte Stehen. Archiv Fuer Anatomie, Physiologie, und wissenschaftliche Medezin, 1853, p 9–48.

Montgomery, PC and Connolly, BH: *Motor Control and Physical Therapy: Theoretical Framework and Practical Applications*. Chattanooga Group, 1991.

Morrey, BF and An, K: Biomechanics of the shoulder. In Rockwood, CA and Matsen, FA (eds): *The Shoulder, Vol 1*, WB Saunders, Philadelphia, 1990.

Morris, JM, Lucas, DB, and Bresler, B: Role of the trunk in stability of the spine. J Bone Joint Surg [Am] 43:327, 1961.

Morrison, JB: The mechanics of the knee joint in relation to normal walking. J Biomech 3:51, 1970.

Mossberg, K and Smith, LK: Axial rotation of the knee in adult females. J Orthop Sports Phys Ther 4:236, 1983.

Murray, MP and Clarkson, BH: The vertical pathways of the foot during level walking: Part I. Range of variability in normal men. Phys Ther 46:585, 1966.

Murray, MP, Drought, AB, and Kory, RC: Walking patterns of normal men. J Bone Joint Surg [Am] 46:737, 1964.

Murray, MP, Gore, DR, Gardner, GM, et al: Shoulder motion and muscle strength of normal men and women in two age groups. Clin Orthop 192:268, 1985.

Murray, MP, Kory, RC, and Clarkson, BH: Walking patterns in healthy old men. J Gerontol 24:160, 1969.

Murray, MP, Kory, RC, and Sepic, SB: Walking patterns of normal women. Arch Phys Med Rehabil 51:637, 1970.

Murray, MP, and Sepic, SB: Maximum isometric torque of hip abductor and adductor muscles. Phys Ther 48:1327, 1968.

Muybridge, E: *The Human Figure in Motion*. New York, Dover Publications, 1955.

Muybridge, E: *Animals in Motion*. New York, Dover Publications, 1957.

Myklebust, J, Pintar, F, Yoganandan, N, et al.: Tensile strength of spinal ligaments. Spine 13:526, 1988.

Nachemson, A: Lumbar intradiscal pressure. Acta Orthop Scand 43:1, 1960.

Nachemson, A: Disc pressure measurements. Spine 6:93, 1981.

Nachemson, A: Lumbar intradiscal pressure. In Jayson, M (ed): *The lumbar spine and back pain*. Churchill Livingstone, Edinburgh, 1987.

Napier, JR: The prehensile movements of the human hand. J Bone Joint Surg [Br] 38:902, 1956.

Neer, CS: *Shoulder Reconstruction*. WB Saunders, Philadelphia, 1990.

Neer, CS and Poppen, NK: Supraspinatus Outlet. Orthop Trans 11:234, 1987.

Neer, CS and Rockwood, CA: Fractures and dislocations of the shoulder. In Rockwood, CA and Green, DP (eds): *Fractures in Adults*. JB Lippincott, Philadelphia, 1984.

Neumann, DA, Soderberg, GL, and Cook, TM: Comparison of maximal isometric hip abductor muscle torques between hip sides. Phys Ther 68:496, 1988.

Neumann, DA, Soderberg, GL, and Cook, TM: Electromyographic analysis of hip abductor musculature in healthy right-handed persons. Phys Ther 69:431, 1989.

Nideffer, RM: *Athletes Guide to Mental Training*. Human Kinetics Publishers, Champaign, IL, 1985.

Nideffer, RM: Concentration and attention control training. In Williams, JM (ed): *Applied Sports, Personal Growth and Peak Performance*. Bayfield Publishing, Mountain View, CA, 1993.

Nilsson, MB: Intra-Individual Variability in Maximal Grip Strength Over a Four Week Period. Unpublished Thesis, Texas Woman's University, Denton, TX, 1978.

Norkin, CC and Levangie, PK: *Joint Structure and Function*. Philadelphia, F.A. Davis, 1992.

Norkin, C and White, D: Measurement of Joint Motion: A Guide to Goniometry, ed 2. FA Davis, Philadelphia, 1995.

O'Brien, SJ, Arnoczky, SP, Warren, RF, et al.: Developmental anatomy of the shoulder and anatomy of the glenohumeral joint. In Rockwood, CA and Matsen, FA: *The Shoulder Vol. I*. WB Saunders, Philadelphia, 1990.

O'Connor, J, Shercliff, T, FitzPatrick, D, et al.: Mechanics of the knee. In Daniel, DM, Akeson, WH, and O'Connor, JJ (eds): *Knee Ligaments: Structure, Function, Injury and Repair*. Raven Press, New York, 1990.

Oatis, CA: Biomechanics of the foot and ankle under static conditions. Phys Ther 68:1815, 1988.

Otis, JC, Warren, RF, Backus, SI, et al.: Torque production in the shoulder of the normal young adult male. Am J Spts Med 18:119–123, 1990.

Ouellet, R, Levesque, HP, and Laurin, CA: The ligamentous stability of the knee: An experimental investigation. Can Med Assoc J 110:45, 1969.

Ouzounian, T and Shereff, M: In vitro determination of midfoot motion. Foot Ankle 10:140, 1989.

Ovesen, J and Nielsen, S: Stability of the shoulder joint: Cadaver study of stabilizing structures. Acta Orthop Scand 56:149, 1985.

Palastanga, N, Field, D, and Soames, R: *Anatomy and Human Movement.* Heinemann Medical Books, United Kingdom, 1989.

Pare, EB, Stern, JT, and Swartz, JM: Functional differentiation within the tensor fasciae latae. J Bone Joint Surg [Am] 63:1457, 1981.

Passmore, R and Durnin, JVGA: Human energy expenditure. Physiol Rev 35:801, 1955.

Pauly, JE: An electromyographic analysis of certain movements and exercises: Part I. Some deep muscles of the back. Anat Rec 155:223, 1966.

Peat, M: Functional anatomy of the shoulder complex. Phys Ther 66:1855, 1986.

Perry, J: Kinesiology of lower extremity bracing. Clin Orthop 102:18, 1974.

Perry, J: Anatomy and biomechanics of the shoulder in throwing, swimming, gymnastics and tennis. Clin Sports Med 2:247, 1983.

Perry, J: Biomechanics of the shoulder. In Rowe, C (ed): *The Shoulder.* Churchill Livingstone, New York, 1988.

Perry, J: *Gait Analysis: Normal and Pathological Function.* Slack, Thorofare, NJ, 1992.

Pocock, GS: Electromyographic study of the quadriceps during resistive exercises. J Am Phys Ther Assoc 43:427, 1963.

Poppen, N and Walker, P: Normal and abnormal motion of the shoulder. J Bone Joint Surg [Am] 58:195, 1976.

Poppen, N and Walker, P: Forces at the glenohumeral joint in abduction. Clin Orthop 135:165, 1978.

Porterfield, JA and DeRosa, C: *Mechanical Low Back Pain Perspectives in Functional Anatomy.* WB Saunders, Philadelphia, 1991.

Powell, S and Burke, AL: Surgical and Therapeutic Management of Tennis Elbow: An Update. J Hand Ther 4:64, 1991.

Pullinger, AG and Monteiro, AA: History factors associated with symptoms of temporomandibular disorders. J Oral Rehabil 15:117, 1988.

Pyykko, I, Aalto, H, Hytonen, M, et al.: Effect of age on postural control. In Amblard, B, Berthoz, G, and Clarac, F (eds): *Posture and Gait.* Excerpta Medica, Amsterdam, 1988.

Pyykko, I, Pirkko, J, and Aalto, H: Age Aging 19:215, 1990.

Rabischong, P: L'innervation proprioceptive et muscles lombric de la main chez l'homme. Rev Chir Orthop 48:234, 1962.

Radakovich, M and Malone, T: The superior tibiofibular joint: The forgotten joint. J Orthop Sports Phys Ther 3:129, 1982.

Ralston, HJ: Some considerations of the physiological basis of therapeutic exercise. Phys Ther Rev 38:465, 1958.

Ralston, HJ: Uses and limitation of electromyography in the quantitative study of skeletal muscle function. Am J Orthop 47:521, 1961.

Ralston, HJ and Libet, B: The question of tonus in skeletal muscle. Am J Phys Med 32:85, 1953.

Ralston, HJ, Polissar, MJ, and Inman, VT,: Dynamic features of human isolated voluntary muscle in isometric and free contractions. J Appl Physiol 1:526, 1949.

Ramsey, RW and Street, SF: Isometric length-tension diagram of isolated skeletal muscle fibers of frog. J Cell Comp Physiol 15:11, 1940.

Ranney, D and Wells, R: Lumbrical muscle function as revealed by a new and physiological approach. Anat Rec 222:110, 1988.

Razemon, JP and Fisk, GR (eds): *The Wrist.* Churchill Livingstone, Edinburgh, 1988.

Reid, DC, Saboe, L, and Burham, R: Current research in selected shoulder problems. In Donatelli, R (ed): *Physical Therapy of the Shoulder.* Churchill Livingstone, New York, 1987.

Reilly, DT and Martens, M: Experimental analysis of the quadriceps muscle force and patellofemoral joint reaction force for various activities. Acta Orthop Scand 43:126, 1972.

Resnick, R and Halliday, D: *Physics for Students of Science and Engineering.* John Wiley & Sons, New York, 1960.

Reuleaux, F: Theoretische Kinematik. Braunschweigh, 1875.

Reys, JHO: Uber Die Absolute Kraft Der Muskeln Im Menchlichenn Korper. Pfleugers Arch 160:183, 1915.

Rietveld, AB, Daanen, HA, Rozing, PM, et al.: The lever arm in glenohumeral abduction after hemiarthroplasty. J Bone Joint Surg [Br] 70:561, 1988.

Ro, CS: Sacroiliac Joint: Part I. Anatomy. In Cox, JM: *Low Back Pain*. Williams & Wilkins, Baltimore, 1990.

Rodenburg, JB, Bar, PR, and DeBoer, RW: Relations between muscle soreness and biochemical and functional outcomes of eccentric exercise. J Appl Physiol 74:2976, 1993.

Rood, M: The use of sensory receptors to activate, facilitate, and inhibit motor response, autonomic and somatic, in developmental sequence. In Satterly, C (ed): *Approaches to the Treatment of Patients With Neuromuscular Dysfunction*. William C Brown, Dubuque, IA, 1962.

Ross, RF: A quantitative study of rotation of the knee joint in man. Anat Rec 52:209, 1932.

Rosse, C and Clawson, K: *The Musculoskeletal System in Health and Disease*. Harper & Row, Hagerstown, MD, 1980.

Sakellarides, HT: Injury to spinal accessory nerve with paralysis of trapezius muscle and treatment by tendon transfer. Orthop Trans 10:449, 1986.

Sale, DG: Neural adaptation to resistance training. Med Sci Sports Exerc 20:S135, 1988.

Sapega, AA: Current concepts review: Muscle performance evaluation in orthopaedic practice. J Bone Joint Surg 72:1562, 1990.

Sarnat, BG and Laskin, DM: *The Temporomandibular Joint: A Biological Basis for Clinical Practice*, ed 4. Philadelphia, WB Saunders, 1992.

Sarrafian, SK: *Anatomy of the Foot and Ankle*. JB Lippincott, Philadelphia, 1983.

Sarrafian, SK: Functional characteristics of the foot and plantar aponeurosis under tibiotalar loading. Foot Ankle 8(4):1, 1987.

Sashin, D: A critical analysis of the anatomy and pathological changes of the sacroiliac joints. J Bone Joint Surg 12:891, 1930.

Saunders, JB de CM, Inman, VT, and Eberhart, HD: The major determinants in normal and pathological gait. J Bone Joint Surg [Am] 35:543, 1953.

Schede, F: *Theoretische Grundlagen fur den Bau von Kunstbeinen*. Ferdinand Enke Verlag, Stuttgart, 1941.

Schenck, J and Forward, E: Quantitative strength gains with test repetitions. Phys Ther 45:562, 1965.

Schleichkorn, J: Signe Brunnstrom: *Physical Therapy Pioneer, Master Clinician and Humanitarian*. Slack Inc., Thorofare, NJ, 1990.

Schlesinger, G: *Der mechanische Aufbau der kuntslichen Glieder. In Ersatzglieder und Arbeitshilfen*. J Springer, Berlin, 1919.

Schlesinger, G: Technische Ausnutzung der kinoplastischen Armstumpfe. Dtsch Med Wochenschr 46:262, 1920.

Schmidt, RA: *Motor Control and Learning: A Behavioral Emphasis*. Human Kinetics Publishers, Champaign, IL, 1988.

Schmidt, RF (ed): *Fundamentals of Neurophysiology*, ed 2. Springer-Verlag, New York, 1978.

Schutte, MJ, Dabezies, EJ, Zimny, ML, et al.: Neural anatomy of the human anterior cruciate ligament. J Bone Joint Surg [Am] 69:243, 1987.

Scott, JJA: Classification of muscle spindle afferents in the peroneus brevis muscle of the cat. Brain Research 509:62, 1980.

Sheffield, FJ: Electromyographic study of the abdominal muscles in walking and other movements. Am J Phys Med 41:142, 1962.

Sherrington, CS: *The Integrative Action of the Nervous System*. Yale University Press, New Haven, CT, 1906, p 7.

Shoemaker, S and Daniel, D: The limits of knee motion. In Daniel, DM, Akeson, WH, and O'Connor, JJ: *Knee Ligaments: Structure, Function, Injury and Repair*. Raven Press, New York, 1990.

Skoglund, S: Anatomical and physiological studies of knee joint innervation in the cat. Acta Physiol Scand (Suppl) 124:1, 1956.

Smidt, GL: Hip motion and related factors in walking. Phys Ther 51:9, 1971.

Smidt, GL: Biomechanical analysis of knee flexion and extension. Biomechanics 6:79, 1973.

Smidt, GL: Aging in gait. In Smidt, GL (Ed): *Gait in Rehabilitation*. Churchill Livingstone, New York, 1990.

Smith, JW: The forces acting at the human ankle joint during standing. J Anat 91:545, 1957.

Smith, LK: Poliomyelitis and the postpolio syndrome. In Umphred, DA (ed): *Neurological Rehabilitation*, ed 2. CV Mosby, St Louis, 1990.

Smith, LK: Unpublished data, 1980.

Soderberg, G: *Kinesiology: Application to Pathological Motion.* Williams & Wilkins, Baltimore, 1986.

Solomonow, M, Baratta, R, Zhou, BH, et al.: The synergistic action of the anterior cruciate ligament and thigh muscles in maintaining joint stability. Am J Sports Med 15:207, 1987.

Spinner, M: *Kaplan's Functional and Surgical Anatomy of the Hand,* ed 3. JB Lippincott, Philadelphia, 1984.

Stanton, P and Purdam, C: Hamstring injuries in sprinting: The role of eccentric exercise. J Orthop Sports Phys Ther 10:343, 1989.

Stauber, WT: Eccentric Action of Muscles. Exerc Sports Sci Rev 17:157, 1989.

Stauffer, RN, Chao, EYS, and Brewster, RC: Force and motion analysis of the normal, diseased and prosthetic ankle joint. Clin Orthop 127:1977.

Steel, FL and Tomlinson, JD: The 'carrying angle' in man. J Anat 92:315, 1958.

Steindler, A: *Kinesiology of the Human Body Under Normal and Pathological Conditions.* Charles C Thomas, Springfield, IL, 1955.

Steiner, LA, Harris, BA, and Krebs, DE: Reliability of eccentric isokinetic knee flexion and extension measurements. Arch Phys Med Rehabil 74:1327, 1993.

Strong, A and Ubell, E: *The World of Push and Pull.* Atheneum, New York, 1964.

Sugi, H and Pollack, GH (eds): *Mechanism of Myofilament Sliding in Muscle Contraction. Advances in Experimental Medicine and Biology, Vol 332.* Plenum Press, New York, 1993.

Sullivan, MS: Back support mechanisms during manual lifting. Phys Ther 69:38, 1989.

Sunderland, S: Actions of the extensor digitorum communis, interosseous and lumbrical muscles. Am J Anat 77:189, 1945.

Sutherland, DH and Hagy, JL: Measurement of gait movements from motion picture film. J Bone Joint Surg [Am] 54:787, 1972.

Sutherland, DH, Olshen, RA, Biden, EN, et al.: *The Development of Mature Walking.* JB Lippincott, Philadelphia, 1988.

Svenningsen, S, Terjesen, T, Auflem, M, et al.: Hip motion related to age and sex. Acta Orthop Scand 60:97, 1989.

Swanson, AB, Matev, IB, and DeGroot, G: The strength of the hand. Bull Prosthet Res BPR 10-14:145, 1970.

Taguchi, K and Tada, C: Change of body sway with growth in children. In Amblard, B, Berthoz, G, and Clarac, F (eds): *Posture and Gait.* Excerpta Medica, Amsterdam, 1988.

Taleisnik, J: Ligaments of the Carpus. In Razemon, JP and Fisk, GR (eds): *The Wrist.* Churchill Livingstone, Edinburgh, 1988.

Taleisnik, J (ed): Management of wrist problems. Hand Clinics 3:31, 1987.

Taylor, A and Prochazka, A (eds): *Muscle Receptors and Movement.* Oxford University Press, New York, 1981.

Taylor, CL and Schwarz, RJ: The anatomy and mechanics of the human hand. Artificial Limbs, 3:22, 1955.

Thorstensson, A: Muscle strength, fibre types and enzyme activities in man. Acta Physiol Scand (Suppl) 443:1, 1976.

Tiberio, D: Pathomechanics of structural foot deformities. Phys Ther 68:1840, 1988.

Tkaczuk, J: Tensile properties of human lumbar longitudinal ligaments. Acta Orthop Scand (Suppl):115:1, 1968.

Toews, JV: A grip-strength study among steelworkers. Arch Phys Med Rehabil 45:413, 1964.

Tornvall, G: Assessment of physical capabilities. Acta Physiol Scand (Suppl) 20:1, 1963.

Travell, JG, and Simons, DG: *Myofascial Pain and Dysfunction.* Williams & Wilkins, Baltimore, 1983.

Valencia, FP, and Munro, RR: An electromyographic study of the lumbar multifidus in man. Electromyogr Clin Neurophysiol 25:205, 1985.

Valenti, V: Proprioception. In Helal, B and Wilson, D (eds): *The Foot, Vol I.* Churchill Livingstone, New York, 1988.

Van Sant, A: Rising from a supine position to erect stance. Phys Ther 68:185, 1988.

Von Recklinghausen, N: *Gliedermechanik and Lahmungsprothesen.* J Springer, Berlin, 1920.

Voss, DE: Proprioceptive neuromuscular facilitation. Am J Phys Med 46:838, 1967.

Voss, DE, Ionta, MK, and Myers, BJ: *Proprioceptive Neuromuscular Facilitation,* ed 3. Harper & Row, Philadelphia, 1985.

Walker, JM, Sue, D, Miles-Elkousy, N, et al.: Active mobility of the extremities in older subjects. Phys Ther 64:919, 1984.

Walker, ML, Rothstein, JM, Finucane, SD, et al.: Relationships between lumbar lordosis, pelvic tilt and abdominal muscle performance. Phys Ther 67:512, 1987.

Waters, RL: Energy expenditure. In Perry, J: *Gait Analysis: Normal and Pathological Function.* Thorofare, NJ: Slack, 1992.

Waters, RL, Campbell, J, Thomas, L, et al.: Energy costs of walking in lower-extremity plaster casts. J Bone Joint Surg [Am] 64:896, 1982.

Waters, RL, Campbell, J, Thomas, L, et al.: Energy costs of three-point crutch ambulation in fracture patients. J Orthop Trauma 1:170, 1987.

Waters, RL and Lunsford, BR: Energy costs of paraplegic locomotion. J Bone Joint Surg [Am] 67:1245, 1985.

Waters, RL and Morris, JM: Electrical activity of muscles of the trunk during walking. J Anat 111:191, 1972.

Waters, RL, Perry, J, and Antonelli, D: The energy cost of walking of amputees: The influence of level of amputation. J Bone Joint Surg [Am] 58:42, 1976.

Weber, EF: Ueber die Langeverhaltnisse der Muskeln im Allgemeinen. Verh Kgl Sach Ges d Wiss, Leipzig, 1851.

Weber, W and Weber, E: *Mechanik der menschlichen Gehwerkzeuge.* Dietarich, Gottingen, 1836.

Weinland, J: A Five-Month Strength Curve. J Appl Psychol 31:498, 1947.

Weisl, H: The Movements of the Sacroiliac Joint. Acta Anat 23:80, 1955.

Wells, PE: Movements of the Pelvic Joints. In Grieve, GF (ed): *Modern Manual Therapy of the Vertebral Column.* Churchill Livingstone, Edinburgh, 1986.

Werner, SL, Fleisig, GS, Dillman, CJ, et al.: Biomechanics of the elbow during baseball pitching. J Sports Phys Ther 17:274, 1993.

Westring, SH and Seger, JY: Eccentric and concentric torque-velocity output comparisons, and gravity effect torque corrections for the quadriceps and hamstring muscles in females. Int J Sports 10:175, 1989.

Westring, SH, Seger, JY, Karlson, E, et al.: Eccentric and concentric torque-velocity characteristics of the quadriceps femoris in man. Eur J Appl Physiol 58:100, 1988.

White, AA and Panjabi, MM: The basic kinematics of the lumbar spine. Spine, 3:12, 1978.

Widmalm, SE, Lillie, JH, and Ash, MM: Anatomical and electromyographic studies of the digastric muscle. J Oral Rehabil 15:3, 1988.

Wikholm, JB and Bohannon, RW: Hand-held dynamometer measurements: Tester strength makes a difference. J Orthop Sports Phys Ther 13:191, 1991.

Wilk, KE, Voight, ML, Keirns, MA, et al.: Stretch-shortening drills for the upper extremities: Theory and clinical application. J Orthop Sports Phys Ther 17:225, 1993.

Williams, M and Lissner, HR: *Biomechanics of Human Motion.* WB Saunders, Philadelphia, 1962.

Williams, M and Stutzman, L: Strength variation through the range of joint motion. Phys Ther Rev 39:145, 1959.

Williams, M and Wesley, W: Hip rotator action of the adductor longus muscle. Phys Ther Rev 31:90, 1951.

Wingstrand, H, Wingstrand, A, and Krantz, P: Intracapsular and atmospheric pressure in the dynamics and stability of the hip. Acta Orthop Scand 61:231, 1990.

Winter, D, Ruder, GK, and MacKinnon, DC: Control of balance of upper body during gait. In Winters, JM and Woo, SL (eds): *Multiple Muscle Systems.* Springer-Verlag, New York, 1990.

Winter, DA, Patala, AE, Frank, JS, et al.: Biomechanical walking pattern changes in the fit and healthy elderly. Phys Ther 70:340, 1990.

Winter, DA and Yack, HJ: EMG profiles during normal human walking: Stride-to-stride and intersubject variability. EEG Clin Neurol 67:402, 1987.

Winters, JM and Woo, SL (eds): *Multiple Muscle Systems.* Springer-Verlag, New York, 1990.

Woodruff, G: Maximum Isometric Torque of the Hip Rotator Muscles in Four Positions of Hip Flexion-Extension. Unpublished Thesis, Texas Woman's University, Denton, TX, 1976.

Woollacott, MH. Posture and gait from newborn to elderly. In Amblard, B, Berthoz, G, and Clarac, F (eds): *Posture and Gait.* Excerpta Medica, Amsterdam, 1988.

Wright, V: Factors influencing diurnal variation of strength of grip. Res Exerc Sport Q 30:110, 1958.

Wyatt, MP: Gait in children. In Smidt, GL (ed): *Gait in Rehabilitation.* Churchill Livingstone, New York, 1990.

Wynn-Parry, CB: *Rehabilitation of the Hand,* ed 4. Butterworths, London, 1981.

Yamamoto, I, Panjabi, M, Osland, T, et al.: The role of the iliolumbar ligament in the lumbosacral junction. Spine 15:1138, 1990.

Yoshioka, Y, Siu, D, and Cooke, D: The anatomy and functional axes of the femur. J Bone Joint Surg [Am] 69:873, 1987.

Zancolli, E: *Structural and Dynamic Bases of Hand Surgery.* JB Lippincott, Philadelphia, 1979.

Zohn, DA and Mennell, J: *Musculoskeletal Pain: Diagnosis and Physical Treatment.* Little, Brown & Co, Boston, 1976, p 123.

Index